Evaluation in health promotion

Principles and perspectives

WHO Library Cataloguing in Publication Data

Evaluation in health promotion : principles and perspectives / edited by Irving
Rootman ... [et al.]

(WHO regional publications. European series ; No. 92)

1.Health promotion 2.Program evaluation – methods
3.Community health services 4.Schools 5.Urban health
6.Workplace 7.Health policy 8.Europe I.Rootman, Irving
II.Goodstadt, Michael III.Hyndman, Brian IV.McQueen, David V.
V.Potvin, Louise VI.Springett, Jane VII.Ziglio, Erio VIII.Series

ISBN 92 890 1359 1   (NLM Classification : WA 590)
ISSN 0378-2255

Text editing: Mary Stewart Burgher

Evaluation in health promotion
Principles and perspectives

Edited by:
**Irving Rootman, Michael Goodstadt,
Brian Hyndman, David V. McQueen,
Louise Potvin, Jane Springett
and Erio Ziglio**

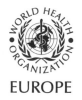

EUROPE

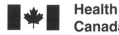

Health   Santé
Canada   Canada

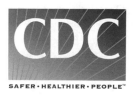

SAFER · HEALTHIER · PEOPLE™

WHO Regional Publications, European Series, No. 92

ISBN 92 890 1359 1
ISSN 0378-2255

Printed in Denmark

Acknowledgements

This book would not have materialized without the strong commitment of the authors, who agreed to develop many drafts of their chapters to fit the overall aim. Special thanks are due to Dr Irving Rootman, Chairman of the WHO European Working Group on Evaluating Health Promotion Approaches. Finally, much appreciated support was received from Health Canada, the Centers for Disease Control and Prevention in the United States of America and the Health Education Authority in the United Kingdom.

Abbreviations

Organizations

BSI	British Standards Institute, United Kingdom
CDC	Centers for Disease Control and Prevention, United States
ENHPS	European Network of Health Promoting Schools
EU	European Union
FAO	Food and Agriculture Organization of the United Nations
ISO	International Organization for Standardization
HEA	Health Education Authority, United Kingdom
NHS	National Health Service, United Kingdom

Specific studies and technical and other terms

4GE	fourth-generation evaluation
CATCH	Child and Adolescent Trial for Cardiovascular Health
CINDI	WHO countrywide integrated noncommunicable disease intervention programme
COMMIT	community intervention trial for smoking cessation
CVD	cardiovascular diseases
DALY	disability-adjusted life year
EIA	environmental impact assessment
GDP	gross domestic product
HIA	health impact assessment
KSDPP	Kahnawake School Diabetes Prevention Project
MATCH	multilevel approach to community health
MRFIT	Multiple Risk Factor Intervention Trial
PATCH	planned approach to community health
NGO	nongovernmental organization
NHEXAS	National Human Exposure Assessment Survey

PRECEDE	predisposing, reinforcing and enabling constructs in ecosystem diagnosis and evaluation
PROCEED	policy, regulating or resourcing, and organizing for educational and environmental development
QALY	quality-adjusted life year

Foreword

Promoting populations' health is an enterprise whose complex and often subtle dimensions challenge scholars and practitioners from diverse disciplines. Epidemiologists, social scientists, educators, policy scientists, economists, urban planners and biomedical scientists (most recently including geneticists) all contribute perspectives that illuminate one aspect or another of health promotion. Each discipline also offers an evaluation scheme appropriate to its strategic focus. It is easy to understand how casual observers may be frustrated in their search for a single, clear analysis to answer the bottom-line question of just how effective health promotion is. As the authors represented in this book attest, the answer very much depends on what aspect of the health promotion initiative is being addressed. Of course, matters of theoretical justification, intervention strategy, adequacy of resources and other issues of quality– the process questions – pertain, but at the end of the day the results should be measured in ways that are consistent with the stated objectives. Who benefits and how, and who is missed and why, are the central evaluation questions.

The genius of this collection of evaluation approaches to diverse health promotion programmes and related policies is what it reveals about the spread of options: options that do not compete but supplement each other. For the builder of a health promotion strategy, the task is to discover the available evaluative technology with the best fit, and to apply it in a way that balances a comprehensive view with a necessary parsimony of effort. Cost–effectiveness must apply to evaluation design as well as programme design.

For organized health promotion efforts to be positioned as key resources in pursuing social and economic goals, there must be evidence of their effectiveness and their relative costs as compared with other health promoting options: for example, approaches targeting reductions in individual risk versus those seeking reductions in risk conditions through policy change.

The requirement for evidence-based health promotion pertains to public health practice in general, from designing an intervention through evaluating its impact. Criteria for such evidence are expanding to include negative impact as well as positive benefits and a wide range of effects on community wellbeing and economic and social development goals.

Until the publication of this book, it was difficult to juxtapose the myriad dimensions of health promotion, the spread of their assumptions and theories, the challenges faced in planning and undertaking evaluations of health promotion initiatives, and the basis for choosing an approach to evaluation. Further, it is now easier to appreciate the value-added potential of combining several measures focused, for example, on personal, community, environmental and political impact. The chapters of this book demonstrate the conundrum that the whole may be greater than the sum of its parts.

As health promotion comes of age as a theory-informed, evidence-based and broadly accountable practice, this book provides a landscape of evalua-

tive issues and options that can help refocus health promotion planning before resources are committed. It is much more than a catalogue of evaluation methods. Implicit in each chapter is a closely argued rationale for the design or choice of a given intervention, a rationale that helps clarify the potential limitations of the method, and the necessity of having a systems-based strategy for promoting the health of populations and individuals. The principal benefit of this book for health promotion practitioners is a sense of how disparate kinds of technology can join together as complementary parts of a strategic whole.

This book – with two shorter companion documents aimed at practitioners and policy-makers – is a major link in a series of developments aimed at strengthening the capacity of national and local resources to broaden the health promoting impact of both programmes and policies. With more powerful evaluation tools, used with greater specificity to pursue diverse objectives, health promotion efforts can be more equitable, more empowering, more participatory, more accountable and more sustainable.

Marc Danzon
WHO Regional Director for Europe

WHO European Working Group on Health Promotion Evaluation

Dr Laurie Anderson
   Health Scientist, Epidemiological Program Office, Urban Health Center, Centers for Disease Control and Prevention, Atlanta, USA

Dr Lynda Anderson
   Health Scientist, Division of Adult and Community Health, National Center for Chronic Disease Prevention and Health Promotion, Centers for Disease Control and Prevention, Atlanta, USA

Mr Nick Doyle
   Head of Policy, Health Education Authority, London, United Kingdom

Dr Brian Flay
   Director, Prevention Research Centre, University of Illinois, Chicago, USA

Dr Michael Goodstadt
   Deputy Director, Centre for Health Promotion, University of Toronto, Canada

Dr Igor Glasunov
   Executive Director, CINDI Russia, Institute of Preventive Medicine, Moscow, Russian Federation

Mr Brian Hyndman
   Consultant, Centre for Health Promotion, University of Toronto, Canada
   (Secretary)

Dr Glenn Irwin
   Senior Policy Analyst, Health Promotion and Programs Branch, Health Canada, Ottawa, Canada

Mr Paul Lincoln
   Director, Health Education Authority, London, United Kingdom

Dr Peter Makara
   Director, National Institute for Health Promotion, Budapest, Hungary

Dr David McQueen
    Assistant Director for Global Health Promotion, National Center for Chronic
    Disease Prevention and Health Promotion, Centers for Disease Control and
    Prevention, Atlanta, USA

Dr Tapani Piha
    Principal Medical Officer, Ministry of Social Affairs and Health, Helsinki,
    Finland

Dr Louise Potvin
    Groupe de recherche interdisciplinaire en santé, Université de Montréal,
    Montréal, Canada

Dr Irving Rootman
    Director, Centre for Health Promotion, University of Toronto, Canada
    (Chairperson)

Dr Tom Schmid
    Evaluator, Division of Nutrition and Physical Activity, Centers for Disease
    Control and Prevention, Atlanta, USA

Dr Sylvie Stachenko
    Director, Department of Health Policy and Services, WHO Regional Office
    for Europe, Copenhagen, Denmark

Dr Jane Springett
    Professor, Health Promotion and Public Health, Institute for Health, Liverpool
    John Moores University, United Kingdom

Dr Erio Ziglio
    Regional Adviser for Social and Economic Development, WHO Regional
    Office for Europe, Copenhagen, Denmark

Contributors

Laurie M. Anderson is a health scientist at the Centers for Disease Control and Prevention (CDC), United States of America. During her participation in the WHO Working Group on Health Promotion Evaluation, she also served as a scientist with the National Center for Chronic Disease Prevention and Health Promotion, working on the Behavioral Risk Factor Surveillance System, a continuous health survey that provides insight into the health behaviour of the adult population of the United States. At CDC she has been responsible for the development, implementation and evaluation of numerous state and national intervention programmes to reduce chronic disease and promote health. Dr Anderson's current work involves conducting evidence-based reviews of community interventions aimed at determinants of health in the broader social environment, within the Community Preventive Services Guide Development Activity of the Epidemiology Program Office, CDC. She holds a B.S. from the University of San Francisco, a Masters degree in public health from Emory University, and a Ph.D. from the University of California, Los Angeles in social behaviour and health and in demography.

Jannette Berkley-Patton, M.A., is pursuing her Ph.D. in developmental and child psychology in the Human Development and Family Life Department at the University of Kansas, United States. She is a research associate of the University's Work Group on Health Promotion and Community Development. Her work involves evaluating and providing technical assistance and community research for community health initiatives. Mrs Berkley-Patton's research interests include community development, adolescent health and the promotion of the personal success of African-American adolescents.

Treena Chomik has a broad record of accomplishment in professional consulting and research services for agencies and governments that seek to advance health, wellness and quality of life. She currently heads Chomik Consulting & Research Ltd, a health consulting practice in health promotion and population health. Dr Chomik's principal areas of interest are health planning, evaluation, programme development and policy. Her doctoral dissertation research, under the direction of Dr Lawrence Green, examined the factors that facilitate and challenge the development of health goals and targets. Recent initiatives include the development of comprehensive agendas for the prevention of cardiovascular diseases and skin cancer, the evaluation of initiatives for tobacco-use cessation and the development of a population health template that provides a framework to define and implement a population health approach. Dr Chomik has co-authored papers and made presentations on health impact assessment, health goals, partnerships in health and community health promotion.

Galen Cole, Ph.D., currently serves as a senior evaluation scientist and health communication analyst in the Office of Communication, Office of the Director, CDC. Before serving in this position, he held other posts at CDC (Chief of Research and Evaluation Branch, National AIDS Information Education Program, and Chief of the Behavioral Studies Section, Division of Sexually Transmitted Diseases and HIV Prevention, National Center for Prevention Services) and served as Assistant Director of Public Health and Director of Epidemiology for Maricopa County, in Phoenix, Arizona, and executive director of a research foundation. He has also served on the faculties of a number of different universities, including his current faculty position at the Rollins School of Public Health, Emory University, Atlanta, Georgia. His areas of expertise include planning and evaluating health communication, evaluating public health interventions and conducting evaluation, behavioural and epidemiological research.

Lisa Curtice is lecturer in community care studies at the Nuffield Centre for Community Care Studies, University of Glasgow, United Kingdom. Her current research interests focus on the social inclusion of people with learning disabilities, and the high support needs of and care at home for older people. She has a particular interest in the role of health promotion in improving the quality of life of users of community care services and their care givers. From 1984 to 1989 she worked at the Research Unit in Health and Behavioural Change, University of Edinburgh, where she was involved in the evaluation of the WHO Healthy Cities project in Europe. She is Chair of Pioneer Health Centre, the charity that established the Peckham experiment, and is now helping to promote the development of healthy living centres.

Evelyne de Leeuw was with the Department of Health Promotion of Maastricht University in the Netherlands. She trained as a health policy scientist in that university and the University of California, Berkeley. She has since moved to the University of Southern Denmark where, as professor of public health and Chair of the Department of Health Promotion, she is developing research and training programmes in the health field. She is also Director of the WHO Collaborating Centre for Research on Healthy Cities. The mission of the Centre is to facilitate research for, on, with and in project cities through the publication of newsletters, bibliographies and monographs that are available on the Internet (http://www.gvo.unimaas.nl/who-city/default.htm, accessed 9 January 2001). Between 1992 and 1998, she was Secretary-General of the Association of Schools of Public Health in the European Region (ASPHER). She has been involved extensively with global and European WHO health promotion programmes, and in 1997 was the General Rapporteur of the 4th International Conference on Health Promotion, Jakarta, Indonesia. Current research interests include not only Healthy Cities matters but also issues in the implementation of health and prevention policy.

Lindsey Dugdill, M.A., M.Phil., is Senior Lecturer in Health, School of Human Sciences in Liverpool John Moores University, United Kingdom. For the last eight years she has worked with businesses and organizations to improve their infrastructures for health at both the local and national levels. Local work has involved improving health and safety support for small businesses. The work in Liverpool has culminated in the production of the Liverpool Health at Work Strategy – the first such strategy in the United Kingdom. Its aim is to provide a coordinated approach to healthy workplaces across the city of Liverpool and to complement the city health plan. Nationally, she has acted as an adviser to the Health Education Authority's research project on health at work in the National Health Service, and contributed to its training programmes. Development and evaluation processes within the workplace are key interests.

Paul Evensen is a doctoral candidate at the University of Kansas, United States, and a research associate in the University's Work Group on Health Promotion and Community Development. Before this, he founded several non-profit community-based organizations that focused on community development approaches to HIV prevention and health promotion for gay/lesbian young people. He has been a consultant to the Services Administration of the National Institutes of Health.

Stephen B. Fawcett holds an endowed professorship at the University of Kansas, United States, where he is Kansas Health Foundation Professor of Community Leadership and University Distinguished Professor of Human Development and Family Life. He is also Director of the University's Work Group on Health Promotion and Community Development. In his work, he uses behavioural science and community development methods to help understand and improve health and social concerns of importance to communities. A former VISTA (Volunteers In Service To America) volunteer, he worked as a community organizer in public housing and low-income neighbourhoods. Dr Fawcett has been honoured as a Fellow in both Division 27 (Community Psychology) and Division 25 (Experimental Analysis of Behavior) of the American Psychological Association. He received the distinguished practice award of the Society for Community Research and Action and the Higuchi/Endowment award for applied sciences. He is co-author of over 100 articles and book chapters and several books in the areas of health promotion, community development, empowerment, self-help, independent living and public policy. Dr Fawcett has been a consultant to a number of private foundations, community partnerships and national organizations, including the John D. and Catherine T. MacArthur Foundation, the Ewing Kauffman Foundation, the California Wellness Foundation, the US Commission on National and Community Service, the Institute of Medicine of the National Academy of Sciences and CDC.

Jacqueline L. Fisher is Coordinator for Site Development for the School/ Community Sexual Risk Reduction Project and a research assistant with the

Work Group on Health Promotion and Community Development at the University of Kansas, United States. She completed her graduate work in public health and health education before joining the Work Group in 1993. Her work involved providing technical assistance and evaluation support to community health initiatives, especially those related to child wellbeing.

Vincent T. Francisco is Associate Director of the Work Group on Health Promotion and Community Development, Courtesy Assistant Professor with the Department of Human Development, and Adjunct Assistant Professor with the Department of Preventive Medicine, University of Kansas Medical School at the University of Kansas, United States. Dr Francisco is primarily interested in research in community development, especially enhancing community integration and support, and work to empower marginalized groups. He is interested in the provision of technical support for the development of coalitions, and evaluation of community-based intervention programmes focusing on adolescent development, the reduction of risk of substance abuse by teenagers, assaultive violence, cardiovascular diseases and teenage parenthood.

C. James Frankish is a Research Scholar of the British Columbia Health Research Foundation, Canada, Associate Director of the Institute of Health Promotion Research and Assistant Professor in the Department of Health Care and Epidemiology at the University of British Columbia. Dr Frankish's research focuses on community participation in health decision-making and includes: participatory research methods, factors influencing and enabling the development and success of community coalitions, citizen participation in health reform, the role of the mass media in health research, measures of health, wellbeing and quality of life, health impact assessment and the dissemination of knowledge of health promotion. He has a broad background in the planning and evaluation of health promotion programmes, and teaches social science applications in health promotion. He is a registered clinical psychologist and has extensive research and clinical experience in employee health, coping with chronic illness and health behaviour change in marginalized groups. He is involved with many organizations for community health and social service. His recent projects include a study of regional health board studies, the implementation of health goals and the development of criteria for health promotion in primary care.

Vicki Freimuth, Ph.D., is the Associate Director for Communication at CDC, United States, and is an internationally recognized leader in health communication. Formerly she was the Director of Health Communication and Professor in the Department of Speech Communication at the University of Maryland, College Park, and taught courses in health communication, diffusion of innovations and research methods. Her research focuses on the role of communication in health promotion in the United States and developing countries. As Associate Director for Communication, she administers the health communication and media relations programmes, and strengthens the science and practice of health communication throughout CDC.

Katherine L. Frohlich is a post-doctoral research fellow in social epidemiology at the School of Public Health, University of California, Berkeley, United States. She currently holds a post-doctoral fellowship award from the Canadian Institutes of Health Research. Her main areas of research include social epidemiology and health promotion.

Sylvie Gendron is a doctoral candidate in public health at the University of Montreal, Canada. She is Fellow of the Conseil québécois de la recherche sociale. Before this, she worked in Montreal's Public Health Department in the field of HIV-related research. Her main areas of interest include the theory and method of participatory practice in public health and women's health.

Christine Godfrey is Professor of Health Economics at the Department of Health Sciences and Clinical Evaluation at the University of York, United Kingdom. She has researched the economics of health promotion since 1984, and heads a small group of researchers at York. With Larry Harrison from the University of York and Slyvia Tilford at Leeds Metropolitan University, she co-directs a WHO collaborating centre in substance abuse. She has acted as an adviser on alcohol and smoking policies to WHO, other international bodies and national governments. She is currently a member of the WHO Expert Committee on Drug Dependence and President of the Society for the Study of Addiction.

Michael Goodstadt is Deputy Director of the Centre for Health Promotion at the University of Toronto, Canada (a WHO collaborating centre in health promotion) and Associate Director of the University's programme for the Master's degree in health sciences. He received degrees in psychology from Stanford University, United States (Ph.D., 1969) and Manchester University, United Kingdom (B.A., 1963). His professional and academic experience has included: 25 years as a Scientist at the Addiction Research Foundation, Toronto, Canada; 3 years at Rutgers University's Center for Alcohol Studies, New Jersey, United States; and faculty positions at the University of Toronto, University of Western Ontario and Rutgers University. His professional life has focused on the prevention of health-related problems among young people, particularly drug use and abuse. Recent interests include the conceptual elaboration and application of the principles of and best practice in health promotion, reducing the impact of personal and environmental risk factors associated with alcohol/drug abuse and other health-related problems, and the development and evaluation of community-based health promotion programmes.

Lawrence W. Green is now Distinguished Fellow in the US National Center for Chronic Disease Prevention and Health Promotion, Acting Director of the

Office on Smoking and Health, and Director of the WHO Collaborating Centre on Global Tobacco Control for CDC. He previously directed the national health promotion programme of the Kaiser Family Foundation as Vice-President of the Foundation, served as professor and director of health education and health promotion programmes at Johns Hopkins University and the University of Texas, and served as Director of the US Office of Health Promotion when the federal initiative on goals and objectives for health promotion and disease prevention was developed. He has received the Award of Excellence and the Distinguished Career Award of the American Public Health Association, the Alumnus of the Year Award of the University of California School of Public Health and the Jacques Perisot Medal of the International Union for Health Promotion and Education.

Slim Haddad is Assistant Professor, Department of Health Administration, University of Montreal, Canada. He is a public health physician with a Ph.D. in health economics. His domain of research is the planning, financing and evaluation of health services in developing and western countries, focusing on evaluation of the quality of primary health care services, patterns of utilization of health care and community health services, and outcome research.

Spencer Hagard is Visiting Professor in the Department of Public Health and Policy at the London School of Hygiene and Tropical Medicine, United Kingdom, and a public health consultant at its London Health Economics Consortium. He works mainly in the development and implementation of effective national systems for health promotion, including the appraisal of national or regional potential for investment for health. Before this, he held a number of positions in the United Kingdom public health system, including Chief Executive of the Health Education Authority for England from 1987 to 1994. He has been a consultant and technical adviser for WHO for a number of years, and is the Hungarian Government's health policy adviser, in association with the WHO Regional Office for Europe and the World Bank. He is the current President of the International Union for Health Promotion and Education (1996–2001).

Kari J. Harris is Research Assistant Professor at the University of Kansas Medical Center, United States, where she is conducting research on smoking cessation among underserved populations. Before joining the Medical Center faculty in 1998, she was a member of the Work Group on Health Promotion and Community Development of the University of Kansas.

Brian Hyndman is a health promotion consultant with the Health Communication Unit, Centre for Health Promotion, University of Toronto, Canada, and a lecturer in the Health Services Management Program at Ryerson Polytechnic University, where he teaches courses in programme planning and evaluation. Since completing his Masters degree in community health at the University of

Toronto, he has been involved in a number of projects for research on and evaluation of health promotion for the Addiction Research Foundation, the City of Toronto Department of Public Health, Health Canada and WHO. He has written and co-authored a number of resource documents and articles on community development, participatory evaluation and health promotion strategies. In addition, he has served as a consultant for a number of research and evaluation initiatives in public health, including the Community Action Program For Children Brighter Futures project, the Royal Commission on New Reproductive Technologies, the National Forum on Health, and the Ontario Task Force on the Primary Prevention of Cancer. From 1997 to 1999, Mr Hyndman was President of the Ontario Public Health Association.

Aine Kennedy is a research fellow at the University of Edinburgh, United Kingdom, and serves as a consultant in community development and health. She is the former Coordinator of the Drumchapel Healthy Cities project in Glasgow.

Susan D. Kirby began her career in business marketing in the United States with Southern Bell in 1980, after earning her degree in business marketing at the University of Alabama. She was an account executive for seven years with Bell, managing state and local government accounts in South Carolina. In 1988, she returned to graduate school to earn a Masters degree in public health and quickly learned that she could integrate her marketing know-how into projects for public health promotion and disease prevention. In 1993, she earned her doctoral degree in public health at the University of South Carolina School of Public Health, concentrating on social marketing and health communication. Dr Kirby is currently a senior health communication scientist with CDC's Office of Communication and consults on many national communication projects on social marketing, formative research and audience segmentation.

Adam Koplan, B.A., has been a health promotion research assistant at Health 2000, in Atlanta, Georgia, United States. He is currently a doctoral student at the University of Washington, in Seattle.

Marshall Kreuter, formerly President of Health 2000, a public health consulting firm in Atlanta, Georgia, United States, is now a Distinguished Scientist/ Fellow in the National Center for Chronic Disease Prevention and Health Promotion at CDC. He has a special interest in the planning, implementation and evaluation of population-based disease prevention and health promotion programmes. He and his colleagues are investigating ways to measure social capital and to explore how social capital may be associated with the effectiveness of community-based interventions. In 1982–1990, Dr Kreuter served as Director of first the Division of Health Education and then the Division of Chronic Disease Control and Community Intervention at CDC.

Craig Larsen has been a policy consultant for the Health Association of British Columbia, Canada, since 1998. Before this, he held a number of positions related to health system reform in British Columbia. He worked at the University of British Columbia's Institute of Health Promotion Research, coordinating research on health impact assessment, health goals and community participation in health system decision-making.

Lowell S. Levin is Emeritus Professor in the Department of Epidemiology and Public Health, Yale University School of Medicine, United States. Professor Levin has served for many years as the Head of the WHO Collaborating Centre for Health Promotion Policy and Research at the Department of Epidemiology and Public Health, and has been a consultant to WHO and, in particular, to its European health promotion and investment-for-health programme from its inception.

Rhonda K. Lewis is an assistant professor in the department of psychology at Wichita State University, Kansas, United States. She received her doctorate from the University of Kansas and her Masters degree in public health from the University of Kansas Medical School. She uses behavioural and community research methodologies to contribute to understanding how communities work, and promotes health strategies to improve the health of people living in Kansas. Dr Lewis has expertise in community organizing and development, and programme development and evaluation. Her research interests include: self-help groups, minority health, disadvantaged populations and issues in adolescent health, such as pregnancy, violence, substance abuse and HIV/AIDS.

Nicole Lezin is President of Cole Communications in Santa Cruz, California, United States. She has a degree in public policy and management from the Yale School of Organization and Management. She designs and manages applied research communication and health policy studies. Ms Lezin has extensive experience in developing and conducting large-scale programme and policy evaluations in a number of public health areas, including HIV/AIDS prevention, injury control, tobacco control and child health.

Christine M. Lopez is a former doctoral student in the Human Development and Family Life Department and was a research associate for the Work Group on Health Promotion and Community Development of the University of Kansas, United States. Ms Lopez is interested in community-based research in the areas of substance abuse, violence by young people and health promotion in rural settings.

David V. McQueen is a Senior Biomedical Research Scientist and Associate Director for Global Health Promotion at the National Center for Chronic Disease Prevention and Health Promotion at CDC, United States. Before this, he had been Director of the Division of Adult and Community Health and Acting

Director of the Office of Surveillance and Analysis at the National Center for Chronic Disease Prevention and Health Promotion. Before joining CDC, he was Professor and Director of the Research Unit in Health and Behavioural Change at the University of Edinburgh, United Kingdom (1983–1992) and, prior to that, Associate Professor of Behavioral Sciences at the Johns Hopkins University School of Hygiene and Public Health in Baltimore. He has served as director of WHO collaborating centres and as a technical consultant with the World Bank.

Nancy Milio, Ph.D., is Professor of Health Policy and Administration at the School of Public Health and Professor of Nursing at the University of North Carolina at Chapel Hill, United States. Her teaching, research and publications centre on policy development and implementation, strategic analysis and evaluation in public health services; food and nutrition; community information technology; and health promotion/education. She has worked with numerous governments (in Scandinavia, eastern and western Europe, Australasia and Latin America), and with WHO and the Pan American Health Organization as policy analyst and consultant for 20 years. Among her publications are 8 books and over 100 articles in 40 health, social science and policy journals in 7 countries. She has been visiting professor at universities in Australia, Brazil, Colombia, Finland, the Netherlands, New Zealand, Spain and the United Kingdom, as well as in the United States. Her most recent book is *Public health in the market: facing managed care, lean government, and health disparities* (Ann Arbor, MI, University of Michigan Press, 2000).

Adrienne Paine-Andrews is Associate Director of the Work Group on Health Promotion and Community Development and Assistant Research Professor of the Schiefelbusch Institute for Life Span Studies at the University of Kansas, United States. She also serves as the programme co-director for the initiative for the prevention of adolescent pregnancy sponsored by the Kansas Health Foundation. She is primarily interested in research that promotes community health and development, and works to empower marginal groups. She conducts collaborative research with a variety of groups, including members of community health initiatives. She is currently involved in several research projects in the areas of health promotion, community development and adolescent health. She is co-author of several articles on self-help, community development, adolescent pregnancy and substance abuse prevention, and health promotion.

Richard Parish is Chief Executive of the Health Development Agency, United Kingdom. Before this appointment, he was Regional Director of Education and Training for Eastern England.

Louise Potvin is Professor of Community Health in the Department of Social and Preventive Medicine, University of Montreal, Canada. She currently holds a Chair/Mentorship from the Canadian Foundation of Health Services Research on community approaches and health inequalities. Her main area of research is the evaluation of community health promotion programmes.

Dennis Raphael received his Ph.D. in educational theory from the Ontario Institute for Studies in Education, University of Toronto, Canada, previously earning a B.Sc. in psychology from Brooklyn College and an M.Sc. in psychology from the State University of New York, Cortland. He is an Associate Professor of Public Health Sciences and a former Associate Director of the Masters of Health Science Program in Health Promotion at the University of Toronto. Dr Raphael is co-director of the Quality of Life Research Unit at the University's Centre for Health Promotion. His areas of expertise are in research methodology and design, quality-of-life research, and the design and evaluation of health promotion activities. Dr Raphael has developed quality-of-life instrumentation for elderly people, adolescents and people with developmental disabilities. He has completed a study of the quality of life of two communities in Metropolitan Toronto and, most recently, a national project, funded by Health Canada, designed to improve the quality of life of older Canadians; information and reports on it are available on the Internet (http://www.utoronto.ca/qol, accessed 9 January 2001).

Pamela Ratner is Assistant Director of the Institute of Health Promotion Research and Associate Professor in the School of Nursing at the University of British Columbia, Canada. Her postdoctoral work, supervised by Dr Lawrence Green, was supported by the Medical Research Council of Canada and the Killam Foundation. She is currently a Health Research Scholar of the Canadian Institutes of Health Research. Her primary research interests are the social and behavioural determinants of health and health promotion. Specific projects have addressed the epidemiology of violence and intentional injury, efforts towards tobacco control and smoking cessation, risk perception and communication, and community participation in health care planning.

Lucie Richard is Assistant Professor, Faculty of Nursing, University of Montreal, Canada. She is currently a Career Award Researcher of the Medical Research Council of Canada. Her main area of research is the professional practice of health promotion practitioners and the theoretical underpinnings of health promotion programmes.

Kimber P. Richter, M.P.H., Ph.D., is a Research Assistant Professor in the Department of Preventive Medicine at Kansas University Medical Center, United States. She is also a faculty fellow in the Center's School of Nursing faculty development programme in substance abuse, funded by the Center for Substance Abuse Prevention of the Substance Abuse and Mental Health Services Administration of the US Department of Health and Human Services. A former doctoral student and member of the Work Group on Health Promotion and

Community Development at the University of Kansas, Dr Richter's current work focuses on developing effective smoking cessation interventions that are tailored to the needs of people in treatment for chemical dependence. Her publications span topics in bioethics, cardiovascular risk reduction, the prevention/ treatment of drug addiction, methodologies used include clinical trials, participatory action research, qualitative research and ecological measurement.

Irving Rootman is Director of the Centre for Health Promotion and Professor in the Department of Public Health Sciences at the University of Toronto, Canada. Before joining the University in 1990, he held a number of positions in Health Canada, including Chief of the Health Promotion Studies Unit in the Health Promotion Directorate, where he was responsible for managing evaluations of health promotion initiatives and for the development of Canada's national health promotion survey. He has been a senior scientist, consultant and technical adviser for WHO, and is currently director of a WHO collaborating centre in health promotion.

Stergios Russos is a research associate of the Work Group on Health Promotion and Community Development and a doctoral student at the Department of Human Development of the University of Kansas, United States. He completed his Masters degree in public health with an emphasis on health promotion at the Graduate School of Public Health at San Diego State University. His research targets clinical and community-based disease prevention and health promotion in areas including cardiovascular diseases, substance abuse, adolescent development and food security. He is author and co-author of several research and conceptual papers in public health and preventive medicine. His work emphasizes understanding and improving how community-based interventions influence population-level health and development outcomes.

Alfred Rütten is Director of the Research Centre for Regional Health Promotion and Professor of Sports Science and Applied Sociology at the Technical University of Chemnitz, Germany. Most recently he has served as Visiting Professor of Public Health at Yale University. He is Director of MAREPS (methodology for the analysis of rationality and effectiveness of prevention and health promotion strategies), an international research project sponsored by the European Commission. Dr Rütten has also worked as temporary adviser for WHO within the activities of the European Committee for Health Promotion Development.

Jerry Schultz is Associate Director of the Work Group on Health Promotion and Community Development and Adjunct Assistant Professor in the Preventive Medicine, Anthropology and Human Development departments at the University of Kansas, United States. Dr Schultz received his Ph.D. in anthropology from the University of Kansas and has taught there and at the University of Nebraska. He is currently directing a rural health promotion initiative in

Kansas and engaged in developing an electronic technical assistance system for health promotion and community development. His primary interest is research in community development, the empowerment of at-risk community groups and participatory action research. Dr Schultz is co-author of several research articles on health promotion and the evaluation of community partnerships. He is a co-author of several manuals for community development in the areas of the strategic planning and evaluation of prevention initiatives. He has been a consultant for a variety of organizations, including private foundations and community coalitions.

Jane Springett is Professor of Health Promotion and Public Health at Liverpool John Moores University, United Kingdom, where she is also Director of the Institute for Health, which publishes the *Journal of contemporary health*. She is actively involved in the development of local healthy public policy, having been a member of the joint public health team that developed the Liverpool City Health Plan. She has a Ph.D. in urban geography, and a longstanding research interest in healthy cities and communities. She is currently a member of the local evaluation team for the new Merseyside Health Action Zone, and involved in the evaluation of the Manchester Salford and Trafford Health Action Zone. Her main research interests are joint work and organizational change, participatory evaluation and action research in a variety of settings. She has considerable experience in curriculum development in health promotion, grounded in a theoretical understanding of the way people learn, and currently teaches in the programme for the M.Sc. in health (promotion, research and policy change) and leads the doctoral programme in that area at Liverpool John Moores University

Sylvie Stachenko is Head, Noncommunicable Diseases and Mental Health in the WHO Regional Office for Europe. Prior to joining WHO in 1997, she held a number of positions in Health Canada, including Director of Preventive Services Division, where she was responsible for the development of national initiatives in heart health, diabetes, and breast and cervical cancer. She was also the Director for the WHO countrywide integrated noncommunicable disease intervention (CINDI) programme in Canada and of the WHO Collaborating Centre in Policy Development in Non-communicable Disease Prevention.

Sarah Stewart-Brown is Reader in Health Services Research in the Department of Public Health at the University of Oxford, United Kingdom. She is also Director of the Health Services Research Unit. Before coming to Oxford, she worked in the National Health Service, first as a paediatrician and subsequently as a public health doctor in London, Bristol and Worcester. She has also held academic appointments at the departments of Child Health and of Epidemiology and Community Health at the University of Bristol. Her past research has been in two fields: community child health and health promotion. Her current research interests centre around the importance of emotional wellbeing for the health of both adults and children. Her recent publications cover the public health implications of parenting programmes, the ethics of childhood screening programmes and the importance of emotional wellbeing for health in adulthood.

Reg Warren carried out the first health promotion survey in Canada and was project director for the 1990 survey. He developed and executed broad-based dissemination strategies for both surveys. Currently, he is a consultant at the Center for Health Promotion, University of Toronto and a member of the Center's Best Practices and Evaluation Unit. He was also the senior consultant on the project to make meaningful the results of health promotion research, and has an extensive background in the dissemination of results from major research projects. Mr Warren also has extensive experience in the analysis, evaluation, development, consolidation and dissemination of complex information. Mr Warren has completed literature reviews and syntheses of available research for a variety of clients, including Health Canada, the Premier's Council of Ontario and the Ontario Ministry of Health. He has extensive experience in the federal Government, and was involved in the national consultation project on healthy aging, the national AIDS phase-III consultation project and the draft framework on the new relationship between Health Canada and national voluntary organizations working in health. Mr Warren has been involved in the evaluation of health promotion strategies in Canada and Europe. He has a graduate degree in international development.

Ella L. Williams is a former doctoral student in the Department of Human Development and was a research associate with the Work Group on Health Promotion and Community Development at the University of Kansas, United States. She has experience in evaluating and providing technical support to community health coalitions, as well as in multicultural issues related to community development and health promotion. Ms Williams is a certified substance abuse counsellor with experience ranging from prevention to treatment and aftercare. She also has expertise in the area of drug-related violence, with a research interest in adolescent health, community psychology and the root causes and prevention of violence by young people.

Rick Wilson acted as project coordinator for the project in Canada to make health promotion research results meaningful. He has also accumulated experience in disseminating information on a wide variety of surveys and on issues such as tobacco and substance abuse. He has extensive experience as an officer and manager in the public sector, combined with practical liaison and consultations with a myriad of user groups. He was also the coordinator for the national consultation project on healthy aging, and participated in the national AIDS phase-III consultation project and the draft framework on the new relationship between Health Canada and national voluntary organizations working in health.

Laura Young, M.P.H., is Senior Program Evaluator, Office of Health Education at the University of Pennsylvania, Philadelphia, United States. Her primary role is designing and implementing evaluation strategies to assess the interactive effects of cognitive and behavioural factors, and social conditions as determinants of the health status of college students.

Erio Ziglio is Regional Adviser for Social and Economic Development at the WHO Regional Office for Europe. Before joining WHO, he worked for 12 years in academia, holding positions in universities in both Europe and North America. He had worked with WHO since 1981.

Contents

Part 1
Introduction and framework

Introduction to the book

Irving Rootman

WHO European Working Group on Health Promotion Evaluation

The WHO Regional Office for Europe and other organizations committed to health promotion have come under increasing pressure to evaluate or support the evaluation of work for health promotion. This pressure has come from both outside and inside the field. Externally, it has come from people involved in health reform, who are anxious to have evidence on the contribution of health promotion to reducing costs, and from the critics of health promotion, who are sceptical of its efficacy. Internal pressure comes from practitioners, who want to document and show the value of their efforts, and improve their practices, policy-makers, who want to defend their investments in health promotion and the Regional Office, which has initiated a series of projects using a health gains framework. This pressure has raised questions about, for example, where are the health investments with the greatest potential benefits, and what new analytical skills will be needed to evaluate the trade-offs involved in and the implications of health investments *(1)*.

The pressure for increased attention to evaluation led the Regional Office to seek partners and funding to support the establishment of a WHO European Working Group on Health Promotion Evaluation. Both were obtained from the Centers for Disease Control and Prevention (CDC) in the United States of America, Health Canada and the Health Education Authority (HEA – now the Health Development Agency) in the United Kingdom. To promote homogeneity, the members of the Group were selected to represent diverse perspectives, and came from Canada, Europe and the United States; from governments, WHO and the academic community; and from different evaluation backgrounds. Membership was limited to western, industrialized countries, however, and the Group focused on evaluation efforts there. Its work began in July 1995, when the purpose of the Working Group was agreed to be *(2)*:

> to stimulate and support innovative approaches to the evaluation and practice of health promotion, by reviewing the theory and best practice of evaluation and by producing guidelines and recommendations for health promotion policy-makers and practitioners concerning evaluation of health promotion approaches.

Its objectives were:

- to examine the current range of evaluation methods, both quantitative and qualitative; and
- to provide guidance to policy-makers and practitioners both to foster the use of appropriate methods for health promotion evaluation and to increase the quality of evaluations.

Process

The following process was adopted to achieve these objectives. Eight meetings of the Working Group, sponsored by CDC, HEA, Health Canada and WHO collaborating centres, were held in North America and Europe. Over 30 background papers were commissioned to address relevant topics. The papers were sent to a range of individuals and groups with stakes in health promotion, including the WHO European collaborating centres for health promotion, the European Committee for Health Promotion Development, the CDC Chronic Disease Conference and the Canadian Consortium for Health Promotion Research. Three reports were planned. The first was a background paper presenting a framework for evaluation of health promotion initiatives, released at the Fourth International Conference on Health Promotion in Jakarta, Indonesia in 1997 (3). The second was a report for policy-makers released at a meeting of the European Committee for Health Promotion Development in 1998 (4). A third report, to provide guidance on evaluation to practitioners interested in health promotion, is being developed with assistance from WHO health promotion collaborating centres in Europe (5).

This book is the fourth product of this collaborative effort. It comprises papers commissioned by the Working Group or submitted for its consideration. Although not all of the background papers submitted were selected for this volume, the Group considered all, and many of their ideas found their way into this book and the above-mentioned documents. The manuscript was produced by an editorial group of seven and reviewed by the full Working Group.

Guiding principles

Early in the discussions of the Working Group, the members agreed that certain basic principles tending to characterize health promotion should guide their work and recommendations. These principles underlie much of the discussion in this book and help to define its content and structure. Specifically, the Group agreed that health promotion initiatives (programmes, policies and other organized activities) should be:

- empowering (enabling individuals and communities to assume more power over the personal, socioeconomic and environmental factors that affect their health);
- participatory (involving all concerned at all stages of the process);
- holistic (fostering physical, mental, social and spiritual health);

4

- intersectoral (involving the collaboration of agencies from relevant sectors);
- equitable (guided by a concern for equity and social justice);
- sustainable (bringing about changes that individuals and communities can maintain once initial funding has ended); and
- multistrategy (using a variety of approaches – including policy development, organizational change, community development, legislation, advocacy, education and communication – in combination).

On the basis of these principles, the Working Group concluded that approaches appropriate for the evaluation of health promotion initiatives share four core features. The first is participation. At each stage, evaluation should involve, in appropriate ways, all with a legitimate interest in the initiative. These can include: policy-makers, community members and organizations, health and other professionals, and local and national health agencies. The participation in evaluation of members of the community whose health is being addressed is particularly important. Second, evaluation should draw on a variety of disciplines, and a broad range of information-gathering procedures should be considered for use. Third, evaluation should build the capacity of individuals, communities, organizations and governments to address important health promotion concerns. Finally, evaluation should be appropriate: designed to accommodate the complex nature of health promotion interventions and their long-term impact.

Limitations and strengths

As noted, this book is limited to evaluation work in western, industrialized societies. This does not make it irrelevant to other parts of the world, but people working in such countries should use judgement and caution in applying the work discussed here. Further, the book does not purport to be a methodology textbook, but considers a whole range of issues pertaining to evaluation of health promotion initiatives, of which methodology is only one. Chapter 1 outlines the types of issues addressed.

This book does not consider in great depth issues in the evaluation of approaches to individual behaviour change. The Working Group felt that other sources provide such discussions, and preferred to focus on issues pertinent to evaluating approaches addressing settings, policies and systems. Similarly, the book does not emphasize the evaluation of traditional work for disease prevention; there is a large literature on this topic. In addition, the Group wanted to focus on evaluation of health promotion efforts consistent with the Ottawa Charter for Health Promotion (6). As the Group believes that a heath promotion approach can strengthen the evaluation of disease prevention efforts, however, the discussion here is relevant to that topic (see Chapter 1).

Finally, the book takes a broad view of what constitutes evidence, which often serves as a code word for accountability and hard science. The Working

Group suggests that a broad view is entirely appropriate to health promotion, given its underlying principles. For example, the Group's report to policy-makers concludes that the use of randomized controlled trials to evaluate health promotion initiatives is "inappropriate, misleading and unnecessarily expensive" in most cases *(4)*. Chapter 2 provides an extended discussion of this issue.

Structure

This book is divided into five parts addressing particular topics. Each contains chapters that identify key issues in relation to the topic, discuss the theory and best practice of evaluation, and suggest guidelines for policy-makers and practitioners. The book is aimed at researchers, students, practitioners, policy-makers and others who want an in-depth understanding of the current issues in evaluating health promotion initiatives. The Working Group hopes that it proves useful.

References

1. *Securing investment in health: Report of a demonstration project in the provinces of Bolzano and Trento. Final report.* Copenhagen, WHO Regional Office for Europe, 1995 (document).
2. *WHO-EURO Working Group on Health Promotion Evaluation: executive summary report of meeting, Atlanta, Georgia, USA, July 27–28, 1995.* Copenhagen, WHO Regional Office for Europe, 1995.
3. *New players for a new era: leading health promotion into the 21st century: 4th International Conference on Health Promotion, Jakarta, Indonesia, 21–25 July 1997.* Geneva, World Health Organization, 1998 (document).
4. *Health promotion evaluation: recommendations to policy-makers: report of the WHO European Working Group on Health Promotion Evaluation.* Copenhagen, WHO Regional Office for Europe, 1998 (document EUR/ICP/IVST 05 01 03).
5. SPRINGETT, J. *Practical guidance on evaluating health promotion: guidelines for practitioners.* Copenhagen, WHO Regional Office for Europe, 1999 (document).
6. Ottawa Charter for Health Promotion. *Health promotion,* **1**(4): iii–v (1986).

1
A framework for health promotion evaluation

Irving Rootman, Michael Goodstadt,
Louise Potvin and Jane Springett

This chapter presents both conceptual and practical frameworks to assist in the evaluation of health promotion initiatives. The first section considers what health promotion is; the second, what evaluation is in general and in the context of health promotion. The third section presents an appropriate and useful framework for evaluating health promotion programmes, policies and other initiatives.

What is health promotion?

To evaluate health promotion initiatives, one needs to be clear about what health promotion is. We attempt to clarify health promotion's meaning in three ways, by examining: its recent origins, including the circumstances and issues to which it is a response; a variety of proposed definitions; and what it seems to constitute in practice.

Recent origins

Although the idea of health promotion is not new, and several attempts were made in the first half of this century to give it prominence *(1,2)*, its rise as an organized field can be traced to 1974 when the Canadian health minister of the time, Marc Lalonde, released a paper entitled *A new perspective on the health of Canadians (3)*. This was the first national government policy document to identify health promotion as a key strategy. It was subsequently used as the basis for similar policy documents in other countries, including Sweden and the United States, and contributed to a growing international enthusiasm for and acceptance of health promotion as both a concept and an approach that could be used by governments, organizations, communities and individuals. In 1986, the first International Conference on Health Promotion captured this growing interest and endorsed the Ottawa Charter for Health Promotion *(4)*, which in turn has reinforced the development of health promotion throughout the world.

The basis for the recent interest in health promotion can be traced to the confluence of a number of disparate forces. Anderson *(5)* considered these under five headings:

1. growing emphasis on positive health and improved quality of life;
2. people's greater desire to exercise control over their lives, associated with trends in consumerism;
3. the limited effectiveness of traditional didactic strategies often associated with health education;
4. recognition that many health problems are related to individual lifestyles; and
5. growing evidence of the weak relationship between health care and health status, especially the poor return on increasingly costly resources invested in health.

Green & Raeburn (6) identified additional, sometimes related, influences, including:

6. the community development and communications movements, which promote grassroots, in contrast to top-down, initiatives;
7. the influence of the self-care and women's movements, which requires a shift in the distribution of power to individuals and communities;
8. the pressure brought to bear on social programmes and high-technology medical care by deterioration in economic conditions around the world;
9. better social, behavioural and educational research on health issues; and
10. greater recognition of the holistic nature of health: that is, the "social, mental and spiritual qualities of life".

(Green & Kreuter (7) and Macdonald & Bunton (8) also discuss such influences.)

Finally, challenging arguments for reorienting public health have come from epidemiological research, which clearly documents the powerful influence of the broader determinants of health. These are factors beyond individual genetic and behavioural characteristics, and are often most strongly associated with socioeconomic conditions, equity and access issues, national wealth, social support and other structural or systemic factors (9–16).

This mixed pedigree has resulted in an understanding of health promotion, sometimes called the new public health (8, 11), that extends beyond health protection to include:

1. strengthening health;
2. redistributing power and control over individual and collective health issues;
3. reducing the negative impact of a broad range of health determinants associated with social, political and economic environments;
4. shifting the allocation of resources upstream, towards preventing problems before they occur;
5. giving attention to the domains of health beyond the physical, including the mental, social and possibly spiritual dimensions;

8

6. taking an ecological approach *(17,18)*; and
7. recognizing community development and involvement as legitimate and effective strategies.

Some of these characteristics are more concerned with the goals of the new public health (1 and 5), while others address the means of achieving these goals (2–6 and 7). Not surprisingly, the various definitions of health promotion that have been proposed reflect these characteristics.

Definitions

Many definitions of health promotion have been proposed over the past two decades. Table 1.1 lists some of the most important. At first glance, these definitions differ in significant ways. Closer scrutiny, however, suggests that the discrepancies represent differences in perspective and emphasis, rather than fundamental conflicts in substance.

A useful distinction has been made between health promotion as an outcome and as a process. Kickbusch *(18)* refers to health promotion in the latter context as "a process for initiating, managing, and implementing change. ... a process of personal, organizational, and policy development". The analysis of other conceptualizations provides further insights into the ways in which health promotion has been understood. What distinguishes health promotion from other approaches is the nature of the expected outcomes (goals and objectives) and the strategies (processes and activities) involved. The nature of these outcomes and processes ultimately determines how one answers the questions of what works in health promotion and how evaluation might best be conducted. (Buchanan *(30)* discusses the "purpose–process gap" in health promotion.)

Borrowing from Rokeach's distinction between terminal and instrumental values *(31)*, one can characterize the goals and objectives of health promotion found in various definitions as falling into two categories: terminal goals and instrumental objectives. Terminal goals refer to the ultimate (usually longer-term) goals of health promotion, or "the desirable end-states" *(31)*, that guide and motivate health promotion strategies and activities. The terminal goal of health promotion most commonly includes a desired end-state of improved health or wellbeing, although WHO has defined health as a resource for living *(4,24)* and therefore not an end in itself. Nevertheless, health clearly has intrinsic value and is a generally accepted outcome for health promotion efforts.

Instrumental objectives refer to the intermediate (usually shorter-term) objectives, the achievement of which is believed to mediate the attainment of the terminal goals. For example, smoking cessation, as an objective, is instrumental in the attainment of improved health or wellbeing, as measured by improvements in life expectancy, reduction in years of life lost, quality of life, etc.

A further distinction can be made between instrumental objectives and the instrumental processes by which they are achieved. For example, the objective of smoking cessation may be achieved through the instrumental process of in-

9

creased self-efficacy (feeling of competence). Finally, one can identify the instrumental activities through which the instrumental processes and hence the
instrumental objectives and terminal goals can be achieved. For example,
participation in a smoking cessation programme can help a smoker come to
experience greater self-efficacy, in being able to take steps that are effective in
quitting.

Table 1.1. Definitions of health promotion

Source and date	Definition (emphasis added)
Lalonde, 1974 (3)	A *strategy* "aimed at informing, influencing and assisting both individuals and organizations so that they will accept more responsibility and be more active in matters affecting mental and physical health"
US Department of Health, Education, and Welfare, 1979 (19)	"A combination of health education and related organizational, political and economic *programs* designed to support changes in behavior and in the environment that will improve health"
Green, 1980 (20)	"Any combination of health education and related organizational, political and economic *interventions* designed to facilitate behavioral and environmental changes that will improve health"
Green & Iverson, 1982 (21)	"Any combination of health education and related organizational, economic, and environmental *supports* for behavior conducive to health"
Perry & Jessor, 1985 (22)	"The implementation of *efforts* to foster improved health and well-being in all four domains of health [physical, social, psychological and personal]"
Nutbeam, 1985 (23)	"The *process* of enabling people to increase control over the determinants of health and thereby improve their health"
WHO, 1984 (24), 1986 (4) and Epp, 1986 (25)	"The *process* of enabling people to increase control over, and to improve, their health"
Goodstadt et al., 1987 (26)	"The maintenance and enhancement of existing levels of health through the *implementation* of effective *programs, services,* and *policies*"
Kar, 1989 (27)	"The advancement of wellbeing and the avoidance of health risks by achieving optimal levels of the behavioral, societal, environmental and biomedical determinants of health"
O'Donnell, 1989 (28)	"The *science* and *art* of helping people choose their lifestyles to move toward a state of optimal health"
Labonté & Little, 1992 (29)	"Any *activity* or *program* designed to improve social and environmental living conditions such that people's experience of well-being is increased"

Definitions and concepts of health promotion have differed in goals, objectives, processes and actions. Table 1.2 analyses the concepts of health promotion as contained in the definitions listed in Table 1.1. These definitions are
deconstructed according to their terminal goals and their instrumental objectives, processes and actions.

Table 1.2. Definitions of health promotion deconstructed

Source and date	Activities (programmes, policies, etc.)	Processes (underlying mechanisms)	Objectives (instrumental outcomes)	Goals (ultimate outcomes)
Winslow, 1920 (2)	"Organized community effort for the education of the individual in personal health, and the development of the social machinery"		"… to ensure everyone a standard of living"	"… the maintenance or improvement of health"
Sigerist, 1946 (1)			"… by providing a decent standard of living, good labor conditions, education, physical culture, means of rest and recreation"	"Health is promoted"
Lalonde, 1974 (3)	"… informing, influencing and assisting both individuals and organizations"	"… so that they [individuals and organizations] will accept more responsibility and be more active in matters affecting mental and physical health"		
US Department of Health, Education, and Welfare, 1979 (19)	"A combination of health education and related organizational, political and economic programs"		"… designed to support changes in behavior and in the environment"	"… that will improve health"
Green, 1980 (20)	"Any combination of health education and related organizational, political and economic interventions"		"… designed to facilitate behavioral and environmental changes"	"… that will improve health"
Green & Iverson, 1982 (21)	"Any combination of health education and related organizational, political and economic supports"		"… for behavior"	"… conducive to health"

Source and date	Activities (programmes, policies, etc.)	Processes (underlying mechanisms)	Objectives (instrumental outcomes)	Goals (ultimate outcomes)
Perry & Jessor, 1985 (22)	"The implementation of efforts"			"... to foster improved health and well-being in all four domains of health [physical, social, psychological and personal]"
Nutbeam, 1985 (23)		"The process of enabling people to increase control"	"... over the determinants of health"	"... and thereby improve their health"
WHO, 1984 (24), 1986 (4) Epp, 1986 (25)		"The process of enabling people to increase control over [their health]"		"... and thereby to improve their health"
Goodstadt et al., 1987 (26)	"... through the implementation of effective programs, services, and policies"			"The maintenance and enhancement of existing levels of health"
Kar, 1989 (27)			"... and the avoidance of health risks by achieving optimal levels of the behavioral, societal, environmental, and biomedical determinants of health"	"The advancement of wellbeing"
O'Donnell, 1989 (28)	"The science and art of helping people choose their lifestyles"			"... to move toward a state of optimal health"
Green & Kreuter, 1991 (7)	"The combination of educational and environmental supports for actions and conditions of living"			"... conducive to health"

As can be seen, most definitions of health promotion express the desired end (terminal goal) in terms of improved health or wellbeing, although several also give health maintenance as a goal. The definitions are more diverse in their identification of objectives, processes and actions; that is, they show greater variability in defining how health promotion is thought to improve health. Some leave components unspecified. This diversity, however, is more apparent than real. The instrumental objectives of the definitions fall into two clusters, clusters that are not mutually exclusive. The first focuses on the environment, and the second, on the individual. Most definitions, however, recognize the need to focus on both.

The instrumental activities vary in their level of specificity and particular elements. For example, some refer to efforts or measures and others to types of intervention, such as programmes, services or policies. Nevertheless, most refer to or imply some sort of action.

Few definitions identify the processes. The exceptions are the WHO definition (4), its elaboration by Nutbeam (23) and the definition put forward by Marc Lalonde (3).

Thus, recent conceptualizations of health promotion differ, but share important elements. Specifically, the makers of definitions see health promotion as involving a diverse set of actions, focused on the individual or environment, which through increasing control ultimately leads to improved health or wellbeing. We nevertheless recognize the pre-eminence of the definition first proposed by the WHO Regional Office for Europe (24), and subsequently endorsed by the first International Conference on Health Promotion and published in the Ottawa Charter for Health Promotion (4); this defines health promotion as "the process of enabling people to increase control over, and to improve, their health".

An expanded version of this definition, used in a glossary of health promotion terms developed by Nutbeam (23), is: "the process of enabling people to increase control over the determinants of health and thereby improve their health". This definition has the merit of making explicit a concern with individuals and communities, what is being controlled and a possible causal mechanism. Nevertheless, there are determinants of health that individuals and communities cannot control, but some of whose negative influences health promotion efforts can help mitigate (such as the establishment of mutual aid among people with genetic disease, and community kitchens for low-income families). In addition, health promotion efforts aim to reinforce or accentuate the positive influences of some determinants of health that cannot be controlled directly (for example, increasing social support – see also Chapter 22). Further, some evidence indicates that increasing personal control or self-efficacy in itself strengthens health (32–34). The Ottawa Charter definition (4), however, captures some of the key elements of health promotion as understood and accepted by many people working in the field.

In particular, it embodies the key underlying concept or cardinal principle of health promotion: empowerment. That is, it suggests that health promotion is fundamentally about ensuring that individuals and communities are able to assume the power to which they are entitled. Thus, we suggest that the primary criterion for determining whether a particular initiative should be considered to be health promoting, ought to be the extent to which it involves the process of enabling or empowering individuals or communities. The absence of empowering activities should therefore signal that an intervention does not fall within the rubric of health promotion. Attempts to encourage public participation are critical to the process of empowerment. Other criteria that help to distinguish health promotion include taking a broad view of health and emphasizing equity or social justice and intersectoral collaboration *(35)*.

Given these criteria, one can argue that a health promotion approach can be applied in a number of domains, including prevention, treatment, rehabilitation and even long-term care. One can also argue that not everything in these domains constitutes health promotion. In particular, health promotion and disease prevention are not synonymous, but complementary. Even so, most if not all activities for prevention (and even treatment and rehabilitation) can be carried out in a health promoting way, by empowering individuals and communities, encouraging public participation, taking a broad view of health and the determinants of health, emphasizing social justice and fostering intersectoral collaboration.

Practice

Notwithstanding these criteria, practitioners have applied the label of health promotion to a wide range of their activities. For example, Downie et al. *(35)* identify seven different types of activities that they consider to fall under this rubric:

1. preventive services (such as immunization, cervical screening, hypertension case-finding and provision of nicotine-containing chewing gum);
2. preventive health education (such as efforts to influence lifestyle and to increase the use of preventive services);
3. preventive health protection (such as the fluoridation of water);
4. health education for preventive health protection (such as lobbying for seat-belt legislation);
5. positive health education (aimed at influencing behaviour on positive health grounds, and including encouraging productive use of leisure time and helping people develop health-related life skills);
6. positive health protection (such as the implementation of workplace anti-smoking policies and provision of leisure facilities); and
7. health education for positive health protection (such as obtaining support for positive health promotion measures).

Whether all of these activities fit the above-noted criteria is a moot point, given the fact that influential organizations in the field, such as HEA in the United Kingdom, support these activities as part of their work for health promotion.

14

In a number of countries, many different types of activities take place under the banner of health promotion, whether they meet the above-noted criteria or not. For example, in Canada, the following activities have been funded and carried out in the name of health promotion: mass-media campaigns to increase awareness of the dangers of smoking and drink–driving; school-based, comprehensive health education programmes; efforts to mobilize community concerns about heart health, low birth weight and other prevention issues; community development projects to enable disadvantaged mothers to strengthen their parenting skills; efforts to enable workplaces to assess and deal with lifestyle and environmental issues that affect them; efforts to build coalitions to respond to cut-backs in services; lobbying for changes in policies on smoking and other issues; and efforts to enhance the preventive practices of physicians and other health care workers.

In addition, health promotion activities are increasingly planned and conducted in combination. A comprehensive approach typically uses a mix of strategies to change individuals' behaviour through environmental and policy changes. The current approach to intervention is to develop multilevel (national, regional, community) action and multidimensional approaches to ensure sustainability. In other words, health promotion initiatives are increasingly complex.

Thus, many different kinds of activities have been called health promotion, whether they fulfil all or any of the criteria derived from theoretical writings. The question is whether all of these activities increasingly should be considered health promotion from an evaluation perspective.

It is tempting to take the view that only the activities that meet at least one of the criteria for health promotion should be included. This, however, might exclude a wide range of interventions, some with very modest scope and objectives, which nevertheless contribute to promoting health. In any case, many of the considerations that apply to evaluation in health promotion also apply to evaluation in other domains, especially prevention. Thus, one should not be too doctrinaire about what health promotion might include for evaluation purposes. At the same time, one should recognize the importance of the principles of health promotion, particularly empowerment, as a means of guiding activities, including those associated with evaluation.

Conclusion

This review of definitions of health promotion from the point of view of the development of the field, theory and current practice shows that health promotion is far from being monolithic. It is multidisciplinary and still full of unresolved tensions. Nevertheless, some areas of broad agreement can form the basis for integrating and resolving some of the existing paradoxes. In particular, there seems to be some agreement that guiding principles such as empowerment and participation are important, and a wide range of activities constitutes health promotion practice aimed at improving the health of individuals and communities. What are the most appropriate ways of evaluating these activities?

Meaning and practice of evaluation in health promotion

Over the last 40 years, many authors have suggested definitions for evaluation. Among the broadest is Green & Kreuter's "comparison of an object of interest against a standard of acceptability" (7). Once this has been said, however, many questions remain. What is the object of inquiry? How is the comparison made? How is the standard defined? For what are evaluation results used? What is the role of evaluators in the life and death of programmes? Evaluation theoreticians and practitioners have proposed many answers. This section presents an overview of development and debate that illustrates the range of possibilities for the evaluation of health promotion.

Fundamental issues and challenges

There are many evaluation textbooks, such as those of Suchman (36) and Wholey et al. (37). Each has proposed a particular set of tools and perspectives for handling the task of evaluating programmes or other kinds of intervention. In addition to the writers of textbooks, many pioneer thinkers have developed their own perspectives in articles published in major peer-reviewed journals of the field, including *Evaluation and program planning, Evaluation review, Evaluation and the health professions and New directions for program evaluation*. Readers should glance through them to capture some of the richness and worth of these scholarly debates.

Evaluation has been enriched by contributions from many disciplines and professional activities. Many evaluators have come from the field of education. Education systems' needs for evaluation are the source of concepts such as summative and formative evaluation (38) and goal-free evaluation (39); these are used to characterize activities aimed at producing, respectively, an overall judgement on a programme, information that helps improve its implementation and delivery, or information on unexpected outcomes.

Social sciences such as social psychology, sociology, social work, political science, anthropology and economic science have also been major sources of input. Taxonomies based on process and impact evaluation (40), the distinction between internal and external validity (41,42), the introduction of cost–benefit and other costing methods (43,44), taxonomies of evaluation based on epistemological paradigms such as "post-positivism", "constructivism" or "critical theory" (45–47) and "empowerment evaluation" (48) are major contributions.

The health sciences have provided another influence. The development of the randomized clinical trial for evaluating medical treatment (49), the use of epidemiological models to take account of population-level variables in evaluation projects (50), the division of programme development into a sequence of evaluative phases that emphasizes the distinction between efficacy and effectiveness (50) and the development and implementation of large-scale preventive programmes (51) have all been integrated into the arsenal of evaluation.

Finally, evaluation has been an important issue outside the academic world. With the adoption of the Planning-Programming-Budgeting-System in all

16

executive-branch agencies of the United States federal Government in the mid-1960s, in an attempt to rationalize its decision-making about social programme issues *(52)*, evaluation became a major preoccupation of public administrators. Evaluators involved with government programmes promoted concepts such as accountability *(53)* and evaluability *(54)* and the emphasis on programme management *(55)* that are now part of the thinking about evaluation.

This broad overview illustrates the multidisciplinary nature of evaluation and the variety of issues and preoccupations that have led to the development of the field. In addition to these contributions, there have been limited efforts to provide analytical frameworks to organize all this activity. Worth noting are House's taxonomy of types of evaluation *(56)*, and Guba & Lincoln's developmental phases of the field *(57)*. Particularly helpful for the present discussion are five fundamental issues, identified by Shadish et al. *(58)*, related to defining and understanding all programme evaluation: social programming, valuing, knowledge construction, knowledge use and evaluation practice. According to these authors, a definition of evaluation:

1. is usually based on a perspective on the way that social programmes develop and improve in regard to the problem they are supposed to address (defining the object of inquiry);
2. should identify how values can be attached to programme descriptions (defining the range of acceptable standards);
3. should reflect evaluators' thinking about the conditions that are necessary to produce knowledge about the programme (helping to identify the comparisons that are allowed);
4. usually reflects how evaluation information can be used and the objectives it helps to pursue; and
5. should identify the approaches and practices evaluators follow in their professional work (determining their role with regard to programmes or other initiatives).

These five issues provide a framework for exploring and clarifying the nature of evaluation in general and in the context of health promotion in particular.

Social programming

Programme evaluation is about the systematic study of programmes. Programmes are not natural objects, but human artefacts composed of resources that are assembled to create activities and services that, taken together, pursue objectives addressing a problem in a given context for a specific population *(59)*. These activities are expected to produce some effects on the situation.

This dimension of evaluation delineates a series of components that can legitimately be assessed, and it encompasses many of the existing typologies. For example, process evaluation *(40)* focuses on resources and activities, while outcome evaluation deals with the relationship between the activities

17

and services and changes in the situation. In the health field, where preoccupations with the efficacy and effectiveness of interventions are paramount, programme evaluation has often emphasized establishing a relationship between the programme or its elements and some aspects of the situation addressed *(60)*. We recommend neither constraining the range of questions that can be addressed nor establishing a hierarchy for valuing the questions. Rather, we suggest that any question that is relevant for the programme or its actors is worth addressing. Any programme has more than one interesting feature.

This aspect of evaluation also emphasizes the fact that programmes are context bound. They are put together as answers to specific problems in specific contexts. Programme evaluators should thus be aware that these programme–context relationships might be crucial in explaining some of the programme's features. Weiss *(61)* and Cronbach et al. *(62)* have been among the strong advocates for a "contextually realistic" theory of evaluation. This means that the information produced by evaluation should be useful for understanding how programmes are designed, implemented and modified, both locally and as generalizable knowledge. In addition, Weiss *(63)* argues that programmes are not static. They are dynamic entities that change as time passes and as information from evaluation is fed back. Thus, no matter what question evaluation addresses, evaluators should remember that the information produced is locally defined by the unique unfolding of the programme in relation to the social problem it addresses.

More recently, Guba & Lincoln's *Fourth generation evaluation (57)* proposes that evaluation should focus exclusively on describing programmes' evolution in relationship to their social context. Without limiting evaluation to that kind of description, we certainly think that there is a gain in understanding the unique dynamic of any single programme. The more complex the programme, the more useful such descriptions are.

Finally, this definition suggests that the relationship between the problem and the programme can be modelled into a programme theory *(64)*. Chen and Rossi *(65,66)* have developed the concept of theory-driven evaluation to exemplify how the effective mechanisms of a programme can be specified from the knowledge of the problem, and how immediate, intermediate and distal outcomes can be identified and then assessed as a test for programme theory. In health promotion, Green & Kreuter's PRECEDE/PROCEED model *(7)* is an example of such a process. Each one of the social, epidemiological, educational, organizational and environmental diagnoses that form the PRECEDE (predisposing, reinforcing and enabling constructs in ecosystem diagnosis and evaluation) part of the model corresponds to specific outcome indicators that form the PROCEED (policy, regulating or resourcing, and organizing for educational and environmental development) or evaluative phases.

Valuing

This is the process by which a value is given to a programme following its evaluation. In the early days, many evaluators thought that facts spoke for themselves and therefore evaluation was value free *(39)*. They were proved wrong on three counts. First, social programmes are themselves value laden. Second, because evaluation data are used to help decision-making that involves the distribution of social resources, they bear value and ethical meanings. Third, data have to be interpreted to gain meaning. As a result, more attention is being devoted to valuing, even though most evaluation thinkers and practitioners do not address this issue *(58)*.

Theories about valuing can be either prescriptive or descriptive. Prescriptive theories promote particular values, such as social justice and equity. These high-priority values provide the standards against which programmes are to be compared. Descriptive theories present the values held by the stakeholders, and these determine the criteria used in judging the programme. Even though most evaluators use this latter form of valuing theory *(58)*, House *(56)* claims that prescriptive ethics are inherent in evaluation because evaluation is a political activity helping decision-makers reallocate resources.

As noted above, health promotion is increasingly defined in terms of values such as empowerment, equity and participation. In this context, holding descriptive theories is very difficult. Evaluators are forced to become active promoters of the values of the field and to use them in assessing the worth of programmes. Evaluation is not politically neutral or ideologically innocent, but well suited to serving political or ideological ends. The question is whose ends it should serve: those who have power or those who lack it, the bureaucracy or the community. Such questions are especially pertinent to health promotion, which is based on a set of values including empowerment, participation and equity, all of which have political consequences.

Thus, evaluation in health promotion is to some degree a political activity and should take account of political issues. Evaluators should understand the political context at the macro, meso and micro levels. At the macro level, evaluators need to take account of the ideology of the powerful and to design their evaluations accordingly without compromising their own principles. Similarly, at the meso level, evaluators and evaluations should be sensitive to the concerns of the people of the community and to their need for information that will provide them with tools for achieving positive social change. At the micro level, evaluators should be aware of the political agendas of the people who participate in evaluations.

Knowledge construction

Knowledge construction is strongly debated in the evaluation literature. Early evaluators assumed that, analogous to treatments, programmes can be studied with the methodological tools of the fundamental natural and social sciences *(67,68)* that are grouped under experimental/quasi-experimental methodology. They saw programmes as complex treatment packages *(69)* the effect of which could be studied by methods akin to those for studying the effects of manipulations *(70)*. Indeed, Campbell's emphasis on internal validity is usually retained as an example of these early days *(67)*. Despite the appeal of the strong

19

research programme advocated by Campbell, it appeared that evaluation results were repeatedly deceptive *(61)*. Programmes were having marginal effects, if any.

Guba *(71,72)* strongly criticized this approach, arguing that causality is a non-issue, and therefore that evaluation cannot demonstrate effect. His position led the way to advocacy of a naturalistic paradigm of evaluation *(73)* in reaction to the prevailing atomistic paradigm. This viewpoint is epitomized in the debate over quantitative versus qualitative methodology.

In this debate, researchers can be characterized (and perhaps stereotyped) as falling into one of three positions. The strong positivist position, claiming that experimental methodology is the royal road to knowledge, has been losing ground. It is rooted in a view that reality can be assessed objectively by a neutral observer and that causality can be demonstrated given that all parameters, except the treatment under study, are kept constant. This view is very attractive for anyone who thinks that hard facts are necessary for making rational decisions. Because most programmes take place in open systems in which control is difficult to achieve *(74)*, however, this position is hardly tenable.

At the other extreme, constructivists claim that all knowledge is local and constructed by an observer. They deny the existence of causality and objectivity, arguing that local constructions reflect the values of the actors in the programme. The evaluator is one of these actors, influencing the unfolding of the programme and the knowledge resulting from the evaluation effort. Evaluators holding this conception have attracted a lot of attention from the people directly involved in programme delivery. This emphasis on unique processes results in information that is usually very helpful for programme improvement, but is seen as difficult to generalize to other programmes or other contexts by many potential funders of evaluation research.

A middle position, called "critical multiplism" *(75)*, claims that methods should be adapted to the question that is being asked. If evaluation can legitimately answer a wide range of questions, it is no surprise that a single method cannot answer them all. Evaluators are thus seen as eclectic methodologists who adapt their practice to the needs of particular initiatives as they are formulated by the decision-makers and the programme workers and participants who comprise the stakeholders *(76)*. One major criticism of this position is that methodologies are rooted in different epistemologies that cannot be reconciled within a single endeavour *(77)*. Even less can they be held by a single evaluator.

As with evaluation in general, evaluation in health promotion must face a number of philosophical issues. Caplan *(78)* identifies two questions in particular that demand attention. The first concerns the evidence on which interventions are planned and revolves around the nature of scientific knowledge; the second concerns assumptions and theories about the nature of society. Caplan goes further, in arguing that the conjunction of these two questions has important implications for evaluation of health education and promotion.

As to the nature of knowledge, one view considers health or illness as the presence or absence of an objective pathological entity. The other is based on less tangible categories of subjective experience, such as meanings ascribed to people's health status. Caplan *(78)* says that "the problem of knowledge on which we base our programmes for action remains *the* fundamental philosophical question of immense practical import in the struggle over competing systems of rationality".

Caplan suggests that assumptions and theories about the nature of society are captured in theories ranging from radical change to social regulation. The former is concerned with change, structural conflict, and modes of domination, contradiction, emancipation, deprivation and potentiality; in contrast, the latter is concerned with the status quo, social order, consensus, social integration and cohesion, solidarity, needs satisfaction and actuality *(78)*.

Caplan *(78)* then combines the two dimensions of subjectivist and objectivist approaches to knowledge with the assumptions of radical change and social regulation about the functioning of society into a typology and suggests that each quadrant "represents a major approach or paradigm to the understanding of health and the practice of health education/promotion". He further suggests that the typology "provides the necessary concepts with which to assess more deeply and fundamentally what the differences are between the various health education/promotion models and what they have in common with each other". He then applies these tools in a reflexive analysis of health education and promotion and concludes that various models of health promotion (educational, self-empowerment, political economy and community development) "have a very similar view of society even though they seem to differ with regard to what they consider to be the *principal sources of health problems,* and the *health education/promotion ends*". He suggests that this analysis demonstrates the need to consider epistemological issues in health-related research. This conclusion certainly can be extended to evaluation in health promotion.

What should be the role of theory in health promotion evaluation and which theories are most appropriate? The difficulty is that, in spite of some efforts to develop a grand theory for health promotion, such as those in *Readings for a new public health (12)*, little success has been achieved. This leaves many different theories, each attempting to explain or predict a limited aspect of the field. This situation is particularly important in evaluation, where calls for "theory-based" evaluation, such as those of Chen *(66)* and Weiss *(79)*, are increasing.

While this problem has no easy answer, one must recognize the need to continue to address it, since theory is extremely helpful in evaluation efforts. For one thing, it provides guidance about the key aspects of programmes on which to focus scarce evaluation resources, thus helping to deal with the need for efficiency. Theory also helps to indicate whether the assumptions on which many specific programme decisions are based are valid, and helps participants reflect on their own assumptions. According to Weiss *(79)*, evaluations that address the theoretical assumptions embedded in programmes can have more influence on both policy and popular opinion. In other words, nothing is as practical as a good theory.

Thus, people evaluating health promotion initiatives should tackle the challenge of learning to develop and use theories within health promotion, as well as to borrow them from other fields in an appropriate manner. Theories on individual, organizational and community change are likely to be especially helpful.

Health promotion, as a developing field, faces a number of conceptual challenges that have implications for evaluation. One set of issues concerns health promotion's emphasis on empowerment. Aside from difficulties in defining empowerment (80), this concept poses unique problems in evaluating health promotion approaches. For example, the tension that has been noted between the goals of efficiency and empowerment in community health programmes (81) requires evaluators to reconcile these conflicting requirements. Similarly, evaluators must struggle with the challenge of evaluating programmes whose stakeholders espouse conflicting values and goals (82).

Boyce (82) describes one approach to meeting this challenge. He puts forward a methodology for the evaluation of community participation, a key element of empowerment. It consists of the development of a code of participatory ethics through a process of public hearings held by a community panel that is representative of key stakeholders. The code would be approved by a public mechanism such as legislation, and be used to guide the collection of information, which might include data relating to fairness, equality and justice. Once these data were collected, evaluators and community assessors would present them to a community forum; there the data would be evaluated using the code of participatory ethics, with the aim of creating public consensus.

While this approach would not necessarily be efficient in terms of the amount of time or effort required, it has the merit of allowing the various stakeholders to reach some consensus on the importance of efficiency as a criterion for evaluating community initiatives, and takes advantage of existing community resources. As Boyce (82) notes, however, "situations in which program efficiency is the primary goal and which do not claim to involve the public should not be evaluated using this model".

Other health promotion concepts, including capacity building and control, also pose challenges for evaluation (see Chapter 11). They are in the early stages of development, making them elusive for evaluation purposes, and requiring the development of new research procedures and technologies.

Knowledge use

Implicit in many definitions of evaluation is an instrumental use of the results for such purposes as helping decision-makers to make decisions about programmes. This is certainly a major use of evaluation results, and several studies have investigated ways to increase the instrumental use of evaluation data (38,61,83,84). Factors generally acknowledged to do so include: identifying potential users early in the process; having frequent meetings with users, especially during the question-definition phase of the evaluation; studying programme features that users can control; providing preliminary and interim reports; translating results into actions; and dissemination through non-technical activities and summaries.

In addition to instrumental use, Rossi & Freeman (40) refer to conceptual and persuasive utilization. Conceptual utilization is defined as using evaluation results to influence thinking about problems in a more general way, without having an impact on specific programmes. For example, researchers in population health make a conceptual use of evaluation results from a variety of sources to generate models on how the health systems in developed countries have reached a point of diminishing returns in terms of population health indicators (10). Rossi & Freeman (40) claim that evaluators should devote as much effort to enhancing conceptual use as instrumental use. Evaluation results provide knowledge about practical solutions in the form of programmes to address contextualized problems. An instrumental use of this knowledge is usually directed at the specific programme under study. The programme is the subject of interest. With conceptual use, a variety of programmes is analysed to elucidate a problem or to generate new hypotheses about how programming should be undertaken to address it more effectively (85). In this case, no specific programme is sufficient in itself, and evaluation results acquire meanings only when they are pooled across programmes.

Presented as being, for the most part, out of the hands of evaluators, persuasive use "refers to enlisting evaluation results in efforts to either defend or to attack political positions" (40). People usually make persuasive use of results when they are in a position to influence political decisions, or political actors themselves. For example, a health officer might use the lack of positive effects on risk factors from community programmes to promote heart health, to argue against community development as a legitimate health promotion strategy.

All three uses of evaluation (instrumental, conceptual and persuasive) are seen as legitimate. Indeed, they serve different purposes for different people, and different theoreticians of evaluation have advocated emphasizing either instrumental (83) or conceptual (85) uses of evaluation. Shadish et al. (58) predict that restricting evaluation to any one use would be fatal for the development of the field of health promotion.

Evaluation practice

Finally, questions about evaluation practice address whether to undertake an evaluation and, if so, what should be its purpose, the role of the evaluator, the questions to be asked, the design to be used and the activities that need to be carried out. According to Shadish et al. (58), very few theories of evaluation are comprehensive enough to encompass all these aspects. Rossi & Freeman's textbook (40) is probably among the most comprehensive, but it falls short of presenting all the diverse positions on each one of these issues.

Shadish et al. (58) claim that a good theory of practice in programme evaluation is mainly about clarifying the trade-offs that go with addressing each issue pertaining to practice. In that sense, evaluation practice highlights the four aspects (social programming, valuing, knowledge construction and knowledge use) discussed above. They are all part of practice. Two questions, however, seem to be unique to practice issues: whether an evaluation should be undertaken and what the role of the evaluator should be.

Authors have taken different approaches to the evaluability of a programme. Campbell *(69)*, for example, has argued that process evaluation aiming at improving programmes should always be undertaken prior to outcome or impact evaluation: "only proud programs should be evaluated", after a debugging period made possible by process evaluation. This is in direct opposition to the Nutbeam et al. *(86)* model for the development of programmes, in which, as programmes evolve from demonstration to dissemination phases, the need for outcome evaluation lessens while the need for process evaluation increases. Others, such as Rutman *(54)*, have been concerned about the conditions and programme characteristics that should be present to increase the likelihood of a successful evaluation, whatever successful evaluation means in terms of producing valid, useful and relevant results.

The last issue to be addressed in this chapter is the role of the evaluator. Conceptualization about the relative positions of the evaluator and the programme participants has evolved over the years, ranging from having evaluators be as separate as possible in an attempt to reach some kind of objectivity *(67)* to advocating daily cooperation and communication, making the evaluator one of the programme's stakeholders *(67)*. The general trend, however, is towards establishing close communication and teamwork between programme and evaluator. (Campbell *(70)* admits that arguing for separate organizations was a mistake.) This trend can also be observed in the health sciences, where clinical researchers evaluate their own treatment or health promotion researchers evaluate their own programmes.

What is the most appropriate methodology to be used in evaluation in health promotion? The American Evaluation Association recognizes more than 100 types of evaluation. Are they all equally appropriate to the evaluation of health promotion initiatives, or are some preferable to others? Moreover, should new methodologies be developed and, if so, how are they to be developed?

Community-based evaluations present a particular challenge. The attributes of community health promotion interventions that make them particularly difficult to evaluate include their complexity, the need to take account of the social and political context, the flexible and evolving nature of interventions, the range of outcomes being pursued and the absence of appropriate control groups for comparison purposes. The measurement of impact or outcome at the level of the community also poses difficult methodological challenges. Any one of these difficulties is daunting.

The increasing complexity of health promotion interventions poses considerable methodological challenges. As noted earlier, initiatives increasingly involve multiple strategies operating at multiple levels. Designing and conducting appropriate evaluations in such circumstances is enormously difficult.

A key challenge is to determine the optimal intervention package and the efficacy of each of its parts.

The long-term nature of health promotion interventions makes it difficult to obtain rapid answers about the ultimate or even the intermediate outcomes of initiatives. This time-lag is often aggravated by the need to develop strategies suited to the requirements of particular evaluations. It also raises the question of whether evaluation efforts should be devoted to process, rather than outcomes, although we think that both are equally needed.

Of the conceptual difficulties mentioned above, measurement is particularly challenging when the concepts are unclear or subject to debate, as is often the case in health promotion. Combining objective and subjective measures is an additional difficulty.

What counts as evidence of effectiveness? Some argue that the only acceptable method of evaluation is the randomized controlled trial, but increasing numbers of researchers and practitioners in health promotion and related fields argue that the nature of health promotion requires a variety of evaluation approaches, and that appropriate techniques need to be developed. We clearly fall into the latter camp, and hope that this book will contribute to a general acceptance of methodological pluralism in health promotion and related fields.

Many methodological issues are associated with evaluation in health promotion, above and beyond the difficulties of programme evaluation in general, which are formidable enough. We hope that this book will contribute to the resolution of at least some of these problems.

In addition, evaluations of health promotion initiatives involve a number of practical issues. For example, what are the appropriate roles for evaluators, practitioners, consumers and funding agencies? This used to be a relatively straightforward matter. The growing emphasis on participatory approaches and utilization-based evaluation, however, has made it more complicated. Certainly, if a participatory approach is to be taken, all parties will have to be more actively involved than before, and their roles will differ. Evaluators, for example, will need to be more respectful of and sensitive to the needs of the practitioners and consumers, and to act more as coaches than experts in control of the process. Practitioners and consumers will have to take more control of the process. Funding agencies will need to recognize the greater power of practitioners and consumers, and to adjust their policies and procedures accordingly.

What should be evaluated? Given the costs involved, it is impossible to evaluate every initiative with the ideal design and maximum effort. Choices must be made about whether and how to invest scarce evaluation resources, but on what basis? Some possibilities include: the cost of the initiative, whether it is evaluable, whether similar initiatives have been well evaluated and whether the technical expertise needed for the evaluation is available. Applying these and related criteria may help in making appropriate decisions on the allocation of evaluation resources. Using an evaluation framework such as the one suggested in the next section of this chapter may also be helpful.

Other practical issues are: how to deal with fuzzy goals and objectives, which unfortunately often characterize health promotion initiatives; how to handle diverse or poorly measured outcomes; how to work with communities in a way that maximizes and builds their own resources; how to ensure that evaluation findings get into the hands of those who need them as soon as possible; how to integrate health promotion and disease prevention efforts at the country, regional and local levels; and how to design appropriate evaluations for them. This book considers such issues.

As do all evaluations, health promotion evaluation faces a number of ethical issues. Aside from the standard ones pertaining to research in general, special ethical issues are associated with participatory approaches to research *(87)*. One type has to do with the potential harm that may come from community members' active involvement in research; for example, information from such research might be used to discredit members of the community. Safeguards should be built into health promotion research to ensure that this does not happen, but it is also important from an ethical point of view that participatory research include built-in procedures to ensure open and honest communication among stakeholders. Unfortunately, appropriate structures to review the special ethical issues associated with this kind of research have not been generally established.

Conclusions

At this point, it should be clear that the field of evaluation contains a plurality of accepted practices, each one contributing to elucidating and developing a particular set of issues and problems. This diversity and richness of conceptualization might be intimidating to anyone who is appraising this field for the first time, either out of curiosity or for planning an evaluation. We think, however, that it is this diversity that makes evaluation such a powerful tool. Depending on the questions of interest, the context, evaluators' own philosophical positions and the characteristics of the other people involved in the initiative, evaluators can call on any combination of stances in relation to the five issues that have been raised, aware that an infinity of different combinations would also be valid. These combinations vary in complexity. We believe that the right level of complexity is the one that can both be handled by the evaluator and satisfy the need for information that has triggered the evaluation process. Thus, sophisticated and costly designs can be a waste of resources if simpler means can answer the question. Further, evaluators dealing with sophisticated tools that they cannot master can hardly produce useful and valid results.

To conclude this overview, evaluation is the systematic examination and assessment of features of a programme or other intervention in order to produce knowledge that different stakeholders can use for a variety of purposes. This provides ample room for accommodating most current definitions, and endorses our belief that a little knowledge is always better than none at all, and that no evaluation can be global enough to answer all relevant questions about a given initiative. Even the simplest evaluation contributes to the incremental process *(88)* of building knowledge about specific programmes or social and health problems.

Evaluation in health promotion shares many issues pertaining to evaluation in general, but needs to consider some issues particular to its domain. We hope that this volume will contribute to identifying these issues and suggesting ways to deal with them, and to specifying the appropriate process for evaluation in health promotion. A general set of processes characterizes or should characterize most evaluations, and should be followed in evaluating health promotion initiatives. Nevertheless, the nature of health promotion suggests other key evaluation elements.

Most importantly, health promotion evaluation should be participatory *(89)*. Community participation is not only a fundamental characteristic of health promotion but also helpful in three other respects. It helps to identify the views of stakeholders, especially the less powerful, increases appreciation of the purpose of the evaluation and understanding and acceptance of the findings, and promotes commitment to act on them. This principle should be followed as far as possible, irrespective of the methodology employed. In using this principle and developing community and individual skills, participatory research has been very successful, and very compatible with health promotion evaluation *(87)*. A second principle is that the evaluation be introduced early and integrated into all stages of the development and implementation of a health promotion initiative. In other words, it should be treated as a continuing activity that includes a monitoring and learning process. Third, evaluation findings should be conveyed to all participants and stakeholders in meaningful, timely and appropriate ways.

The potential to empower individuals and communities is a powerful rationale for evaluating health promotion activities. This potential can be realized by involving community members at all stages of the process. In addition to informing the community, evaluation can help in developing skills that in turn will allow community members to increase control over and improve their lives. These include skills in logical thinking, communication and interpersonal relations, as well as specific research skills. In this way, evaluation can both be personally rewarding and contribute to the creation of resources within the community. As well as increasing the legitimacy of health promotion activities and the power of those involved, evaluations can assist in developing networks and contacts, and provide feedback to practitioners and participants. As a means of empowering individuals and communities, evaluation in health promotion is an important tool, one that is often overlooked or misused.

The next section presents a framework based on these and related principles that can serve as a useful guide in evaluating health promotion initiatives. It is not intended to be a handbook for evaluating health promotion; it does not provide the level of practical detail required. Springett *(89)* gives more fully developed guidance for practitioners on evaluating health promotion programmes.

A framework for the evaluation of health promotion initiatives

Springett et al. *(90)* have suggested that a model originally proposed to help evaluate workplace programmes *(91)* can be transferred to other health promotion settings. The model draws heavily on the work of Patton *(76)* and forms the basis, along with other considerations discussed above, for a framework for the evaluation of health promotion initiatives. This framework is based on the following six principles, which reflect the key ideas already discussed; it should:

1. be applicable to all evaluation approaches, but ensure that the most appropriate method is used for the programme or policy being assessed;
2. be consistent with health promotion principles, in particular empowering individuals and communities by emphasizing participation;
3. focus on collective as well as individual accountability: that is, be designed to apply to both institutional and individual and both synergistic and single outcomes;
4. be flexible in its application, able to respond to changing circumstances, opportunities, challenges and priorities;
5. cover all stages of the evaluation process, from setting the agenda to using the results; and
6. apply to all levels of evaluation: that is, be helpful no matter the level at which the evaluation takes place.

Based on these principles, evaluations in health promotion should include eight steps. The first is describing the proposed programme, policy or initiative. This includes clarifying the initiative's mandate, aims and objectives, linkage with other initiatives, procedures and structures. A programme logic model is often helpful in this process. This step also includes getting people on board, establishing a group to oversee and undertake the evaluation, examining the health issues of concern, and collecting baseline information.

Next is identifying the issues and questions of concern. This includes deciding on the purpose(s) of the evaluation, clarifying the issues that are likely to concern all of the stakeholders, including the potential users of the results, and specifying evaluation questions about the aims and objectives of the programme or other initiative. These aims and objectives should be clarified before the evaluators decide how to measure the extent to which they have been achieved. There is a danger that, if measurement dictates the aims of an initiative, only quantifiable objectives will be pursued.

Third, the process for obtaining the required information is designed. This includes deciding on the kind of evaluation to be carried out, the objects to be assessed, measurement methods, for whom the evaluation is undertaken, and when the data are to be collected. This step should also include choosing the best approach for the questions being asked, as well as a plan for implementing the design. Ensuring maximum participation in this process ensures that all experience is valued, and that information is collected from all credible sources.

Step four is to collect the data by following the agreed-on data collection methods and procedures, and step five, to analyse and to evaluate the data. The latter includes interpreting the data, and comparing observed with expected outcomes.

Sixth, recommendations are made. All the stakeholders should be involved in interpreting the results. This includes clarifying the short- and long-term implications of the findings, and identifying the costs and benefits of implementing recommendations and of ignoring them.

Step seven is to disseminate the findings to funding agencies and other stakeholders in a meaningful and useful form. Taking action is the last step. Action is much more likely to occur if the people who need to act on the evaluation findings have been part of the process.

These steps are iterative and, as Springett et al. *(90)* note:

> At each stage there are … questions and key issues that need to be considered explicitly. These questions ensure that the aims of the project and the evaluation are clear, the objectives are set, the correct data are collected in the most appropriate way so as to measure the right outcomes in relation to the original objectives, all within the resources available.

Finally, to be consistent with the principles of health promotion, all relevant stakeholders must be involved in a meaningful way at every step in the process. The more detailed discussion below emphasizes considerations that are particularly important for the evaluation of health promotion activities.

Step 1. Describing the programme

As suggested above, logic models provide a helpful tool in describing the initiative. A logic model is merely a diagrammatic representation of the logical connections among the various elements of a programme or initiative, including its activities, outputs, impact, effects, objectives and goals.

Developing a logic model for any health promotion initiative should involve all key stakeholders, including both those whose health is of concern and those responsible for the programme or initiative to be evaluated. Ideally, they should also be involved in examining the health issue of concern and collecting the baseline data. Springett et al. *(90)* note:

> The importance of spending time on this ground work cannot be overemphasized. Involvement of the right people will ensure commitment, use of information generated and a good response to any questionnaires. The evaluation group (minimum of 3) should reflect the range of interests. Proper clarification makes the evaluation straightforward.

Patton *(76)* suggests setting up an evaluation task group as a vehicle for: actively involving the key stakeholders in the process of decision-making, providing a forum for the political and practical aspects to be taken into account, and increasing commitment to the results, knowledge about the evaluation and ability to interpret the results. Members should include representatives of the various groups and constituencies that: have a stake in the information generated, have the authority and power to use the findings or the ability to influence the powerful, believe that the evaluation is worth doing, care about how the results should be used and are willing to make a firm commitment of time to the process.

Step 2. Identifying the issues and questions

Thompson *(92)* has identified three issues of concern in a health promotion evaluation: concept and design, processes and impact. Other important issues concern: the operation of the initiative, the effects, the achievement of objectives and goals, and alternatives to the intervention.

Numerous questions about each of these issues are worth addressing. For example, in relation to the issue of health promotion concept and design, one might assess whether a programme is consistent with the concepts and principles of health promotion, or ask whether the implemented processes were delivered in a participatory and empowering manner. As to impact, one might examine the extent to which the initiative produced the expected effects, as shown in the logic model. Here, too, issues of equity can be addressed.

Questions about the operation of the initiative might include whether the programme was delivered efficiently and as intended. Although at first sight this might appear to be merely an issue of audit or quality control, it is important in assessing effectiveness. An unsuccessful outcome may have more to do with the way a programme was implemented than anything inherently wrong with its content. Further, one might want to examine the extent to which the intervention produced the effects indicated in the logic model and achieved the specified objectives and goals. Finally, with regard to alternatives, one might want to assess the effectiveness of the mixture of activities used by the initiative, and determine the best combinations and relative emphasis of components.

In other words, the consideration of a logic model raises many key issues and questions – hence the importance of consensual development. The identification of issues and questions and the specification of purposes of the evaluation should also be a consensual process involving key stakeholders. This will empower the stakeholders and bring into the open for debate any conflicting expectations and paradigms. It will provide an opportunity for each set of stakeholders to understand each other's paradigms and perspectives better, thereby reinforcing the learning process that is inherent in any effective evaluation.

Step 3. Designing the data-collection process

The design of the data-collection process depends on the issues and questions selected for study and the users of the evaluation's findings. The users will also be the stakeholders involved in the evaluation process if the right people have been invited to participate. If the process is truly participatory, the actual choice of information to be collected will be one of its outcomes. While policy-makers and managers might be chiefly interested in cost–effectiveness and the bottom line, one of the main purposes of evaluation is to enable practitioners to discover what worked, what did not work and why. Establishing the value of different types of initiative so that other practitioners can replicate them is as important as accountability. Thus, stakeholder involvement will ensure the choice is made through an open debate between the different priorities and paradigms. It will also ensure that successful interventions are not judged ineffective because inappropriate criteria are used to assess them. Moreover, shared decision-making on what to measure and what questions to ask will ensure commitment to both making the evaluation and acting on the results. It will also mean that everyone involved understands the inevitable trade-offs in terms of feasibility and practicality and their impact on validity and reliability.

Among the important decisions made by the evaluator are those related to the kind of data required. These decisions are complex and fraught with challenges. The choice depends on:

1. the goals and objectives of the intervention
2. the criteria for their successful achievement
3. the indicators of successful achievement
4. the perspectives and needs of the different stakeholders
5. the level at which the information is required.

Much could be written concerning the problems related to each of these factors and they are elaborated in the guidelines for practitioners (89). Here it is sufficient to emphasize some of the major difficulties they present in determining the nature of the data to be collected in evaluating health promotion initiatives.

First is the issue of what kind of data should be collected. In part, this depends on the evaluation paradigm, with positivist approaches preferring quantitative data and hermeneutic, qualitative. One can argue that this is a false dichotomy, however, and the selection of data is not necessarily linked to the selection of the paradigm, but rather to the nature of the information required to answer the questions asked (93). Meaningful soft measures are better than meaningless hard ones (76).

Second, health promotion initiatives tend to have multiple goals and objectives, which are often ill specified and/or lack consensus, and can refer to a wide range of desired outcomes related to a variety of domains (individual, social and societal). As suggested earlier, some desired outcomes are instrumental in achieving the intervention's ultimate goals and objectives. Where evaluation focuses on outcomes, data should be obtained on the achievement of both instrumental and ultimate goals.

Third, identifying goals and objectives is relatively easy; they usually flow readily from the intervention's overall purpose (vision and mission). Specifying the criteria for and indicators of success, however, is more difficult.

Evaluation poses two questions. First, what are the criteria for success in achieving the goals and objectives? In this context, the term *criteria* refers to the standards against which success will be assessed, such as a 50% reduction in smoking by young people. Second, what indicators will be used to measure performance against the criteria for success? Here, *indicators* refer to the data or measures used to determine success as measured against the criteria: for example, self-reported daily smoking, as measured by a school-based survey of young people aged 15–18 years. The challenges involved in these processes include: the multiplicity of criteria required to assess success in achieving a range of goals and objectives, lack of clarity and/or agreement concerning criteria, and the absence of valid and appropriate indicators of success. In some cases, proxy measures will need to be used.

Step 4. Collecting the data

The collection of information raises fundamental and sensitive issues. That all procedures should be followed in a rigorous and ethical manner is axiomatic. Confidentiality and the need to use information about non-participants in a programme may generate problems. Some of these problems can be resolved if the evaluation process has been participatory, if more than one form of data collection is used and if the people from whom the data are obtained are given some feedback. By endorsing and facilitating the active involvement of stakeholders, all participants will be aware of the constraints on the process and the validity and reliability of the results.

Step 5. Analysing and interpreting the data

If all the stakeholders are involved in analysis and interpretation, they will understand the strengths and limitations of the data and be more receptive to qualitative data. Statistics have varying degrees of error, and numbers are only one form of indicator of what the world is like. Stakeholders also need to understand what is being compared with what and why. In addition, the way results are presented can affect their impact.

Step 6. Making recommendations

Stakeholder participation is especially critical in developing recommendations from the evaluation of health promotion initiatives, as Springett et al. *(90)* argue: "if people have been involved in the process, they will already be committed to acting on the findings and be receptive to the results". Participation also increases the accountability of policy-makers. Recommendations should cover the immediate practical changes needed, clarify what is useful, challenge existing beliefs and include the costs and benefits of not implementing the findings, as well as those of implementing them.

Step 7. Dissemination

Evaluation findings and recommendations are often disseminated in an *ad hoc* fashion, if at all, without much thought or resource investment. Nevertheless, investment in dissemination is extremely important, particularly in health promotion, where information can be a powerful tool in empowering communities and individuals *(94)*. Effective dissemination can reduce the need for additional time-consuming evaluation. Guidance should be disseminated not only on evaluation but also on how practitioners can make the best use of it. Such a process will affect quality standards in the execution of programmes, so that practitioners may realize the same benefit as the evaluated programmes they wish to replicate. Thus, developing a marketing or dissemination plan should be a required activity for most, if not all, evaluations of health promotion interventions. It has even been suggested that the effort and resources devoted to disseminating evaluation findings and recommendations should match those spent on creating them.

Step 8. Taking action

Too often, the lessons learned from one short-term project are not translated into action on the next one. Key decisions in taking this step include identifying the resources required for change and developing appropriate action plans. This both completes the cycle and begins it again. This step automatically becomes the first in the next evaluation planning cycle, through which evaluation is integrated into the culture of health promotion.

References

1. SIGERIST, H.M. *The university at the crossroads.* New York, Henry Schuman, 1946.
2. WINSLOW, C.E.A. The untilled fields of health promotion. *Science,* **51**: 23 (1920).
3. LALONDE, M. *A new perspective on the health of Canadians: a working document.* Ottawa, Canada Information, 1974.
4. Ottawa Charter for Health Promotion. *Health promotion,* **1**(4): iii–v (1986).
5. ANDERSON, R. *Health promotion: an overview.* Edinburgh, Scottish Health Education Group, 1984 (European Monographs in Health Education Research, No. 6).
6. GREEN, L.W. & RAEBURN, J. Contemporary developments in health promotion: definitions and challenges. *In:* Bracht, N., ed. *Health promotion at the community level.* Thousand Oaks, Sage, 1990.
7. GREEN, L.W. & KREUTER, M.M. *Health promotion planning: an educational and environmental approach,* 2nd ed. Mountain View, Mayfield, 1991.

8. MACDONALD, G. & BUNTON, R. Health promotion: discipline or disciplines. *In:* Bunton, R. & MacDonald, G., ed. *Health promotion: disciplines and diversity.* London, Routledge, 1992.

9. EVANS, R.G. & STODDART, G.L. Producing health, consuming health care. *Social science and medicine,* **31**(12): 1347–1363 (1990).

10. EVANS, R.G. ET AL., ED. *Why are some people healthy and others not? The determinants of health of populations.* New York, Walter de Gruyter, 1994.

11. *Knowledge development for health promotion: a call for action.* Ottawa, Health and Welfare Canada, 1989.

12. MARTIN, C.J. & MCQUEEN, D.V., ED. *Readings for a new public health.* Edinburgh, Edinburgh University Press, 1989.

13. ROSE, G. *The strategy of preventive medicine.* Oxford, Oxford University Press, 1992.

14. SYME, S.L. Control and health. *Advances,* **7**(2): 16–27 (1991).

15. TERRIS, M. Determinants of health: a progressive political platform. *Journal of public health policy,* **15**(1): 5–17 (1994).

16. WILKINSON, R.G. *Class and health.* London, Tavistock, 1986.

17. CHU, C. & SIMPSON, R., ED. *Ecological public health: from vision to practice.* Toronto, Centre for Health Promotion & Participation, 1996.

18. KICKBUSCH, I. Introduction: tell me a story. *In:* Pederson, A. et al., ed. *Health promotion in Canada: provincial, national and international perspectives.* Toronto, W.B. Saunders, 1994, pp. 8–17.

19. GREEN, L.W. National policy in the promotion of health. *International journal of health education,* **22**: 161–168 (1979).

20. GREEN, L.W. Current report: Office of Health Information, Health Promotion, Physical Fitness and Sports Medicine. *Health education,* **11**(2): 28 (1980).

21. GREEN, L.W. & IVERSON, D.C. School health education. *Annual review of public health,* **3**: 321–338 (1982).

22. PERRY, C.L. & JESSOR, R. The concept of health promotion and the prevention of adolescent drug abuse. *Health education quarterly,* **12**(2): 169–184 (1985).

23. NUTBEAM, D. *Health promotion glossary.* Copenhagen, WHO Regional Office for Europe, 1985 (document ICP/HBI 503 (GO 4)).

24. *Discussion document on the concept and principles of health promotion.* Copenhagen, WHO Regional Office for Europe, 1984 (document).

25. EPP, J. *Achieving health for all: a framework for health promotion.* Ottawa, Health and Welfare Canada, 1986.

26. GOODSTADT, M.S. ET AL. Health promotion: a conceptual integration. *American journal of health promotion,* **1**(3): 58–63 (1987).

27. KAR, S.B., ED. *Health promotion indicators and actions.* New York, Springer, 1989.

28. O'DONNELL, M.P. Definition of health promotion. Part III. Expanding the definition. *American journal of health promotion,* **3**(3): 5 (1989).

29. LABONTÉ, R. & LITTLE, S. *Determinants of health: empowering strategies for nurses.* Vancouver, Registered Nurses Association of British Columbia, 1992.

30. BUCHANAN, I. The purpose–process gap in health promotion. *In:* Liss, P.-E. & Nikku, N., ed. *Health promotion and prevention: theoretical and ethical aspects.* Stockholm, Forskningsradsnamnden, 1994.

31. ROKEACH, M. A values approach to the prevention and reduction of drug abuse. *In:* Glynn, T.J. et al., ed. *Preventing adolescent drug abuse: intervention strategies.* Rockville, US Department of Health and Human Services, 1983, pp. 172–194.

32. LANDAU, R. Locus of control and socioeconomic status: does internal locus of control neglect real resources and opportunities of personal coping abilities? *Social science and medicine,* **41**(11): 1499–1505 (1995).

33. MARMOT, M.C. ET AL. Socioeconomic status and disease. *In:* Badura, B. & Kickbusch, I., ed. *Health promotion research: towards a new social epidemiology.* Copenhagen, WHO Regional Office for Europe, 1991, pp. 113–146 (WHO Regional Publications, European Series, No. 37).

34. MIROWSKY, J. & ROSS, C. Control or defense? Depression and the sense of control over good and bad outcomes. *Journal of health and social behavior,* **31**(1): 71–86 (1990).

35. DOWNIE, R.S. ET AL. *Health promotion: models and values.* Oxford, Oxford University Press, 1990.

36. SUCHMAN, E.A. *Evaluation research. Principles and practice in public service and social action programs.* New York, Russell Sage Foundation, 1967.

37. WHOLEY, J.S. ET AL., ED. *Handbook of practical program evaluation.* San Francisco, Jossey-Bass, 1994.

38. WEISS, C.H. *Evaluation research. Methods for assessing program effectiveness.* Englewood Cliffs, Prentice Hall, 1972.

39. SCRIVEN, M. Goal-free evaluation. *In:* House, R.E., ed. *School evaluation: the politics and process.* Berkeley, McCutchan, 1973, pp. 319–328.

40. ROSSI, P.H. & FREEMAN, H.E. *Evaluation: a systematic approach,* 5th ed. Thousand Oaks, Sage, 1993.

41. CAMPBELL, D.T. & STANLEY, J.C. *Experimental and quasi-experimental designs for research.* Chicago, Rand McNally, 1963.

42. CRONBACH, L.J. *Designing evaluation of educational programs.* San Francisco, Jossey-Bass, 1982.

43. DRUMMOND, M.F. ET AL. *Methods for the economic evaluation of health care programs.* Toronto, Oxford University Press, 1987.

44. LEVIN, L.S. & ZIGLIO, E. Health promotion as an investment strategy: consideration on theory and practice. *Health promotion international,* **11**(1): 33–40 (1996).

45. GUBA, E.G. & LINCOLN, Y.S. Competing paradigms in qualitative research. *In:* Denzin, N.K. & Lincoln, Y.S., ed. *Handbook of qualitative research.* Thousand Oaks, Sage, 1994, pp. 105–117.

46. LINCOLN, Y.S. & GUBA, E.G. *Naturalistic enquiry.* Thousand Oaks, Sage, 1985.

47. REICHARDT, C.S. & COOK, T.D. Beyond qualitative versus quantitative methods. *In:* Reichardt, C.S. & Cook, T.D., ed. *Qualitative and quantitative methods in evaluation research.* Beverly Hills, Sage, 1979, pp. 7–32.

48. FETTERMAN, D.M. ET AL., ED. *Empowerment evaluation: knowledge and tools for self-assessment and accountability.* Thousand Oaks, Sage, 1996.

49. POCOCK, S.J. *Clinical trial. A practical approach.* New York, Wiley, 1983.

50. SUSSER, M. Epidemiological models. *In:* Struening, E.L. & Guttentag, M., ed. *Handbook of evaluation research.* Beverly Hills, Sage, 1975, pp. 497–517.

51. BRAVERMAN, M.T. & CAMPBELL, D.T. Facilitating the development of health promotion programs: recommendations for researchers and funders. *In:* Braverman, M.T., ed. *Evaluating health promotion programs.* San Francisco, Jossey-Bass, 1989, pp. 5–18 (New Directions for Program Evaluation, No. 43).

52. O'CONNOR, A. Evaluating comprehensive community initiatives: a view from history. *In:* Connell, J.P. et al., ed. *New approaches to evaluating community initiatives: concepts, methods and contexts.* New York, Aspen Institute, 1995, pp. 23–63.

53. CHELIMSKY, E. What have we learned about the politics of program evaluation? *Evaluation news,* **11**: 5–22 (1987).

54. RUTMAN, L. *Planning useful evaluations.* Beverly Hills, Sage, 1980.

55. WHOLEY, J.S. *Evaluation and effective program management.* Boston, Little, Brown, 1983.

56. HOUSE, E.R. *Evaluating with validity.* Beverly Hills, Sage, 1980.

57. GUBA, E.G. & LINCOLN, Y.S. *Fourth generation evaluation.* Thousand Oaks, Sage, 1989.

58. SHADISH, W.R. ET AL. *Foundations of program evaluation.* Thousand Oaks, Sage, 1991.

59. PINEAULT, R. & DAVELUY, C. *La planification de la santé: concepts, méthodes, stratégies.* Montréal, Agence d'Arc, 1986.

60. FLAY, B.R. Efficacy and effectiveness trials (and other phases of research) in the development of health promotion programs. *Preventive medicine,* **15**: 451–474 (1986).

61. WEISS, C.H. The politicization of evaluation research. *In:* Weiss, C.H., ed. *Evaluating action programs: readings in social action and education.* Boston, Allyn and Bacon, 1972, pp. 327–338.

62. CRONBACH, L.J. ET AL. *Toward reform of program evaluation.* San Francisco, Jossey-Bass, 1980.

63. WEISS, C.H. Evaluating educational and social action programs: a treeful of owls. *In:* Weiss, C.H., ed. *Evaluating action programs: readings in social action and education.* Boston, Allyn and Bacon, 1972, pp. 3–27.

64. LIPSEY, M.W. Theories as methods: small theories of treatment. *In:* Seechrest, L. et al., ed. *Research methodology: strengthening causal*

interpretations of non-experimental data. Washington, DC, US Department of Health and Human Services, 1990, pp. 33–52.

65. CHEN, H. & ROSSI, P.H. The theory-driven approach to validity. *Evaluation and program planning,* **10**: 95–103 (1987).
66. CHEN, H.T. *Theory-driven evaluation.* Thousand Oaks, Sage, 1990.
67. CAMPBELL, D.T. Reforms as experiments. *American psychologist,* **24**: 409–429 (1969).
68. COOK, T.D. & CAMPBELL, D.T. *Quasi-experimentation: design and analysis issues for field settings.* Chicago, Rand McNally, 1979.
69. CAMPBELL, D.T. Guidelines for monitoring the scientific competence of prevention intervention research centers. *Knowledge: creation, diffusion, utilization,* **8**: 389–430 (1987).
70. CAMPBELL, D.T. Can we be scientific in applied social science? *In:* Connor, R.F. et al., ed. *Evaluation studies review annual.* Thousand Oaks, Sage, 1984, pp. 26–48.
71. GUBA, E.G. The failure of educational evaluation. *In:* Weiss, C.H., ed. *Evaluating action programs: readings in social action and education.* Boston, Allyn and Bacon, 1972, pp. 25–266.
72. GUBA, E.G., ED. *The paradigm dialogue.* Thousand Oaks, Sage, 1990.
73. PATTON, M.Q. *Qualitative evaluation methods.* Beverly Hills, Sage, 1980.
74. POTVIN, L. & MACDONALD, M. *Methodological challenges for the evaluation of the dissemination phase of health promotion programs.* Montreal, University of Montreal, 1995.
75. COOK, T.D. & MACDONALD, M. Postpositivism critical multiplism. *In:* Shortland, L. & Mark, M.M., ed. *Social science and social policy.* Beverly Hills, Sage, 1985, pp. 21–62.
76. PATTON, M.Q. *Practical evaluation.* Beverly Hills, Sage, 1982.
77. HALDEMAN, V. & LEVY, R. Oecomenisme méthodologique et dialogue entre paradigmes. *Canadian journal on aging,* **14**: 37–51 (1995).
78. CAPLAN, R. The importance of social theory for health promotion: from description to reflexivity. *Health promotion international,* **8**(2): 147–156 (1993).
79. WEISS, C.H. Nothing as practical as good theory: exploring theory-based evaluation for comprehensive initiatives for children and family. *In:* Connel, J.P. et al., ed. *New approaches to evaluating community initiatives: concepts, methods, and contexts.* Washington, DC, Aspen Institute, 1995.
80. RISSELL, C. Empowerment: the Holy Grail of health promotion? *Health promotion international,* **9**(1): 39–47 (1994).
81. FOSTER, G. Community development and primary health care: their conceptual similarities. *Medical anthropology,* **6**(3): 183–195 (1982).
82. BOYCE, W. Evaluating participation in community programs: an empowerment paradigm. *Canadian journal of program evaluation,* **8**(1): 89–102 (1993).

83. PATTON, M.Q. *Utilization-focused evaluation.* Beverly Hills, Sage, 1978.

84. LEVITON, L.C. & BORUCH, R.F. Contributions of evaluation to educational programs and policy. *Evaluation review,* **7**: 563–599 (1983).

85. WEISS, C.H. Research for policy's sake: the enlightenment function of social research. *Policy research,* **3**: 531–545 (1977).

86. NUTBEAM, D. et al. Evaluation in health education: a review of progress, possibilities, and problems. *Journal of epidemiology and community health,* **44**: 83–89 (1990).

87. GREEN, L.W., ET AL. *Study of participatory research in health promotion. Review and recommendations for the development of participatory research in health promotion in Canada.* Ottawa, Royal Society of Canada, 1995.

88. WEISS, C.H. Improving the linkage between social research and public policy. *In:* Lynn, L.E., ed. *Knowledge and policy: the uncertain connection.* Washington, DC, National Academy of Science, 1978, pp. 20–39.

89. SPRINGETT, J. *Practical guidance on evaluating health promotion: guidelines for practitioners.* Copenhagen, WHO Regional Office for Europe, 1999 (document).

90. SPRINGETT, J. ET AL. Towards a framework for evaluation in health promotion: the importance of the process. *Journal of contemporary health,* **2**: 61–65 (1995).

91. SPRINGETT, J. & DUGDILL, L. Workplace health promotion programmes: towards a framework for evaluation. *Health education journal,* **55**: 91–103 (1995).

92. THOMPSON, J.C. Program evaluation within a health promotion framework. *Canadian journal of public health,* **83**(Suppl. 1): S67–S71 (1992).

93. BAUM, F. Researching public health: behind the qualitative–quantitative debate. *Social science and medicine,* **40**(4): 459–468 (1995).

94. CROSSWAITE, C. & CURTICE, L. Disseminating research results – The challenge of bridging the gap between health research and health action. *Health promotion international,* **9**(4): 289–296 (1994).

Part 2
Perspectives

Introduction

Louise Potvin

Chapter 1 presented five issues that were identified by Shadish at al. *(1)* as fundamental to defining and understanding programme evaluation: social programming, valuing, knowledge construction, knowledge use and evaluation practice. Articulating a position on these related issues leads to the formation of a coherent approach to evaluation.

The field of health promotion, still struggling to define its theoretical underpinnings *(2)*, is not yet ready to propose such an approach, but a number of current debates in the social sciences and the health research literature can be called upon to investigate these five fundamental issues. Examining these debates through the lens of health promotion provides useful perspectives for discussing evaluation. Each of the eight chapters forming Part 2 of this book develops a perspective on the fundamental issues identified by Shadish et al.

In Chapter 2, Potvin, Haddad and Frohlich focus primarily on social programming and secondarily on knowledge use. To identify the range of questions that can legitimately be asked in an evaluation study, the authors develop a schematic view of what constitutes a health promotion programme. Their concept takes account of two characteristics of health promotion that distinguish it from the more general approach of management by objective usually found in public health programmes. First, health promotion interventions are complex packages of multilevel, multistrategy, population-based approaches that focus on a broad range of environmental changes. Second, some intervention goals may be better described as broad societal changes than as precisely defined health improvements. This leads to conceptualizing health promotion programmes using three dimensions: interaction with the environment, components and evolution. This allows the mapping of relevant evaluation questions, making the usual dichotomy between process and outcome evaluation mostly irrelevant.

In their provocative chapter, McQueen and Anderson develop an argument highly relevant to the issues of valuing and knowledge construction. Reviewing how the concepts of evidence and its corollary, evidence-based practice, are being borrowed from biomedicine, the authors warn practitioners against the potentially misleading attractiveness of the evidence-based argument for valuing health promotion interventions. It is tempting to think that good, solid, quantitative and scientific evidence of programme effectiveness is a prerequisite for decision-making on the planning and implementation issues in health promotion. The authors discuss the methodological and epistemological problems that are linked with the somewhat false reassurance provided by the evidence-based argument in the field of health promotion. They argue that, because health promotion is largely based on knowledge resulting from social sciences, it cannot count on theories that are agreed by large segments of practitioners to create a repertoire of evidence from which to draw when valuing or creating programmes.

Chapter 4 is primarily concerned with evaluation practice. Springett develops the argument that evaluation in health promotion is different from other evaluation endeavours. Because health promotion is value laden and directed towards ideologically defined objectives, programme evaluation should ideally be health promoting in itself. At least it should not promote values at odds with those pursued in health promotion. This challenging agenda, Springett argues, can only be met through the participation of the programme's targeted recipients in the evaluation process. Evaluation approaches based on the assumption that programme participants are objects to be studied are inherently disempowering and therefore counterproductive. In addition, the chapter positions participatory research as a general approach to evaluation, instead of a methodology, and presents six issues to be addressed when conducting participatory evaluation.

In the next chapter, Gendron examines the epistemological and methodological implications of the debate about qualitative versus quantitative methods in the social sciences, and develops an argument that is highly relevant to the issue of knowledge construction. She argues that quantitative methods are associated with the production of generalizable knowledge. This kind of knowledge is made possible under the assumption that an objective reality exists and that it can be assessed by means of quantifiable dimensions. Gendron argues that the complexity of projects aimed at social transformation or reform requires the use of a qualitative approach to apprehend the constructed reality to be transformed by the programme. Because health promotion is concerned with both producing generalizable knowledge and transforming reality, qualitative and quantitative methods should be viewed as complementary in health promotion research.

Chapters 6–9 broadly address the issue of knowledge use in health promotion evaluation. Each explores a feature of evaluation research relevant to answering the following question: for what could the information produced by evaluation studies be used? Rejecting the easy answer – to make decisions about the future of programmes – the authors discuss how evaluation results can be used in the debates over what constitute relevant and legitimate outcomes for health promotion programmes. Issues such as quality of life, economic evaluation, auditing and quality control, and policy impact are increasingly relevant for health promotion. The four chapters provide the reader with introductory syntheses of these issues.

Raphael addresses the issue of quality of life as an outcome indicator of health promotion interventions. During the last decade or so, many areas discussed in the health and biomedical literature have designed and used measures of quality of life to evaluate interventions. Health promotion has not escaped this tendency. The multiplicity of definitions used in designing these measures has created a fair amount of confusion and debate. Raphael presents a conceptual map of the issues related to the assessment of quality of life based on the four scientific paradigms identified by Guba and Lincoln. His main argument is that these issues are not concerned only with the development of indicators, such as quality-adjusted life years (QALYs) and disability-adjusted life years (DALYs), as shown in the health economics literature. Rather, indicators of quality of life for evaluating health promotion outcomes should be based on explicit definitions of positive health, the social determinants of health and the aspect of quality of life that is relevant to the programme under study.

In Chapter 7, Godfrey introduces the main concepts in economic evaluation and discusses how they can be adapted for evaluation in health promotion. She presents economic evaluation as an aid to decision-making. Economic evaluation provides data that allow for the comparison of different programmes or of programmes with different types of outcome. Most of this chapter provides an introduction to the jargon used in economic evaluation. What distinguishes it from others and makes it a valuable contribution to this book is the discussion of five burning issues at the heart of potential attempts to use economic evaluation in health promotion. Given the purpose of health promotion, these issues mainly are related to the nature of its outcomes and to the ethical considerations of using economic indicators.

In Chapter 8, Parish describes quality assurance as a monitoring and evaluation mechanism to ensure that explicit quality standards are defined and implemented in all iterations of a programme. He reviews the objectives and principles underlying the quality assurance movement and goes on to discuss how the principles of the Ottawa Charter for Health Promotion *(3)* can be used as a starting point for defining standards of quality.

In the last chapter of Part 2, de Leeuw examines the link between evaluation research and policy development and research. Two propositions underline this chapter: that healthy public policy is made largely outside the health sector and that policy is developed in situations in which vastly different players are interdependent. These lead to a perspective in which policy development follows an interactive networking process. This process, de Leeuw argues, is similar to the one described by Guba & Lincoln in their fourth-generation evaluation methodology *(4)*. It aims at rendering explicit the values and stakes involved in programme or policy development.

References

1. SHADISH, W.R. ET AL. *Foundations of program evaluation.* Thousand Oaks, Sage, 1991.
2. MCQUEEN, D.V. The search for theory in health behaviour and health promotion. *Health promotion international,* 11: 27–32 (1996).
3. Ottawa Charter for Health Promotion. *Health promotion,* 1(4): iii–v (1986).
4. GUBA, E.G. & LINCOLN, Y.S. *Fourth generation evaluation.* Thousand Oaks, Sage, 1989.

2

Beyond process and outcome evaluation: a comprehensive approach for evaluating health promotion programmes

Louise Potvin, Slim Haddad and Katherine L. Frohlich

Health promotion is an applied field of knowledge and practice. As mentioned in Chapter 1, it borrows theories and methods from the fields of psychology, sociology, anthropology, geography, education and epidemiology *(1)* to elaborate an understanding of the ways in which populations' health is maintained and strengthened. A common way of building on this applied knowledge is by designing, implementing and evaluating programmes. In this chapter we use the term *programme* with the understanding that it also includes what others have labelled *intervention, initiative* or *action aimed at promoting health*. Examining health promotion in action – by assessing the links between programme activities and services, the environment in which they are implemented and the resulting changes – is an important means of knowledge accumulation. The knowledge ensuing from any single evaluation may contribute to the improvement of the programme. In addition, evaluations that identify intrinsically health promoting collective processes have the potential to expand the broader knowledge base of health promotion.

The literature describes many types of evaluation questions (see Chapter 1). One of the most widely used distinctions is between process and outcome evaluation. Although process evaluation has been defined in many different ways, the health promotion literature tends to place it in opposition to outcome evaluation *(2–4)*. For Green & Lewis *(2)*, process and formative evaluations are equivalent and relate to the control and assurance of quality of practice. For Nutbeam et al. *(3)*, process evaluation can be used to assess how a programme is implemented: what activities are provided, under what conditions, by whom, to what audience and with what level of effort. Nutbeam et al. *(3)* add that it can assist in attributing causality.

In this chapter we argue that relevant evaluation questions should be based on a comprehensive conceptualization of health promotion programmes. Because health promotion programmes form complex packages that evolve in interaction with their context, their assessment requires a broad range of evalu-

45

ation questions. Indeed, the capacity of evaluation results to contribute both to the improvement of a given programme and to the accumulation of knowledge in the field lies in an in-depth understanding of how programmes evolve and interact with their environments to achieve their outcomes. Our conceptualization of both health promotion programmes and evaluation questions renders obsolete the prevailing distinctions between programme monitoring, process evaluation and outcome evaluation.

Programmes

Our conceptualization of health promotion programmes expands the approach of management by objectives that is frequently adopted in public health. A public health programme is commonly described as a coordinated set of activities or services, organized within a particular time frame, which aims to modify a difficult situation affecting a targeted segment of the population *(5)*. A public health programme is thus an institutional or community response to a difficult situation. Both the situation and the programme are embedded in a broader environment.

Health promotion programmes expand this definition in two major ways. First, they have moved away from high-risk approaches (which seek to identify people at high risk through screening and to provide them with health services, as in the Multiple Risk Factor Intervention Trial *(6)*) to broader, multilevel, multistrategy, community-based approaches. Using such an approach, programmes target for intervention whole populations, broad segments of a community or an organizational setting such as a workplace or school *(7,8)*. An assumption underlying this approach is that programmes that employ multiple strategies targeting the physical, regulatory and socioeconomic environments are more supportive of healthful behaviour *(9–12)*. Health promotion programmes are thus increasingly characterized by their complexity and their focus on a broad range of environmental changes *(13)*(see Chapter 10).

Second, health promotion programmes are not always designed to respond to specific problems, such as cardiovascular diseases or diabetes. Indeed, health promotion has been defined as "a process for initiating, managing and implementing changes" *(14)*. When such changes aim at community development, they may embrace broad societal issues such as poverty or sexism, which become health promotion issues in their own right *(15)*. Because these issues are related to health in a non-specific way *(16)*, some health promotion programmes' goals may be better described as targets of change than as problems.

Programmes as living systems

The primary assumption underlying our conceptualization of programmes is that they cannot be seen as kits to be distributed to and used by health professionals with minimal reference to the environment in which they are implemented. Instead, each health promotion programme constitutes a social organization and as such should be characterized as a living, open system *(10–17)*.

Le Moigne defines five dimensions of a system *(18)*. The first is structural; a system is made up of components. The second is functional; a system performs operations that can be observed as transformation processes. The third dimension is evolutionary; a system evolves through life cycles. Although it changes as time goes by, a system maintains its identity. The fourth dimension is contextual; a system interacts with other systems in its environment. These interactions contribute to the individual evolution of all. The fifth dimension is teleological; a system has aims and objectives.

Complex community health promotion programmes can be modelled according to these dimensions *(18)*. Like any public health programme, they can be characterized by their objectives (teleological dimension), their activities (functional dimension), their components (structural dimension), their life cycle (evolutionary dimension) and their relationship with their environment (contextual dimension). In our conceptualization, health promotion programmes extract information, material and human resources from their environment. These are transformed into services or activities aimed towards a previously determined set of objectives. All dimensions of the programme, in turn, evolve through its various phases, responding throughout to the feedback provided by the environment.

Our conceptualization collapses Le Moigne's five dimensions into three. The first, which parallels Le Moigne's contextual dimension, comprises the interactions between the programme and its environment. There is a dialectical relationship between a programme and its environment; the programme aims to modify some aspect of the environment – the target of change – and is in turn modified by contextual elements. The second dimension is a programme's internal features: its objectives, structural components (resources and services provided) and transformation processes *(19)*. The third dimension is the evolution of the programme. At any given moment, a programme can be characterized as going through a particular phase in its life cycle.

Programme–environment interactions

By environment we mean all aspects of the social system in which a programme is implemented, such as social actors, resources and systems of meaning. These social systems can be organizational settings, communities, municipalities, provinces or a country *(11)*. For clarity of presentation we distinguish somewhat artificially between two subcategories of environmental elements. First, as can be noted in Fig. 2.1, we create a category called target of change, which includes the environmental conditions or relations that are targeted by the programme's objectives. These targets of change are further divided into initial and resulting conditions. The environmental conditions are those aspects of the programme's setting that are neither part of the programme itself, nor part of the target of change.

Fig. 2.1. programme components and evaluation questions

Environmental conditions

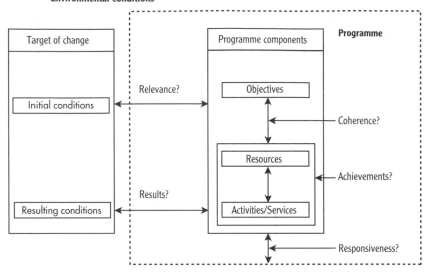

Source: adapted from Contandriopoulos et al. *(19)*

One key element of most community health promotion programmes is the use of participation *(20)* or other collective mechanisms that are thought to be health promoting in themselves (see Chapter 1). In fact, Stokols *(12)* suggests that what distinguishes health promotion from disease prevention is the emphasis of the former on the role of people, groups and organizations as active agents in shaping health practices and policies. While community participation can be understood as a means to increase the effectiveness of intervention and hence to achieve better health outcomes at an individual level, it can also be seen to have intrinsic health benefits *(21)*.

Current practice in health promotion values a participatory approach in which practitioners work in partnership with the primary beneficiaries of the programme through all its phases *(22)*. This reliance on collective processes has two implications. First, processes occurring in the programme's environment create a dense network of relationships between the programme and its environment. Thus, in health promotion, more than in other types of public health programme, the environment cannot be dissociated from the programme. Second, because of these processes' importance in modifying the programme's components, they should be included in theories of treatment.

Programme components
Like most programme planning models *(5,23)*, ours divides health promotion programme components into three broad categories, as illustrated in Fig. 2.1.

The objectives or expected results are the driving force of the programme. In principle, these objectives are formulated in terms of particular changes in the environment. Resources are the raw materials – usually knowledge, money, staff and physical infrastructure – necessary for a programme to operate. The activities/services are the means by which the programme pursues its objectives, and comprise the intervention strategy *(11)*. These three categories are linked together by a chain of events *(24,25)*. As noted above, the chain of events should include the elements of the environment that are thought to be interacting with any of the programme components.

When based on systematic knowledge about factors associated with the target of change, a formalization of this chain of events may lead to the formulation of a theory of treatment *(26,27)*. Theories of treatment are often opposed to a black-box conception of evaluation that seeks to establish a input–output link between a programme and its effects *(28)*. For programme planning a theory of treatment provides a framework that ensures the congruence of the sequence of activities and services with the objectives, and the type and quantity of resources that are needed to implement activities and services.

The PRECEDE/PROCEED model is an example of a framework for formulating a theory of treatment *(13)*. This model leads programme planners to establish a series of diagnoses of a situation. Essentially, the task is to identify the behaviour and environmental features that are causally related to a given health problem. Then the programme planner determines which predisposing, enabling and reinforcing factors are associated with these causes. The final task is to mobilize the necessary resources to develop and implement activities.

Programme evolution

Programmes change over time. Three broad phases are commonly identified, as shown in the top section of Fig. 2.2, with development as the first. The major tasks in this phase are to identify the target of change, to study the feasibility and acceptability of different intervention strategies, to set objectives, to elaborate the theory of treatment, to plan the sequence of activities and to estimate the nature and amount of resources needed to carry out the activities and deliver the services. In this phase, the programme receives resources and extracts information from the environment. Most activities consist of gathering the necessary resources to launch and operate the programme and selecting, collecting and analysing information about the target of change and other relevant elements of the environment.

The second phase is implementation, in which resources are channelled through activities and services delivered to the targeted population. While the objectives, activities and resource estimates may be revised during the implementation phase as a by-product of evaluation, such revisions are not the primary task in this phase. This phase is the longest; it requires the greatest effort, as shown in Fig. 2.2, and sees the most intensive exchanges between the programme and its environment. The programme directs its activities and services towards elements of the environment. Evaluation activities, for their part, extract information from the environment, process it and feed it back to programme staff, the targeted population or other stakeholders.

Fig. 2.2. Programme phases and evaluation questions

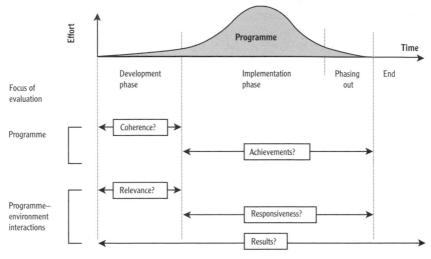

Source: adapted from unpublished course material developed by S. Haddad and L. Albert, University of Montreal, 1997.

Finally, the programme is phased out, because either it has been transformed into another cycle, with another set of activities pursuing different objectives, or the original objectives have been attained and the resources exhausted. Some evaluation activities, such as data collection, can be scheduled to occur after the end of the programme.

No single evaluation project is likely to address all dimensions and components of health promotion programmes. The scope of an evaluation is usually limited by the components of interest, the timing of the project with regard to the programme's evolution and the degree of focus on the interaction between the programme and its environment. Possible evaluation questions can be categorized and labelled in a variety of ways. Some are based on the potential use of the evaluation results, as in formative versus summative evaluation *(29)*, and others are based on the type of performance indicators used, as in process versus outcome evaluation *(3)*. We think that our conceptualization of health promotion programmes provides a theoretically sound starting point for organizing evaluation questions in health promotion.

Evaluation questions

The evaluation of a programme may be called a subproject within a project. Like a programme, an evaluation project comprises resources and activities organized to reach previously determined objectives. Evaluation objectives are concerned with the production of programme knowledge, and the questions asked determine the nature of this knowledge. Based on our conceptualization of a health promotion programme, we propose five evaluation questions.

Questions may focus on the programme or its interaction with its environment. Two questions can be asked about programme components.

- How coherent is the theory of treatment linking the programme's objectives, resources and activities/services?
- What are the achievements of the programme's activities and services?

We suggest three questions about programme–environment interactions.

- How relevant are the programme's objectives to the target of change?
- How responsive are the programme's components to environmental conditions?
- What are the indications of the programme's results in the environment?

These questions should be considered during specific phases of a programme's life cycle. Fig. 2.2 shows that questions of relevance and coherence are usually examined during the development phase, while the programme's achievements and responsiveness should be studied during the implementation phase. We do not think that the question of results is intrinsically linked to any one specific programme phase. To illustrate how each type of evaluation question may be used, we employ the example of the Kahnawake School Diabetes Prevention Project (KSDPP) *(30)*, a description of which can be found in Box 2.1.

Analysing programme coherence

As shown in Fig. 2.1 and 2.2, the analysis of coherence focuses solely on programme components and is usually conducted during the development phase. These evaluations tend to examine primarily the correspondence between programme objectives, planned activities and services, and resources, by unveiling the underlying theory of treatment in part or as a whole. When the programme planners have spelled out the theory of treatment in detail, the task of the evaluator is to determine whether the programme plan corresponds with the most up-to-date professional knowledge. Often, however, the theory of treatment has not been made explicit or at best has been only briefly sketched. In such cases the evaluator's main task is to render it explicit. Chen *(28)* and Sheirer *(25)* discuss at length the components of a theory of treatment and how to recover them from programme plans.

When addressing the question of coherence in participatory programmes, evaluators should pay attention to programme–environment interactions. In participatory programmes, the collective processes triggered may not be directly related to the risk factors and behaviour targeted by the intervention.

51

Box 2.1. The Kahnawake School Diabetes Prevention Project

The Kahnawake School Diabetes Prevention Project (KSDPP) was a community health promotion programme implemented in a native Mohawk community in Canada. Its objectives were to promote an active lifestyle and healthy dietary habits among young people to prevent the onset of non-insulin-dependent diabetes mellitus.

KSDPP was developed as a school-based programme, coupled with community development and activation, with the themes of active lifestyle and healthy eating. The intervention model combines elements from social learning theory, the PRECEDE/PROCEED model, the Ottawa Charter for Health Promotion and traditional learning techniques that emphasize the oral tradition and the involvement of the entire community. Activities were designed around four elements of the Ottawa Charter: developing personal skills, strengthening community action, creating supportive environments and lobbying for healthy public policy.

The activities developed during the demonstration cycle of KSDPP included the implementation of an in-class health promotion curriculum for all children in the two community elementary schools (aged 6–12 years), lobbying for the creation of a recreation path and the enactment of policies for a healthy school environment. The underlying principle was that schoolchildren can acquire and maintain knowledge, attitudes and healthy habits if their parents and other adults in the community convey the same message and practise what they preach. The activities carried out in the community aimed to inform adults about KSDPP and diabetes prevention in general. In addition, activities provided families with the opportunity to try out new, healthy ways of living.

KSDPP was developed as an equal partnership between the community of Kahnawake, researchers and academics. Members of the community comprised both a community advisory board and all KSDPP staff. The community's strong presence in all structural elements and phases of KSDPP created a dense network of relationships and mutual feedback between the programme and many organizations and individuals.

The demonstration phase provided the resources to launch a full-scale evaluation study based primarily on the principles of participatory research. The evaluation and the intervention teams worked together to create a knowledge base:

- to disseminate information to the community on the evolution of KSDPP, the changes in the community environment and the prevalence of diabetes risk factors in the population;
- to provide feedback to the intervention team on various aspects of KSDPP; and
- to make a convincing case for arguing that community activation and development on issues such as diabetes prevention can create opportunities for community empowerment and improvements to living conditions in native communities.

Health promotion programmes cannot therefore be seen as simple standardized sequences of events; the black box between an intervention and its outcome(s) is complex *(31)* and constantly modified by its interactions with environmental conditions.

During its development phase, KSDPP developed a sophisticated and complex theory of treatment, drawing from four domains of knowledge and defining four areas of action. The literature on community intervention shows that such comprehensive strategies can have effects extending far beyond the targeted health problem. For instance, KSDPP could move beyond diabetes to other lifestyle related diseases such as heart disease or stroke. It could also affect health in a broader fashion by helping the community experience success in dealing with a public health issue and thereby contributing to its empowerment. An interesting coherence analysis might examine the broad array of potential health outcomes, which may lead to redesigning programme objectives accordingly. A coherence question might address how the four domains of knowledge were used in each one of the action areas of KSDPP.

Analysing programme achievements

Achievement questions focus on the programme itself, but are asked during the implementation phase. This type of evaluation usually seeks to answer questions related to whether the programme is succeeding in achieving its plan of action. Achievement questions address two issues: the resources and the services/activities produced (quality issues) and the links between resources and activities (productivity issues). Quality issues may be related to organizational and structural features of the programme's delivery system, such as availability, accessibility and technical quality, or to some descriptive features of the results, such as the coverage of the targeted population or clients' satisfaction *(26)*. Productivity analysis seeks to estimate the amount of resources necessary to produce given units of activity. Programme achievement questions are usually addressed by what has been called programme monitoring *(32)*, process evaluation *(25)* or formative evaluation *(3)*. Achievement analyses require the collection of empirical data. The choice of methods for collecting and analysing lies with the evaluator, in consultation with the relevant stakeholders. These methods may be quantitative, qualitative or a mixture of both.

In health promotion, interest is increasing in describing and analysing programme achievements. The Pawtucket Heart Health Program gives a good example of an achievement analysis. Through the years during which the interventions were implemented, a sophisticated tracking system recorded all contacts between individual members of the community and the Program *(33,34)*. This system allowed the evaluators to report on the types of people reached by various Program components *(35)*. The evaluators were also able to analyse the evolution of the public's participation in the activities *(36)*. This preoccupation with analysing achievement questions culminated in the Child and Adolescent Trial for Cardiovascular Health (CATCH), which applied a series of assessments to every programme component that was part of the theory of treatment *(37)*.

The evaluation of KSDPP addressed numerous achievement questions. The core component of KSDPP was the delivery of a health promotion curriculum to elementary school children. Data on the acceptability of KSDPP and teachers' agreement with its objectives were gathered and analysed annually. Each year a cross-sectional sample of teachers was selected and individual semi-structured interviews were conducted. Interview recordings were briefly analysed and the results were reported to both the community advisory board and the intervention team. A second question focused on the acceptability of KSDPP to community members. The data used for this analysis were collected by a telephone survey of a representative sample of the community adult population midway through KSDPP. A third question related to whether an equal partnership between various groups had been constituted: a cardinal principle of KSDPP *(38)*. A programme ownership survey was thus conducted during the second year of KSDPP. The results were reported to the relevant groups and used to enhance the participation of community advisory board members.

Analysing programme relevance

Questions of relevance are asked during the development phase and address the relationship between the programme and the target of change. This form of evaluation assesses the appropriateness of the objectives, given the health problems and living conditions of the target population. Some authors have labelled it strategic evaluation *(19)*. Two issues may be of interest: whether the target of change is a relevant issue for the intervention, given the local conditions, and whether the choice of the target population for the intervention is relevant to local people. The method is usually to analyse the process in which the programme objectives were defined. Two sources of information are often available for this task: the scientific literature, which gives justifications for the objectives and target population, and the expressed concerns of the local population.

Evaluations of community health promotion interventions rarely address both of the relevance issues. Further, the reports of such evaluations in the literature indicate that programme designers seem to value only information on the scientific bases of programmes as shedding light on relevance. Needs assessments are almost never conducted before the launching of projects, and targeted populations are rarely consulted about either the hypotheses or the implementation of intervention. This lack of consultation may at least partly explain the absence of effect observed in many community heart health promotion trials *(39)*.

The evaluation of KSDPP did not include an analysis of relevance. Had one been done, however, it could have raised the problem of targeting elementary school children for diabetes prevention when non-insulin-dependent diabetes is known to affect adults. It could also have raised the question of the importance of dealing with this particular health issue when native communities throughout Canada have multiple public health problems, many of which are associated with poor living conditions *(40)*. Evaluators could have found data for this type of relevance analysis in the literature on the etiology and epidemiological aspects of diabetes and on public health problems among native populations. Evaluators could have used this information to analyse the process by which objectives were set and the target population selected.

Analysing programme responsiveness

Responsiveness questions are investigated during the implementation phase. These evaluations examine how environmental conditions modify various programme components. Any component can be evaluated this way. Discussions of this question in the literature mainly cover ways of standardizing programme delivery processes. The three issues in responsiveness analysis *(41)* are: variations in programme delivery as a function of environmental conditions (for instance, the variation across implementation sites likely in complex programmes that rely on citizen participation); variation in programme results as a function of environmental conditions; and variation in results due to the delivery system.

When addressing programme components (the content of the black box), evaluations of health promotion programmes have tended to have a narrow focus *(42)*, merely describing how a programme was implemented, how well the activities fit the original design, to whom services were delivered, the extent to which the target population was reached and the external factors that may compete with the programme's effects. Too often, evaluations have neglected the interactions between programme components and exogenous factors *(26)*. One step that could be taken to study responsiveness would be to examine how the theory of treatment interacts with health promoting environmental conditions. Rather than attempting to enhance the design of future evaluations by identifying key intervening variables and processes (to increase internal validity) and then controlling for them, evaluators might integrate these variables and processes into new theories of treatment *(37)*. This notion of health promoting process, which is equally endorsed by Hoffman *(43)* and McQueen *(44)*, raises the critical point that behaviour takes place in a context, a context that is a combination of social and environmental factors.

Theory-oriented treatment research should value information that is gathered from testing the fit between prior theoretical frameworks and the empirical world. To comprehend behaviour and change, one must therefore examine the process during which behaviour is modified, as well as the factors that influence this process. This implies that any evaluation endeavour must study and take account of the dependence of any health promotion programme on its context.

An analysis of the responsiveness of KSDPP would have addressed questions about the extent to which environmental conditions modified the planning and implementation of the activities. An important source of data for such an analysis is the minutes of meetings held during the implementation phase; the KSDPP community advisory board, for example, studied all propositions for action and rated their acceptability. Another potential source of information is documents produced during the planning phase. Analysing information from both sources would reveal how input from the community is sought and taken into account. A further step is to examine how the intervention team modifies its theory of treatment according to what is learned from day-to-day programme management. Studying how the participatory nature of KSDPP interacted with the planned chain of events could lead to useful insights concerning theories of intervention.

Analysing programme results

Finally, by result analysis we mean an evaluation that examines the changes in the environment associated with a programme. Results may include both expected and unforeseen outcomes. Many sources of data may be used for these analyses and a variety of research designs may be created to provide valid answers. Numerous textbooks on health promotion *(3,45)* and evaluation *(46)* deal with the problems associated with assessing programme results. These problems may be divided into two general categories: those related to the validity of the causal link between the programme and the observed effects and those concerned with the type of indicators selected to assess the effects.

The main problem in result analysis is the attribution of the observed changes to the programme. The literature shows heated debate over the appropriate research designs for evaluating health promotion programmes. Chapters 3 and 10 address this issue at length. Many authors have recently argued that, in community programmes and other complex, multistrategy programmes, observational methods may be more suitable for providing valid results than reliance on randomization and experimental control *(47,48)*.

The second category of issues relates to the confusion created by giving different labels to evaluations according to the result indicators used. For example, some authors oppose outcome and impact (or process) evaluations *(2,3)*, where the former is concerned with the ultimate outcome of a programme and the latter focuses on changes in intermediate processes of the theory of treatment. These processes are thought to be triggered by programme activities or services and in turn affect the ultimate outcome.

The objective of health promotion is not simply to produce changes in individuals' health behaviour but also to induce or modify intermediate outcomes in communities. The practice in evaluation, however, has been to neglect intermediary processes and to concentrate on assessing individual-level outcomes. To move beyond this, one can employ theories of treatment *(21,26)*. In a community programme, a theory of treatment would include the key inputs, outputs and the sequence of events or processes connecting them *(31)*.

Because KSDPP was funded as a demonstration project, the evaluation emphasized results analysis. It did so, however, in relationship with a theory of treatment formulated at the start of the programme. The evaluation assessed most elements of the theory of treatment. It measured the behaviour and anthropometric characteristics of elementary school children, as well as community and organizational processes thought to contribute to changes in diabetes risk factors. By helping identify these processes, the data facilitated decisions about programme management, and allowed the revision of some of the theoretical propositions upon which KSDPP was founded.

Beyond process and outcome evaluation

Our conceptualization of health promotion programmes and the evaluation questions to which it leads differ markedly from a more traditional view of evaluation, based on a distinction between process and outcome evaluation and administrative monitoring. In this traditional perspective, monitoring is an administrative function that ensures that programme resources are transformed into services and activities. The aim is to document and justify programme expenditures. To support management and daily decision-making, such monitoring is usually very broad in scope and covers the crucial components of programmes. The knowledge produced by monitoring systems is viewed as having limited usefulness for programmes in other contexts.

Outcome evaluation traditionally seeks to find out whether a programme produces the changes intended. The evaluator's task is to provide valid data establishing causal links between the programme and observed changes in its environment. This focus on causal relationships often leads outcome evaluations to formulate narrow questions. This type of evaluation is associated with research and scientific activities, and, it has been argued, therefore requires expert methodological skills and knowledge (4). It is intended to produce knowledge that can be used to deal with similar situations in other contexts.

From a traditional viewpoint, process evaluation analyses programme activities as they were implemented. It may serve three purposes: to improve the capacity of programme components to reach the targeted population, to document any discrepancy between the programme as planned or adopted from another context and as implemented, and to provide the information required for the interpretation of outcomes. In all cases it is thought to result in local knowledge.

Such an approach – making epistemological, conceptual and methodological distinctions between various forms of programme evaluation and monitoring – might be tenable for simple programmes composed of a limited number of standardized activities and targeting a precise segment of the population within a relatively closed system (49). Implicit in such programmes is a top-down philosophy of implementation in which health planners and practitioners select the best available programme for a diagnosed population health problem. In public health and particularly in health promotion, where programmes are complex, the separation between programme monitoring, process evaluation and outcome evaluation may impede the production of useful knowledge.

In our view, evaluation is a feedback system between the programme and its environment. An important purpose of this system is to produce information that helps to improve local programmes. No less important, however, is to produce knowledge that improves theories of treatment and consequently the understanding of how health promotion works more generally. All five questions presented in this chapter contribute to both of these aims. Ideally, programme evaluations should address them all and share the results with everyone concerned.

In practice, however, no single evaluation may have the resources to address all five questions. We therefore advocate the creation and coordination of broad evaluation agendas *(50)*. The evaluation of different programmes with similar theories of treatment could be coordinated to address issues covering the whole range of evaluation questions discussed in this chapter. Every programme provides an opportunity to replicate and to refine theories and models of health promotion. To the extent that programme evaluation concentrates solely on showing differences between experimental and control groups, the cross-fertilization between programmes addressing similar health issues is limited.

Conclusion

We propose that evaluations of standardized programmes are not the sole source of generalizable knowledge. Like all empirical knowledge, that resulting from an evaluation is indeed local *(51)*; that is, it is rooted in a particular object and produced in a very specific context. Knowledge from any one evaluation, however, contributes to a more comprehensive learning endeavour. Any programme can be viewed as an element of a universe of action, to the understanding of which any evaluation project contributes *(52)*. The knowledge produced can be used to modify theories in health promotion. Using programmes as reforms *(53)*, evaluators thus extract as much information as possible from these social trials to construct a knowledge base that improves with each iteration and is useful to practitioners and decision-makers *(54)*. The more comprehensive and encompassing this knowledge base, the more useful it will be for improving the practice and theory of health promotion.

References

1. MACDONALD, G. & BUNTON, R. Health promotion: discipline or disciplines. *In*: Bunton, R. & MacDonald, G., ed. *Health promotion: disciplines and diversity.* London, Routledge, 1992.
2. GREEN, L.W. & LEWIS, F.M. *Measurement and evaluation in health promotion.* Palo Alto, Mayfield, 1986.
3. NUTBEAM, D. ET AL. Evaluation in health education: a review of progress, possibilities, and problems. *Journal of epidemiology and community health,* **44**: 83–89 (1990).

4.   MITTLEMARK, M.B. ET AL. Realistic outcomes: lessons from community-based research and demonstration programs for the prevention of cardio-vascular diseases. *Journal of public health policy,* **14**: 437–462 (1993).

5.   PINEAULT, R. & DAVELUY, C. *La planification de la santé: concepts, méthodes, stratégies.* Montréal, Agence d'Arc, 1986.

6.   BENFARI, R.C. ET AL. The Multiple Risk Factor Intervention Trial (MRFIT). III. The model for intervention. *Preventive medicine,* **10**: 426–442 (1981).

7.   ROSE, G. *The strategy of preventive medicine.* Oxford, Oxford University Press, 1992.

8   PATRICK, D.L. & WICKISER, T.M. Community and health. *In:* Amick, B.C., III et al., ed. *Society and health.* New York, Oxford University Press, 1995, pp. 46–92.

9.   BRESLOW, L. Social ecological strategies for promoting healthy life-styles. *American journal of health promotion,* **10**: 253–257 (1996).

10.   GREEN, L.W. ET AL. Ecological foundations of health promotion. *American journal of health promotion,* **10**: 270–281 (1996).

11.   RICHARD, L. ET AL. Assessment of the integration of the ecological approach in health promotion programs. *American journal of health promotion,* **10**: 318–328 (1996).

12.   STOKOLS, D. Translating social ecological theory into guidelines for community health promotion. *American journal of health promotion,* **10**: 282–298 (1996).

13.   GREEN, L.W. & KREUTER, M.M. *Health promotion planning: an educational and environmental approach,* 2nd ed. Mountain View, Mayfield, 1991.

14.   KICKBUSCH, I. Introduction: tell me a story. *In:* Pederson, A. et al., ed. *Health promotion in Canada: provincial, national and international perspectives.* Toronto, W.B. Saunders, 1994, pp. 8–17.

15.   LABONTÉ, R. Death of a program, birth of a metaphor: the development of health promotion in Canada. *In:* Pederson, A. et al., ed. *Health promotion in Canada: provincial, national and international perspectives.* Toronto, W.B. Saunders, 1994, pp. 72–90.

16.   LINK, B.G. & PHELAN, J. Social conditions as fundamental causes of disease. *Journal of health and social behavior,* Special issue, 1995, pp. 80–94.

17.   SOUBHI, H. ET AL. Repères pour une conceptualisation systémique des programmes communautaires en promotion de la santé. *In:* Soubhi, H. *Une vision systémique de la famille et de la promotion de la santé – Un exemple avec l'activité physique de loisir* [Dissertation]. Montréal, Université de Montréal, 1999.

18.   LE MOIGNE, J.-L. *La théorie du système général. Théorie de la modélisation,* 4ième édition. Paris, Presses universitaires de France, 1994.

19.   CONTANDRIOPOULOS, A.-P. ET AL. L'évaluation dans le domaine de la santé: concepts et méthodes. *In:* Lebrun, T. et al., ed., *L'évaluation en*

matière de santé: des concepts à la pratique. Lille, Crege, 1992, pp. 14–32.

20. MINKLER, M. Challenges for health promotion in the 1990s: social inequities, empowerment, negative consequences, and the common good. *American journal of health promotion,* **8**: 273–274 (1994).

21. WEISS, C.H. Nothing as practical as good theory: exploring theory-based evaluation for comprehensive community initiatives for children and families. *In:* Connell, J.P. et al., ed. *New approaches to evaluating community initiatives: concepts, methods and contexts.* New York, Aspen Institute, 1995, pp. 65–92.

22. GREEN, L.W., ET AL. *Study of participatory research in health promotion. Review and recommendations for the development of participatory research in health promotion in Canada.* Ottawa, Royal Society of Canada, 1995.

23. REINKE, W.A. An overview of the planning process. *In:* Reinke, W.A., ed. *Health planning for effective management.* New York, Oxford University Press, 1988, pp. 57–74.

24. DONABEDIAN, A. The quality of care. How can it be assessed? *Journal of the American Medical Association,* **260**: 1743–1748 (1988).

25. SHEIRER, M.A. Designing and using process evaluation. *In*: Wholey, J.S. et al., ed. *Handbook of practical program evaluation.* San Francisco, Jossey-Bass, 1994, pp. 40–63.

26. LIPSEY, M. Theory as method: small theories of treatment. *In*: Sechrest, L. et al., ed. *Research methodology: strengthening causal interpretations of nonexperimental data.* Washington, DC, US Department of Health and Human Services, 1990, pp. 33–52.

27. CHEN, H. & ROSSI, P.H. Issues in the theory-driven perspective. *Evaluation and program planning,* **12**: 299–306 (1989).

28. CHEN, H.T. *Theory-driven evaluation.* Thousand Oaks, Sage, 1990.

29. SCRIVEN, M. The methodology of evaluation. *In*: Weiss, C.H., ed. *Evaluating action programs: readings in social action and education.* Boston, Allyn and Bacon, 1972, pp. 123–136.

30. MACAULAY, A.C. ET AL. The Kahnawake School Diabetes Prevention Project: intervention, evaluation, and baseline results of a diabetes primary prevention program with a Native community in Canada. *Preventive medicine,* **26**: 779–790 (1997).

31. KOEPSELL, T.D. ET AL. Selected methodological issues in evaluating community-based health promotion and disease prevention programs. *Annual review of public health,* **13**: 31–57 (1992).

32. ROSSI, P.H. & FREEMAN, H.E. *Evaluation: a systematic approach,* 5th ed. Thousand Oaks, Sage, 1993.

33. ASSAF, A.R. ET AL. The Pawtucket Healt Health Program. II. Evaluation strategies. *Rhode Island medical journal,* **70**(12): 541–546 (1987).

34. McGRAW, S.A. ET AL. Methods in program evaluation: the process evaluation system of the Pawtucket Heart Health Program. *Evaluation review*, **13**: 459–483 (1989).

35. LEFEBVRE, R.C. ET AL. Characteristics of participants in community health promotion programs: four years' results. *American journal of public health*, **77**: 1342–1344 (1987).

36. ELDER, J.P. ET AL. Organizational and community approaches to community-wide prevention of heart disease: the first two years of the Pawtucket Heart Health Program. *Preventive medicine*, **15**: 107–117 (1986).

37. McGRAW, S.A. ET AL. Design of process evaluation within the Child and Adolescent Trial for Cardiovascular Health (CATCH). *Health education quarterly*, **Suppl. 2**: S5–S26 (1994).

38. MACAULAY, A.C. ET AL. Participatory research with Native community of Kahnawake creates innovative code of research ethics. *Canadian journal of public health*, **89**: 105–108 (1998).

39. POTVIN, L. ET AL. Le paradoxe de l'évaluation des programmes communautaires multiples de promotion de la santé. *Ruptures, revue transdisciplinaire en santé*, **1**: 45–57 (1994).

40. MACMILLAN, H.L. Aboriginal health. *Canadian Medical Association journal*, **155**: 1569–1578 (1996).

41. DENIS, J.L. & CHAMPAGNE, F. L'analyse de l'implantation: modèles et méthodes. *Canadian journal of program evaluation*, **5**: 47–67 (1990).

42. TAGGART, V.S. ET AL. A process evaluation of the District of Columbia "Know Your Body" project. *Journal of school health*, **60**: 60–66 (1990).

43. HOFFMAN, K. The strengthening community health program: lessons from community development. *In*: Pederson, A. et al., ed. *Health promotion in Canada: provincial, national and international perspectives*. Toronto, W.B. Saunders, 1994, pp. 123–138).

44. McQUEEN, D.V. The search for theory in health behaviour and health promotion. *Health promotion international*, **11**: 27–32 (1996).

45. WINDSOR, R.A. ET AL. Evaluation of health promotion and education programs. Palo Alto, Mayfield, 1984.

46. COOK, T.D. & CAMPBELL, D.T. Quasi-experimentation: design and analysis issues for field settings. Chicago, Rand McNally, 1979.

47. FISHER, E.B. The results of the COMMIT trial. *American journal of public health*, **85**: 159–160 (1995).

48. SUSSER, M. The tribulations of trials – Interventions in communities. *American journal of public health*, **85**: 156–158 (1995).

49. FLAY, B.R. Efficacy and effectiveness trials (and other phases of research) in the development of health promotion programs. *Preventive medicine*, **15**: 451–474 (1986).

50. POTVIN, L. Methodological challenges in evaluation of dissemination programs. *Canadian journal of public health*, **87**(Suppl. 2): S79–S83 (1996).

51. CAMPBELL, D.T. Relabeling internal and external validity for applied social scientists. *In*: Trochim, W.M.K., ed. *Advances in quasi-experimental design and analysis*. San Francisco, Jossey-Bass, 1986, pp. 67–77 (New Directions for Program Evaluation, No. 31).

52. CRONBACH, L.J. ET AL. *Toward reform of program evaluation*. San Francisco, Jossey-Bass, 1980.

53. CAMPBELL, D.T. Reforms as experiments. *American psychologist*, **24**: 409–429 (1969).

54. CAMPBELL, D.T. The experimenting society. *In*: Campbell, D.T. & Overman, E.S., ed. *Methodology and epistemology for social science*. Chicago, University of Chicago Press, 1988, pp. 290–314.

3

What counts as evidence: issues and debates

David V. McQueen and Laurie M. Anderson[1]

In general, unscientific beliefs are held independently of anything we should regard as evidence in their favor. Because they are absolute, questions of evidence are regarded as having little or no importance.

– Irving M. Copi, *Introduction to logic*

The rise of the evidence discussion

Today, in both medicine and public health, practitioners are urged to base their decisions on evidence. In health promotion, an interdisciplinary field that overlaps substantially with public health, the issue of evidence has recently received considerable attention. In May 1998, for example, the Fifty-first World Health Assembly *(1)* urged all Member States "to adopt an evidence-based approach to health promotion policy and practice, using the full range of quantitative and qualitative methodologies".

In the discussions that went into the preparation of this book, many themes repeatedly arose. Many issues were resolved and integrated into Chapter 1, and others are taken up in subsequent chapters. One theme, however, continued throughout the discussions and remains as an area of debate: evidence, its meaning and its importance to evaluation.

At first glance, the discussion of evidence might appear to be merely an academic problem, one that turns on questions of epistemology and logic, a subject for debating halls and philosophers of science. Sober reflection shows that the idea of evidence is intimately tied to very pragmatic issues. One wants evidence to take action, spend money, solve problems and make informed decisions. The use of the word *evidence* is at the very heart of current discussions in public health *(2)*:

---

[1]   For their sage advice, editorial comments, and reflections on earlier drafts of this paper, we are especially indebted to Michael Hennessey, Matt McKenna and Marguerite Pappaioanou, CDC, United States; Don Nutbeam, University of Sydney, Australia; and Alfred Rütten, Technical University of Chemnitz, Germany. The opinions expressed are ours.

A piece of evidence is a fact or datum that is used, or could be used, in making a decision or judgement or in solving a problem. The evidence, when used with the canons of good reasoning and principles of valuation, answers the question why, when asked of a judgement, decision, or action.

This chapter explores the discourse on evidence in health promotion and the evaluation of interventions. It does not provide a set of tools or principles on how to establish evidence for health promotion. This task is taken up in numerous documents and is the subject of many workshops and presentation at professional meetings *(3)*. Here, we examine some of the many assumptions underlying the nature of evidence and so raise issues and provide background for later chapters' discussions of evaluation and evidence.

Defining evidence

Evidence commonly denotes something that makes another thing evident: for example, the fact that a lake is frozen solid is an indication or sign of low temperatures. Words such as *apparent, manifest, obvious, palpable, clear* or *plain* may also be used when describing evident things or events, and all share the characteristic of certainty. In many ways this is a very strict definition. No one can fail to perceive what is evident. In brief, the everyday use of the word *evidence* carries very high expectations. If one has evidence, can there be any doubt?

In legal terms, evidence has a different meaning. In a criminal trial, for example, evidence is introduced to prove, beyond a reasonable doubt, that something has occurred. Juries and judges weigh the strength of evidence before a finding of guilt or innocence. Evidence is said to be overwhelming, to convince beyond the shadow of a doubt. Such language seems foreign to the field of health promotion, but this is exactly the framework espoused by Tones *(4)* in a recent editorial:

> Accordingly, I would argue that we should assemble evidence of success using a kind of *"judicial principle"* – by which I mean providing evidence which would lead to a jury committing themselves to take action even when 100% proof is not available.

Evidence presented in a western legal setting, however, is often a mixture of stories: witness accounts, police testimony and expert opinions, including those of forensic scientists. In short, it frequently comes from multiple sources and people of widely varying expertise. In this sense, determining the value of evidence requires the interpretation of accounts.

Evidence can also be understood as the product of observation or experiment, sometimes over a long period. Such evidence may be described as empirical. In some cases, observation has an underlying theoretical perspective,

64

as with Darwin's observations leading to a theory of evolution. Observation as evidence is often tied to the notion of data as evidence, and this usage is quite common in public health.

Weiner's recent book *(5)*, winner of a Pulitzer prize, explores the notion of observation as evidence in great depth; it uses research on the beak of the finch to tell the story of evolution. Weiner illustrates how modern observational techniques and data collection can reveal the operational mechanism of natural selection. He shows how years of repeated, careful measurement built the evidence base to show that the process of selection is both measurable and observable.

Two critical points might be inferred from this. First, there is no implied hierarchy of sources of evidence; evidence is convincing, whether it comes from forensic pathology or witness accounts. Second, evidence is often the result of a complex mixture of observation, experiment and theoretical argument.

The problem of defining health promotion

When health promotion came into prominence in the 1970s and 1980s, considerable time and effort had to be spent on defining the field. Documents, such as the WHO discussion of the concepts and principles of health promotion *(6)*, attested to the need to make maps and set boundaries. The ensuing and continuing debate about definitions largely focuses on issues of inclusion and exclusion. Every branch of knowledge has probably had such a debate. The end result is usually a more precisely bounded definition of a discipline. Thus, the established discipline of physics has certain characteristic concepts, principles, rules and other agreed features. Eventually, through long years of established use, the field yields textbooks, training programmes, certification, etc. Scholars universally recognize and distinguish a physics text from a biology text, for example. In spite of some shared edges with other disciplines, yielding subdisciplines and specialties such as biophysics, what constitutes physics is clear and largely agreed by all who practise in the discipline and regard themselves as physicists.

In contrast to physics, health promotion is probably not yet a discipline, and lacks an easily distinguishable paradigm. Rather, it sits inside a larger universe of disciplines. When health promotion takes on a particular task – say, advocacy for higher taxation on health damaging substances such as tobacco, alcohol and air pollutants – the appropriate evaluation paradigms may therefore not be found in the health promotion literature, but in other areas, such as the literature of political science and the study of advocacy. In brief, much of the practice of health promotion consists of looking outside the field for models, evidence of what works and the best methods. This wide-ranging, multidisciplinary approach is not only valuable but necessary at this stage of development. This implies a very broad understanding of how evidence is gathered and appreciated in many different disciplines.

Health promotion and the discussion on evidence

While defining health promotion remains difficult, listing its characteristics is relatively easy. The field includes a wide range of research, programmes and interventions, and it has a profound ideological component. It also has a broad theoretical underpinning, which includes contextualism, dynamism, participation and an interdisciplinary approach. Further, it is assumed that relevant theory would arise from multiple disciplines and represent research from diverse traditions. Finally, it is often argued that health promotion theory, research and practice should reflect the expressed needs of communities, groups and consumers *(7)*.

A recent view holds that practice should depend less on quantitative analyses and more on qualitative approaches. Sophisticated data analysis, it is argued, may provide too much unnecessary detail for policy-makers, who may not be sufficiently familiar with the complexity of multivariate analyses and how they should be interpreted. Paradoxically, in a multidisciplinary field such as health promotion, analyses often need to be complex, and a qualitative analysis may be as difficult to grasp as a quantitative one. In fact, complexity is a strong theme in the realm of population health research *(8)*; it reflects much of the current work in health promotion interventions that consider the combined effects of educational, political and social action on the health of individuals, groups and communities. How the debates over qualitative versus quantitative approaches and simple versus complex analyses are resolved should have important implications for the use of evidence in health promotion.

A major viewpoint incorporates the definition of the Ottawa Charter for Health Promotion *(9)* quoted in Table 1.1, Chapter 1 (p. 10). How exactly the specified control and improvement of health are to be obtained remains a subject of considerable research. A key factor, however, is the role of the context for action and, for many in the field, the appropriate setting is the community. Indeed, Green & Kreuter *(10)* call the community the "center of gravity" for health promotion and cite an extensive literature to support their assertion (see also Chapter 19). In the past decade, this notion has been sustained. It appears to derive from the convergence of sources including health promotion ideology, theory, policy and practice. In addition, the idea is tied into the notions of control and empowerment, thus leading to community participation as a fundamental principle of health promotion. The active, participating community is not a new idea in public health *(11)*, but it is a core principle for health promotion.

The concept of community comes with much ideological baggage, but, if one accepts its centrality in health promotion, what does one need as evidence that the community has been engaged appropriately? In answering this question, one must understand that communities cannot be conceptualized as individuals, and should not be reified as such. While members of a community vary in attitudes, opinions and behaviour, communities have collective behaviour. Communal behaviour has to be seen as the outcome of collective deci-

66

sion-making processes, which have a theoretical basis that is largely distinct from that of individual decision-making *(12,13)*. It follows that many evaluation considerations, including the role and nature of evidence, need to be conceptualized accordingly.

Though health promotion is characterized by its complicated socioenvironmental setting, theories of health promotion have seldom started with phenomena. They have started with ideology disguised as theory: ideologies based on beliefs and cognitive understandings of the world *(14)*, ideologies derived from the behavioural and social sciences that make up part of the ethos of health promotion. This heritage has come from the belief that knowledge is a product of social, historical, cultural and political processes. Similarly, a notion such as evidence cannot be separated from the processes in which it developed.

Health promotion is widely assumed to be based on science and a scientific basis for human behaviour. One could assert, however, that a strictly scientific paradigm does not underlie this scientific basis. In other words, the view that human behaviour is simply a response to physiological and neural processes is largely rejected in favour of characterizing human beings as organisms that live and operate within a society that is a product of human behaviour. Further, a strong case would be made that cognition is important and that human behaviour operates under a general concept of free will. Thus, if this behaviour is to be understood in terms of an underlying scientific paradigm, this paradigm would not be deterministic but probabilistic, in which statistical approaches to methods would be appropriate.

Given the diversity of research and practice in health promotion, another issue to consider is who asks the question: "What do we mean by evidence?". In many sciences the question is moot. The answer refers to established researchers in the discipline, carrying out research in a paradigmatic fashion. Further, the answer is the same for similar audiences. For example, the answer to the question of the type and amount of fuel needed to get a spacecraft from the earth to the moon would be the same for all engineers and advocates of space programmes. The most efficacious way to get funding for this space mission, however, is a very different question, highly contextual and specific to the characteristics of the politics of the country in question.

One could further explore the above example in the light of health promotion concerns. The role of disagreement, difference and dialogue would be critical. In the first part of the example, disagreement and difference are not essential elements. While there might be probabilistic arguments on the fuel type and tonnage necessary to obtain escape velocity, engineers from different countries would be relatively close in their estimates. They would use the same calculating equations, address the same gravitational forces and consider the same propellant alternatives. Differences, if they arose, would be explained as errors of calculation; consensus would be the most likely outcome. In short, disagreement, difference and dialogue would be minimal. In sharp contrast, similar strategies to seek funds are difficult to imagine, and there would undoubtedly be disagreement, difference and dialogue among many different groups and people unconnected with the science of the voyage.

Defining evidence in the context of health promotion

Evidence and *evidence-based* are popular terms and the whole area of evidence-based medicine may be considered a hot topic *(15)*. Both terms are regularly invoked in health promotion and population health discussions. Why should this be so? The literature on the history and philosophy of science does not show an extensive discussion of evidence. The word is seldom used and often appears only in the context of a broader discussion on data, observation, contexts and other aspects of scientific inquiry *(16)*. Perhaps the best reason for the present interest in evidence-based practice is that the sociopolitical climate has permitted it to flower, with emphasis on health care as one enabling element. Although this interest has had a relatively brief career in public health, people working in this domain must now deal with the proliferation of workshops and seminars on and rising expectations for an evidence-based approach. For example, papers commissioned by the national forum on health evidence and information in Canada have recently been published *(17)* and, in the United States, CDC has taken the lead in assisting the independent Task Force on Community Preventive Services to produce a guide to community preventive services. The document is intended to define, categorize and rate the quality of evidence on the effectiveness of population-based interventions in contributing to the achievement of specific outcomes. It will summarize what is known about the effectiveness and cost–effectiveness of population-based interventions for prevention and control, make recommendations on these interventions and methods for their delivery based on the evidence, and identify a prevention research agenda *(18)*.

Descriptions of the Task Force and its work on the planned guide are available on the Internet (http://www.health.gov/communityguide, accessed 29 February 2000). The recommendations on interventions will be based on the strength of evidence of their effectiveness, their beneficial and harmful effects and their generalizability. To categorize the strength of a body of evidence, the Task Force considers the following factors: the suitability of an evaluation study design to provide convincing evidence of effectiveness, the number of studies made, the quality of study execution, the consistency of their findings, the size of observed effects and, in rare circumstances, expert opinion. The Task Force regards as most suitable studies for which there are concurrent comparison groups and prospective measurements of exposure and outcome (such as randomized or non-randomized clinical or community trials, designs with multiple measurements of concurrent comparison groups before and after intervention, and prospective cohort studies). All designs that are retrospective or have multiple before-and-after measurements but no concurrent comparison groups (such as retrospective cohort studies and case–control studies) are called moderately suitable. Least suitable are designs with single before-and-after measurements and no concurrent comparison group or with exposure and outcomes measured in a single group at the same point in time. The Task Force has noted that population-based prevention strategies are frequently multiple component and complex, and that randomized controlled trials may not be feasible or desirable to evaluate the effectiveness of community interventions. What is noteworthy about this undertaking is the time and effort that have gone into establishing a way to categorize and define evidence. The Task Force has devoted much effort to defining evidence in terms of intervention design.

Indicators and evidence

To provide a background for understanding the relationship between types of evidence and evaluation issues in health promotion programmes, we look at several basic epistemological questions. What is the nature of evidence, science and proof? What is the relationship between health promotion theory and the rules of evidence? How does surveillance as a methodological approach relate to evidence? How is rigour defined in evaluation? Where do the concepts of error and the immeasurable enter into evaluation, and how does the issue of causation play a role? As an exemplar we consider the lessons learned in the failure of attempts to build satisfactory social indicators to illustrate how the epistemological issues intertwine with reality.

Assigning a numerical value to a construct is at the heart of measurement in the social sciences. For example, most people would agree that the concept of social status is a construct with multiple dimensions. It is commonly seen as both determined by concrete factors, such as income, level of education and occupation, and related to many contextual and cultural factors, such as age, race, gender, ethnic and family background, and attractiveness. In short, it is a very complex construct. A general approach taken by those who measure it is to develop and elaborate a scheme to classify all the gradations of relevant factors, and then to select the number of parts to the construct and how they should be mixed or valued. In the end, numbers are assigned to the weighted factors; in brief, the complexity of social status has been reduced to a scale of measurement. This is done to create a numerical assignment to each value of the construct that can be manipulated mathematically. The underlying epistemological assumption is that manipulating the numerical assignment sets up a method for manipulating the construct. Researchers often assume that these assigned numbers are linear and ordinal. Thus, a person with a social status score of 4 conceptually has twice the social status of a person whose score is 2. In common usage, a social indicator is essentially a construct that can have a numerical assignment.

Health promotion researchers have laboured valiantly to develop social indicators, with evaluation as a driving force. Because many both inside and outside the field see numbers as the hallmark of proof, they see quantitative social indicators as the best evidentiary base for illustrating the success of interventions. In the case of a health promotion programme to reduce smoking among young adults, for example, one would like to see a decrease in the rate of smoking over time in that population group commensurate with the introduction and application of interventions to it. Here the indicator, the rate of smoking, is simple, clear and easily measurable.

In many ways the search for indicators as a solution to the problem of obtaining evidence reflects the general idea that evidence can be conceptualized in terms of design structures. MacDonald *(19,20)* has suggested combining three evaluative strands in a complementary fashion to provide an appropriate overall design for evidence. The first strand would involve qualitative research methods that focus on process or formative evaluation. The second strand involves developing intermediate and indirect indicators of the delivery of interventions, and the third combines intermediate indicators of success with measures of outcome effectiveness. Thus, indicators play a key role in MacDonald's design for evaluation that provides the evidence for successful health promotion. This multifaceted, composite approach to evidence has been further elaborated by many who have argued that adding a mixture of designs, including qualitative approaches and process evaluation, to the focus on indicators will provide evidence of success in health promotion *(4,21,22)*.

History and philosophy of science and the nature of evidence

Science can be quite simply defined as the best explanation for phenomena at any given point in time. Such a definition integrates a historical context into the definition. Under such a definition, Aristotle's biology or Ptolemy's explanation of planetary motion, despite being discarded explanations for present-day purposes, are clearly scientific. They reigned supreme for millennia: hardly a minor achievement for humanity. Even according to a more rigorous definition – such as that provided by Webster's *(23)*: "a branch or department of systemized knowledge that is or can be made a specific object of study" – the ancient scientists hold up extremely well. They also provided the evidential basis for proof of phenomena in the context of their science.

Any definition of science contains many challenging words; complications arise from words such as *systemized*, *knowledge*, *observation* and *nature*. Each of these provides a cascade of additional concepts and issues to be addressed. Even if the additional issues are resolved satisfactorily, a larger question remains. Is health promotion a science and are the activities of science applicable to the health promotion endeavour? For the purposes of this discussion, we say, "Yes".

The literature supports the argument that many people view health promotion research as a science. For example, the *American journal of health promotion*, a leader in the field in the United States, has published since its inception a series of reviews arguing that health promotion research should adhere to rigorous scientific principles. The opening issue in 1986 included "Evaluation model: a framework for the design of rigorous evaluation of efforts in health promotion" *(24)*. Almost a decade later, the editor and publisher announced a series of systematic reviews of the literature, conducted by qualified scientists, on the effects of specific types of health promotion intervention on specific outcomes *(25)*. Since then, the journal has continued to review the state of the science of health promotion *(26)*. The noteworthy characteristic of the series is the classification of interventions according to a rating system for research evidence. The rating runs from five stars (conclusive evidence) to one star (weak evidence). Conclusive evidence shows a "cause-effect relationship between intervention and outcome supported by substantial number of well-designed studies with randomized control groups", and weak evidence is based on "research evidence supporting relationships [that] is fragmentary, nonexperimental and/or poorly operationalized"; evidence warranting two stars is characterized by "multiple studies consistent with relationship, but no well-designed studies with randomized control groups" *(25)*. Clearly, the *American journal of health promotion* has attached great importance to randomized controlled trials.

Although considered a science by many, health promotion is also a technical field of practice. This duality has implications for evidence. Historically, technology has been seen as distinct from science, as the application of science. In reality, however, there has always been a continuum between the pure and the applied. Thus, theoretical physics tends to merge into experimental physics and, further, into engineering; psychological theory yields to clinical psychology. Similarly, the field of health promotion shows a continuum between theory and research and intervention. This is important because evidence may vary with its purpose.

Overall, the evidence for a theory may be seen as more abstract and difficult to conceptualize than evidence to show that something works. In general, evidence is seen as easier to find when it is based on a controlled experiment. In the physical and biological sciences, such as astronomy, geology and evolutionary biology, where experimentation is very difficult, evidence must be based on complex, detailed observation of uncontrolled events. Thus, evolutionary theory remained unproven experimentally until the late twentieth century because of the complexity and multivariate nature of the observations needed to obtain proof *(5)*. Even relativity physics has relied less on actual experiment than on the classic *Gedankenexperiment (16)*.

Health promotion theory should define the methods

In contrast to the relatively tidy laboratory world of molecular genetics, the territory of health promotion is the community, steeped in historical and political context and consisting of intricate, fluid social relationships. In a laboratory, the observer can manipulate variables, but health promotion is social action through community participation, in an environment with a myriad of mediating and interacting factors that bear on health and are quite difficult to account for, much less control. Darwin's theory of evolution by natural selection provided scientists with a framework to make sense out of observed phenomena that allowed them to move to the next level: new discovery. Health promotion, while multidisciplinary in character, has primarily relied on cognitive-based behavioural theories, with few well developed structural theories of social change and health *(14)*.

As discussed in chapters 1 and 22, health promotion initiatives involve multiple strategies operating at multiple levels. Measurement in particular is challenging when the concepts are unclear or subject to debate, discourse and speculation. When evidence for the effects of a programme on community health is needed, how does one sort out the relevant phenomena? When competing suggestions for action are proposed, what underlying logic guides decision-making? Ultimately, what new knowledge can one provide about successful practices in community health promotion?

E.O. Wilson recently said, "Scientific evidence is accretionary, built from blocks of evidence joined artfully by the blueprints and mortar of theory" *(27)*. Knowledge must be placed in context to communicate meaning. Bringing together experience and knowledge gained in community interventions requires some logical underpinning. As noted in Chapter 2, theory provides a framework. In participatory models of health promotion, making explicit theoretical assumptions is essential to reaching a shared understanding of ways to promote community health. Without theory, how can one evaluate evidence? Evidence is only meaningful in light of the theory that led to its production. People construct models of phenomena from observations in an attempt to explain the phenomena in a broader sense. This is the first step in putting observations together in a coherent pattern. Further elaborations, using inductive and deductive reasoning, attempt to discern consistent patterns or laws that apply to the phenomena, and to construct a theory. A theory is superior to a model because it not only explains observations related to the phenomena but predicts events.

We use the theory of rational action described by Coleman to illustrate the distinction between theory and models. He refers to this theory as the dynamic between social structure and actors within it, in which "each actor has control over certain resources and interests in certain resources and events" *(28)*. One conceptual component of this theory is social capital and its underlying assumptions. Social capital refers to the relationships and norms in a community that are exemplified by trust, cooperation and civic engagement for mutual benefit (see Chapter 19). Parallel to the concept of financial capital, social capital assumes that investment will yield benefits: in this case, public good. A second assumption is that, as social capital increases through civic engagement, public institutions will better serve the community. Coleman *(28)* describes a model of schools that foster the completion of secondary education as a function of social capital. He asserts that social capital in both the family and the community surrounding a school increases the likelihood that students will achieve this goal. The model describes a specific set of interactions that result in schools that foster completion, while the theory provides a framework for explaining the broader relationships between civic engagement and the social institutions that benefit communities. The phenomenon of civic engagement, while complex, can be observed more simply through some of its elements (such as attending church and doing volunteer work). Thus, a model would provide the links to combine the discrete observations into a richer description of the phenomenon of civic engagement. In summary, a theory (such as that of rational action) provides the foundation to for a model of a variety of complex social relationships and outcomes (such as community programmes for young people, voting behaviour and community use of leisure time).

Unfortunately, many heath promotion researchers put the cart before the horse when choosing research methods. They let research methodology drive the investigation, rather than allowing theory and models to provide the conceptual underpinnings for the advancement of knowledge. With such conceptual understanding, investigators can then seek appropriate methods. For instance, many researchers inappropriately use randomized controlled trials in health research. Although valid and appropriate for testing many hypotheses about the physiological phenomena for which models describe simple and direct relationships, such as the relationship between a drug and a physical reaction, such trials are inappropriate for many of the complex social phenomena that are often encountered in health promotion research. Before choosing a methodology, researchers should gain a conceptual understanding from theory and models of the phenomena being investigated. This approach has the potential not only to increase knowledge but also to lead to better theories and models.

Scientific rigour

Challenges to the scientific status of the field of health promotion often rest on questions of the rigour of methods used to accumulate knowledge within the discipline. These challenges often imply that any discipline worthy of being called scientific must uncover universal generalizations about its subject matter by employing a strict, systematic, consistent approach. Unfortunately, much confusion and misdirection result from the mistaken idea that the scientific method is first and foremost about doing controlled experiments with statistical rigour. In fact, it is largely about the attempt to transform perceived patterns into something of meaning. At the point where controlled experiments are possible and standard statistics apply, a great deal has already been learned *(29)*.

Health promotion is a rather new, multidisciplinary field in public health. The methods and aims of health promotion scientists have varied widely. This raises the question: is such pluralistic activity within the field inconsistent with the notion of scientific rigour? In considering the history of the sciences, Fiske & Shweder *(30)* note:

> Clarity of aim is an uncertain virtue in a healthy science: some activities that turn
> out to be important seemed aimless originally, and scientists who do have clear

aims in mind are often aimed in different directions or at each other. Typically, in a healthy, developing science, the work at the growing edge is highly contested.

Thus, there is a cautionary note to using standardized, explicit, and precise criteria for judging and regulating the development of a science. Rigour should not be confused with convention.

The methods of evaluating evidence in health promotion are many and varied. They include case studies, correlation studies, narrative analyses, experimental and quasi-experimental studies, interviews and surveys, epidemiological studies, ethnographic studies and others. The nature of the question guides the choice of research techniques. The need to study phenomena in their natural setting is of particular relevance. Some phenomena may be investigated satisfactorily in the laboratory, but generalizations from laboratory results may not be valid due to features of the setting. Studying certain social phenomena outside their natural setting may be impossible, and thus considering samples representative of situations or settings, rather than subjects, may be more important. The consequences of certain phenomena (such as population density, community social cohesion and income equality) may not be addressed adequately outside the natural setting. Reducing social phenomena to individual-level variables (such as annual income and years of education) limits the ability to understand their effects on a community.

Why evidence is so critical to clinical medicine

The idea of error is anathema to modern clinical medicine. In his book on human experimentation, Silverman (31) relates many examples of the disasters and deaths caused by the ritualistic application of treatments that were unscientific and of unproven value. Particularly noteworthy is the long and sad history of therapies applied enthusiastically and without observation and recognition of their untoward results. The history of bloodletting, purging and the use of heavy metals and poisons in both heroic and routine patient care is well known. Indeed, even the twentieth century was replete with treatment disasters, such as the inappropriate use of radiation for enlarged tonsils and high concentrations of oxygen for premature infants.

Evidence-based medicine may be viewed as a scientifically agreed protection from error. Sackett et al. (15) and the Evidence Based Care Resource Group (32) argue that evidence-based medicine is the "conscientious, explicit, and judicious use of the current best evidence in making decisions about the care of individual patients" (15). This conceptualization has several notable features. First, *evidence* remains a primitive term, without further specification and definition. Second, the legalistic term *judicious* implies that the practitioner judges the evidence. Third, and most critical, the terms relate to the care of and outcome for the individual patient. These are not the grounds for determining the best evidence; rather, the experimental evidence provided by the randomized controlled clinical trial gives final confirmation.

74

This is the case in ideal circumstances; in reality, decisions related to risk–benefit analyses of treatment and cost–effectiveness considerations also drive patient care.

Nevertheless, clinicians and others with medical training use the word *evidence* within a broad context of a hierarchy of proof resting on experiment in general and the randomized controlled trial in particular. The idea is that a strong research history underlies the acceptance of any procedure or technique used in clinical practice. Those not supported by many rigorous trials should be regarded as weaker on a scale of evidence anchored by research that is not in dispute. Subtlety of findings is not a characteristic of evidence-based medicine. Consensus on and similar interpretations of findings are its hallmarks.

The medical community contains critics of the pursuit of evidence-based medicine. In his Cochrane lecture at the Society for Social Medicine meeting in 1997, Hart took a very sceptical look at the notion *(33)*. He reflected on the importance and impact of Cochrane's original work, *Effectiveness and efficiency (34)*. He argued that the advocates of evidence-based medicine *(33)*:

> accept uncritically a desocialised definition of science, assume that major clinical decisions are taken at the level of secondary specialist rather than primary generalist care, and ignore the multiple nature of most clinical problems, as well as the complexity of social problems within which clinical problems arise and have to be solved.

Hart's position parallels much of the participatory research perspective of health promotion practitioners *(33)*: "We need to work within a different paradigm based on development of patients as coproducers rather than consumers, promoting continuing output of health gain through shared decisions using all relevant evidence, within a broader, socialised definition of science". Hart thinks that evidence-based medicine is heavily influenced by underlying assumptions of economic theory and recent market-driven decision-making strategies in managed care. This counteracts efforts to bring the patient into a more active role in decision-making about care. Thus, a major part of the context of care, the patient's knowledge and experience, tends to be lost in the search for evidence-based medicine.

Problems with evidence in health promotion

The underlying epistemological basis for health promotion is not experimental science but the social and behavioural sciences. To a degree, some subgroups of the latter (such as clinical psychology) model their research and practice on the former. Nevertheless, most social science is non-experimental. Even in the very quantitative domains of sociology and economics, researchers' manipulation of variables is not characteristic, and experiment is largely absent in disciplines such as anthropology and political science. One could argue that most of the social and behavioural sciences are highly empirical: characterized by observation and classification, rather than any effort to manipulate the subject of study.

When intervention is intended to manipulate variables (to change knowledge, attitudes and behaviour, for example), the design can rarely possess the rigorous structure of an experiment. As pointed out elsewhere, researchers cannot control all the relevant variables or have a control group for comparison. The most that can be obtained is the oft-cited quasi-experimental design.

As participation is the chief characteristic of health promotion interventions, an ideal design would involve the collapse of the artificial dichotomy between researchers and the researched. This characterization and the attendant assumptions would make a rigorous experimental design totally inappropriate. Because evidence is so closely associated with rigorous experimental designs, the use of the term in health promotion becomes highly questionable.

For all the reasons given above, it is time to assert that the careless application of this term will deflect health promotion practice from concentrating on how best to design and evaluate interventions. It may mislead those who are not familiar with the epistemological base of health promotion into expectations deriving from a clinical science base. People in biomedicine are often criticized for having inappropriate expectations for health promotion research, but one could argue that these expectations result from the failure those in health promotion to provide an understanding of the theoretical foundation and epistemology of the field.

Three critical and unresolved issues
Rules of evidence
Three critical issues await resolution. The first is establishing a basis for the rules of evidence. To begin with, the rules of evidence appear to be tied to disciplines, not projects. Over the years, scientific disciplines have developed their standards for what constitutes proof in observation and experiment. Thus, the appropriate scientific method is both a product of historical development and the characteristic observables in the discipline, and rules of evidence differ between disciplines. Many community-based disease prevention and health promotion projects are not based on a discipline, but represent a field of action. No discipline-based epistemological structure therefore underlies the evaluation of effort. Underlying rules of evidence needed to be distinguished for the disciplines of public health that are related to community-based research and intervention: specifically, epidemiology, social psychology, sociology, anthropology and health education. Similarities and differences should be specified, and rules for fields of action should be considered.

Part of the problem of developing a basis for rules of evidence is the unresolved issue of a hierarchy of evidence. Within the general area of community research, intervention and evaluation, great debate focuses on what constitutes knowledge in the field, what evidence is and even whether the notion of evidence is applicable to the evaluation of interventions in communities. Researchers and practitioners have not reached consensus on any hierarchy of evidence, and international groups have asserted that it is premature to prioritize types of evidence in a linear hierarchy (35). There remains a need to document this lack of consensus, to consider the pros and cons of consensus in the context of community intervention and to suggest directions for the future.

Finally, the complexity of multidisciplinary, compound interventions makes simple, universal rules of evidence untenable. Rules of evidence are often based on interventions that have relatively simple, demonstrable chains of causation, where the manipulation of single factors produces single, easily measured outcomes. Many community-based health interventions include a complex mixture of many disciplines, varying degrees of measurement difficulty and dynamically changing settings. In short, understanding multivariate fields of action may require a mixture of complex methodologies and considerable time to unravel any causal relationships. New analyses may reveal some critical outcomes years after an intervention. Thus, there is a need to recognize the complexity of community interventions and to suggest areas needing development to reach a better understanding of the analytical challenges. More appropriate analytical methods and evaluation designs should be developed and supported.

Indicators

The second unresolved issue is the search for and identification of indicators in health promotion. Despite years of what might be called indicator scepticism by positivists and indicator bashing by anti-positivists (21), two salient factors remain: decision-makers expect and often demand numbers derived from indicators, and most public health and health promotion practitioners and researchers have been trained to produce quantitative data and to respect them and the value of the associated indicators. Indicators and reports based on them often seem to galvanize interest and resources. An example is the strong current interest in general health indicators such as QALYs and DALYs. WHO is undertaking and supporting a large-scale project using DALYs to measure the global burden of disease (36). Individual countries are also taking up this task.

Appropriate theoretical basis

The third issue is the development of an appropriate theoretical basis for health promotion. This chapter has highlighted only a few of the many thorny theoretical issues that influence practice and the evaluation of initiatives. Lively discussion in the past two decades (8,10,37) has not led to a general theory of health promotion. Theory provides the foundation for the research and practice paradigms of the field, and one could assert that the more substantial and coherent the theory base, the more credible research and practice will be for the simple reason that the theoretical base establishes the parameters for what constitutes evidence.

Health promotion initiatives draw on a variety of disciplines and employ a broad range of ways to accumulate data. Since the field uses mixed methods to deliver interventions, it should develop a number of design strategies for evaluation. Health promotion is a relatively young approach, which has not had time to establish a deep theoretical base *(14)* or the accompanying methodology. This forms a marked contrast to the history of clinical medicine, with hundreds of years of development accompanied by a century of experimental rigour. Even the social sciences forming the base for health promotion (sociology, anthropology, etc.) are relatively new, arising mainly in the middle of the nineteenth century and developing strong interest in methodology only in the past 50 years. Thus, the lack of a widely accepted paradigm for the conduct of health promotion research and therefore of consensus on the best evaluation strategies is not surprising.

Conclusions: optimism and the way forward

Despite its apparently critical tone, this chapter is much more a discussion of the issues than a condemnation of the current state of methodology in health promotion evaluation.

There is reason for optimism. First, the recognition of the complexity of the evidence debate reveals that researchers and practitioners cannot apply standard evaluation approaches to population-based community interventions. A need is now recognized for the careful design of evaluation strategies that take account of diversity, multidisciplinarity and local contexts. Thus, the emerging theoretical perspective of health promotion, which embraces participation, context and dynamism, is being brought into the thinking on evaluation design.

Rigour in health promotion research requires the use of methods appropriate to the theoretical issues at hand, which may well mean avoiding one-shot studies in order to emphasize systematic replication in the appropriate setting. The result may be more integrated and productive studies and less fragmented and irrelevant research. Scientific disciplines and the theories upon which they are built require epistemologies and accompanying methodologies that open the doors to new knowledge, rather than barring them.

A second reason for optimism is that the continuing search for appropriate indicators for health promotion success is now better informed, and only naive practitioners would believe that there are simple, single solutions to developing appropriate indicators. Further, the recognition of the need for appropriate indicators has reinforced the awareness that health promotion efforts affect the basic infrastructure of public health. For example, the tracking of behavioural risk factors, the number of health promotion surveys and the general concern with monitoring lifestyles have developed markedly in recent years in the western industrialized world. This development is coupled with the desire that these surveillance systems extend beyond traditional concerns with etiology to address public awareness and expectations. There is an increasing desire to use these systems to assist the evaluation of population-based programmes and changes resulting from health promotion interventions. The positive aspect of this is the shift of focus towards population health and away from the individual.

Most significant, the debate on evidence has led to a broadening of the base of appropriate evaluation in health promotion and particularly community-based programmes. This debate has always recognized that health promotion interventions could not be separated from issues of policy, resources, community interests, ideologies and other difficult-to-measure parameters, and that many interventions succeeded or failed owing to intangible factors that were known anecdotally but difficult to document. Thus, researchers and practitioners were often forced to rely on traditional evaluation approaches that stressed inappropriate design strategies. The current debate recognizes the many possible directions in which to seek appropriate evidence. Although no perfect designs have yet been found, the accumulating scientific literature promises to identify the best possible.

References

1. *World Health Assembly resolution WHA51.12 on health promotion* (http://www.who.int/hpr/docs/index.html). Geneva, World Health Organization, 1998 (accessed on 8 December 2000).
2. BUTCHER, R.B. Foundations for evidence-based decision making. *In*: *Canada health action: building on the legacy. Vol. 5. Evidence and information*. Quebec, Editions Multimondes, 1998, pp. 259–290.
3. NUTBEAM, D. & Vincent, N. *Evidence-based health promotion: methods, measures and application*. 16th World Conference on Health Promotion and Health Education, San Juan, Puerto Rico, 23–26 June 1998.
4. TONES, K. Beyond the randomized controlled trial: a case for "judicial review". *Health education research*, **12**(2): 1–4 (1997).
5. WEINER, J. *The beak of the finch: a story of evolution in our time.* New York, Random House, 1995.
6. *Discussion document on the concept and principles of health promotion.* Copenhagen, WHO Regional Office for Europe, 1984 (document).
7. MCQUEEN, D.V. A methodological approach for assessing the stability of variables used in population research on health. *In*: Dean, K., ed. *Population health research: linking theory and methods*. London, Sage, 1993, pp. 95–115.
8. DEAN, K., ET AL. Researching population health: new directions. *In*: Dean, K., ed. *Population health research: linking theory and methods*. London, Sage, 1993, pp. 227–237.
9. Ottawa Charter for Health Promotion. *Health promotion*, **1**(4): iii–v (1986).
10. GREEN, L.W. & KREUTER, M.M. *Health promotion planning: an educational and environmental approach*, 2nd ed. Mountain View, Mayfield, 1991.

11. WINSLOW, C.E.A. *The evolution and significance of the modern public health campaign*. New Haven, Yale University Press, 1923.
12. COLEMAN, J.S. Collective decisions. *Sociological inquiry*, **34**: 166–181 (1964).
13. COLEMAN, J.S. Foundations for a theory of collective decisions. *American journal of sociology*, **71**: 615–627 (1966).
14. MCQUEEN, D.V. The search for theory in health behaviour and health promotion. *Health promotion international*, **11**(1): 27–32 (1996).
15. SACKETT, D. ET. AL. Evidence-based medicine: what is it and what isn't? *British medical journal*, **150**: 1249–54 (1996).
16. SUPPE, F., ED. *The structure of scientific theories*, 2nd ed. Urbana, University of Illinois Press, 1977.
17. *Canada health action: building on the legacy. Vol. 5. Evidence and information*. Quebec, Editions Multimondes, 1998.
18. PAPPAIOANOU, M. & EVANS, C. Development of the guide to community preventive services: a U.S. Public Health Service Initiative. *Journal of public health management practice*, **4**(2): 48–54 (1998).
19. MACDONALD, G. Where next for evaluation? *Health promotion international*, **11**(3): 171–173 (1996).
20. MACDONALD, G. ET. AL. Evidence for success in health promotion: suggestions for improvement. *Health education research: theory and practice*, **11**(3): 367–376 (1996).
21. MCQUEEN, D.V. & NOVAK, H. Health promotion indicators. *Health promotion*, **3**(1): 73–78 (1998).
22. SANSON-FISHER, R. ET AL. Developing methodologies for evaluating community-wide health promotion. *Health promotion international*, **11**(3): 227–236 (1996).
23. *Webster's third new international dictionary*. Springfield, MA, G. & C. Merriam, 1981, p. 2032.
24. GREEN, L. Evaluation model: a framework for the design of rigorous evaluation of efforts in health promotion. *American journal of health promotion*, **1**(1): 77–79 (1986).
25. O'DONNELL, M. & ANDERSON, D. Toward a health promotion research agenda: state of the science reviews. *American journal of health promotion*, **8**(6): 462–465 (1994).
26. ANDERSON, D.R. Database: research and evaluation results. *American journal of health promotion*, **13**(1): 52–56 (1998).
27. WILSON, E.O. *Consilience*. New York, Alfred Knopf, 1998.
28. COLEMAN, J.S. Social capital in the creation of human capital. *American journal of sociology*, **94**: 95–120 (1988).
29. LOEHLE, C. *Thinking stratgically*. Cambridge, Cambridge University Press, 1996.
30. FISKE, D.W. & SHWEDER, R.A., ED. *Metatheory in social science*. Chicago, University of Chicago Press, 1986.

31. SILVERMAN, W.A. *Human experimentation: a guided step into the unknown.* Oxford, Oxford University Press, 1985.

32. EVIDENCE BASED CARE RESOURCE GROUP. Evidence-based care. 1. Setting priorities: how important is this problem? *Canadian Medical Association journal*, **15**: 1249–1254 (1994).

33. HART, J. What evidence do we need for evidence-based medicine? *Journal of epidemiology and community health*, **51**: 623–629 (1997).

34. COCHRANE, A. *Effectiveness and efficiency.* London, Nuffield Provincial Hospitals Trust, 1972.

35. *Health promotion evaluation: recommendations to policy-makers: report of the WHO European Working Group on Health Promotion Evaluation.* Copenhagen, WHO Regional Office for Europe, 1998 (document EUR/ICP/IVST 05 01 03).

36. WORLD HEALTH ORGANIZATION & WORLD BANK. *The global burden of disease: a comprehensive assessment of mortality and disability from diseases, injuries and risk factors in 1990 and projected to 2020: a summary edited by Christopher J.L. Murray, Alan D. Lopez.* Cambridge, Harvard School of Public Health, 1996 (Global Burden of Disease and Injury Series, Vol. 1).

37. ANDERSON, R. ET AL., ED. *Health behaviour research and health promotion.* Oxford, Oxford University Press, 1988.

Participatory approaches to evaluation in health promotion

Jane Springett

A participatory approach to evaluation attempts to involve all who have a stake in the outcome in order to take action and effect change. Some argue that this is more a way of working than a methodology, and that it reflects the nature of health promotion practice, particularly in community settings *(1,2)*. Its philosophical and epistemological base lies in a hermeneutic tradition of knowledge creation *(3,4)*. Its methodological and ideological roots lie in participatory action research, which has been used extensively in developing countries and is increasingly adopted in the developed world *(5–9)*. Health promotion practitioners see it as playing a particular role in knowledge development *(2,10)* and use it most commonly in communities and disadvantaged groups where there is a grassroots tradition *(11–15)*. The strength of participatory approaches lies in their contribution to empowerment and social change *(16)*. In other words, participatory evaluation is a health promotion strategy.

This chapter examines the nature and origins of participatory evaluation, its strengths and weaknesses, the challenges it faces and how it might be undertaken in the context of health promotion. Only a few published sources relate specifically to the participatory evaluation of health promotion, but an increasing literature addresses evaluation and the social sciences in general. This literature reflects the growing disillusionment at a number of levels with approaches to research and evaluation derived from methodologies originating in the natural sciences. It also represents a philosophical debate that challenges thinking about how and by whom knowledge is created. On a practical level, the literature is a response to the great divide between research and practice, which is maintained by the tendency of those who commission most evaluation studies to ignore the results *(17)*.

Nature and origins of participatory evaluation
Roots
The roots of participatory evaluation lie in the notion of action research developed by Lewin in the 1940s *(18)*. Since then it has been pursued in a variety of contexts. It is well established as an approach and methodology in three areas: development research, management science and education. Within these areas,

the approach has shown tremendous variety in form and has been applied to increasingly complex problems *(7,18–24)*.

In development research, action research has been extensively used as a vehicle for rural development and is closely associated with approaches to popular education stemming from the work of the Brazilian educator Paulo Freire *(8,12)*. This southern focus, as Brown & Tandon *(19)* call it, emphasizes mobilizing, raising the consciousness of and empowering the oppressed to achieve community transformation and social justice, notions that have much in common with those of community development and empowerment in health promotion. Indeed, in the 1960s and 1970s, action research was seen in western Europe as an important feature of community development approaches, but differed from the southern tradition in being seen more as the involvement of the local community in research initiated by others than as real collaborative inquiry in which the community leads in identifying the problem and producing knowledge. The latter has been widely used in primary health care and public health, particularly for assessing health needs in developing countries *(11,12)*.

The increasing adoption of participatory principles stems from the southern tradition of aid agencies' use of action research for the evaluation of development projects *(25,26)*. Such principles have appeared, for example, in the guise of "beneficiary or user assessment" in the work of the World Bank *(27)*. Agencies see participatory approaches as a management tool, and increasingly use them to avoid the inherent weaknesses of conventional evaluation methods *(9)*, especially when clear objectives have not been set at the outset of a project. While the principles are better established in aid work than many other areas, the practices are taking longer to establish and have been found to challenge many fundamental ideas, including the notion of the project itself. Some see the persistence of the project cycle, with relatively fixed procedures for the individual steps, as an obstacle to the full adoption of participatory principles *(28)*.

Mikkelsen *(28)* distinguishes participatory evaluation in the development context from fourth-generation and utilization-focused evaluation, arguing that the latter are more concerned with establishing final conclusions and the former, with adapting and adjusting a project in progress to conditions set by the participants. Such an approach to evaluation is seen as a prerequisite to ensuring project sustainability because of the focus on learning from experience. It serves, then, as both a management tool to enable people to improve their efficiency and effectiveness, and an educational process in which the participants increase their understanding of factors affecting their situation. Particularly in development work, it ensures that those locally involved in the project, rather than outsiders, learn the lessons provided by evaluation. Fuerstein has written a seminal work on participatory evaluation *(29)*, and suggests that a participatory evaluation in the development context include certain steps *(30)*.

1. All those involved in a programme decide jointly to use a participatory approach.
2. They decide exactly what the objectives of the evaluation are. This can turn out to be far harder than originally thought.
3. When agreement is reached, a small group of coordinators is elected to plan and organize the details.
4. The best methods for attaining the objectives are chosen. The capabilities of the people involved and the available time and other resources will influence this choice.
5. Decisions are recorded in a written plan, specifying why, how, when and where the evaluation will take place and who will be involved.
6. The methods are prepared and tested. Selected participants will need training (for example, in interviewing). The objectives and methods should be explained to all participants; the more they understand, the better their participation will be.
7. The methods are used to collect information.
8. The participants, mainly the coordinators, analyse the information.
9. They present the results in written, oral or pictorial form.
10. The programme participants decide how the results will be used, especially to improve the effectiveness and performance of the programme.

In addition, the Food and Agriculture Organization of the United Nations (FAO) has suggested a whole range of appropriate techniques *(31)*:

1. making of a community map
2. preparation of a group resource matrix
3. participatory monitoring wall charts
4. active learning techniques by participants
5. educational games and role playing
6. practical group exercises
7. presentation of findings through stories and drama
8. group field visits and study tours
9. use of real case studies
10. group presentation of meaningful data
11. group analysis of research reports
12. trend and change analysis
13. causal diagramming.

In management science, action research has come to be seen as a form of learning that encourages the systematic collection of data and information, combining rigour and relevance in moving towards high levels of performance in organizations and leading to innovation *(32)*. It is therefore geared to use groups, particularly of decision-makers, to solve major problems with jobs or in organizations. A key feature of recent research in this area is the emphasis on participation, the use of action research to generate networks to support economic development, and change in multilevel systems rather than single units or organizations (20). Such work has considerable relevance for the evaluation of cross-sectoral work.

Participatory evaluation in organizations draws on this action research tradition to build on the notion of stakeholder involvement. This differs from the stakeholder tradition in evaluation practice (33,34), however, by engaging the primary users in all stages of the process. In addition, rather than being the principal investigator, the evaluator acts as a coordinator of the project. He or she is responsible for technical support, training and quality control but shares the responsibility for conducting the inquiry. The evaluator becomes a partner in a process in which everyone involved is committed to change. Such partnerships may continue to develop beyond the duration of one project. An additional advantage is that managers are less likely to coopt or manipulate the evaluator to support their own agenda (35). Participatory evaluation has thus been defined as (36):

> Applied social research that involves a partnership between trained evaluation personnel, and practice based decision makers, organisation members with programme responsibility or people with a vital interests [sic] in the programme or – in Alkin's terms – primary user.

Underpinning the rationale is the notion of learning, particularly by organizations. This reflects the increasing emphasis of management literature on the importance of participatory decision-making in changing organizations (37).

While education research has an organizational focus, action research in this area gives greater emphasis to practitioners' becoming researchers in order to become more reflective and to improve their practice (38). Researchers pursue this aim by systematically collecting evidence, through collaborative and collective inquiry, in a quest to learn how to make improvements by examining the effects of changes made, particularly in the classroom (39). Similarly, nursing action research has tended to focus mainly on day-to-day practice on the ward (40). This notion of reflective practice is increasingly a feature of health promotion research (41).

From these different traditions and the research literature, one can identify three types of action research that are relevant to the evaluation of health promotion but differ according to their participants:

- participatory action research, which usually involves a community that, in theory, identifies the problem to be studied and a researcher who acts as a facilitator;
- action research, which involves a practitioner and a researcher, usually with the former determining the agenda; and
- collaborative inquiry, in which the researcher, practitioners and the community are equal partners who generate the initial agenda in the process of inquiry.

86

In each of these categories, practitioners could include policy-makers or the key managers implementing policy within organizations that affect health. Other authors have made different distinctions; for example, Fetterman et al. *(5)* have recently coined the term "empowerment evaluation". The categories identified here reflect the traditions of thought that have developed in the last 50 years.

These traditions have influenced evaluation theory and practice as more participatory approaches have been adopted in a whole range of fields relevant to health promotion, including policy analysis, social work and urban planning. A common factor has been an increasing concern about the variability in evaluation utilization, as well as the failure to develop useful indicators using conventional approaches. Another concern has been the high failure rate of some types of evaluation to affect policy implementation in the public services. For example, a recent study of the evaluation of urban regeneration policies implemented in the United States of America in the1980s found considerable disillusionment with large-scale external evaluation studies using sophisticated methods, such as mathematical modelling, often to answer questions that had not been asked. Evaluations were rarely driven by systems or concepts, but often developed inappropriate indicators that were difficult to measure and failed to influence policy. In response, participatory approaches to evaluation involving learning networks have been developed. The demand for universal indicators has given way to involving users and managers in developing locally sensitive indicators, often of a soft type *(42)*. In the United States, in this area at least, narrowly defined empirical evaluation is retreating before a movement towards an eclectic mix of methods involving the people who manage programmes.

In general, the failure to develop appropriate performance indicators has led to involving the user in evaluation *(43)*:

> There is a tendency in both the public and private sectors to develop indicators which reflects [*sic*] the performance that the provider thinks the public wants. Evaluation must, therefore, attempt to confront the dysfunction, which can sometimes arise, between user perceptions of their own wants and professional judgement as to their needs.

Relationship between action research, participatory research and participatory evaluation

The research and evaluation literature makes a subtle and perhaps semantic distinction between participatory research and participatory evaluation. Some consider the latter to be one aspect of the cycle of the former *(44)*; others see it as a distinctive approach to evaluation. The two share the key principles of the active involvement of various parties in the work of and decisions about the evaluation process, requiring the continuous exchange of knowledge, skills and resources *(36)*. Some argue that the two are the same if participation takes place throughout a project cycle *(28,45)*. Others say that action research differs from participatory research or evaluation only in not viewing power and its relationship to knowledge as a central issue. For example, action research is seen as a process evolving from negotiation, dialogue, learning and change among the participants.

Advocates of participatory evaluation often emphasize the distinction between evaluation and research *(46)*, as well as that between participatory evaluation and participatory action research, which is seen as "explicitly normative and ideological in form and function" *(35)*. Participatory evaluation here is linked directly to participatory decision-making *(36)*. It is distinctive in changing the relationship between the evaluated and the evaluator *(47–49)*, and thus challenges evaluation based on the authority of the outside observer and independent assessor. Similarly, participatory action research challenges the scientific notion of an independent and objective researcher *(50)*.

Given these nuances, practitioners' confusion about participatory research and participatory evaluation is not surprising, and leads to wide variation in practice *(2)*. Wadsworth *(45)* has tried to resolve the dilemma by combining the two, calling for an action evaluation research process; she has summarized the basics of the process in a visual model that forms a useful wall chart accompanying her practical book, *Everyday evaluation on the run*. Except in very few circumstances, however, this model is an ideal to pursue, not a reality. Levels of participation vary widely, and small groups of people still set most agendas. At best, practice is consultative, rather than really participatory *(51)*. Opinion in this debate, however, depends on ideological perspective and context. People concerned with the evaluation of community-based projects will be attracted to the ideology underpinning participatory research, which was developed to empower the oppressed, while those evaluating organization-based programmes and policies will emphasize the decision-making aspects of participatory evaluation.

While the distinctions between participatory research, participatory evaluation and action research are blurred, all three differ fundamentally from conventional research in health promotion. Evaluation in this field continues to be dominated by epidemiologists, demographers and biomedical experts with a positivist view of the world that conflicts with the hermeneutic perspective that underpins action research; Table 4.1 contrasts the characteristics of positivism and hermeneutics. Moreover, some studies bear the label of participatory action research but lack its underlying ideological, methodological and epistemological basis, reflecting the appropriation of the term by positivist science *(52–54)*. Participation means engaging in a dialogue at all stages of the process of evaluation and shifting power in favour of those who are being researched: what Vanderplaat *(47)* calls "evaluation for empowerment".

Philosophical and epistemological basis of participatory evaluation
What unites the definitions of action research and participatory evaluation is their focus on knowledge creation in the context of practice, the development of local theory *(55)* and capacity building. Such a perspective is based on a

Table 4.1. Characteristics of positivism and hermeneutics

Positivism	Hermeneutics
Objective observation	Critical subjectivity
Explanation and prediction	Understanding and finding meaning
Search for general knowledge and standardization	View of every situation as unique
View of social organization as combinations of similar things Surface view	Stress on richness, variety and depth
Hypothesis testing through formal definition of ideas and measurement	Dialectical cycle to gain knowledge
Mechanistic, with a focus on an object that has no voice and is submissive	Dialogue and subjective participation (understanding is not real unless it is mutual)
Aim: the power to control the collection of facts	Aim: enlightenment, edification, enrichment, personal growth
Emphasis on quantity	Emphasis on quality

Source: adapted from Dahlbom & Mathiassen *(4).*

completely different conception of the relationship between science, knowledge, learning and action from that of positivist methods in social science *(50).* It assumes that people can generate knowledge as partners in a systematic inquiry based on their own categories and frameworks. This, one can argue, enhances scientific validity, producing richer and more accurate data, and creates active support for the results and therefore greater commitment to change *(56).*

Learning is the *raison d'être* of action research, which draws heavily on the notions about the way adults learn that form the basis of the Kolb learning cycle *(3)* (Fig. 4.1). For learning to take place, all elements of the cycle must be present. Traditional research and practice emphasize the creation and testing of theory and action, respectively. Action research addresses the entire cycle, with the collaboration between insider (practitioner) and outsider (evaluator or researcher) producing knowledge.

The emphasis on change is another distinguishing feature. People engaged in traditional health research and evaluation rarely link their work to action; making use of the findings is primarily the responsibility of others. Further, action research rejects the positivist assumption that researchers' involvement in the research setting is incompatible with good science *(57).*

Participatory evaluation aims to make change and learning a self-generating and self-maintaining process that continues after the evaluator/researcher has left. It seeks change with a positive social value: for example, a healthy community. Moreover, the process is as important a product as any evaluation

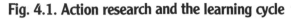

Fig. 4.1. Action research and the learning cycle

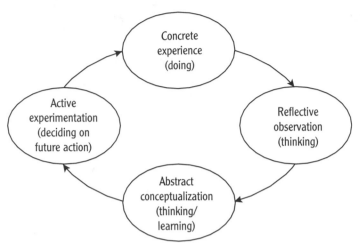

report. This type of evaluation is an emergent process controlled by local conditions. It involves the collective production of knowledge and seeks to empower the participants in a way that encourages endogenous change. While this approach is particularly appropriate to community-based projects, it also has value for those at the other end of the spectrum: policy development and implementation *(58,59)*. It appears to be an excellent vehicle for breaking down the boundaries between research and policy. No longer would experts produce knowledge that is shelved in offices and libraries but not applied to day-to-day practical problems. Instead, participatory evaluation would involve policy-makers in the research process, which would change the way they act and what they believe. Their involvement would ensure that they own both the ideas of the research and its results, and thus that they would be ready to take appropriate action. The key to this process is dialogue *(48)*. The exchange of ideas starts to shape a new social reality *(60,61)*; the role of the evaluator is to create situations for such exchanges through, for example, workshops and to allow the joint product, a more integrated and better understanding of the situation, to emerge *(62)*. This process creates a new set of social relations, as well as new knowledge.

This approach represents a challenge to the conventional scientific view of the way knowledge is constructed. Conventional science is predicated on the principle of objectivity, inherited from the positivist natural sciences, but it is an illusion to assume that people can conduct objective, value-free research that will yield immutable facts about the way things really are throughout the social world, particularly in complex social systems. As Schultz *(63)* argues, what distinguishes people from electrons and subatomic particles as research subjects is that being researched means something to the former. The social sciences thus examine reflective subjects: other thinking, feeling human beings who construct meanings, hold values and have a dynamic relationship with those studying them. If so, the relationship between the researcher and the researched must be central to the research process, not excluded from it (Table 4.2).

Table 4.2. Differences between the natural and social sciences in approach to and methods of programme evaluation

Question	Natural sciences	Social sciences
Who performs evaluation?	External experts	Community, project staff facilitator
What is examined?	Predetermined indicators of success, principally cost and health outcomes/gains	Indicators of success identified by participants, which may include health outcomes and gains
How?	Focus on objectivity, distancing evaluators from other participants; uniform, complex procedures; delayed, limited distribution of results	Self-evaluation, simple methods adapted to local culture; open, immediate sharing of results through local involvement in evaluation processes
When?	Usually at programme completion; sometimes also mid-term	Merging of monitoring and evaluation; hence frequent small-scale evaluation
Why?	To ensure accountability, usually summative, to determine whether funding continues	To empower local people to initiate, take and control corrective action

The tenets of participatory evaluation therefore appear counterintuitive to researchers schooled in conventional research methods. Action research urges that the dichotomy between researcher and researched be abandoned and that all programme participants be co-researchers and co-subjects producing the data that constitute the object of research, with even measurement being the product of a negotiated process. Further, analysis of the data would be no longer the sole domain of the researcher but a collaborative venture of all the participants.

Participatory evaluation in health promotion

The lack of reports of participatory approaches to evaluation in health promotion is not surprising, given the general lack of evaluation in health promotion and the paucity of outlets, until recently, for reporting this type of research. In addition, this type of study takes time both to conduct and to report in the literature; reports go to funding agencies first. The dominance of medicine in the health field and the resulting sanctity of the randomized controlled trial, traditional epidemiology and the conventional scientific method, however, are major factors. Objections to the approach – lack of scientific rigour and generalizability, validity of the results and replicability – stem from its perceived failure to be objective *(57)*.

Other issues, which do not stem from this perspective, affect the amount of participatory evaluation that takes place. These include the resources needed and the messiness of the process, even if it has clear steps, which conflicts with the desire for clarity, control, and logical and planned activities. Further, funding is hard to secure for an emergent and often indefinable outcome, as well as an unpredictable process *(64)*. Moreover, researchers lack the skills required, and the community, capacity for critical thinking *(30)*. When policy and multifaceted health promotion programmes are involved, participants must deal with the potential complexity of the process *(65)*. All these barriers are reinforced by the tradition of evaluating health promotion projects from the outside and often in inappropriate ways *(66)*. These issues are discussed in more detail below.

Participatory evaluation or action research in health promotion has rarely risen to true collaborative inquiry. Formative evaluation or needs assessment has overshadowed summative evaluation, particularly for projects aimed at disadvantaged groups *(12)*. Nevertheless, the value of participatory approaches to health promotion research is increasingly recognized, and they have formed the focus of a major study for the Royal Society of Canada *(2)*. They are gaining substantial popularity in research on primary care and health promotion in developing countries, and in nursing research, particularly in the community *(67)*.

Participatory evaluations of community-based programmes stem from the central role of empowerment in health promotion. The process is seen to contribute to the elimination of social inequality, the intended outcome of many programmes. It openly addresses issues of power, bringing social action and community development methods to evaluation. It also makes explicit the values and interests involved in evaluation, thus asking whose interests are being served. It allows participants to engage in democratic dialogue and thus creates new social knowledge *(61,62,68)*. Additional advantages include an increased likelihood that evaluation results will be used. This, according to Patton *(69)*, is the greatest benefit of participation, alongside the avoidance of orthodoxy and the encouragement of the use of a range of methods and tools in data collection and analysis. Participation also creates in people a critical awareness of their problems, an important part of capacity building. In effect, the process is the creation of knowledge on its own battleground, from the conflict inevitable in participatory evaluation *(70)*.

Further benefits arise from the sharing of lay and expert knowledge and the pooling of resources and strengths. For example, if the participants are involved in decision-making, they may even carry out the survey themselves, thus reducing the cost of evaluation. Finally, participatory evaluation is likely to produce relevant results, which can help achieve more traditional goals of behavioural change, as well as social change *(71)*: "When long term behavioural change, self sustaining capacity and universal coverage is [*sic*] desired, community participation is essential".

In the United States, empowerment was a feature of the evaluation of the Alcohol and Substance Abuse Prevention Program in New Mexico *(72)*. Freirean ideas of empowerment education formed a crucial role both in the Program and in its evaluation. Operating since 1982, it has sought to empower young people from high-risk populations to make healthier choices using Freire's three-stage methodology of listening, dialogue and action. Programme evaluation and policy implementation were undertaken by ensuring the same process is built into the organization of the Program. The evaluation has involved both quantitative and qualitative methods, alongside the participatory methods.

In addition, participatory evaluation was applied to the Partners for Improved Nutrition and Health, implemented in 1988 as a five-year collaborative programme by Freedom From Hunger, the Mississippi State Department of Health and the Mississippi Co-operative Extension Agency. Evaluation was an integral part of the agenda for an action research programme that involved developing community competence and was based on outreach programmes with community-determined goals. All stakeholders participated in defining and constructing measures of competence and deciding on the selection of interviewers and respondents, even though they were not involved in selecting community competence as the outcome to be measured. Nevertheless, decisions on what to evaluate were grounded in the experiences and visions of people living and working in the three areas of the programme *(15)*.

The failure to ground evaluation indicators in the needs of local workers and the community led the people in the Drumchapel section of Glasgow, United Kingdom to develop their own evaluation of their project (see Chapter 14 for information on the project). Disillusioned with an externally commissioned evaluation driven by the agenda of a university, they adopted a truly participatory approach that enabled a whole range of innovative methods to be used. These included reporting the results through art and a video *(66)*. The use of art was also a feature of the evaluation of the Healthy Cities Noarlunga Project, in South Australia, which used a participatory approach somewhat constrained by the requirements of the evaluation *(73)*. Roebottom & Colquhoun *(74)* used participatory action research when working on environment and health issues with a group of adolescents in the Bellarine Youth Network in Australia. They have noted some of the issues (such as the right to privacy) that need to be addressed when working with young people in this way.

The tendency for agencies with direct experience in developing countries to be involved in participatory evaluation is probably no coincidence. For example, charities such as Save the Children, which are working on health promotion in poor areas of the developed world, have spearheaded the use of participatory approaches and action research in needs assessment and programme evaluation in the United Kingdom. Bang & Bang *(75)* document the benefits of such an approach; they contrast the lack of impact of a traditional epidemiological study of sickle cell disease in the Gadchioli district in India with participatory action research on alcoholism prevention in the same district, which led to collective action both at the local and state levels.

Participatory evaluation has been applied to health promotion programmes in the workplace, particularly those dealing with stress *(76)*. Studies have tended to use organizational rather than programme-based approaches to health promotion. Action research is required, it is argued, because organizations can undergo many changes (such as layoffs and changes in product line and personnel) that can undermine the use of control and experimental groups. Studies have used statistical control techniques and time-series design, which demonstrates that participatory evaluation entails not just qualitative techniques but the eclectic use of appropriate methods. The culture of the organization, however, can limit the extent of participation in both action and intervention; cooption and manipulation can take the place of true participation in evaluation projects *(34,77)*.

There is less experience with participatory evaluation of policy development and implementation. Springett & Leavey *(78)* used action research to evaluate health promotion clinics in primary health care. While making every effort to encourage participation through creating arenas for dialogue, they struggled constantly to engage the general practitioners in the process. Action was restricted to the development of guidelines for primary health care teams that were circulated locally *(79)*.

The development of a tool was also the focus of a participatory approach to developing indicators to evaluate multisectoral collaboration. This project, funded by HEA, is a good example of how the characteristics of the participants affect the outcome. The research involved 200 people and was conducted in three stages. The first began with a telephone survey, which was conducted through the use of the snowball technique to gain an overview of work for alliances for health. Then followed a series of 6 workshops, involving 38 representatives from the sample gained, many of whom were members of the United Kingdom Health for All Network or, the Healthy Cities network of the United Kingdom and employed as Health For All or Healthy Cities coordinators. These workshops generated definitions of the characteristics of alliances for health and measures of success. The results were used to develop process and outcome indicators, which were then critically examined in a consensus forum.

Stage two involved refining the indicators by applying them in three test sites. The results were fed back into the process though a focus group, and then discussed in a workshop of 20 participants, which included some representatives of purchasers of health care services; afterwards, the indicators pack was modified *(80)*. Opportunities for dialogue between the practitioners and decision-makers and resource holders were limited and did not occur until the end of the process, so the final indicators very much reflected the views of the dominant group, practitioners, rather than those of the other key stakeholders.

Moreover, when tested, the pack was found to be inappropriate for small-scale community-based projects, particularly in the early stages of development, and was criticized by community participants. The pack's main advantage was that it helped to provide a framework for discussion of more relevant local indicators. Despite these drawbacks, the project was an unusually well funded attempt at true participation in indicator development.

Such work has great potential in health promotion. Just as participatory evaluation encourages empowerment, a collaborative problem-solving approach encourages intersectoral collaboration by forcing the participants to make conscious choices on how to collaborate and reflect on practice *(81)*.

The difficulty of developing indicators in complex projects, such as those for healthy public policy, is well illustrated by the development of an evaluation and monitoring framework and indicators for the city health plan in Liverpool, United Kingdom *(82)*. An attempt was made to satisfy a range of stakeholders while incorporating evaluation into the implementation process. The interplay between an ideal model and reality in a particular context produced a pragmatic approach. Costongs & Springett *(83)* have developed a framework using a participatory approach to policy evaluation.

Guidelines for engaging in participatory evaluation in health promotion

We see participatory evaluation as a cyclical process that is based on the action research cycle but contains a series of steps involving decisions in which all stakeholders participate (see Table 13.1, Chapter 13, pp. 298–299). Evaluators can use these steps as a checklist when engaging in the process. Although participatory evaluation can be called a process, not a technique, the methodological issues involved are concerned with how participants engage in the process, ensure it is systematic, and adhere to basic principles. A key focus is how opportunities for dialogue are created *(35)*. Many issues stem from the need to balance the requirements of participation, the use of appropriate, rigorous, verifiable and valid tools and techniques, and the practical demands of the real world, while retaining the values of social action *(84)*. Participatory evaluation is not clearly understood and is context driven, so it varies considerably in practice. Nevertheless, the following issues need to be addressed.

The first issue concerns the level and cyclical nature of participation. It is a spiralling process, rather than a series of static episodes. In practice, who participates is the product of the negotiated situation. While the ideal is total participation by all stakeholders, the distribution of power and resources between them and the time and other resources available for the evaluation are the determining factors. Inevitably, difficult decisions will have to be made, since who participates affects both the process and the results. Greenwood et al. *(55)* argue, "the degree of participation achieved in any particular project is the joint result of the character of the problems and environmental conditions under study, the aims and capacities of the research team, and the skills of the professional researcher".

Couto *(52)* notes that this balancing act can have different outcomes in different contexts, and medical hegemony in the health field often tips the balance towards traditional approaches. In addition, participation may change during the process. The larger the reach of a project, the more difficult it is to ensure a democratic process. A great deal of creativity is required. Small-scale community-based programmes are thus easier to manage. In all cases, involving managers and funding agencies is quite important. While managers may try to limit participation, preferring to exercise control, they often see no need to be involved in the process and fail either to attend workshops and meetings or to send representatives. This means that they do not own or understand the results at the end of the process.

Another difficulty in this context is the rapid turnover of project managers and other staff, a particular problem when dealing with a bureaucracy such as a government department. A recent evaluation of the potential for introducing more community participation in decision-making in federal government policy on health and human service delivery in Australia noted the high turnover of career staff as a major barrier to change (F. Baum et al., personal communication, 1995). The facilitator of the evaluation needs to ensure that arenas for dialogue are created and there is feedback at every stage of the process. She or he also needs to be aware of and try to reduce the inequalities in power between the participants. Arenas for dialogue should be varied and include workshops and other meetings varying in formality. While formal meetings can be barriers to effective communication, they are nevertheless necessary.

A second issue is the relationship between the evaluator and the evaluated, and the balance between expert and lay involvement and particularly between insider and outsider evaluation. Each has advantages and disadvantages (Table 4.3). Outside evaluators still have the greatest credibility. At a minimum, an external evaluator can act as facilitator at workshops, writer of the report and controller of quality. Both layperson and expert have something to offer. Indeed, the value of participatory action research is that it adds the technical expertise of the evaluator and the local knowledge of the lay participants to create a whole greater than the sum of its parts. Tied up with this issue is the need to gain the commitment of busy professionals and to negotiate who owns the findings. This is a particular problem for academics; the question of the authorship of research papers is important to them but difficult to settle when participation is broad. A lack of participation flies in the face of the concept of participatory evaluation and reinforces academic hegemony *(85)*. All these issues need to be negotiated at the beginning and the agreements written down, so that all are clear about their roles and responsibilities.

A third issue is the inherent contradiction that is a feature of participatory evaluation's dialectical nature. The bringing together of different agendas inevitably results in conflict and power struggles. This makes skills in conflict

Table 4.3. The advantages and disadvantages of external and internal evaluators

External evaluators	Internal evaluators
Can take a fresh look at the programme	Know the programme well
Are not personally involved	Find it harder to be objective
Are not part of the programme's normal power structure	Are part of the programme's normal power structure
Gain nothing from programmes, but may gain prestige from evaluations	May be motivated by hopes of personal gain
Are trained in evaluation methods, may have experience with other evaluations, are regarded as experts by programme participants	May not be trained in evaluation methods, have little or no more training than others in the programme
Are outsiders who may not understand programmes or the people involved	Are familiar with and understand programmes and can interpret personal behaviour and attitudes

Source: Fuerstein *(29).*

resolution as important to a good evaluator as knowledge of data collection and analysis techniques. Evaluators have competing and often contradictory tasks to fulfil. For example, an evaluation of health promotion policy and its implementation must be both useful to the policy initiative and relevant to external interest groups and policy-makers. The evaluator should be involved with the policy initiative in order to collaborate effectively with local workers, while keeping enough distance to be critical and ask the right questions *(86).* Also, the evaluator must strike a balance between the public's right to know and the individual's right to privacy, and be discreet *(34).* Evaluators therefore need a whole range of skills in, for example, communication, negotiation, motivation, politics and facilitation *(87).* As Long & Wilkinson *(88)* point out, evaluators "must have the ability to carry out an evaluation, while coping with the complexities of social programmes and conflicting personalities in a less than friendly environment". Means & Smith *(89)* reached the same conclusion when they involved stakeholders in their research into a regional alcohol education programme in south-western England.

In addition, evaluators should play a more active role in the policy process *(34),* going beyond evaluation to sell their ideas to policy-makers *(90).* Simply publishing in journals is not enough, particularly for qualitative evaluations, which are often less widely read than the compact reports of quantitative work *(91).* Evaluators must present their ideas and recommendations clearly and attractively to make an impact. Ham *(90)* remarks that communication and salesmanship must go hand in hand with good academic techniques if the evaluator wants to influence policy.

A fourth issue is the emergent nature of the process, which can have a number of effects. First, those who fund and make evaluations feel a lack of control. Participatory evaluation does not always fit into a neat project cycle; funds can be cut off at crucial moments, and reports can miss their deadlines. Having a committed project manager in the funding agency helps. Particularly relevant to health promotion is the fact that most projects address single issues, reflecting the disease and lifestyle model that still dominates the sector. Thus, evaluators must apply for funds on the basis of single issues, such as the prevention of coronary heart disease, reduction of alcoholism or cessation of smoking. The lay perspective is very different and reflects a more holistic approach to life. Programme outcomes may include raised self-worth and better quality of life, while still retaining high levels of smoking. The aims, objectives and outcomes that the participants value may therefore differ widely from the originals. Moreover, as action and change are central, the programme might change direction. This is another reason why the participation of the funding agencies and initiators of the evaluation is vital. Keeping the process going and ensuring appropriate communication and feedback at every stage are essential, although difficult to achieve during a participatory evaluation in a complex environment with different interest groups and multicausal effects (65).

A fifth issue concerns funding. Participatory evaluation receives less funding than more traditional forms of assessment. Funding agencies lack expertise in participatory approaches and chiefly demand short-term, task-oriented approaches to evaluation (2), even though partcipation offers greater potential for change because the evaluation results are more likely to be implemented. Evaluators depend for effective follow-through on a sympathetic fund-holder project officer who understands the unpredictability of the process and is willing to go along with it. Evaluators should form a good relationship with project officers at the beginning.

The evaluator's task often becomes more difficult because many health promotion practitioners think about evaluation only when a programme's end is in sight. This is too late to adopt a truly participatory approach. Health promotion has the added problem of being poorly resourced in general. Some organizations and funding agencies, however, now approve programmes only if a sum is allocated to evaluation; this is the case with health projects funded by the tobacco levy in Australia.

A sixth issue is choosing the appropriate tools and techniques both for data collection and for dissemination of results at each stage in the feedback cycle: a traditional methodological issue with a particular action research slant. Tools should be simple but effective, understandable but relevant. Often a community group may be forced to defend its findings before people trained in traditional epidemiology, as did the Yellow Creek Concerned Citizens their evaluation of the impact of waste dumping on health. This resulted in the use of quantitative methods within a scientific framework (52).

As mentioned, the choice of tools should emphasize eclecticism and appropriateness (51,92,93). Training is almost certainly required and should be included in the budget. The aim is to create a process that is sustainable and concludes with added knowledge. A health project in China used photographs as a form of data collection that provided a valuable and effective alternative to the graphs and other presentation methods demanded by decision-makers, who want concrete measures *(94)*. The information gained from the evaluation process should probably be presented in more than one form, as in the Drumchapel and Noarlunga projects *(66,73,95)*, and this needs to be taken into account in the work plan.

Conclusion and recommendations

Participatory action research is increasingly used in evaluating health promotion, but is far less widely accepted than in other areas, where the failure of conventional methods to bring about change has been openly acknowledged. The dominance in the health field of medical science, with methods rooted in the natural sciences, is a major factor in the slow adoption of this potentially fruitful approach to change. Ironically, participatory evaluation is the central feature, although not named as such, of clinical audit. The recent review by Cornwall & Jewkes *(12)*, demonstrating the strong influence of development work on those working in primary health care and public health in developing countries, and the Royal Society of Canada study *(2)* should give much needed impetus to the acceptance of this form of evaluation in the developed world. Here, other countries should follow Canada's lead. Action on the following recommendations would assist the process.

Policy-makers should:

- provide greater funding support for participatory evaluation;
- participate more in evaluation themselves;
- produce guidelines that encourage good practice and give funding agencies a standard against which to measure applications;
- support the development of skills training both for researchers and practitioners; and
- recognize the value of participatory evaluation in the long term and in building capacity, and its contribution to knowledge development and effective change, rather than the completion of specific and often inappropriate short-term tasks.

Practitioners should:

- accept that a participatory approach is inherently and overtly political and accept the resulting conflict;
- have faith in the approach;
- take part in evaluation because it can change the views of policy-makers;
- acquire the necessary skills; and

- ensure that the process is systematic and encourages participation and communication.

There is still a long way to go before so-called participatory evaluations are truly so; most are still controlled by the funding agencies and evaluators, and are more consultative than participatory. At its best, participatory evaluation provides a solution to the practical problem of crossing the boundaries between theory and practice and the competing cultures of research and policy-making. While it can be a real catalyst for change *(14,55,83,96)*, it is profoundly challenging in execution.

References

1. BEATTIE, A. Evaluation in community development for health: an opportunity for dialogue. *Health education journal*, **64**: 465–472 (1995).
2. GREEN, L.W., ET AL. *Study of participatory research in health promotion. Review and recommendations for the development of participatory research in health promotion in Canada.* Ottawa, Royal Society of Canada, 1995.
3. KOLB, D.A. *Experiential learning: experience as a source of learning and development.* Englewood Cliffs, Prentice Hall, 1984.
4. DAHLBOM, B. & MATHIASSEN, L. *Computers in context: the philosophy and practice of systems design.* Oxford, Blackwell, 1993.
5. FETTERMAN, D.M. ET AL., ED. *Empowerment evaluation: knowledge and tools for self-assessment and accountability.* Thousand Oaks, Sage, 1996.
6. BARNETT, L. & ABBATT, F. *District action research and education.* London, Macmillan, 1994.
7. ELDEN, M. & CHISHOLM, R.F. Emerging varieties of action research: an introduction. *Human relations*, **46**(2): 121–141 (1993).
8. KROEGER, A. & FRANKEN, H.P. The educational value of participatory evaluation of primary health care programmmes: an experience with four indigenous populations in Ecuador. *Social science and medicine*, **15**(4): 535–539 (1981).
9. ROVERS, R. The merging of participatory and analytical approaches to evaluation: implications for nurses in primary health care programs. *Nursing studies*, **23**(3): 211–219 (1986).
10. BOUTILIER, M. & MASON, R. *Community action and reflective practice in health promotion research.* Toronto, University of Toronto, 1994 (document).
11. DE KONING, K. & MARTIN, M. *Participatory research in health.* London, Zed Books, 1996.
12. CORNWALL, A. & JEWKES, R. What is participatory research? *Social science and medicine*, **41**(12): 1667–1676 (1995).
13. STANDISH, M.A. View from the tightrope: a working attempt to integrate research and evaluation with community development. *In*: Bruce, N. et

al., ed. *Research and change in urban community health*. Aldershot, Avebury, 1995, pp. 259–262.

14. SARRI, R.C. & SARRI, C.M. Organsiational and community change through participatory action. *Administration in social work*, **16**(3–4): 99–122 (1992).

15. ENG, E. & PARKER, E. Measuring community competence in the Mississippi Delta: the interface between programme evaluation and empowerment. *Health education quarterly*, **21**(2): 199–220 (1994).

16. LABONTÉ, R. Health promotion and empowerment: reflections on professional practice. *Health education quarterly*, **21**(2): 253–268 (1994).

17. WEISS, C.H. Evaluation for decisions. Is there anybody there? Does anybody care? *Evaluation practice*, **9**(1): 15–20 (1988).

18. LEWIN, K. Action research and minority problems. *Journal of social issues*, **2**(4): 34–46 (1946).

19. BROWN, L.D. & TANDON, R. Ideology and political economy in inquiry: action research and participatory action research. *Journal of applied behavioural science*, **3**: 277–294 (1983).

20. LEDFORD, G.E. & MOHRMAN, S.A. Looking backwards and forwards at action research. *Human relations*, **46**(11): 1349–1359 (1993).

21. REASON, P., ED. *Participation in human inquiry*. London, Sage, 1994.

22. REASON, P. Three approaches to participative inquiry. *In*: Denzin, N.K. & Lincoln, Y.S., ed. *Handbook of qualitative research*. Thousand Oaks, Sage, 1994, pp. 324–339.

23. WHYTE, W.F., ED. *Participatory action research*. London, Sage, 1991.

24. WINTER, R. *Action research and the nature of social inquiry*. Aldershot, Avebury, 1990.

25. WORLD CONFERENCE ON AGRARIAN REFORM AND RURAL DEVELOPMENT. *Guidelines on socioeconomic indicators for monitoring and evaluating agrarian reform and rural development*. Rome, Food and Agriculture Organization of the United Nations, 1988.

26. DEVELOPMENT ASSISTANCE COMMITTEE. *Sustainability in development programmes: a compendium of evaluation experience*. Paris, Organisation for Economic Co-operation and Development, 1989.

27. SALMEN, L.F. *Beneficiary assessment: an approach described*. Washington, DC, Poverty and Social Policy Division, World Bank, 1992 (Working Paper, No. 1).

28. MIKKELSEN, B. *Methods for development work and research. A guide for practitioners*. New Dehli, Sage, 1995.

29. FUERSTEIN, M.T. *Partners in evaluation*. London, Macmillan, 1986.

30. FUERSTEIN, M.T. Finding methods to fit the people: training for participatory evaluation. *Community development journal*, **23**: 16–25 (1988).

31. *Participatory monitoring and evaluation. Handbook for training field workers*. Bangkok, Food and Agriculture Organization of the United Nations, 1990.

101

32. MAGERISON, C.J. Integrating action research and action learning in organsiational development. *Organisational development*, Winter, pp. 88–91 (1987).

33. FRICKE, J.G. & GILL, R. Participative evaluation. *Canadian journal of program evaluation*, **4**(1): 11–25 (1989).

34. GREENE, J.C. Qualitative program evaluation, practice and promise. *In*: Denzin, N.K. & Lincoln, Y.S., ed. *Handbook of qualitative research.* Thousand Oaks, Sage, 1994.

35. MATHISON, S. Rethinking the evaluator role: partnerships between organsiations and evaluators. *Evaluation and planning*, **17**(3): 299–304 (1994).

36. COUSINS, J. ET AL. The case for participatory evaluation. *Educational evaluation and policy analysis*, **14**(4): 397–418 (1992).

37. SENGE, P. *The fifth discipline: the art and the practice of the learning organization.* New York, Doubleday, 1990.

38. McTAGGART, R. Principles of participatory action research. *Adult education quarterly*, **41**(3): 168–187 (1991).

39. KEMMIS, S. Improving education through action research. *In*: Winter, R. *Action research and the nature of social inquiry.* Aldershot, Avebury, 1990, pp. 57–74.

40. MEYER, J.E. New paradigm research in practice – The trials and tribulations of action research. *Journal of advanced nursing*, **18**: 1066–1072 (1993).

41. HART, E. & BOND, M. *Action research for health and social care.* Buckingham, Oxford University Press, 1995.

42. BARNEKOV, T. ET AL. *US experience in evaluating urban regeneration.* London, H.M. Stationery Office, 1990.

43. KNOX, C. & McALISTER, D. Policy evaluation: incorporating user views. *Public administration*, **73**: 413–415 (1995).

44. ISRAEL, B. ET AL. Health education and community empowerment: conceptualising and measuring perceptions of individual, organisational and community control. *Health education quarterly*, **21**(2): 149–170 (1994).

45. WADSWORTH, Y. *Everyday evaluation on the run.* Melbourne, Melbourne Action Research Issues Incorporated, 1991.

46. SPRINGETT, J. & DUGDILL, L. Workplace health promotion programmes: towards a framework for evaluation. *Health education journal,* **55**: 91–103 (1995).

47. VANDERPLAAT, M. Beyond technique: issues in evaluating for empowerment. *Evaluation*, **1**(1): 81–96 (1995).

48. HAZEN, M.A.A. Radical humanist perspective of interorganisational relationships. *Human relations*, **47**(4): 393–415 (1994).

49. GUSTAVSEN, B. *Dialogue and development.* Assen, Van Gorcum, 1992.

50. PEILE, C. Theory, practice, research: casual acquaintances or a seamless whole? *Australian social work*, **47**(2): 17–23 (1994).

51. BAUM, F. Research and policy to promote health: what's the relation-ship? *In*: Bruce, N. et al., ed. *Research and change in urban community health*. Aldershot, Avebury, 1995, pp. 11–31.

52. COUTO, R.A. Participatory research: methodology and critique. *Clinical sociology review*, **5**: 83–90 (1987).

53. LAWELL, A.C. ET AL. Participatory research on worker health. *Social science and medicine*, **34**(6): 603–613 (1992).

54. DOCKERY, G. Rhetoric or reality? Participatory research in the NHS UK. *In*: De Koning, K. & Martin, M. *Participatory research in health*. London, Zed Books, 1996, pp. 164–175.

55. GREENWOOD, D. ET AL. Participatory action research as a process and as a goal. *Human relations*, **46**(2): 171–191 (1993).

56. REASON, P. & ROWAN, J. *Human inquiry: a sourcebook of new paradigm research*. London, Wiley, 1981.

57. SUSMAN, G.I. &.EVERED, R.D. An assessment of the scientific merits of action research. *Administrative science quarterly*, **23**: 582–602 (1978).

58. WINJE, G. & HEWELL, H. Influencing public health policy through action research. *Journal of drug issues*, **22**: 169–178 (1992).

59. LIPMAN-BLUMEN, J. The dialectic between research and social policy. *In*: Bernard, J.L.B. & Bernard, J., ed. *Sex roles and social policy*. London, Sage, 1979.

60. HABERMAS, J. *The theory of communicative action*. London, Polity Press, 1984, Vol. 1.

61. HABERMAS, J. *The theory of communicative action*. London, Polity Press, 1987, Vol. 2.

62. REASON, P., ED. *Human inquiry in action: developments in new paradigm research*. London, Sage, 1988.

63. SCHULTZ, A. Concept and theory formation in the social sciences. *Journal of philosophy*, **51**: 257–273 (1954).

64. MACLURE, R. The challenge of participatory research and its implica-tions for funding agencies. *International journal of sociology and social policy*, **10**(3): 1–21 (1990).

65. COSTONGS, C. & SPRINGETT, J.A. *Conceptual evaluation framework for health related policies in the urban context*. Liverpool, Institute for Health, Liverpool John Moores University, 1995 (Occasional Paper 2).

66. KENNEDY, A. Measuring health for all – A feasibility study of a Glasgow community. *In*: Bruce, N. et al. *Research and change in urban community health*. Aldershot, Avebury, 1995, pp. 199–217.

67. ABBOTT, K. ET AL. Participatory research. *Canadian nurse*, **89**(1): 25–27 (1993).

68. BARNES, M. Introducing new stakeholders – User and researcher inter-ests in evaluative research. *Policy and politics*, **21**(1): 47–58 (1993).

69. PATTON, M.Q. *Practical evaluation*. Beverly Hills, Sage, 1982.

70. RAHMAN, M.D. *People's self-development: perspectives on participatory action research: a journey through experience.* London, Zed Books, 1993.

71. PYLE, D.F. *Framework for the evaluation of health sector activities by private voluntary organisations receiving matching grants.* Washington, DC, US Agency for International Development, 1982, p. 64.

72. WALLERSTEIN, N. & BERNSTEIN, E. Empowerment education: Freire's ideas adpated to health education. *Health education quarterly,* **15**(4): 379–394 (1994).

73. BAUM, F. ET AL. *Healthy Cities Noarlunga Project evaluation.* Adelaide, South Australian Community Health Research Unit, 1990.

74. ROEBOTTOM, I. & COLQUHOUN, D. Participatory research, environmental health education and the politics of methods. *Health education research, theory and practice,* **7**(4): 457–469 (1992).

75. BANG, A.T. & BANG, R.A. Community participation in research and action against alcoholism. *World health,* **12**(1): 104–109 (1991).

76. ISRAEL, B. ET AL. Action research in occupational stress: involving workers and researchers. *International journal of health services,* **19**: 135–155 (1989).

77. BAKER, E. ET AL. A participatory approach to worksite health promotion. *Journal of ambulatory care management,* **17**(2): 68–81 (1994).

78. SPRINGETT, J. & LEAVEY, C. Participatory action research: the development of a paradigm: dilemmas and prospects. *In*: Bruce, N. et al. *Research and change in urban community health.* Aldershot, Avebury, 1995, pp. 57–66.

79. LEAVY, C. & THOMAS, P. *Improving health promotion in primary health care: a health professional's guide to increasing well woman clinic attendance.* Liverpool, Institute for Health, Liverpool John Moores University, 1995 (Research Report 1).

80. FUNNELL, R. ET AL. *Towards healthier alliances – A tool for planning, evaluating and developing healthier alliances.* London, Health Education Authority, Wessex Institute of Public Health Medicine, 1995.

81. CLARK, N.M. ET AL. Sustaining collaborative problem solving: strategies from a study of six Asian countries. *Health education research, theory and practice,* **8**(3): 385–402 (1993).

82. SPRINGETT, J. & LUCY, J. *In search of the Holy Grail: towards a participatory approach to the development of indicators for healthy public policy at the city level.* Liverpool, Institute for Health, Liverpool John Moores University, 1998 (Occasional Paper 11).

83. COSTONGS, C. & SPRINGETT, J. Towards a framework for the evaluation of health-related policies in cities. *Evaluation,* **3**(3): 345–362 (1997).

84. HOGGART, R. ET AL. Reflexivity and uncertainty in the research process. *Policy and politics,* **22**(1): 59–70 (1994).

85. GARANTA, J. The powerful, the powerless and the experts. Knowledge struggles in an information age. *In*: Park, P, et al., ed. *Voices of change:*

participatory research in the United States and Canada. Toronto, Oise Press, 1993.

86. SWEEP, A. Proces-evaluatie [Process evaluation]. *In*: Ten Dam, J. & de Leeuw, E., ed. *Gezonde Steden en onderzoek: reikwijdte, methoden, toepassingen* [Healthy Cities and evaluation: scope, methods, implementation]. Assen, Van Gorcum, 1993.

87. QUELLET, F. ET AL. Preliminary results of an evaluation of three Healthy Cities initiatives in the Montreal area. *Health promotion international,* **9**(3): 153–159 (1994).

88. LONG, R.J. & WILKINSON, W.E. A theoretical framework for occupational health program evaluation. *Occupational health nursing,* **32**(5): 257–259 (1984).

89. MEANS, R. & SMITH, R. Implementing a pluralistic approach to evaluation in health education. *Policy and politics,* **16**(1): 17–28 (1988).

90. HAM, C. Analysis of health policy – principles and practice. *Scandinavian journal of social medicine,* **Suppl. 46**: 62–66 (1991).

91. RICHARDSON, L. Writing: a method of inquiry. *In*: Denzin, N.K. & Lincoln, Y.S., ed. *Handbook of qualitative research*. Thousand Oaks, Sage, 1994.

92. BAUM, F. Research for Healthy Cities: some experiences from down under. *In*: de Leeuw, E. et al., ed. *Healthy Cities research agenda. Proceedings of an expert panel*. Maastricht, University of Maastricht, 1992 (Research for Healthy Cities Monograph Series, No. 2.).

93. EVERITT, A. Values and evidence in evaluating community health. *Critical public health,* **6**(3): 56–65 (1995).

94. WANG, C. & BURRIS, M.A. Empowerment through photo novella: portraits of participation. *Health education quarterly,* **21**(2): 171–186 (1994).

95. BAUM, F. & COOKE, D. Healthy Cities Australia. The evaluation of the pilot project in Noarlunga, S. Australia. *Health promotion international,* **7**(3): 181–193 (1992).

96. CHARLES, C. ET AL. Involving stakeholders in health services research: developing Alberta's resident classification system for long-term care facilities. *International journal of health services,* **24**(4): 749–761 (1994).

5

Transformative alliance between qualitative and quantitative approaches in health promotion research

Sylvie Gendron

Introduction

Research and evaluation in health promotion invite researchers – practitioners and their various partners, as well as research professionals and specialists – to consider complex phenomena *(1,2)*, to develop within a multidisciplinary context *(3–5)* and to participate in a process intended to give individuals and communities the means to improve their wellbeing *(6,7)*. These circumstances, which are further conditioned by the requests of public health authorities and funding agencies seeking a broader perspective on the impact and effectiveness of health promotion initiatives, inevitably influence researchers. More specifically, while planning and carrying out their studies, researchers often find themselves discussing the role of qualitative and quantitative approaches and their possible combination. Consequently, the practice of research is called into question and transformed.

For a better understanding of this transformation, this chapter considers the principal views on combining qualitative and quantitative research approaches held in the last 20 years by researchers involved in programme evaluation. These approaches call upon different philosophies, the former being essentially interpretive and associated with constructivist and naturalist paradigms and the latter, analytical and associated with realist and positivist paradigms. Moreover, either approach can use qualitative and quantitative methods. This examination extends beyond methodological considerations, however, to examine the approaches not only as processes but also in terms of their purposes and underlying ideas. The chapter concludes by proposing that research practice be shaped in accordance with the tenets of contemporary health promotion.

To establish common ground for further discussion, I highlight the important elements of contemporary health promotion, and present three perspectives indicating a potential alliance between qualitative and quantitative approaches. First is the debate on the incommensurability of qualitative and quantitative approaches; second, current discussions among health promotion researchers imply that these approaches are compatible and making distinctions between them is unnecessary. Third, a view of the approaches as complementary needs development; action should be taken to reconcile these approaches and use them to enrich understanding of the world. This vision extends beyond the first two perspectives. Paradoxically, it favours the simultaneous use of both qualitative and quantitative approaches, while acknowledging their incommensurability. In the end, this can bring research practice into alignment with the tenets of contemporary health promotion. This transformation promises novel contributions to the development of health promotion theory, which in turn could enhance the credibility of a discipline in the process of defining itself.

Contemporary health promotion

Chapter 1 discusses the origins of health promotion in detail. Despite Lalonde's *A new perspective on the health of Canadians (8)* and the understanding that achieving optimal health requires changing lifestyles and environmental conditions *(3)*, until the late 1980s the most widely used definition merely referred to "the science and art of helping people change their lifestyle to move toward a state of optimal health" *(9)*. Biomedical and epidemiological research models, as well as quantitative approaches, thus dominated early health promotion research; the goal was to identify risky behaviour and associated factors, and to determine which strategies to use against them *(10)*. Lalonde's report, however, was the basis for a series of initiatives by the WHO Regional Office for Europe that led to the Ottawa Charter for Health Promotion *(6)*, which set the starting point for contemporary health promotion practice *(7)*. This chapter is based on a WHO definition of health promotion as "the process of enabling individuals and communities to increase control over the determinants of health and thereby improve their health" *(11)*.

Three points deserve specific attention. First, the notion of health is complex and rather subjective: understood as a resource of everyday life, it refers to the extent to which a group or individual can realize aspirations, satisfy needs and take up the challenges presented by the environment *(6)*. Optimum health therefore evolves from a dynamic interaction between individuals and their environments; this highlights the relative nature and the complexity and subjectivity of health, since individuals and groups are greatly influenced by the context in which they develop.

Second, health has many determinants whose interaction is complex. The Ottawa Charter *(6)* proposes that economic, political, social, cultural, environmental, behavioural and biological factors can all affect health. Tackling such diverse factors can be considered as an ecological approach to health *(12)*. For a better understanding of these multiple determinants and their interdependence, researchers must call upon partners from various disciplines. Thus, contemporary health promotion goes beyond the single consideration of healthy habits and lifestyles and fosters the conduct of research within a multidisciplinary context *(13)*.

Finally, at the core of the definition lie two complex and interrelated concepts: the participation and empowerment of individuals and communities. Empowerment can pertain to both individuals and communities, be either a means or an end and undergo qualitative and quantitative assessment *(14–16)*. Through participation, health promotion starts a cycle of transformation of participants, their environments and their relationships with others, including various health promotion agents. As the cycle progresses, these changes are most likely to occur through the establishment of new partnerships, as health promotion professionals are increasingly asked to serve as more active mediators between the divergent interests that affect the health and impede the empowerment of individuals and communities. In the end, researchers who wish to contribute to the development of knowledge in the field must take account of this new context of partnership. In so doing, they begin to redefine their role to take better account of the ideology and aims of contemporary health promotion.

To conclude, researchers in health promotion study complex phenomena and should consider the contribution of various disciplines and their participation in health promotion's work to change societies within a context requiring the establishment of new partnerships. These are stimulating challenges. The three perspectives on qualitative and quantitative approaches may indicate how researchers can meet these challenges by transforming their practice.

Incommensurability

Elements considered to be different, having no common measure, are incommensurable *(17)*. For example, material interests are incommensurable with moral obligations; each is measured in a different way. The issue of incommensurability is part of a long debate between the partisans of qualitative and of quantitative approaches *(18)*, to which a widespread reconsideration of modern scientific culture and the emergence of a pluralist and relativist view of knowledge seem to add animation *(19,20)*.

The core of the debate is the supposedly incommensurable paradigms involved, which I delineate according to four interconnected axes proposed by Levy *(21)*: ontological, epistemological, methodological and teleological. The proponents of incommensurability argue that the internal coherence between the axes required to make up a paradigm excludes the integration of differing visions *(22,23)*.

Thomas Kuhn defines a paradigm as a general conceptual framework that reflects a set of scientific and metaphysical beliefs within which theories are tested, evaluated and revised if necessary *(24)*. It guides people within a discipline in formulating questions deemed to be legitimate, identifying appropriate techniques and instruments and building explanatory schemes for the phenomena under consideration. A paradigm thus provides a field within which individuals or groups opt for certain research directions and approaches to accomplish their discipline's normal work *(21,25,26)*. The central point of the concept is the notion of belief, which is the most significant determinant in choosing a paradigm *(18,21,23)*. The difficulty here, however, is the absence of any tangible proof of the truth and legitimacy of a belief system. People's choices of paradigm depend on their values and convictions, and are influenced by historical context.

The issue of incommensurability thus brings researchers back to the paradigms that guide their practice. This investigation addresses the constructivist and realist paradigms, those usually chosen by the adherents of qualitative and quantitative approaches, respectively.

The ontological axis describes the nature, constitution and structure of reality, and what one may know about existing entities *(24)*: the range of entities or beings considered to be physically or mentally manipulable during the research process *(21)*. Constructivist ontology recognizes the existence of multiple perceptions of a plurality of world views that can best be represented as an intricate network of human constructs. In contrast, realist ontology contends that there is only one independent and ordered reality, whose elements are governed by immutable natural laws and which is the ultimate focus of all research activities.

The epistemological axis describes the defining features, the substantive conditions and the structural limits of knowledge, as well as the justifications people use to legitimize knowledge *(24)*. This axis helps people substantiate the type of questions they ask, circumscribe their vision of the world and establish the boundaries of the research approach *(21)*. The constructivist paradigm stems from a pluralist and subjectivist epistemology, in which the researcher is a non-neutral creator inseparable from created or observed phenomena. Knowledge is then a constructed representation subject to continual change. Realist epistemology has a dual and objectivist nature; the researcher attempts to remain separate from the observed object or the studied phenomena, aiming for neutrality. Knowledge is meant to reflect a world regulated by causal laws.

The methodological axis describes the methods, procedures and techniques that people use to perceive the world and that allow them to generate findings and derive conclusions. The constructivist paradigm brings into play methods based on processes of association and relationships, taking into account the whole as it influences the parts, from which emerge multiple representations of perceived world views *(27)*. Adherents of this paradigm seek to engender meaning in the world and negotiate with the various actors involved in a project. The realist paradigm focuses on reductive methods to analyse the whole by its parts in order to describe, predict and control. The manipulation of observable and measurable facts and the demonstration of their convergence and potential replication lead the way towards expressions of natural truth, the single reality postulated by a realist ontology.

Finally, the teleological axis originates from a philosophical doctrine stipulating that all nature or at least intentional agents are self-organized to gain their ends *(24)*. Levy *(21)* describes this axis as vital because it determines the course along which projects develop, and reveals the interests of their adherents. It reveals, among other things, what researchers see as their responsibility in knowledge development and intervention. Constructivist teleology asserts the necessity to identify, interpret and give meaning to the multiple intentions and purposes underlying a given project and its concurrent process of knowledge construction. Researchers share responsibility for the meanings and interpretations derived from and the impact of their projects, and are considered accountable for the use or misuse of any resulting knowledge. In this way, they not only produce knowledge but also participate directly in the transformation of world views. Because of its assumption of neutrality, the realist paradigm eschews any purpose for a study other than the production of objective knowledge that can be generalized and used by others. This distinguishes researchers/producers from users/actors, and can cause problems for the latter. Because the process of knowledge production may not fully consider the multiple purposes of users/actors, the results may prove useless to them.

A paradigm's coherence results from the interdependence of these axes and the overlapping of their respective domains. Accordingly, the orientation of one axis will situate the others within a given paradigmatic field. For instance, the practice of measurement, which occupies a central role in the quantitative approach, must rest on the ontological postulate of the existence of a single reality to achieve its ends. Otherwise, how can the dedication to prediction and replication be justified? Moreover, since reality is deemed independent of researchers, they have little choice but to call upon a dualist and objectivist epistemology.

What are the repercussions of the incommensurability standpoint for health promotion researchers? On the one hand, it helps them clarify and articulate their paradigmatic assumptions, and understand better the potential sources of discordance between qualitative and quantitative approaches. On the other hand, the debate may cause a power struggle among people with divergent views. Thus, the working partnerships required by the multidisciplinary nature of health promotion may become difficult, and researchers may be less able to grasp the complexity of the phenomena under study. Of even greater concern, however, is the paradox raised by the teleological axis. For the most part, health promotion research rests on an essentially quantitative approach with a neutral researcher, separate from the subjects and their projects. A researcher with such attitudes is less likely than one taking a qualitative approach to answer the call of contemporary health promotion to take part in a transformation intended to contribute to the health of individuals and communities.

In short, calling the approaches incommensurable creates an impasse, but suggests that a qualitative approach may more readily bring the researcher's practice in alignment with the ideology and aims of contemporary health promotion. The compatibility perspective attempts to address the issue of irrevocable dualism.

Compatibility

Several authors argue that the incommensurability debate exaggerates the differences between the approaches, and creates a false dichotomy between paradigms and stereotypes that must be transcended *(28–31)*. Shadish *(32)* calls the debate "paradigmism" and not very useful in practice. Reichardt & Rallis *(33)* suggest that qualitative and quantitative approaches share many more common points than portrayed in the debate; partisans of both approaches recognize the complexity of world views, acknowledge the necessity of a rigorous approach to research and appreciate that human beings construct their understanding of reality. (Supporters of quantitative approaches may agree with the notion of a constructed understanding of reality because it implies the existence of a single reality. If proponents of qualitative approaches deny any kind of external, independent reality of the subject, however, Reichardt & Rallis *(33)* acknowledge that the approaches are deeply incompatible.)

The issue of methods is the core of the discussion of the compatibility of approaches. Methodological choices do not depend entirely on underlying ontological and epistemological considerations; they also hinge on the characteristics of the phenomenon under study, as well as the context *(28–30)*. Given the complexity of the projects and programmes considered for evaluation in health promotion and the many methods available to grasp the various issues at hand, this argument resonates among researchers, who invariably face all sorts of technical and political considerations in the field *(1,18,34)*. Researchers must cope with the burden of selecting and combining the methods most suited to both the goals of their study and local circumstances, within the limits imposed by available resources and their own abilities. Different designations are used to label this task: *critical multiplism (35)*, the *paradigm of choice (36)* and *methodological pluralism (31,37)*. Other names include: the *concept of appropriate methodology*, derived from the concept of appropriate technology *(2)*, *methodological ecumenism (38)* and *technical eclecticism (18)*.

The compatibility perspective gives rise to the practice of combining multiple methods, qualitative or quantitative, to triangulate the information obtained. Campbell & Fiske *(39)* first proposed the concept of triangulation: they applied more than one method to measure psychological traits (quantitatively), therefore ensuring that the variance detected was an outcome derived from the object under consideration, not the measurement procedure. Denzin *(40)* later illustrated multiple applications of this concept in social science research. Triangulation is now commonly described as the joint use of different qualitative or quantitative methods to attempt to cancel the errors inherent in each and thus obtain the best description of the object studied. Moreover, through replicated measurements, the multimethod approach maintained by triangulation purports to ensure a greater validity of conclusions, provided that the results converge.

To a certain extent, methodological pluralism has facilitated the recognition of qualitative research methods. Campbell *(41)* legitimized this recognition by portraying qualitative knowledge ("commonsense knowledge") as the foundation of all quantitative knowledge, when he suggested that quantitative knowing depends on qualitative knowing. He has argued that qualitative methods supply the preliminary measures for the more sophisticated quantitative measures, allow the interpretation of quantitative data and explore the various threats to their validity, and play a role in eliminating rival hypotheses. Further, qualitative data are useful to set the limits of a study's generalizability *(42)*.

Given such terms, qualitative approaches, although deemed compatible with quantitative approaches, seem often to be given a subordinate role *(1,2,25,41)*. Of course, quantitative approaches sometimes facilitate the implementation of primarily qualitative studies by allowing, for example, the establishment of a sampling frame, but this is rather rare *(43)*. Interestingly, a search on computer for public health and health promotion studies that were published between 1986 and 1995 and reported combined use of qualitative and quantitative approaches, indicated a widespread endorsement of methodological pluralism *(44–49)*. As can be expected, this search also showed an apparent preponderance of studies whose main purpose was the production and understanding of quantitative data. For instance, of the studies discussed in seven articles in a special edition of *Health education quarterly* on the integration of qualitative and quantitative research methods *(48)*, two used qualitative approaches to help develop quantitative measures and instruments *(50,51)* and three used qualitative approaches to interpret and contextualize quantitative data *(52–54)*. Similarly, evaluations of health promotion programmes, whether at the demonstration or dissemination phases, appear to use qualitative methods mainly to enrich interpretations and validate quantitative measures *(55,56)*. Although the value of qualitative data is appreciated, the organization of evaluations of large-scale community-based programmes has tended to preclude the use of qualitative methods, as these often require more direct observation and contact with participants, a potentially less feasible and economical avenue *(55)*.

Given the indubitable importance of quantified data, to what extent are the quantitative and qualitative approaches compatible? Since the latter seems subservient to the requirements of the former, the assumption of a harmonious balance between them seems puzzling. Further, four issues require clarification.

First, the dismissal of the paradigmatic debate suggests that these deliberations are of secondary importance or have somehow been resolved *(57)*. On the contrary, methodological pluralism appears essentially to support a quantitative approach, in accordance with the axioms of Cartesian science. The ascendancy of quantitative methods *(41,58)*, the central role ascribed to triangulation to delineate better one underlying reality *(31)* and knowledge production as a principal motivation *(33)* leave little room for the development of the qualitative approach.

Second, the concept of triangulation rests on the assumptions that different methods do not share the same biases and that these various biases can somehow cancel each other. This has yet to be confirmed *(59)*. Moreover, it is improbable that the triangulation of methods based on different paradigmatic postulates allows the probing of the same aspects of a given phenomenon *(28,38)*. At best, triangulation helps recognize the limits of interpretations, rather than giving a measure of validity *(43,60,61)*.

Third, methodological pluralism allows the use of all available methods without clearly discussing the quality standards to adopt. Are they the same for all methods? What should researchers do to make the best choices from among the various methods and techniques available *(18,28)*?

Finally, although the compatibility perspective opens the door to the contributions of multiple disciplines to the study of complex issues, it raises a particular concern for health promotion research. Eluding the paradigm debate and increasingly focusing on methods avoid posing the teleological question. In fact, the seventeenth-century scientific revolution, whose postulates still inspire researchers advocating methodological pluralism, disposed of this Aristotelian concept *(62)*. Thus, the compatibility discussion leaves little room for transformation originating in the notions of participation and empowerment. How, then, can researchers align their practice with the tenets of contemporary health promotion?

In the end, arguing for compatibility, like defending incommensurability, leads to an impasse. The latter fosters a duality between qualitative and quantitative approaches; the former fails to resolve this duality while concealing a certain subordination of the qualitative to the quantitative approach. Thus, from duality emerges a trend towards assimilation that retains the components of duality. This leads to a cycle of constructive feedback *(63)*, which in turn introduces the notion of complementarity.

Complementarity

In calling for the development of a paradigm of complexity, the French philosopher Edgar Morin *(63)* suggests the re-examination of the issue of incommensurability, as it could open the way to novel conceptions and insights. From here emerges the notion of complementarity, which implies that, at the heart of any phenomenon, fundamentally different, even antagonistic, elements interact. (Morin cites the notion of light consisting of waves and particles as an example. Although widely different, both are parts of the same phenomenon, presenting its two contradictory sides.) Morin argues that denying or reducing these contradictions restricts the development of innovative knowledge, so he proposes a new way of thinking about incommensurability that takes advantage of the richness of the many paradoxes that arise in the human quest to understand and transform the world. Although they do not refer directly to such terms, Reichardt & Rallis *(33)* call for a new partnership between qualitative and quantitative approaches, and even for a new paradigm *(64)* whereby each approach is valued and fully used; this has established the foundation for a dialogue on the complementarity of approaches.

A mixed-methodology research design *(65)*, also called a multiparadigm inquiry *(66)*, plays on the complementarity of approaches, realizing the full potential of each. It enables researchers to combine features of qualitative and quantitative approaches at each step of the research process, while clearly outlining the postulates that guide their decisions. This combination of paradigms, however, interweaves the approaches, rather than fusing them: the elements composing each paradigm remain distinct and operational. This approach allows the broadening of the scope of a study and examination of the different facets of a phenomenon, and fosters the emergence of contradictions that may lead to new perspectives and knowledge. The need to know and to merge two different approaches can make the development and implementation of such a research design complex and challenging tasks. Failure here often results in the simultaneous conduct of two separate but linked studies, with the risk that the connections are not adequately elucidated by the researchers or even detected by the various stakeholders *(28,43)*. Researchers should thus consider using a sequential, interactive approach, in which each study acts as a springboard for the next *(59)*. At present, experience with this type of research design is unfortunately too limited to indicate clear lines of conduct or standards of practice.

This presents health promotion researchers with a challenge; successfully meeting it can lead to the transformation of their practice in alignment with the tenets of contemporary health promotion. As they deal with complex issues and develop within a multidisciplinary context, researchers must eventually understand the various principles and processes of both qualitative and quantitative approaches. This provides an excellent opportunity for the development and testing of novel multiparadigm research designs that support the complementary use of qualitative and quantitative approaches. Thus, contemporary health promotion places researchers in a position in which they can contribute to the development of new research models, which can bring their practices in line with the evolving terms of the discipline and pave the way to original knowledge. For example, inquiry into the concept of empowerment as a determinant of health already calls on diverse qualitative and quantitative approaches, but integrating these approaches would lead to a broader understanding of this complex notion.

Meeting this challenge, however, requires the clarification of the researcher's role in health promotion's transformative project. Here again the teleological question arises; researchers must clearly articulate the purpose underlying their projects and activities.

Seeking transformation

What should be the purpose of health promotion research: the development and production of knowledge (the ultimate aim of the quantitative approach) or the transformation of world views (the ultimate aim of the qualitative approach)? From a perspective of complementarity, these two projects coexist, although this coexistence has a particular significance in light of the notions of contemporary health promotion. The production of knowledge is, to some degree, a necessary but not sufficient pursuit for health promotion research *(67–69)*; the notions of participation and empowerment harbour a political agenda that seeks change. To contribute to the agenda of contemporary health promotion, researchers could choose to develop their new multiparadigm research models in line with participatory research traditions *(70–72)* (see Chapter 4). For example, a successful approach in health promotion that has generated new insights, contributed to the empowerment of individuals and communities through participation and thus led to improved living conditions, is based on the participatory action research methodology of Brazilian educator Paulo Freire *(73–76)*. Interestingly, such approaches redefine the role of the researcher as that of partner with the various actors involved, a redefinition similar to that proposed for health promotion agents by the Ottawa Charter *(6)*.

The further elaboration of the complementarity perspective opens the way to the alignment of research practices with the tenets of contemporary health promotion. It suggests the development of novel multiparadigm research designs, within a participatory research perspective, to deal with complexity, integrate the contributions of various disciplines and support health promotion's work for change.

Conclusion: challenges ahead

Health promotion researchers face many questions when they consider the diverse contributions of qualitative and quantitative approaches, and their attempts to find answers inevitably transform their practices. This transformation must be in line with the tenets of contemporary health promotion if researchers wish to solidify the foundations of their discipline and secure greater credibility for their assessments of health promotion initiatives.

Now is the time to elaborate and experiment with novel multiparadigm research designs to determine their parameters and terms of implementation, and to establish criteria and quality standards to determine the value of the various study outcomes. This requires that health promotion researchers' training be adapted to ensure a deeper knowledge of and expertise in the use of both qualitative and quantitative approaches, and that the purposes and intentions underlying research and evaluation be more closely examined to clarify the roles and missions of researchers in relation to their various partners.

Beyond these rather pragmatic considerations, health promotion researchers should continue to reflect on and contribute to the discussion of complementarity. By using it to renew research and evaluation practices, researchers could acquire an unprecedented ability to combine incommensurable approaches and to process divergent or inconsistent study outcomes. Researchers should seize this opportunity.

References

1. BAUM, F. Researching public health: behind the qualitative–quantitative debate. *Social science and medicine,* **40**(4): 459–468 (1995).
2. MCKINLAY, J.B. The promotion of health through planned sociopolitical change: challenges for research and policy. *Social science and medicine,* **36**: 109–117 (1993).
3. BUNTON, R. & MACDONALD, G., ED. *Health promotion: disciplines and diversity.* London, Routledge, 1992.
4. KICKBUSCH, I. Health promotion: a global perspective. *Canadian journal of public health,* **77**: 321–326 (1986).
5. TILFORD, S. & DELANEY, F.F. Editorial. Qualitative research in health education. *Health education research,* **7**: 451–455 (1992).
6. Ottawa Charter for Health Promotion. *Health promotion,* **1**(4): iii–v (1986).
7. ROBERTSON, A. & MINKLER, M. New health promotion movement: a critical examination. *Health education quarterly,* **21**: 295–312 (1994).
8. LALONDE, M. *A new perspective on the health of Canadians: a working document.* Ottawa, Canada Information, 1974.
9. O'DONNELL, M. Definition of health promotion. *American journal of health promotion,* **1**: 4–5 (1986).
10. MINKLER, M. Health education, health promotion and the open society: an historical perspective. *Health education quarterly,* **16**: 17–30 (1989).
11. NUTBEAM, D. *Health promotion glossary.* Copenhagen, WHO Regional Office for Europe, 1985 (document ICP/HBI 503 (GO 4)).
12. MCLEROY, K.R. et al. An ecological perspective on health promotion programs. *Health education quarterly,* **15**: 351–377 (1988).
13. GREEN, L.W. & KREUTER, M.M. *Health promotion planning: an educational and environmental approach.* Mountain View, Mayfield, 1991.
14. ISRAEL, B.A. ET AL. Health education and community empowerment: conceptualizing and measuring perceptions of individual, organizational, and community control. *Health education quarterly,* **21**: 149–170 (1994).
15. PURDEY, A.F. ET AL. Participatory health development in rural Nepal: clarifying the process of community empowerment. *Health education quarterly,* **21**: 329–343 (1994).
16. WALLERSTEIN, N. Powerlessness, empowerment and health: implications for health promotion programs. *American journal of health promotion,* **6**: 197–205 (1992).
17. LALANDE, A. *Vocabulaire technique et critique de la philosophie.* Paris, Quadrige/Presses Universitaires de France, 1993.
18. KRANTZ, D.L. Sustaining vs. resolving the quantitative–qualitative debate. *Evaluation and program planning,* **18**: 89–96 (1995).
19. EISNER, W.E. The meaning of alternative paradigms for practice. *In*: Guba, E.G., ed. *The paradigm dialogue.* Thousand Oaks, Sage, 1990, pp. 88–102.

20. PHILLIPS, D.C. Postpositivistic science: myths and realities. *In*: Guba, E.G., ed. *The paradigm dialogue*. Thousand Oaks, Sage, 1990, pp. 31–45.

21. LEVY, R. Croyance et doute: une vision paradigmatique des méthodes qualitatives. *Ruptures, revue transdisciplinaire en santé*, **1**: 92–100 (1994).

22. GUBA, E.G. & LINCOLN, Y.S. Competing paradigms in qualitative research. *In*: Denzin, N.K. & Lincoln, Y.S., ed. *Handbook of qualitative research*. Thousand Oaks, Sage, 1994, pp. 105–117.

23. LINCOLN, Y.S. & GUBA, E.G. *Naturalistic enquiry*. Thousand Oaks, Sage, 1985.

24. AUDI, R., ed. *The Cambridge dictionary of philosophy*. Cambridge, Cambridge University Press, 1995.

25. FILSTEAD, W.J. Qualitative methods: a needed perspective in evaluation research. *In*: Cook, T. & Reichardt, C., ed. *Qualitative and quantitative methods in evaluation research*. Beverly Hills, Sage, 1979, pp. 33–48.

26. PATTON, M.Q. *Qualitative evaluation methods*. Beverly Hills, Sage, 1980.

27. LEVY, R. Critical systems thinking: Edgar Morin and the French school of thought. *Systems practice*, **4**: 87–99 (1991).

28. BRYMAN, A. Quantitative and qualitative research: further reflections on their integration. *In*: Brannen, J., ed. *Mixing methods: qualitative and quantitative research*. Aldershot, Avebury, 1992, pp. 57–77.

29. HAMMERSLEY, M. Deconstructing the qualitative–quantitative divide. *In*: Brannen, J., ed. *Mixing methods: qualitative and quantitative research*. Aldershot, Avebury, 1992, pp. 39–55.

30. REICHARDT, C. & COOK, T. Beyond qualitative versus quantitative methods. *In*: Cook, T. & Reichardt, C., ed. *Qualitative and quantitative methods in evaluation research*. Beverly Hills, Sage, 1979, pp. 7–32.

31. SECHREST, L. & SIDANI, S. Quantitative and qualitative methods: is there an alternative? *Evaluation and program planning*, **18**: 77–87 (1995).

32. SHADISH, W.R. The quantitative–qualitative debates: "DeKuhnifying" the conceptual context. *Evaluation and program planning*, **18**: 47–49 (1995).

33. REICHARDT, C.S. & RALLIS, S.F., ED. *The qualitative–quantitative debate: new perspectives*. San Francisco, Jossey-Bass, 1994.

34. BRANNEN, J. Combining qualitative and quantitative approaches: an overview. *In*: Brannen, J., ed. *Mixing methods: qualitative and quantitative research*. Aldershot, Avebury, 1992, pp. 3–37.

35. COOK, T.D. & MACDONALD, M. Postpositivism critical multiplism. *In*: Shortland, L. & Mark, M.M., ed. *Social science and social policy*. Beverly Hills, Sage, 1985, pp. 21–62.

36. PATTON, M.Q. *How to use qualitative methods in evaluation*. Newbury Park, Sage, 1987.

37. MCLEROY, K. ET AL. Editorial. *Health education research*, **7**: 1–8 (1992).

38. HALDEMANN, V. & LEVY, R. Oecoménisme méthodologique et dialogue entre paradigmes. *Canadian journal on aging,* **14**: 37–51 (1995).
39. CAMPBELL, D.T. & FISKE, D.W. Convergent and discriminant validation by the multitrait-multimethod matrix. *Psychological bulletin,* **59**: 81–105 (1959).
40. DENZIN, N.K. *The research act in sociology: a theoretical introduction to sociological methods.* London, Butterworths, 1970.
41. CAMPBELL, D.T. Qualitative knowing in action research. *In*: Brenner, M. et al., ed. *The social contexts of method.* London, Croom Helm, 1978, pp. 184–209.
42. CRONBACH, L.J. Beyond the two disciplines of scientific psychology. *American psychologist,* **2**: 116–127 (1975).
43. DRYMAN, A. *Quantity and quality in social research.* London, Unwin Hyman, 1988.
44. CAPARA, A. ET AL. The perceptions of AIDS in the Bete and Baoule of the Ivory Coast. *Social science and medicine,* **36**: 1229–1235 (1993).
45. CAREY, J.W. Linking qualitative and quantitative methods: integrating cultural factors into public health. *Qualitative health research,* **3**: 298–318 (1993).
46. DENNIS, M.L. ET AL. Integrating qualitative and quantitative evaluation methods in substance abuse research. *Evaluation and program planning,* **17**: 419–427 (1994).
47. STECKLER, A. The use of qualitative evaluation methods to test internal validity: an example in a work site health promotion program. *Evaluation and the health professions,* **12**: 115–133 (1989).
48. STECKLER, A. ET AL. Integrating qualitative and quantitative methods. *Health education quarterly,* **19**(1): 46 (1992).
49. YACH, D. The use and value of qualitative methods in health research in developing countries. *Social science and medicine,* **35**: 603–612 (1992).
50. BAUMAN, L.J. & ADAIR, E.G. The use of ethnographic interviewing to inform questionnaire construction. *Health education quarterly,* **19**(1): 9–23 (1992).
51. DE VRIES, H. ET AL. The utilization of qualitative and quantitative data for health education program planning, implementation, and evaluation: a spiral approach. *Health education quarterly,* **19**(1): 101–115 (1992).
52. GOTTLIEB, N.H. ET AL. The implementation of a restrictive worksite smoking policy in a large decentralized organization. *Health education quarterly,* **19**(1): 77–100 (1992).
53. HELITZER-ALLEN, D.L. & KENDALL, C. Explaining differences between qualitative and quantitative data: a study of chemoprophylaxis during pregnancy. *Health education quaterly,* **19**(1): 41–54 (1992).
54. HUGENTOBLER, M.K. ET AL. An action research approach to workplace health: integrating methods. *Health education quarterly,* **19**(1): 55–76 (1992).

119

55. PIRIE, P.L. ET AL. Program evaluation strategies for community-based health promotion programs: perspectives from the cardiovascular disease community research and demonstration studies. *Health education research*, **9**: 23–36 (1994).

56. POTVIN, L. Methodological challenges in evaluation of dissemination programs. *Canadian journal of public health*, **87**(Suppl. 2): S79–S83 (1996).

57. GLASSNER, B. & MORENO, J.D. Quantification and enlightenment. *In*: Glassner, B. & Moreno, J.D., ed. *The qualitative–quantitative distinction in the social sciences*. Dordrecht, Kluwer Academic Publishers, 1989, pp.1–13

58. CAMPBELL, D.T. Can we be scientific in applied social science? *In*: Connor, R.F. et al., ed. *Evaluation Studies Review Annual, Vol. 9*. Beverly Hills, Sage, 1984, pp. 26–48.

59. BLAIKE, N.W.H. A critique of the use of triangulation in social research. *Quality and quantity*, **25**: 115–136 (1991).

60. FIELDING, N.G. & FIELDING, J.L. *Linking data*. Beverly Hills, Sage, 1986 (Qualitative Research Methods, Vol. 4).

61. HAMMERSLEY, M. & ATKINSON, P. *Ethnography: principles in practice*. London, Tavistock Publications, 1983.

62. CHECKLAND, P. *Systems thinking, systems practice*. Chichester, John Wiley & Sons, 1981.

63. MORIN, E. *Science avec conscience*. Paris, Fayard, 1982.

64. DETTA, L. Paradigm wars: a basis for peaceful coexistence and beyond. *In*: Reichardt, C.S. & Rallis, S.F., ed. *The qualitative–quantitative debate: new perspectives*. San Francisco, Jossey-Bass, 1994, pp. 53–70.

65. CRESWELL, J.W. *Research design: qualitative and quantitative approaches*. Thousand Oaks, Sage, 1994.

66. LINCOLN, Y.S. & GUBA, E.G. RSVP: we are pleased to accept your invitation. *Evaluation practice*, **15**: 179–192 (1994).

67. EAKIN, J.M. & MACLEAN, H.M. A critical perspective on research and knowledge development in health promotion. *Canadian journal of public health*, **83**(Suppl. 1): S72–S76 (1992).

68. POLAND, B.D. Learning to "walk our talk": the implications of sociological theory for research methodologies in health promotion. *Canadian journal of public health*, **83**(Suppl. 1): S31–S46 (1992).

69. STEVENSON, H.M. & BURKE, M. Bureaucratic logic in new social movement clothing: the limits of health promotion research. *Health promotion international*, **6**: 281–289 (1991).

70. WHYTE, W.F. *Participatory action research*. Thousand Oaks, Sage, 1991.

71. REASON, P., ED. *Participation in human inquiry*. London, Sage, 1994.

72. GREEN, L.W. ET AL. *Study of participatory research in health promotion. Review and recommendations for the development of participatory re-*

search in health promotion in Canada. Ottawa, Royal Society of Canada, 1995.

73. FREIRE, P. *Education for critical consciousness.* New York, Continuum Press, 1983.

74. FREIRE, P. *Pedagogy of the oppressed.* New York, Continuum Press, 1988.

75. MINKLER, M. & COX, K. Creating critical consciousness in health: application of Freire's philosophy and methods to the health care setting. *International journal of health services,* **10**: 311–322 (1980).

76. WALLERSTEIN, N. & BERNSTEIN, E. Empowerment education: Freire's ideas adpated to health education. *Health education quarterly,* **15**(4): 379–394 (1988).

6
Evaluation of quality-of-life initiatives in health promotion

Dennis Raphael

Overview

The concept of the quality of life has only recently been considered within contemporary health promotion approaches consistent with WHO definitions of health *(1)* and health promotion *(2)* and visions of achieving health for all *(3)*. This delineation is necessary, as the recent explosion of interest in issues of quality of life by medical and nursing workers in the areas of disability and aging *(4)* could easily be seen as pertaining to health promotion. Adding to the conceptual confusion is the continuing emphasis on quality of life among workers in the social indicators tradition. Although the social indicators approach stems, not from health or health promotion, but from the social policy and development literature, it has much to offer to contemporary health promotion.

Many debate the boundaries between health and the quality of life. Michalos *(5)* argues that health professionals see health as a requirement for living a life of high quality, while people focusing on, for example, social support or financial security use quality of life as a predictor of health status and outcomes. In some cases, the promotion of a high-quality life and the promotion of health are indistinguishable, as in the 1952 report of a United States presidential commission on health needs *(5)*. Rootman *(6)* and Raeburn & Rootman *(7)* have considered the relationship between quality of life and health promotion. Concepts of quality of life and health have different sources. The former have come from the social sciences, which have been concerned with levels of functioning ranging from exemplary to poor, while the latter have been rooted in concerns with illness and death. Recent WHO definitions of health as a resource for daily living notwithstanding, this divide remains, even though the two areas of health promotion and quality of life are complementary. Health promotion can be seen as a process of improving the quality of life, while quality of life can be seen as the preferred outcome of health promotion.

This chapter considers evaluation issues related to health promotion initiatives to improve the quality of life and the related areas of health and social indicators. After a brief overview of the roots of quality of life in contemporary social and health sciences inquiry, I review emerging issues that have implications for the evaluation of quality-of-life initiatives in health promotion, and consider the various health-related concepts of quality of life that health promotion practitioners are likely to encounter in the contemporary literature. The contributions from the social indicators tradition are presented, with emphasis on those conceptually related to health and wellbeing. The chapter considers the conceptual roots of each approach and the associated evaluation issues.

Two models are directly relevant to health promotion practitioners working within WHO definitions: those of Bengt Lindström of the Nordic School of Public Health and those of Rebecca Renwick, Ivan Brown, Irving Rootman and Dennis Raphael of the Centre for Health Promotion at the University of Toronto. The discussion covers key evaluation issues and problems, and options for response, and concludes with the presentation of a community project that builds on and extends these models.

Nature of and intellectual underpinnings of quality of life

Although the quality of life has been an important human concern since antiquity, social science research into the concept gained prominence following Thorndike's work on life in cities (8). Despite the concept's long history in the literature, debate on how it should be defined and measured continues in every discipline that uses it (9). The lack of agreement arises from the complexity of the concept. Further, the quality of life has an intuitive importance that makes it vulnerable to influence and manipulation by social and political trends and policies (10), and it is used in extremely diverse contexts (11). Quality of life is a social construct, "the essential meaning [of which] may be understood by all, but when it is related to real people's lives, it is interpreted in any number of ways" (12).

Until quite recently, sociologists, social psychologists and economists dominated empirical research on quality of life, but interest in the concept has exploded among health workers. While these differing approaches are more fully discussed elsewhere (13), most health-related approaches emphasize the effects of ill health and associated treatment on quality of life. These approaches are not particularly attractive to health promotion practitioners working within either the framework of the Ottawa Charter for Health Promotion (2) or population-based health initiatives such as that of the Canadian Institute for Advanced Research (14).

Such work addresses the broader determinants of health, so its consideration of quality of life could be expected to focus on community and societal factors that support or harm health. Interestingly, the work in the social indicators area has primarily sought to identify such factors, but the indicators have not, until recently, been specifically related to health and health promotion. Not surprisingly, then, health promotion practitioners have looked to the social science literature with its focus on dimensions of functioning in the general population.

Michalos (15) made a thoughtful analysis of the various uses of the word *quality*. It can describe the characteristics of a population, such as gender, income, age, etc., and depict something's value or worth. Michalos terms the former the descriptive use, and the latter the evaluative use of the word. He makes further distinctions, but two main ideas seem especially relevant: the strong evaluative component of the term *quality* and the potential for work on the quality of life to have a strong prescriptive (or advocacy) emphasis. In general, such reflections on the nature and use of the term are rare in the literature *(16,17)*.

Paradigms of inquiry and quality of life

The extensive and contentious literature on evaluation issues has implications for the evaluation of quality-of-life initiatives in health promotion. While many practitioners may find these issues rather esoteric, they have profound implications for the development, implementation and use of evaluation and its results. These issues include:

- the differing views on the nature of reality and the appropriate research and evaluation methods for understanding it *(18)*;
- the nature of rigour in research and evaluation, and how differing paradigms have different criteria for truth; and
- the emerging conceptions of truth criteria that integrally link inquiry methodology with issues of ethics, sharing commitment and information with participants, and social responsibility *(19)*.

Lincoln & Guba's *Naturalistic inquiry (20)* and Guba's *Paradigm dialogue (17)* discuss these issues at length. An additional emerging literature addresses the importance of participatory research as a means of addressing societal power imbalances and the marginalization of particular groups and individuals *(21–23)*. These conceptual issues are especially important in evaluation, with its explicit notion of judgment of worth. The importance of quality of life as a focus of health promotion initiatives adds urgency to the discussion.

The nature of knowledge and the knowable

Debates about the nature of reality and methods for understanding it usually take place in debates about quantitative versus qualitative research methods (see Chapter 5), but their implications go deeper than simply choosing a method of inquiry. A paradigm is "a basic set of beliefs that guides action, whether of the everyday garden variety or action taken in connection with a discipline inquiry" *(18)*. Adherents to different paradigms answer the following questions on the nature of disciplined inquiry in different ways *(18)*:

What is the nature of the knowable; what is the nature of reality?	Ontological
What is the nature of the relationship between the knower (the inquirer) and the known (or knowable)?	Epistemological

How should the inquirer go about finding out about   Methodological
the world?

As discussed in Chapter 1, commitment to a paradigm determines the issues
that research should address and how to define and examine them. Researchers
and practitioners all adhere to paradigms, although many do not make their
allegiance explicit. Wilson *(24)* outlines three paradigms in the social science
literature while Guba *(18)* considers four; the latter are the basis for the four
approaches that follow.

First, positivist approaches predominate among all approaches to quality of
life. Not surprisingly, then, evaluation activity in the field usually emphasizes
traditional approaches to scientific inquiry: focusing on observable phenomena, favouring careful experimental design and using traditional quantitative
approaches to information. This is especially true of health-related approaches. Wilson *(24)* suggests that this tradition contains a strong tendency
towards individual-level measurement.

Second, idealist or interpretive approaches see the individual as an active
creator of the social world, and society as resulting from the actions of individuals within social structures. Since social acts result from the intentions of
individuals, understanding social reality is ultimately an attempt to understand the meanings that individuals place on their dealings in the world. The
quality-of-life literature increasingly emphasizes idealist approaches. Evaluations carried out within this paradigm make their values explicit, show a
strong tendency towards individual-level focus with some emphasis on system-level issues, include ethnographic and phenomenological analyses, and
emphasize emergent design and the qualitative analysis and reporting of information.

Third, realist approaches are less frequently considered, and differ in
many ways from positivist and idealist approaches. Like positivists, realists
believe that objects and events exist in the world independent of the meanings created by individuals, but, like idealists, they believe that human beings
can create and modify the realities within which they live. Social realists seek
to identify the underlying societal mechanisms that regulate social behaviour
and determine social realities. Unlike positivists, who base models and theories on observable phenomena, realists use models to understand society and
behaviour. Evaluations within this approach emphasize analyses of power relations within society, models of economic activity and resource distribution,
and a search for underlying structures influencing societal and individual
wellbeing. The critical approach *(18,21)* adds an action component to the realist analysis.

Fourth, participatory approaches oppose traditional ones. The latter have
been harshly criticized by people who think that much medical and social science research, in addition to its announced aims, has maintained the marginal
status of those who are poor, have disabilities or need services *(23,25)*. Oliver
(26) argues that traditional research in disability has tended to reduce the prob-

lems of disabled or handicapped people to their own inadequacies or functional limitations, failed to improve their quality of life and been so divorced from their everyday experience that many rightly feel victimized by researchers.

Woodill *(23)* develops this theme by arguing that, in a society in which categorization is common and frequently related to inequality, the disability category is used to isolate populations from the mainstream. Proponents of action or participatory research, which denies the common distinction between scientist and subject and is overtly political in values and orientation, argue that such research could equalize the power relationships in social science research and is more likely to empower people and thus improve their lives (see Chapter 4).

The paradigm debate should profoundly influence the aims, methods and evaluation of initiatives focusing on the quality of life. In addition, I have identified no less than 11 debates on defining and measuring of quality of life in health promotion and rehabilitation *(16)*. When issues related to the definition of health and health promotion are added to the debates on paradigms and quality of life, it is a wonder that any agreement can be reached on how to evaluate quality-of-life initiatives in health promotion.

Areas of quality-of-life activity

Many disciplines take great interest in the quality of life, particularly those concerned with the medical and health sciences, disability and traditional social indicators. This section suggests relevant contributions for those working within WHO principles of health promotion.

Health-related models

Medical and health workers consider quality of life an outcome variable useful in evaluating the effectiveness of medical treatment *(27)* and rehabilitation efforts *(28)*. Nevertheless, medicine-based approaches can be distinguished from those based on health. Both emphasize the outcomes of medical and health service interventions, but they differ in emphasis on the type and content of indicators.

Spilker's approach illustrates the medical view *(29)*: in theory, quality of life should be assessed through examination of physical status and functional abilities, psychological status and wellbeing, social interactions, and economic status and factors. Both objective and subjective assessments should be made. In addition, the patient should provide an overall subjective assessment of his or her quality of life: "an individual's overall satisfaction with life, and one's general sense of personal well-being" *(29)*. Such an approach is closely tied to the traditional biomedical view of health and illness. Schipper et al. *(30)* consider the WHO definition of health – "a state of complete physical, mental and social well-being and not merely the absence of disease or infirmity" *(1)* – to inform their model of quality of life, but conclude:

This is a commendable definition, but it includes elements that are beyond the purview of traditional, apolitical medicine. Opportunity, education, and social security are important overall issues in the development of community health, but they are beyond the immediate goal of our assessment, which is treating the sick.

These approaches are closely linked to the effects of illness upon individuals and the measurement of day-to-day competences and abilities. *Quality of life in clinical trials (29)* is an excellent introduction to the medical approach – discussing instrumentation, special populations and applications to specific problems and diseases – and an entire special supplement of *Medical care (31)* is devoted to it. In practice, most medical quality-of-life assessments are limited to measures of physical functioning and reports of psychological and sometimes social wellbeing.

Research uses a medical measure of quality of life, the QALY, to provide a value or weighting to various states of living and to assess treatments with different outcomes *(32)*. These values can then be used to rationalize medical decision-making, possibly including the allocation of resources or rationing of services. Two main QALY approaches, those of Kaplan & Bush *(33)* and Torrance *(34)*, reject the WHO definition of health. The inquiry and measurement approaches within this tradition are clearly positivist, frequently biomedical and virtually always oriented to individuals.

More recently, the related concept of the DALY has gained some prominence. It was developed to take account of degrees of disability, in addition to mortality. Fernandez et al. *(35)* summarize the concept: "The experts of WHO and the World Bank elaborated a new measurement of the global burden of disease, the Disability-Adjusted Life Year (DALY). It's an indicator that summarizes the health status of a population, combining mortality, morbidity and disability data".

The concept has been used to measure the burden of disease in developing countries *(36,37)*. Nevertheless, objections have been raised *(38,39)* concerning the complexity of measuring the many dimensions of morbidity, the ethics of placing values on quality of life and the need to take account of specific cultural contexts. Using DALYs, as with QALYs, may also require the balancing of efficiency with equity, although this is rarely discussed in the literature. Clearly, the DALY and the QALY are embedded in medical concepts of health; the former emphasizes morbidity and the latter, mortality.

Recently, a literature on quality of life has appeared that tries to focus on health, rather than illness, and the positive, rather than the negative, aspects of behavioural functioning. Bowling *(40)* draws on the *International classification of impairments, disabilities, and handicaps (41)* to move beyond a limited focus upon disease by stressing how environmental contexts can help to determine whether disease and disorder become impairment, disability and handicap. Bowling *(40)* and McDowell & Newell *(42)* provide indices focusing on disability and the illness-related aspects of wellbeing and adaptive behaviour.

128

The medical outcomes study *(43)* is a large-scale application of the health-related quality-of-life approach to a variety of medical conditions.

Health-related approaches have a clearly positivist emphasis, extend beyond the biomedical and stress individual measurement. For them, quality of life represents individual responses to the physical, mental and social effects of illness on daily living, which influence the extent to which personal satisfaction with life circumstances can be achieved *(40)*.

Social indicators approaches

For a number of reasons – including interest in the social determinants of health *(14)*, the impact of the Healthy Cities and Healthy Communities movement *(44,45)* and increased focus on inequalities in health *(46)* – health workers are paying more attention to environmental indicators of the quality of life. Well prior to this recent concern, workers within the social indicators tradition identified many system-level indicators of societal functioning and wellbeing. Many of these efforts have clear implications for the health and health promotion agenda.

The social indicators approach differs from health-related approaches in its rationale for developing measures, level of focus and emphasis on social policy and change *(47–49)*. The early work did not explicitly link social indicators with quality of life or health, but more recent work almost always makes this link and, to a lesser extent, acknowledges that between social indicators and health.

Rationale

During the 1960s in both North America and Europe, interest surged in social indicators as a means of providing evidence on the impact of government social programmes *(48)*. Three factors gave impetus to the development of systems of social indicators: recognition of the problems of relying on economic indicators *(49)*, the obvious problems of environmental degradation and economic and social inequities associated with developed economies and the need for assessing the impact of social programmes *(50)*. An initial definition was *(51)*:

> A social indicator ... may be defined to be a statistic of direct normative interest which facilitates concise, comprehensive and balanced judgments about the conditions of major aspects of a society. It is in all cases a direct measure of welfare and is subject to the interpretation that, if it changes in the "right" direction, while other things remain equal, things have gotten better, or people are "better off." Thus, statistics on the number of doctors or policemen could not be social indicators, whereas figures on health or crime rate could be.

Early work *(52)* suggested that the following could constitute the content categories of a social report using indicator systems: socioeconomic welfare (including the composition, growth and distribution of the population), labour force and employment, income, knowledge and technology, education, health, leisure, public safety and legal system, housing, transport, physical environment, and social mobility and stratification. In addition, assessment should cover social participation and alienation (focusing on family, religion, politics and voluntary associations) and the population's use of time, consumption patterns, aspirations, satisfaction, morale and other characteristics.

To collect these data, objective measures of system functioning, drawn from system-level data on physical conditions, for example, could be used. Individual-level measures, in the form of subjective measures (of, for example, aspirations and expectations) or subjective wellbeing indices (of, for example, life satisfaction, specific satisfactions and alienation) could be used. A systems-level approach could include data on, for example, the number of items of legislation considered by a parliament, the style of government, government expenditure, gross national product or rates of deforestation (49). Indicators could include the availability of housing for elderly people, meeting the transport needs of people with disabilities and providing opportunities for people with mental handicap to live in the community. For example, an important theme in the emerging literature on the social determinants of health is the equitable distribution of economic resources (53). Raphael et al. (13) give further details on the implications of the social indicators tradition.

Some recently identified indicators

The four-volume global report on student wellbeing (5) provides an impressive example of the range of possible indicators, including general satisfaction and happiness with life; satisfaction with family, friends and living partner, and self-esteem; employment, finances, housing and transport; and religion, education, recreation and health. The Swedish surveys of level of living (54) are a contemporary individual-level approach, in which the indicators used include health and access to health care, employment and working conditions, economic resources, and education and skills. Each issue of *Canadian social trends (55)* provides a system-level example, measuring population (annual growth, immigration and emigration), families (birth rate and marriage and divorce rates), the labour force (unemployment, part-time employment and women's participation), income (median family income, women's full-time earnings as a percentage of men's), education (government expenditure and number of doctoral degrees awarded) and health (government expenditure and deaths due to cardiovascular disease). *Social indicators research: a multidisciplinary journal of quality of life* is a rich source of potential indicators.

Using social indicators to document the health effects of economic inequality

Since the publication of the so-called Black report and the follow-up report on the health divide in the United Kingdom (56,57), economic inequality and its contribution to health inequities have attracted increased attention. For example, Lee & Townsend *(58)* have documented the effects on individuals' lives of economic policy and associated unemployment levels. Similarly, Wilkinson *(46)* has recently summarized much of the research, both British and international, showing how increasing economic inequality is related to poor health outcomes and increasing societal disintegration. Clearly, such research touches on issues of the quality of life.

Healthy Cities and Healthy Communities approaches

Not usually associated with the social indicators tradition but showing strong similarities with it is the Healthy Cities and Healthy Communities movement: community health promotion focused on the development of healthy public policy *(44,45)*. It involves municipal governments, community residents and the environmental, economic and social services sectors in projects to address health issues (see Chapter 14). Its method is to enable people to take control of their health as agents for change. While academics and practitioners are concerned about appropriate indicators for the movement *(59)*, an impressive amount of documentation has begun to identify them. *City health profiles: how to report on health in your city (60)* suggests a number of wide-ranging indicators, including: health status, lifestyles, living conditions, socioeconomic conditions, physical environment, inequalities, physical and social infrastructure, and public health services and policies. Similarly, Flynn & Dennis *(61)* have compiled a number of tools for documenting urban health. While not explicitly working within a quality-of-life perspective, these works can contribute to initiatives.

Other areas relevant to health and health promotion

Work on developmental disabilities has proved very useful in work on the quality of life *(62)*, as is Green & Kreuter's model of health promotion *(63)*.

Developmental disabilities

Especially thoughtful work has tried to define and measure the quality of life of people with developmental disabilities. The impetus came from a realization of the poor quality of many aspects of their lives. For people with developmental disabilities, the divergence between the reality of and the potential for their living conditions was so great as to require identification of broad areas of life functioning in need of attention.

Borthwick-Duffy *(64)* categorizes quality-of-life aspects across three dimensions: independence (living environment), interpersonal and community relationships and productivity. Other examples of variables in the literature include: physical environment, home and family, neighbourhood quality, access to services (independence and living environment), social support, activity patterns, community integration, leisure, friends (interpersonal and community relationships), and employment, income and work status (productivity) *(13)*. Clearly, these issues play a role in the health of populations, as well as individuals.

The social diagnosis approach

In Green & Kreuter's model of health promotion *(63)*, assessing quality of life is part of the social diagnosis phase of programme development, carried out through such means as focus groups, community fora and community surveys. The authors argue that health outcomes are embedded in the broader concerns encompassed by quality of life. Thus, the community's concerns about quality of life provide the context for understanding how health promotion practitioners could raise health-related issues in communities. Green & Kreuter *(63)* focus on issues of behavioural change that fall within the purview of traditional health workers: illness prevention, health status, lifestyle and health education. By understanding the quality-of-life concerns of the community, the health promotion practitioner demonstrates the connections between these concerns and health issues. The authors highlight the need to involve the community in the development, implementation and evaluation of health services and health promotion programmes. They contend that changes in health and health behaviour ultimately affect the quality of life, but do not define the latter except as possible concerns of community members.

Work on the quality of life that is relevant to health promotion activities has raised some issues and controversies. Two research programmes on the quality of life are clearly relevant to those working within WHO health promotion concepts. These case studies illustrate how paradigm and definitional issues merge.

Quality-of-life issues: levels and focus of inquiry and measurement

The broad debates on the nature of the knowable have only recently begun to intrude on the literature *(16)*; while largely absent from the traditional literature on health-related quality of life, they have been most apparent in that on disabilities *(25)*. More apparent in the literature have been concerns with the level and focus of inquiry and measurement *(9)*. Should quality-of-life initiatives focus on effecting change in individuals, communities or social structure and policies *(65)*? These discussions are related to those on assessing the effects of initiatives. Should initiatives be assessed for their effects on the behaviour of individuals, the development of communities or the development of healthy public policies?

The issue of where to intervene to improve the quality of life clearly parallels debates underway in health promotion as a whole. In general, health promotion activities are aimed at social policy, communities and individuals. Although the pendulum of popularity swings back and forth among them, each clearly seems to have some role in promoting health. The same issues arise when discussing how to define and influence the quality of life.

Many approaches that consider the quality of life emphasize measurement at the individual level to assess either subjective life satisfaction or objective

132

functioning. An incredibly wide range of measuring instruments for such assessments is available from the literature on psychology, nursing and occupational therapy. As mentioned, the medical approaches to quality of life strongly emphasize measurement at this level, as do the health- and disability-oriented approaches. An individual emphasis is not inconsistent with WHO principles, which include aspects of individual coping and wellbeing *(2)*.

Much of this work, however, does not present the conceptual basis for the usefulness of indices in measuring quality of life. Many approaches simply gather a range of indices and redefine them as measuring quality of life. Working at the individual level only may ignore important societal determinants.

Workers within the social indicators tradition have usually measured quality of life at the community level. An extensive literature reports scores on researcher-designed instruments measuring community members' perceptions of neighbourhood quality and positive community aspects, and objective measures of neighbourhood quality, usually relying on professionals' views *(13)*. The approaches and indicators of the Healthy Cities and Healthy Communities movement can easily be seen as consistent with a framework seeking improved quality of life.

The quality of life is also analysed at the societal level. The social indicators literature takes a system-level approach, but until very recently this approach was not part of health and health promotion analyses. The increasing emphasis on population-based approaches to health has led to greater attention being paid to system-level indicators of quality of life. Clearly, the work in the United Kingdom on economic inequalities can contribute to analyses at this level.

Quality-of-life models consistent with WHO approaches to health promotion

I have been able to identify only two quality-of-life approaches that explicitly draw on contemporary notions of health and health promotion.

Lindström's model

Lindström *(53)*, working within a health promotion approach, has outlined a wide range of system-level indicators of quality of life for children in the Nordic countries. These concern income distribution, type of housing, education and employment levels and availability of parental leave for family-related matters.

Lindström sees his model as a means of assessing health as a resource for daily living and quality of life as an indicator of healthy functioning *(66)*: "The potential of the quality of life concept lies in its basically positive meaning and interdisciplinary acceptance. This can be used to develop health into a resource concept, as is the intention of the WHO health for all strategy.". Lindström's model highlights the importance of considering the societal and structural determinants of health. Lindström defines quality of life as the "total existence of an individual, a group or a society" *(66)*. More specifically, his model *(53,66)* examines four spheres of life:

- the personal, including physical, mental and spiritual resources;
- the interpersonal, including family structure and function, intimate friends and extended social networks;
- the external, including aspects of work, income and housing; and
- the global, including the societal environment, specific cultural aspects and human rights and social welfare policies.

The first two cover areas usually considered in discussions of quality of life and health, and Lindström examines them through large-scale surveys. Work on the fourth sphere, usually through policy analysis of the distribution of societal resources and general social welfare approaches, may uncover some of the most interesting determinants of health.

Lindström *(53,66)* analyses Nordic children's health in the external and global spheres. Such policy analysis is infrequently made within a quality-of-life framework and offers areas for potential multidisciplinary integration. Lindström uses a variety of methods of assessment. His empirical research uses survey instruments utilizing self-report, and his policy analyses highlight distinctive aspects of Nordic societies. Lindström has not elicited information directly from children, but relied on the views of parents to inform his social and welfare policy analyses. Table 6.1 summarizes Lindström's model.

Table 6.1. Lindström's model for the quality of life of children in Nordic countries

Spheres	Dimensions	Examples
Global	1. Macro environment	Physical environment
	2. Culture	Responsiveness to the United Nations
	3. Human rights	Convention on the Rights of the Child
	4. Welfare policies	Welfare distribution
External	1. Work	Parental education and satisfaction with employment
	2. Income	Income distribution
	3. Housing	Quality of and satisfaction with housing
Interpersonal	1. Family structure and function	Satisfaction with family, lack of negative events
	2. Intimate friends	Support from friends, neighbours and
	3. Extended social networks	society
Personal	1. Physical	Growth, activity
	2. Mental	Self-esteem and mood
	3. Spiritual	Meaning of life

Source: Lindström *(66)*.

Lindström has made extensive surveys of citizens across the Nordic countries that examine these issues. He uses traditional approaches to data collection; his surveys focus on individual aspects of functioning and wellbeing, and components of the immediate environment, including employment, housing and family life. He has not used qualitative approaches to data collection, or made naturalistic analyses of individuals' quality of life. His main contribution, a terribly important one, is his expansion of the concept of the quality of life to include the entire range of components and determinants of health, from the individual through the societal, within a health promotion approach that is based on WHO policy statements.

Lindström reports that his full model and related research have influenced efforts to develop a national child ombudsman office in Sweden, and the content of the national child public health reports of Finland, Norway and Sweden *(53)*. In addition, his work has provided a basis for courses in adolescent health at the Nordic School of Public Health in Gothenburg, Sweden, and the content of the *European textbook on social paediatrics (67)*.

Key issues
Lindström's approach uses traditional methods to collect questionnaire and survey data. The model includes a very wide range of objective and subjective indicators of self-reported functioning and satisfaction. The scope of the model suggests policy analysis at societal levels. I drew on the model to outline some unexplored determinants of adolescent health *(68)*. The model's value lies in its suggestion that intervention occur at a wide range of levels, even though the assessments are made at the individual level. Further, social policy analysts can draw on the model to illuminate areas of key concern.

Centre for Health Promotion approach
The other model consistent with WHO thinking is that developed by researchers at the Centre for Health Promotion, University of Toronto. It builds on the WHO emphasis on health as a resource for daily living *(2)* and work in the developmental disabilities field. It takes a holistic approach to conceptualizing and measuring quality of life that stresses the importance of personal control and opportunities to improve the quality of life by changing the environment. This approach seeks the perspective of the individual, but also uses other data sources *(69)*.

The conceptual approach is influenced by the humanist–existential tradition *(70–74)*. More detailed discussion of these philosophical foundations appears elsewhere *(69)*, but this tradition recognizes that people have physical, psychological and spiritual dimensions, and acknowledges their needs both to belong to physical places and social groups and to distinguish themselves as individuals by pursuing their own goals and making their own choices and decisions. Quality of life is defined as the degree to which a person enjoys the important possibilities of his or her life. This enjoyment takes place in three major domains of life: being, belonging and becoming. Being reflects who one is; belonging concerns one's fit with environments, and becoming refers to one's activities for self-expression and the achievement of personal goals and aspirations. Each domain has three subdomains (Table 6.2).

Table 6.2. The Centre for Health Promotion's domains of quality of life

Domains	Subdomains	Contents
Being	Physical	Physical health, mobility, nutrition, exercise, fitness and appearance
	Psychological	Independence, autonomy, self-acceptance and freedom from stress
	Spiritual	Personal values and standards and spiritual beliefs
Belonging	Physical	Physical aspects of the immediate environment
	Social	Relationships with family, friends and acquaintances
	Community	Availability of societal resources and services
Becoming	Practical	Home, school and work activities
	Leisure	Indoor and outdoor activities, recreational resources
	Growth	Learning things, improving skills and relationships, adapting to life

Instrumentation has been developed for and applied to populations: people with physical disabilities *(75)*, adolescents *(76)*, elderly people *(77)* and adults in general *(78)*. In these applications, self-report inventories are applied through traditional survey methods.

Key issues
This approach uses qualitative methods to develop appropriate instrument items; these items are then used to collect data according to traditional instrument and survey methods. The approach is oriented towards subjective indicators of individual functioning. These measures have the potential to examine the effects of interventions at individual, community and social policy levels. Instruments for people with developmental disabilities are used to assess the effects of provinces' policies on the disabled; potential uses of the instruments for other populations continue to be explored. Those for elderly people are used to assess interventions that involve both individual and community services. In addition, the model has used constructivist approaches to help study the quality of life of communities.

The community quality-of-life project: understanding communities through a health promotion approach
The purpose of the community quality-of-life project in Canada is to develop a process to increase community-based health workers' understanding of com-

136

munities' needs. Asking community members to identify aspects of their neighbourhoods and communities that increase the quality of life is expected to indicate needs and help to develop solutions. The expected outcomes of the study are:

- the development of a process to identify community factors that affect the quality of life;
- the development of resource materials that will allow other communities to carry out similar activities;
- the evaluation of the usefulness of the Centre for Health Promotion's model of quality of life for considering community needs; and
- the identification of the strengths and drawbacks of participatory approaches in assessing the quality of life of communities.

A number of Metropolitan Toronto organizations are participating: four community health centres, two public health departments, the District Health Council, the Canadian Mental Health Association and the University of Toronto. The project is taking place in two communities and focusing on elderly people, teenagers and people receiving social assistance. Data are being collected through community meetings and interviews in which community members are being asked: what factors in their neighbourhood or community make life good for them and the people they care about, and what factors do not do so. Data are also being collected through interviews with community workers, local politicians and the managers of service agencies.

Key issues
This initiative explicitly draws on the principles of the Ottawa Charter for Health Promotion (2). It views "health as a positive concept emphasizing social and personal resources, as well as physical capacities", and defines health promotion as "the process of enabling people to increase control over, and to improve, their health" (2). An important aspect of its approach is the focus on the unique perceptions of community members. In one sense, this gives a human face to the determinants of health. These perceptions are being considered in relation to a model of human functioning: the quality-of-life model of the Centre for Health Promotion.

Summary of key issues
The nature of quality of life and how to define and measure it are key issues in the evaluation of health promotion initiatives. Research in this field has focused on determining the appropriate level of analysis and measurement. Should quality-of-life initiatives attempt primarily to benefit individuals? Should they address the more immediate determinants of health at the neighbourhood and community levels or system-level indicators of quality? Not surprisingly, these issues parallel similar ones in health promotion.

Evaluation issues

In the literature, the main issue in the evaluation of quality-of-life initiatives is the appropriateness of using various paradigms. Qualitative methods have an obvious and compelling potential in evaluating the quality of life of individuals and the effects of initiatives.

Since quality-of-life measurement is so embedded within subjective perceptions and values, the paucity of work using qualitative methods is surprising. This deficiency is especially important in view of the potentially powerful effects of the implementation and evaluation of initiatives to improve the quality of life of vulnerable people, such as the elderly, ill, disabled and poor. Means should be developed that allow people to tell their own stories in ways that are meaningful to them. Any evaluation of a quality-of-life initiative should have a qualitative component to supplement the quantitative measurements made (see Chapter 5).

A lively debate has emerged that is moving beyond the discussion of quantitative versus qualitative methods. It asks whether researchers have a responsibility to consult and collaborate with the participants in the research, and about the utility of research endeavours. Advocates of participatory action research have argued that most research brings limited or no benefit to the participants, although it often furthers the careers of researchers (see Chapter 4).

Quality-of-life issues

The issues specific to quality of life concern the focus of initiatives and the appropriate level of measurement. Should quality-of-life initiatives focus on individuals' coping behaviour and skills, community-level processes or the development of healthy public policies? Should interventions be assessed by measurement at the individual, community or societal level? The two issues are related but not necessarily synonymous. For example, community-level initiatives can be assessed through measurement of community members' characteristics, and the impact of social policy changes through measurement at both the individual and community levels. Other combinations are not only possible but probable.

Many health promotion practitioners continue to work with individuals. People are treated for illness or disability; public health departments identify individuals at risk, and physicians continue to see clients one at a time. Such one-on-one opportunities can be used to identify a range of issues that affect individuals' lives, inquire into their quality of life and work with them to improve it.

Community development approaches organize members of a common geographical, social or cultural unit for health promotion activities, and stress the strengthening of communities through their members' identification and solution of self-defined problems. Community-level approaches address the connection of individuals with their environments and developing community structures and organizations. Assessing the effects of such interventions may not require measurement at the individual level.

Social policy approaches to health promotion are defined as "ecological in perspective, multisectoral in scope and participatory in strategy" *(79)*. The Ottawa Charter *(2)* calls for the advocacy and development of healthy social policy: interventions at the legislative level that may have obvious effects on quality of life. The main contemporary issues concern the distribution of economic resources, the availability of social and health services on an equitable basis and the development of health promoting environments.

The assessment of quality-of-life initiatives at any level can involve individual-level measurement. Combining such measurement with intervention at the individual level, however, can create problems. Societal factors may be neglected, or attention may focus solely on individual adjustment. Robertson *(80)* suggests that an individual-level approach towards the lives of elderly people, for example, may lead to seeing aging as individual pathology to be treated by health professionals, thereby ignoring societal determinants such as poverty, isolation and the loss of role and status. Obviously, interventions at the community level should focus on measurement at this level, supplemented by individual-level measurement. Societal-level initiatives could be assessed at the societal, community and individual levels.

Guidelines for evaluations of health promotion initiatives

These guidelines for evaluations of health promotion initiatives highlight the importance of expressing assumptions about the quality of life, justifying the choice of approach and examining the implications of initiatives for the theory and practice of health promotion. Implicit in all of these activities is an awareness of the various agendas behind initiatives and their evaluations. The agenda of the initiator of an evaluation may not be obvious, and may conflict with those of various stakeholders. Identifying the clients – that is, the person or persons whom the evaluation must satisfy – is important. Evaluators of a health promotion initiative should:

- make explicit their assumptions about the quality of life
- determine their evaluation approach
- determine their measurement focus
- determine the nature of the outcome measures of quality of life.

Explicit assumptions

As indicated earlier, *quality of life* has become an almost ubiquitous term in the health sciences. The reasons for this probably involve health professionals' perceived need to be seen as focusing on clients and moving beyond a strict biomedical approach to health, the increasing awareness of the effects of environments on health and the attractiveness of quality of life as a way to address these concerns. While not denying the importance of these developments, this chapter argues that quality-of-life initiatives should be based on WHO definitions of health, health promotion and societal functioning and wellbeing *(1–3)*.

The case studies presented here show how a WHO-informed view can lead to quality-of-life initiatives that are likely to capture the complex components of health and move to improve them.

Evaluation approach

The choice of an approach to evaluation goes beyond choosing the methods to use, to determining the issues that will be addressed and the kinds of data to collect. Evaluations conducted within the traditional paradigm emphasize traditional approaches to design and instrument development, quantitative data analysis and easily measurable and quantifiable outcomes. Lincoln & Guba (20) summarize the nature of the reality consistent with these approaches.

Similarly, a constructivist approach emphasizes the perceptions of individuals, the use of phenomenological and ethnographic methods, and the qualitative analysis and reporting of data. The issues examined will be concerned with personal meanings. As realist approaches emphasize the functioning of society and the analysis of societal structures, policy analyses, perhaps from a radical or critical perspective, are the norm.

Further, the nature of collaboration and participation is an increasingly important issue in community-based research that has implications for both the implementation and evaluation of programmes. Quality-of-life research cannot ignore these recent developments.

Measurement level

As noted, Lindström's model suggests that attention be paid to the effects of quality-of-life initiatives at all levels. While it can be seen as exhaustive, addressing all levels will not usually be practical. One rule of thumb could be that the assessment of effects could include the main level of focus and all levels below it. This suggests that an initiative focused on social policy could theoretically assess effects at this level and in the community and individuals. An initiative at the individual level could assess effects at this level and those above it, but this appears unlikely in practice.

Outcome measures of quality of life

Related to measurement focus is the content of outcome measures for assessing initiatives. A useful taxonomy concerns attitudes, beliefs, intentions and behaviour at the individual level. Additional outcome measures should include personal control and/or empowerment. There is lively debate about the measures appropriate at the community level, including those outlined in recent WHO Healthy Cities documentation. The indicators chosen should reflect the purpose and content of the initiative.

To determine the appropriate societal-level indicators for assessing initiatives, evaluators can draw on the extensive work in the social indicators tradition (12) and WHO documents. The approaches of Lindström and the Centre for Health Promotion are important starting points.

Equity and the quality of life

The concept of equity is an important WHO principle, enshrined in the Ottawa Charter *(2)* and elsewhere *(1,3,81)*, and applied in discussions of access to health care and health outcomes *(82,83)*. Much attention focuses on barriers to receiving health services *(84)*. More recently, research has examined inequities in organ transplants, particular types of surgery and the allocation of health resources *(85,86)*.

The identification of systematic differences in health outcomes between and within societies has eclipsed the initial concern with access to health care. Reports in the United Kingdom *(56,57)* highlighted the role of social status in determining health. A wealth of recommendations followed from these reports, and how to reduce inequities in health through social welfare policy has been a lively issue in Europe.

The focus of debate has shifted to the role of economic inequalities in promoting health inequities. The publication of Wilkinson's *Unhealthy societies (46)* will certainly further spur discussion concerning the distribution of wealth and resources within societies and how increasing inequality increases inequity of health outcomes. Further, the debate can be expected to begin to have a higher profile in Canada and the United States, where it has been relatively muted. Research on inequalities in health has exploded. Politically, some governments in developed countries that were seen as increasing inequality have been removed from office. Whether this trend will continue is uncertain.

This discussion has far-reaching implications for people implementing quality-of-life initiatives in health promotion. At one level, those focusing on individuals or communities cannot easily ignore the strong role of societal inequalities in supporting health inequities. Any attempt to improve quality of life by relying upon relatively individualized approaches will surely run up against the important role of the societal determinants of health. At another level, those concerned with health promotion initiatives may be emboldened to tackle the quality-of-life issues identified by societal analyses: equalizing distribution of economic resources, advocating health promoting policies and fighting problems such as unemployment, food insecurity and inadequate housing.

One should remember, however, that a stance on the quality of life frequently has as much to do with one's values as with any objective truth that may exist. While health promotion may be used to advocate greater economic equality within a society *(87)*, such advocacy is ultimately a political statement whose motive may simply and justifiably be a belief in a just society. Such a stance is becoming increasingly common in public health circles *(88)*.

Adopting such a stance requires a number of strategic decisions, beginning with a greater reliance on the social indicators tradition described earlier to help identify relevant indicators for health promotion initiatives. It will require that health policy-makers recognize the key issues being raised by those working on social policy. One interesting example of this occurred in Canada,

141

where Linda McQuaig, the author of books critical of increasing economic inequality in Canada *(89,90)*, addressed the 1997 convention of the Canadian Public Health Association on economic inequality and health.

Such a broadened approach to the quality of life may be a welcome balance to the increasing emphasis on QALYs and DALYs *(39,91)*. The latter represent a medicalization of quality of life. An emphasis on equity in health, however, draws one back to the broader determinants of health, and a discussion of a just society and the means to work towards it. Such an approach seems especially timely given the current evidence of increasing economic inequality in societies. As Geoffrey Rose points out *(92)*: "The primary determinants of disease are mainly economic and social, and therefore its remedies must also be economic and social. Medicine and politics cannot and should not be kept apart".

References

1. Constitution of the World Health Organization. *In*: *Basic documents*, 42nd ed. Geneva, World Health Organization, 1999.
2. Ottawa Charter for Health Promotion. *Health promotion*, **1**(4): iii–v (1986).
3. *HEALTH21: the health for all policy framework for the WHO European Region*. Copenhagen, WHO Regional Office for Europe, 1999 (European Health for All Series, No. 6).
4. ROMNEY, E. ET AL., ED. Improving the quality of life of people with and without disabilities. *Social indicators research*, **33**: 1–3 (1994).
5. MICHALOS, A.C. *General report on student well-being*. New York, Springer, 1993.
6. ROOTMAN, I. How is quality of life related to health and health promotion? *In*: Liss, P. & Nikku, N., ed. *Health promotion and prevention: theoretical and ethical aspects*. Linköping, Department of Health and Society, University of Linköping, 1994.
7. RAEBURN, J.M. & ROOTMAN, I. Quality of life and health promotion. *In*: Renwick, R. et al., ed. *Quality of life in health promotion and rehabilitation: conceptual approaches, issues, and applications*. Thousand Oaks, Sage 1996.
8. THORNDIKE, E.L. *Your city*. New York, Harcourt, Brace and Company, 1939.
9. NAESS, S. *Quality of life research: concepts, methods and applications*. Oslo, Institute of Applied Social Research, 1987.
10. TURNBULL, H. & BRUNK, G. Quality of life and public philosophy. *In*: Schalock, R., ed. *Quality of life: perspectives and issues*. Washington, DC, American Association on Mental Retardation, 1990.
11. SCHALOCK, R. Where do we go from here? *In*: Schalock, R., ed. *Quality of life: perspectives and issues*. Washington, DC, American Association on Mental Retardation, 1990.

12. BROWN, I. Promoting quality within service delivery systems. *Journal on developmental disabilities*, **3**(2): i–iv (1994).

13. RAPHAEL, D. ET AL. Quality of life indicators and health: current status and emerging conceptions. *Social indicators research*, **39**: 65–88 (1996).

14. EVANS, R.G. ET AL. *Why are some people healthy and others not? The determinants of health of populations*. New York, Aldine de Gruyter, 1994.

15. MICHALOS, A.C. *North American social report. Volume 1. Foundations, population, and health*. Boston, Reidel Publishing Company, 1980.

16. RAPHAEL, D. Defining quality of life: eleven debates concerning its measurement. *In*: Renwick, R. et al., ed. *Quality of life in health promotion and rehabilitation: conceptual approaches, issues, and applications*. Thousand Oaks, Sage 1996.

17. RAPHAEL, D. Quality of life of persons with developmental disabilities: five issues concerning its nature and measurement. *Journal on developmental disabilities*, **5**(2): 44–66 (1997).

18. GUBA, E. The alternative paradigm dialogue. *In*: Guba, E.G., ed. *The paradigm dialogue*. Thousand Oaks, Sage, 1990.

19. LINCOLN, Y.S. Emerging criteria for quality in qualitative and interpretive research. *Qualitative inquiry*, **1**: 275–290 (1995).

20. LINCOLN, Y.S. & GUBA, E.G. *Naturalistic inquiry*. Thousand Oaks, Sage, 1985.

21. FAY, B. The elements of critical social science. *In*: Hammersley, M., ed. *Social research: philosophy, politics, and practice*. Newbury Park, Sage, 1993.

22. PARK, P. What is participatory research? A theoretical and methodological perspective. *In*: Park, P. & Hall, B., ed. *Voices of change: participatory research in the United States and Canada*. Westport, Begin & Garvey, 1993.

23. WOODILL, G. *Independent living and participation in research: a critical analysis*. Toronto, Centre for Independent Living, 1992.

24. WILSON, J. *Social theory*. Englewood Cliffs, Prentice Hall, 1983.

25. RIOUX, M.H. & BACH, M., ED. *Disability is not measles: new research paradigms in disability*. North York, Roeher Institute, 1994.

26. OLIVER, M. *The politics of disablement*. London, Macmillan, 1990.

27. HOLLANDSWORTH, J. Evaluating the impact of medical treatment on the quality of life: a 5-year update. *Social science and medicine*, **26**: 425–434 (1988).

28. LIVNEH, H. Rehabilitation goals: their hierarchical and multifaceted nature. *Journal of applied rehabilitation counselling*, **19**(3): 12–18 (1988).

29. SPILKER, B. *Quality of life in clinical trials*. New York, Raven, 1990.

30. SCHIPPERS, H. ET AL. Definitions and conceptual issues. *In*: Spilker, B., ed. *Quality of life in clinical trials*. New York, Raven, 1990.

31. SPILKER, B. ET AL. Quality of life bibliography and indexes. *Medical care*, **28**(Suppl. 12) (1990).

32. LAWTON, M.P. A multidimensional view of quality of life in frail elders. *In*: Birren, J. et al., ed. *The concept and measurement of quality of life in the frail elderly.* New York, Academic, 1991.

33. KAPLAN, R.M. & BUSH, J.W. Health-related quality of life measurement for evaluation research and policy analysis. *Health psychology*, 1: 61–80 (1982).

34. TORRANCE, G.W. Multiattribute utility theory as a method of measuring social preferences for health states in long-term care. *In*: Kane, R.L. & Kane, R.A., ed. *Values and long-term care.* Lexington, MA, Lexington Books, 1982.

35. FERNANDEZ, M.J. ET AL. An agenda to debate: the World Bank report *Investing in health. Revista espanola de salud publica*, **69**(5): 385–391 (1995).

36. MARSEILLE, E. Cost–effectiveness of cataract surgery in a public health eye care programme in Nepal. *Bulletin of the World Health Organization*, **74**(3): 319–324 (1996).

37. PRABHAKAR, R. Tuberculosis – The continuing scourge of India. *Indian journal of medical research*, **103**: 19–25 (1996).

38. BARKER, C. & GREEN, A. Opening the debate on DALYs. *Health policy and planning*, **11**(2): 179–183 (1996).

39. MORROW, R.H. & BRYANT, J.H. Health policy approaches to measuring and valuing human life: conceptual and ethical issues. *American journal of public health*, **85**(10): 1356–1360 (1995).

40. BOWLING, A. *Measuring health.* Philadelphia, Open University Press, 1991.

41. *International classification of impairments, disabilities, and handicaps: a manual of classification relating to the consequences of disease published in accordance with resolution WHA29.35 of the Twenty-ninth World Health Assembly, May 1976.* Geneva, World Health Organization, 1980.

42. MCDOWELL, I. & NEWELL, C. *Measuring health.* New York, Oxford University Press, 1987.

43. STEWART, A. & WARE, J. *Measuring functioning and well-being: the medical outcome study approach.* Durham, NC, Duke University Press, 1992.

44. ASHTON, J. *Healthy Cities.* Philadelphia, Open University Press, 1992.

45. DAVIES, J.K. & KELLY, M.P. *Healthy Cities: research and practice.* New York, Routledge, 1993.

46. WILKINSON, R. *Unhealthy societies: the afflictions of inequality.* New York, Routledge, 1996.

47. FINSTERBUSCH, K. ET AL., ED. *Social impact assessment methods.* Newbury Park, Sage Publications, 1983

48. LAND, K.C. Social indicator models: an overview. *In*: Land, K.C & Spilerman, S., ed. *Social indicator models*. New York, Russell Sage Foundation, 1975.

144

49. MILES, I. *Social indicators for human development*. London, Frances Pinter Publishers, 1985.

50. WOLF, C.P. Social impact assessment: a methodological overview. *In*: Finsterbusch, K. et al., ed. *Social impact assessment methods*. Newbury Park, Sage Publications, 1983, pp. 15–33.

51. US DEPARTMENT OF HEALTH, EDUCATION, AND WELFARE. *Towards a social report*. Washington, DC, US Government Printing Office, 1969.

52. SHELDON, E. & LAND, K.C. Social reporting for the 1970's: a review and programmatic statement. *Policy sciences*, **3**: 137–151 (1972).

53. LINDSTRÖM, B. *The essence of existence: on the quality of life of children in the Nordic countries*. Gothenburg, Nordic School of Public Health, 1994.

54. ERIKSON, R. Descriptions of inequality: the Swedish approach to welfare research. *In*: Nussbaum, M. & Sen, A., ed. *The quality of life*. Oxford, Clarendon Press, 1993.

55. STATISTICS CANADA. *Canadian social trends*, **33** (1994).

56. TOWNSEND, P. & DAVIDSON, N., ED. The Black report. *In*: *Inequalities in health*. Harmondsworth, Penguin, 1992.

57. WHITEHEAD, M. The health divide. *In*: *Inequalities in health*. Harmondsworth, Penguin, 1992.

58. LEE, P. & TOWNSEND, P. A study of inequality, low incomes and unemployment in London, 1985–92. *International labour review*, **133**(5-6): 579–595 (1994).

59. HANCOCK, T. The healthy city from concept to application: implications for research. Kelly, M. & Davies, J., ed. *Healthy Cities: research and practice*. London, Routledge, 1994.

60. *City health profiles: how to report on health in your city*. Copenhagen, WHO Regional Office for Europe, 1994 (document ICP/HSIT/94/01 PB 02).

61. FLYNN, B.C. & DENNIS, L.I. *Documenting the urban health situation: tools for Healthy Cities*. Copenhagen, WHO Regional Office for Europe, 1995 (document EUR/ICP/HCIT 94 07/PB01).

62. RAPHAEL, D. ET AL. Quality of life: what are the implications for health promotion? *American journal of health behavior*, **21**: 118–128 (1997).

63. GREEN, L.W. & KREUTER, M.M. *Health promotion planning: an educational and environmental approach*, 2nd ed. Mountain View, Mayfield, 1991.

64. BORTHWICK-DUFFY, S.A. *Quality of life of mentally retarded people: development of a model* [Dissertation]. Riverside, University of California, Riverside, 1986.

65. RAPHAEL, D. ET AL. Assessing the quality of life of persons with developmental disabilities: description of a new model, measuring instruments, and initial findings. *International journal of disability development and education*, **43**: 25–42 (1996).

145

66. LINDSTRÖM, B. Quality of life: a model for evaluating health for all. *Sozial und praventivmedizin*, **37**: 301–306 (1992).
67. LINDSTRÖM, B. & SPENCER, N. *European textbook of social paediatrics*. Oxford, Oxford University Press, 1994.
68. RAPHAEL, D. The determinants of adolescent health: evolving definitions, recent findings, and proposed research agenda. *Journal of adolescent health*, **19**: 6–16 (1996).
69. RENWICK, R. & BROWN, I. Being, belonging, becoming: the Centre for Health Promotion model of quality of life. *In*: Renwick, R. et al., ed. *Quality of life in health promotion and rehabilitation: conceptual approaches, issues, and applications*. Thousand Oaks, Sage, 1996.
70. BAKAN, D. *The duality of human existence: isolation and communion in western man*. Boston, Beacon, 1964.
71. BECKER, E. *The birth and death of meaning*, 2nd ed. New York, Free Press, 1971.
72. MERLEAU-PONTY, J. *The visible and the invisible*. Evanston, Northwestern University Press, 1968.
73. SULLIVAN, E. *A critical psychology: interpretation of the personal world*. New York, Plenum, 1984.
74. ZANER, R. *The context of self: a phenomenological inquiry using medicine as a clue*. Athens, Ohio University Press, 1981.
75. RUDMAN, D. ET AL. The quality of life profile for adults with physical disabilities. *Canadian journal of occupational therapy*, **62**: 25 (1995).
76. RAPHAEL, D. ET AL. The quality of life profile – Adolescent version: background, description, and initial validation. *Journal of adolescent health*, **19**: 366–375 (1997)
77. RAPHAEL, D. ET AL. The quality of life of seniors living in the community: a conceptualization with implications for public health practice, *Canadian journal of public health*, **86**: 228–233 (1995).
78. RAPHAEL, D. ET AL. *The quality of life profile: a generic measure of health and well-being*. Toronto, Centre for Health Promotion, 1997.
79. MILIO, N. Making healthy public policy; developing the science by learning the art: an ecological framework for policy studies. *Health promotion international*, **2**(3): 263–274 (1987).
80. ROBERTSON, A. The politics of Alzheimer's disease: a case study in apocalyptic demography. *International journal of health services*, **20**: 429–442 (1990).
81. EPP, J. *Achieving health for all: a framework for health promotion*. Ottawa, Health and Welfare Canada, 1986.
82. DEPPE, H.U. Health and society in times of change. *World health forum*, **17**(2): 194–196 (1996).
83. KRASNIK, A. The concept of equity in health services research. *Scandinavian journal of social medicine*, **24**(1): 2–7 (1996).

146

84. LILLIE-BLANTON, M. ET AL. Latina and African American women: continuing disparities in health. *International journal of health services*, **23**(3): 555–584 (1993).

85. GRYTTEN, J. ET AL. Can a public health care system achieve equity? The Norwegian experience. *Medical care*, **33**(9): 938–951 (1995).

86. KESKIMAKI, I. ET AL. Socioeconomic equity in Finnish hospital care in relation to need. *Social science and medicine*, **41**(3): 425–431 (1995).

87. GLYN, A. & MILIBRAND, D. *Paying for inequality: the economic costs of social injustice*. London, Oram Press, 1994.

88. *Action statement on health promotion*. Ottawa, Canadian Public Health Association, 1996.

89. MCQUAIG, L. *The wealthy banker's wife: the assault on equality in Canada*. Toronto, Penguin, 1993.

90. MCQUAIG, L. *Shooting the hippo: death by deficit and other Canadian myths*. Toronto, Viking, 1995.

91. MOATTI, J.P. ET AL. QALYS or not QALYS: that is the question? *Revue d'epidemiologie et de santé publique*, **43**(6): 573–583 (1995).

92. ROSE, G. *The strategy of preventive medicine*. New York, Oxford Books, 1992.

7
Economic evaluation of health promotion

Christine Godfrey

Introduction

Resources for health promotion are frequently limited, and ensuring value for money is an important objective for those delivering interventions and those providing the funding. Although these issues are of considerable interest, specific applications of economic techniques to the evaluation of health promotion interventions remain limited.

Economic evaluations involve identifying, measuring and valuing both the inputs (costs) and outcomes (benefits) of alternative interventions. The inputs and outcomes included in a study depend on both the question being addressed and the perspective of the study. The question might be quite specific. For example, which interventions (or mix of interventions) would achieve some target for reducing smoking among pregnant women, given a set budget? A more general question would be how available resources should be divided among different health promotion activities. Further, the total level of resources available for these activities must be set. In this case, the task may be to compare health promotion activities to treatment or rehabilitation approaches as candidates for health-sector funding. Alternatively, in the education sector, a health promotion intervention may be compared to other uses of teachers' time, or the purchase of alternative equipment in terms of value for money. Different questions set the alternatives to be considered and hence the costs and outcomes that need to be identified, measured and valued.

This perspective is also important in determining the scope of a study. Some may be interested only in the costs and outcomes that directly affect their service or budget. Thus, the health promotion practitioner may be concerned with the costs of services directly provided, but not the time and other resources contributed by others. For example, interventions with pregnant women may involve input from midwives, physicians and other health workers. A narrow perspective on the evaluation would include only the resources used by the health promotion agency, but most economists would argue that a narrow approach has great limitations and would tend to favour programmes with the most cost shifting: those with the smallest direct input from the health promotion practitioner and the largest input from other groups. The ranking of projects in terms of value for money may be very different if the analysis in-

149

cludes all costs and benefits, whoever incurs them. In general, economists favour a societal perspective, in which all costs and consequences are considered, no matter who pays the costs or gains the benefits.

Clearly, economic evaluations attempt to address questions set in real situations, rather than theoretical abstractions. They build upon and frequently use other evaluation methods. In particular, economic evaluations include outcome or effectiveness approaches as one component of the analysis. No intervention can be considered more cost-effective than the alternatives unless it is effective. Assessing the effectiveness of many health promotion interventions is challenging. A clear hierarchy of evidence has been accepted for medical care interventions, but such a hierarchy will be more difficult to establish for the range of health promotion interventions.

In addition, economic evaluations belong in a much larger evaluation toolbox. Their blind use, when other qualitative and quantitative techniques have not been employed to understand how health promotion activities work, can be very misleading. Generalizing the results is a particular problem because of the small volume of literature. For example, the results of a study evaluating the costs and benefits of a mass-media intervention cannot be generalized to apply to all similar mass-media campaigns without a far greater body of research. More problematically, such studies are sometimes used to make even broader generalizations: for example, about the type of health promotion programmes in related areas. More high-quality economic evaluations are needed, with economists working in partnership with health promotion specialists, to overcome these problems. With greater knowledge of both the advantages and limitations of economic evaluation techniques, progress can be made.

Economic evaluation requires quantification and comparison. So far, very few have been undertaken, and health promotion interventions having an economic component as an integral part of a more general evaluation package are difficult to find. This chapter outlines economic evaluation approaches and how they could be applied to health promotion activities, while recognizing the need for a greater body of studies. It outlines the different types of economic evaluation, with examples from the literature where available, and gives some guidance on the steps required in an economic evaluation of health promotion activities. Economic evaluations require a number of assumptions and choices. The chapter reviews the many issues being debated, both among health economists and between them and health promotion specialists.

Types and uses of economic evaluation

The type of economic evaluation technique adopted is strongly related to the question addressed, but terms can be confusing. *Cost–effectiveness* is frequently used as a generic term covering all types of economic evaluation. Further, authors misclassify some types. The first distinction is between full and partial economic evaluations. The former have two main characteristics: consideration of both inputs (costs) and outcomes (benefits), and a comparison of both over several alternative interventions. Partial evaluations include only some of these elements. Full evaluations include several distinct types characterized by how the principal outcome is measured and valued (1).

Some of the published economic evaluations of health promotion activities have followed the conventions of health care evaluations, and can be criticized for their narrow perspective on health (2). Most focus on disease, rather than adopting a broader concept of health. Of course, health promotion interventions that can compete with many health care interventions – and indeed win in value-for-money terms, even when some potential benefits are ignored – deserve strong support. Not all health promotion interventions, however, are funded or undertaken by people in the health sector (see Chapter 22). For example, transport agencies may try to prevent accidents by changing road layout or introducing legislation. Environmental interventions may offer important lessons. In general, the diverse benefits from environmental interventions undergo some money valuation, and cost–benefit techniques are more common than in the health care sector. While some of the conventions used in economic evaluations by transport or environmental economists may differ slightly from those described here, the theoretical basis is the same. Also, in most cases, the final result and policy recommendations would be the same, even if results were presented slightly differently.

Types of partial economic evaluation

Outcome description, costing analysis or cost–outcome descriptions can be undertaken on single interventions or programmes. Costing analysis may clearly be seen as the special preserve of the economist, while outcome and cost–outcome studies are more likely to be undertaken in cooperation with other evaluators.

Costing health promotion interventions presents problems. Many interventions involve time and other resources from a range of individuals and agencies that may be engaged in numerous activities in addition to the health promotion intervention of interest. In costing, economists use the notion of opportunity costs, and not necessarily financial value. The opportunity cost is based on the value of the resource (raw materials, land, labour or capital) in terms of the opportunity for using it for some other purpose. The problem of shared resources, tracing all inputs and finding adequate valuations for some types of resources used in health promotion interventions are the major issues in costing health promotion interventions.

Shipley et al. (3) conducted a cost–outcome study examining the relationship between costs and participation across 26 different community smoking cessation (quit-and-win) contests. This study included the contributions of the community in time, money or materials, as well as the direct health promotion input, which included the total media and personnel costs. Data were collected by means of a questionnaire, but few details are given about the methodology used. The objective was to examine the relationship between outcomes and level of resources.

Comparing just the outcomes of alternative interventions has limited usefulness. From an economic perspective, this amounts to a partial evaluation, with no account taken of the resources required to achieve the different outcomes. Clearly the most economically efficient intervention is not necessarily the one that yields the greatest outcomes. Equally, comparing only costs would not yield sufficient information to judge economic efficiency, and would favour the cheapest option. In fact, only evaluations that consider both outcomes and resource use can be considered full economic evaluations, capable of answering the types of questions outlined in the introduction.

Costing analysis, however, may be performed for descriptive rather than analytic purposes. It may be possible to use the information to explore the factors influencing the costs of different interventions. This information can in turn be used to design new interventions or to help monitor existing ones.

Full economic evaluations

There are four distinct types of full economic evaluation:

- cost-minimization
- cost–effectiveness
- cost–utility
- cost–benefit.

All measure the inputs or costs in monetary units; they differ in how the principal outcome is measured. This issue is one of the main areas that require development before economic evaluations can gain wider support from health promotion specialists. Most existing measures focus on disease or saving lives, rather than the broader principles of the Ottawa Charter for Health Promotion (4). Many people ask whether experts should value health-related quality of life even when measures are used that attempt to do so, such as DALYs and QALYs (5) (see Chapter 6). In addition, there is the question of who benefits from health promotion interventions. The main outcomes of health care interventions are their effects on the health of the individuals directly receiving them. The subjects of health promotion interventions may be more difficult to identify. The target of legislation, protection or even education may be the whole community or population, and assessing the actual reach of the programme may be difficult. The choice of evaluation type and how the principal outcomes are measured is therefore crucial. Table 7.1 gives the main features of each type of economic evaluation technique.

Cost-minimization analysis

Cost-minimization analysis involves the comparison of two or more alternative interventions, whose outcomes are assumed to be exactly the same. If this can be assumed, the intervention that minimizes costs is judged to give the best value for money.

152

Table 7.1. Different types of full economic evaluation

Type of study	Treatment of alternatives		
	Measurement/ Valuation of costs in alternatives	Identification of consequences	Measurement/ Valuation of consequences
Cost-minimization analysis	Monetary terms	Identical in all relevant respects	None
Cost–effectiveness analysis	Monetary terms	Single effect of interest, common to both alternatives, but achieved to different degrees	Natural units (life years gained, numbers stopping smoking, etc.)
Cost–utility analysis	Monetary terms	Single or multiple effects, not necessarily common to both alternatives	Healthy years or (more often) QALYs
Cost–benefit analysis	Monetary terms	Single or multiple effects, not necessarily common to both alternatives	Monetary terms

Source: adapted from Drummond et al. *(1).*

A strong assumption would be that all consequences of all the alternative interventions were the same. For example, as well as direct benefits, some health promotion interventions may have consequences, or additional benefits, in reducing future demands on health care resources. Interventions could have a number of additional effects, however, and assuming equality of outcomes may be difficult. In some cases, the individual benefits may be assumed to be the same, but attempts are made to measure and include all other consequences in monetary terms. The net costs (resource costs less the other beneficial consequences) could then be compared. In practice, this latter type of cost-minimization study is often wrongly labelled as a cost–benefit study.

The advantage of this approach is that it avoids the problems of measuring and valuing the individual outcomes of the interventions. Such outcomes, however, can seldom be safely assumed to be equal across interventions. In general, standard texts and guidelines therefore do not recommend this method *(1)*.

Cost–effectiveness analysis

Cost–effectiveness analysis is by far the most common type of economic evaluation of health care, and has comprised most published economic evaluations of health promotion interventions. The individual benefit is usually measured as some sort of quantifiable unit, either behavioural (such as numbers who stopped smoking) or health outcome (such as life years saved, coronary heart disease events averted, etc.). Obviously, such analyses can be criticized for taking a very narrow measure of outcome and failing to include many of the potential benefits of the health promotion intervention. Their main advantage, however, is that they allow quantification.

153

A few examples illustrate some of the different measures used and methodologies adopted. Langham et al. *(6)* considered the costs per percentage-point reduction in a coronary risk score, using data on costs and outcomes from a trial. The intervention under consideration was a health check programme, with a control group being used. Field et al. *(7)* used data from the same trial and an epidemiological model to translate reductions in risk factors into estimates of life years gained, with the cost–effectiveness in terms of net costs per year gained. Kahn *(8)* considered the targeting of HIV prevention, using epidemiological models and reviews of effectiveness data to simulate the number of HIV infections averted with US $1 million additional spending on prevention programmes. Similarly, Buck et al. *(9)* used modelling and review evidence to consider the broad costs and life years gained of different coronary heart disease strategies, although this was not a formal cost–effectiveness study.

In planning a specific economic intervention, the choice of main outcome measure may be obvious. For example, the numbers who quit as a result of antismoking interventions are a measurable and useful endpoint. It would be impossible, however, to use a common behavioural measure to compare a smoking programme with, say, one on skin cancer. Without a common health measure, cost–effectiveness analysis cannot be used. Such analysis is most suitable when programmes with health aims are being compared and these objectives are the primary outcomes of interest.

Cost–utility analysis

Cost–utility studies identify, measure and value individual health outcomes using a measure that reflects how individuals value or gain utility from the quality and length of life. While actual measures differ in practice, QALYs *(10)* and DALYs (a variant of QALYs) *(11)* are used, although some have criticized them *(12)* (see Chapter 6).

One means of comparing interventions that have a number of health effects is to devise a composite health measure. This was the starting point for developing utility-based measures of health outcome. If a generic health measure is available, comparisons could be made over a wide range of interventions, between different health promotion programmes or, say, between a health promotion intervention and a treatment approach. Clearly, if economic evaluations are to become more routine and results collated to answer some of the higher-level questions about allocating resources between different activities, using the same generic health outcome measure offers many advantages to evaluators.

A generic measure obviously needs to cover all the dimensions of health. The changes in different health states before and after an intervention then need to be valued. What value is given, for example, to decreasing pain, but not relieving stress or increasing mobility? Also, the measures of health-related quality of life attributable to an intervention need to be combined with life expectancy to arrive at QALYs. For example, if health-related quality of

154

life is valued on a scale from 0 (death) to 1 (perfect health), an intervention increases the quality of life for an individual from 0.5 to 0.9 for 10 years and the individual would otherwise have a quality of life of 0.5 for those 10 years without the intervention, then the intervention yields a health gain of 4 QALYs (10 x (0.9 – 0.5)).

The next section discusses these and other outcome measures in more detail. While utility-type measures have been recommended for health care interventions, their usefulness for all health promotion interventions is open to question. Cribb & Haycox *(13)*, for example, argue that this type of measure can identify only relatively large changes in health states. Health promotion may improve the health of the population, but the individual changes, especially for those who currently experience generally good quality of life, may be small and difficult to quantify. Further, health promotion may have non-health benefits for individuals and communities. Interventions may, for example, increase self-worth and confidence. Such empowerment may translate to healthier choices but not necessarily to changes in health-related quality of life.

Fiscella & Franks *(14)* and Holtgrave & Kelly *(15)* provide two recent examples of studies using QALYs. Fiscella & Franks *(14)* considered the cost for additional QALYs gained from physicians prescribing the nicotine patch, compared to a base case of counselling for smokers. They drew data on benefits from reviews of the literature, and based the costs on an estimate of the physicians' time spent and the retail price of the patches. They made assumptions about the numbers of smokers who would accept prescriptions for patches and the compliance of those accepting them. Quality-of-life gains from stopping smoking were based on a population survey. Holtgrave & Kelly *(15)* based their analysis on a randomized controlled trial of an HIV prevention programme for women. Behavioural outcomes from the trial were translated by modelling into the number of HIV infections averted. Another model allowed the conversion of HIV infections averted into QALYs saved.

Cost–benefit analysis

In cost–benefit analysis, all outcomes are measured in monetary terms. This method is useful in evaluations of interventions with many diverse outcomes. This is likely for health promotion interventions, which may address communities rather than individuals and involve a number of different agencies, not all of them in the health sector, with different priorities and principal outcomes of interest. Currently available utility-based health measures are unlikely to capture all these outcomes, even measuring at the community level.

Drummond & Stoddart *(16)* suggest that cost–benefit analysis would be the obvious method to adopt in the economic evaluation of intersectoral interventions. Ginsberg & Silverberg *(17)* provide an example (Table 7.2). They estimated the expected costs and benefits from legislation requiring bicycle-helmet use in Israel, calculating all costs and benefits over a five-year period and discounting them at 5% per annum. The costs included those of an education campaign and of the helmets, but not those involved in changing legislation or enforcing the law when enacted. Nevertheless, the benefits are considerable; the social benefits exceed the costs by a ratio of 3:1.

Table 7.2. An example of cost–benefit analysis: legislation for bicycle helmets in Israel

Benefits and costs	Values (US $)
Benefits	
Value of lives saved	8 939 979
Reduced health care costs	17 412 622
Reduced long-term care costs	25 263 243
Reduced need for special education	1 527 131
Productivity gain from reduced disabilities	7 545 779
	60 688 754
Costs	
Health education programme and helmets	(20 143 984)
Total social benefits	40 544 770

Source: adapted from Ginsberg & Silverberg *(17)*.

The study also illustrates one of the problems of using cost–benefit analysis, however: that some monetary value must be given to the loss of life and life quality. Ginsberg & Silverberg *(17)* approximated the value of a year of life by gross national product per head for the population. Thus, in this example, each potential life year gained was valued by the same amount and no discrimination was made between individuals. Other methods attempt to value life by asking individuals to give valuations. These methods usually yield higher values than productivity measures. For example, in the United Kingdom, the Department of Transport moved from a productivity-based measure of valuing loss of life to a willingness-to-pay measure. This change more than doubled the value of a lost life *(18)*.

The choice of type of economic evaluation is linked to the specific study question and to the planned use of the results. The next section explores these and other issues in conducting an actual economic evaluation.

Steps in undertaking an economic evaluation

Several general texts give guidance on undertaking economic evaluations. Drummond et al. *(1)* provide a number of case studies and examples of health care evaluations. Cohen & Henderson *(19)* discuss prevention and health promotion examples in more detail. Tolley *(20)* gives a specific guide to applying cost–effectiveness analysis to health promotion interventions. These guides can help people plan economic evaluations or critically analyse published studies. Many issues arise in any evaluation of health promotion interventions, however, and a multidisciplinary team, containing both economists and health promotion specialists, is clearly necessary to undertake a high-quality study. The main steps in an economic evaluation are:

- defining the economic question and perspective of the study
- determining the alternatives to be evaluated
- choosing the study design
- identifying, measuring and valuing the costs
- identifying, measuring and valuing the benefits
- adjusting costs and benefits for differential timing
- measuring the incremental costs and benefits
- putting the costs and benefits together
- testing the sensitivity of the results
- presenting the results to the users.

Defining the study question

Economic evaluations of health promotion interventions could address many different questions. The choice of study and perspective depend on the policy question being addressed. Tolley *(20)* suggests that the study questions can be seen as a number of levels. The first would involve a comparison of two or more health promotion interventions. For example, nicotine patches might be compared to counselling only, as done by Fiscella & Franks *(14)*. A second-level evaluation would involve a comparison of health education with alternative health promotion interventions; Buck et al. *(9)* examined this type of evaluation framework. A third-level evaluation would involve comparing a health promotion intervention to a treatment alternative. For example, Williams *(21)* examined a range of options for coronary heart disease and found physician advice to stop smoking more cost-effective than any treatment option. The final level of evaluation involves comparing health promotion interventions to other public-sector services as recipients of resources, such as education and defence. This level of evaluation is rare, although Graham & Vaupel *(22)* examined the cost per life year saved of a wide range of interventions from environmental measures such as road safety measures, through immunization programmes to coronary heart disease screening programmes.

The second important aspect of the design is the perspective taken for the study. A health promotion practitioner interested in comparing two alternative ways of delivering an HIV prevention programme may be concerned only with the costs and benefits directly affecting the agency. The intervention that yields the most benefit for the least cost from this narrow perspective, however, may be the one that involves the highest contribution from other agencies. Other agencies' resources are not without value. Taking a wider perspective could change the economic ranking of the alternative interventions being evaluated.

Economists usually recommend that the widest societal perspective be taken, but a narrow health service or public-financed resource perspective is frequently adopted. Fiscella & Franks' study (14) took a payer's perspective in the United States. Field et al. (7) used a National Health Service perspective for their study of health checks in the United Kingdom. Health promotion activities can affect many agencies, particularly in the longer term. For example, extending the length of life would have harmful consequences for the pension industry, if it failed to adjust contributions and payments. Similarly, life insurers should respond to increasing quality and length of life by lowering premiums, rather than increasing profits, if markets are competitive. Such consequences are usually outside the scope of an economic evaluation, even though economic groups that are adversely affected may influence policy-makers, as shown in the long history of measures to reduce smoking. The general advice for economic evaluators is not only to calculate the net results in terms of cost per effect but also to consider who gains and who loses, as this may influence policy decisions.

One common fault of economic evaluations is that attempts to address more than one question compromise the study design. Some trade-off is likely to result from designing an evaluation to answer a very specific question, rather than a more general one. With so few published studies, there is a tendency to attempt to generalize from specific evaluations. Drummond et al. (23) explore some of the difficulties of comparing results across studies, especially when compiled into cost-per-QALY league tables.

Determining the alternatives

Full economic evaluations require two or more alternatives to be compared. Choosing these alternatives is a very important part of the process. An economic evaluation would not be informative if it omitted an intervention with potentially greater benefits and lower costs from consideration. In some circumstances, a prior option appraisal may be undertaken, looking at costs and benefits in broad terms, to create a short list of options. Health promotion initiatives can clearly vary in setting, target area and intervention type. Tolley (20) explores illustrations of different options.

One potential option is to do nothing. In this case, the additional benefits and costs of some health promotion intervention(s) could be compared with the status quo. Obviously, evaluating the do-nothing alternative may involve the prediction of adverse consequences for the health and wellbeing of the population.

More complex designs may be involved in evaluating multicomponent programmes. This may entail comparing the results of adding different components to some core activities. An alternative design may involve more intense interventions with certain groups after some initial screening procedures.

Choosing the study design

Economic evaluations require the establishment of the effectiveness of interventions. As suggested earlier, this is only part of a much broader range of

158

evaluations that can be undertaken. In general, full economic evaluations would take place at the end of this evaluation process. The most rigorous designs for evaluating health care interventions are based on the random allocation of individuals to alternative interventions. This would not always be possible with health promotion interventions. The people comprising the targets of some types of intervention may not be specifically identified, such as those receiving a media message, or the intervention may focus on the community. Other types of controls are available in quasi-experimental studies. The purpose of controls is to determine that the outcomes can be adequately attributed to the intervention and not to other factors. The scientific rigour of some designs, however, can detract from the evaluation in practice. The solution is to devise pragmatic designs including rigour, but approximating as nearly as possible to the situation in normal circumstances. In addition, data from different sources may need to be combined to estimate the effects of complex interventions.

Ideally, economic data would be collected concurrently with the effectiveness data, but costs may be estimated retrospectively, as in the study by Holtgrave & Kelly *(15)*. Some studies, such as that by Fiscella & Franks *(14)*, base both costs and effects on literature reviews, combined with modelling techniques.

Part of the study design involves the choice of evaluation method: cost-minimization, cost–effectiveness, cost–utility or cost–benefit analysis. The appropriate choice depends on the study question and the alternatives being evaluated.

Identifying, measuring and valuing costs
The full range of costs to be identified for a health promotion intervention would include: the direct costs of the intervention to the health promotion agency, the other agencies involved in delivering the intervention and the people who participate, and productivity costs.

The direct costs incurred by the health promotion agency cover direct consumables (such as leaflets, etc.), staff costs and overhead expenditure on, for example, rent and general administration and management costs. While overheads are sometimes called indirect costs, in health care interventions these are more generally taken to be the productivity costs.

The direct costs to other agencies often include staff time but can cover other items. Time and other resources from these agencies have opportunity costs. Tracing these inputs would be important in any but the narrowest of economic evaluations of health promotion interventions.

The direct costs to the people participating in the intervention may involve travel or other expenses. There may be difficult-to-measure costs in terms of stress, worry or distress. This phenomenon has been observed with some disease screening programmes and some media campaigns, and is associated with the worried well syndrome.

Productivity costs are the value of the time spent participating in the health programme. An intervention that takes place in working hours obviously results in a loss of productivity. The time of the unemployed and leisure time also have value. Productivity costs can be high for treatment in hospital, and small for most health promotion interventions. In addition, the common practice of valuing by the participants' earning capacity can introduce distortions. The usual advice is to show these types of costs separately, so that readers of the study can examine the results including or excluding this item.

The costs measured depend on the perspectives and the alternatives being considered. Some costs, for example, may be the same across the alternatives. These will not need to be considered, as they will not affect the choice between the programmes. While there is some limit to tracing all the effects, especially in the level of detail in costing, any study should justify any decisions to exclude costs.

Several issues arise in measuring and valuing different costs. The process has two parts: measuring the resource use and valuing that resource. The time of personnel is an important resource in health promotion, although determining an appropriate method for allocating individual staff members' time to the different interventions in their work programme is sometimes difficult. Allocation is usually based on time diaries kept by staff over a sample period, or more direct monitoring of the time spent on a specific intervention.

Time is not the only resource; many programmes have material costs. Allowance must be made for capital resources consumed, including space and a share of overhead costs. Capital costs need to be valued in a specific way (1). Overhead costs may be easier to identify in total, but both types of cost are more difficult to allocate to specific units of activity of the interventions, for example, per leaflet distributed, health check completed, etc. Different methods of allocating these shared resources could be appropriate for different resources. For example, the proportion of floor space used by one programme in a larger unit could be used to estimate the share of heating, lighting and cleaning services. For management costs, an allocation based on the proportion of the total specialist staff time spent on the intervention could be used.

Most resources have a market value, but the value of some is not obvious. For example, staff time would be valued at the full employment costs, salary and employers' costs, but how should the time of the unwaged or volunteer workers be valued? There is no agreed formula, and often a range of values is used to test the sensitivity of the results to different assumptions. The values would usually take on some percentage of a like market price, such as some percentage of employment costs.

Identifying, measuring and valuing benefits

Economic evaluations principally focus on the effects of alternative interventions on their targets. How these effects are measured, identified and valued varies with the type of evaluation undertaken.

With cost–effectiveness analysis, depending on the evaluation question, a range of effect measures may be available. Some studies may use a process measure (for example, the number of leaflets distributed) rather than a true outcome measure. Process is far easier to measure than outcomes. A process measure, however, could only be used with confidence if it were an adequate proxy of all the outcomes that would be expected from all the alternative interventions being evaluated. In addition, process measures may not be convincing to the agencies funding health promotion, who face many demands on their resources.

In cost–utility studies, broad health outcome measures are used. The QALY is the most popular, although other methodologies exist *(10)*. QALYs are made up of a set of descriptors of different health states, measurement of changes of health states as a result of the intervention and a valuation of the different health states. The health descriptors vary across different measures. The EQ-5D, for example, considers five dimensions: mobility, self-care, usual activity, pain/discomfort and anxiety/depression *(24)*. For each dimension, there are three possible states. These descriptors may be adequate for acute or chronic illness, but less useful for health promotion interventions. Because of their use in health care, these measures were devised to examine acute and chronic ill health, rather than positive health. Population surveys suggest they are applicable to the general population *(24)*. Further primary research is required to judge their applicability in health promotion settings.

Different methods are available to measure how people value changes in health states *(10)*. The valuations are generally scaled between 0 and 1, with 1 representing perfect health. The final step is estimating how long the changes will last. Obviously, the health benefits of some health promotion interventions, such as those for smoking cessation, may last a long time.

Cost–benefit analysis values health outcomes in monetary terms; the methodologies available range from using some sort of market valuations to asking people about their willingness to pay. This may be thought to be more useful than existing or adapted QALYs in gauging the more subtle changes that may result from health promotion interventions. Obtaining values on sensitive issues such as loss of life or health quality of life, however, poses obvious difficulties.

As well as direct health benefits, health promotion activities can have a number of other consequences. Rosen & Lindholm *(2)* suggest that evaluations have usually ignored the latter and paid too much attention to individual health outcomes, and that the following areas need to be considered:

- consumption benefits of health promotion
- other non-health benefits
- social diffusion effects
- effects on future resource use, such as health care and other costs.

Consumption benefits refer to the reduction of anxiety at which some health promotion interventions may aim. Cohen *(25)* cites the example of smoke detectors, which yield direct benefits in reducing health risks and anxiety about fires in the household.

Interventions may bring non-health benefits to individuals. The prime outcome of some may be argued to be increasing knowledge to use in

161

making choices. In this model of health promotion, changes in behaviour and consequently health outcomes are secondary. Similar arguments suggest that health promotion should be directed at raising self-esteem to enable people to make better choices. These are valid concepts, although measurement may be difficult. The most obvious method, discussed by Rosen & Lindholm *(2)*, is to employ some willingness-to-pay methodology to capture these effects.

Traditional economic evaluations in health have focused measurement effort on the individuals directly affected by the intervention, but many types of health promotion intervention may have social diffusion effects. For example, the effects of a primary care intervention to change the lifestyle of individuals may spread to these people's families, friends and colleagues. Interventions aimed at communities directly attempt to foster such diffusion. Evidence for such diffusion effects is drawn mainly from population studies of mass changes in habits, rather than attempts to estimate this effect from individual studies. Shiell & Hawe *(26)* outline in more detail some of the challenges of undertaking economic evaluations of community development projects. They emphasize the need to measure community cohesion and wellbeing, which are of central importance in such programmes but not necessarily captured by individual-based outcome measures.

The potential for health promotion to result in medium- or long-term savings in expenditure on health care or other welfare services is more controversial. Some interventions, such as influenza vaccinations for older people, may have a clear link with a reduction in a specific disease and associated health care costs. Other interventions, such as any intervention with younger smokers, may reduce future ill health, but over a much longer time period. Estimating such consequences obviously raises a considerable measurement problem. In general, direct observation would be extremely difficult, as the effects may occur over too long a period for most evaluations. In the absence of direct observation, some sort of modelling is needed to estimate these effects. A further issue is whether any potential saving in costs from one disease needs to be adjusted for the higher health care costs that may arise from extending people's lives *(27)*.

Adjusting benefits and costs for differential timing

Some individual health benefits and health care savings will occur at a different time than the direct costs of the health promotion intervention. The time dimension of any study is important. Over what period should costs and consequences be measured, and how should effects that occur in different periods be treated? In general, economists try to consider costs and benefits over as long a period as practicable, but discount all belonging to the first period of the study. This method follows most commercial practice. In general, people value future benefits or costs less than those that occur at present. There has been considerable debate, however, as to whether health benefits should be treated in the same way as financial costs and benefits. No agreement has been

162

reached, and most advice suggests that a range of discount rates (different weights to future benefits) be used, including the case in which health benefits are not discounted *(28)*.

Discounting can make a difference to the choice between alternative interventions. Drummond & Coyle *(29)*, for example, consider the cost per QALY of different blood pressure programmes for different gender and age groups. With discounting, the programmes seemed most cost-effective for older and male groups; without discounting, programmes for women and younger groups appeared more cost-effective. As an illustration, Drummond & Coyle *(29)* estimate that, with discounting, stepped care cost £12 000 per QALY for a 30-year-old woman, and £3000 for a 60-year-old woman. Without discounting, care for both groups seemed more cost-effective: £800 per QALY for the 30-year-old and £900 for the 60-year-old.

Similar changes in ranking may occur if a health promotion intervention is compared to a treatment for the same condition. The intervention is likely to seem more cost-effective if health or other benefits are not discounted, as most benefits are likely to occur in the future. Discounting also gives a lower weight to potential health care savings that may occur well into the future. Nevertheless, many health promotion interventions, even with discounting, have been judged to be very cost-effective, especially when compared to treatment options *(21)*.

Measuring incremental costs and benefits

The comparison of the alternatives has so far been considered as if there were a simple choice between a set of alternatives. In reality, the question may not be choosing between A and B so much as choosing how much of A and how much of B. One should know how both costs and benefits change as the scale of activity changes. For example, mass-media campaigns may be less effective than, say, a direct mailing at low levels of expenditure, but have much greater reach and effectiveness at higher levels of expenditure.

Economists stress the importance of margins, or the extra costs or benefits for one extra unit of the activity. In health promotion, units of activity may be hard to define. Clearly, average costs for each unit vary with the level of the fixed costs. For example, the set-up costs for producing, say, 1000 leaflets for a campaign would involve all the design and preparatory costs, but printing an extra 200 leaflets may cost just a little more.

Putting costs and benefits together

Once all the costs and benefits have been measured, valued and discounted to present values, the results can be put together. They can be presented in several different ways. In some cases, one of the alternative interventions could clearly dominate, with greater effects and lower costs. In other cases, however, one intervention may have both higher costs and higher benefits. In this case, marginal analysis is clearly important to ascertain the amount of extra benefit for each extra increase in the overall resources available.

With cost–effectiveness ratios in particular, results can differ because of the way the ratios are compiled. The question is, what items make up the numerator and which the denominator of the ratio? To aid clarity, most guidelines suggest that results should be presented as the net costs per main effect. Ideally, these ratios should be presented in incremental form, as well as the average or baseline figure.

To some extent, this dilemma does not occur for cost–benefit analysis, as all effects have been valued in themselves. Hence the analysis should yield the net social worth (benefits less costs) for each unit of the intervention compared to some alternative. Some care should be taken with studies labelled as cost–benefit analyses, however, as they are often partial evaluations and do not value the main effects.

Testing the sensitivity of results to assumptions and dealing with uncertainties

Most evaluations of health promotion interventions involve some estimates of future gains in health. Models to estimate such gains involve uncertainties, so the sensitivity of any economic evaluation results should be tested by using different estimates of the gains. This can often be done by using statistical properties of the estimated effects, such as the confidence intervals around the estimate. Similarly, one could explore some major element of cost. In addition, the sensitivity analysis usually includes varying discount rates.

Presenting the results to the user

Economic evaluation is a powerful tool and, may result in very clear policy guidance in some circumstances. It will not do so in most cases, however. In addition, policy-makers may have other objectives than maximizing population wellbeing. Some may be financial, having to do with the level and timing of required funding, and others may relate to specific groups of the population or certain geographical areas. The results of economic evaluation will be useful only if they can address aspects of interest to the decision-maker. Ensuring that such subanalyses can be made, however, requires good communication between the evaluators and the intended users of the results throughout the planning and execution of the evaluation.

Even if only the main results are of interest, the results need to be presented with clarity and transparency, given the number of assumptions that may have been made at different points of the study. As noted earlier, avoiding inappropriate generalizations from the very limited number of published studies is very important. Several publishing guidelines have been constructed to aid this process (30). Any report should include the following areas:

- the background and importance of the question considered
- the perspective of the study
- the reasons for choosing the particular form of economic analysis used
- the population to which the analysis applies

- the alternatives being considered
- the source of the effectiveness data
- measurement of costs in physical and money terms
- measurement of benefits in economic terms
- methods for discounting, incremental analysis and sensitivity analysis
- the overall results and limitations of the study.

Drummond et al. *(1)* give more formal questions on how to interpret published or commissioned studies.

Current debates in using economic techniques to evaluate health promotion

This chapter has already mentioned many issues that lead to disputes between economists. Health promotion specialists may raise some additional issues, and question the whole philosophy of applying economic techniques to health promotion *(31)*. This chapter cannot address all these issues. Clearly some concerns arise, not from economic techniques, but from their poor or inappropriate use. For example, Rosen & Lindholm *(2)* comment on effects omitted from evaluations. Other criticism stems from the incorrect generalization of the results of one evaluation, especially when conclusions are based on inadequate research on how and why some interventions work and others do not. Economic evaluations clearly focus on outcome and hence are only one part of a larger evaluation toolbox.

As mentioned, texts are available to guide those undertaking economic evaluations and attempting to use the results. Critical appraisal of the techniques, especially by referees for journals, should limit problems that have occurred in the past. Raising the standards for and providing clarity in published studies should help resolve some of the more technical issues. Other, more fundamental issues remain; some of these are discussed briefly below.

What are the principal outcomes of health promotion?

Health promotion practitioners, and practitioners and funding agencies, disagree about the principal outcomes of health promotion interventions. While economists may contribute to the debate, they cannot and should not resolve it on their own. Economists should identify the alternative programmes with which health promotion interventions may be competing for resources. In some settings, such as the school, the outcomes may focus narrowly on health but be framed in a more general life-skill and quality approach. In many other settings, however, at least some resources for health promotion come from health budgets and there are questions about the division of funds between health promotion, prevention and treatment options. Even within this framework, other outcomes can be considered with the health outcomes of principal interest.

The increasingly general use of health measures based on acute and chronic health conditions may hamper health promotion evaluations. Some of the wider benefits of health promotion, which are more focused on the principles of the Ottawa Charter *(4)*, require further research so that adequate quantifiable measures can be constructed. Willingness-to-pay methodology may be a useful way to explore some of the wider benefits of health promotion. This could include the consideration of social benefits, as well as effects on individuals' quality of life. Applying economic techniques to other problems, such as environmental assessments, may offer useful lessons.

Can the effects of health promotion be quantified?

Economic evaluation is quantitative, based on the principle that effects can be measured and attributed to different interventions. Some have argued that this is not feasible, and economic evaluations are not worth doing *(31)*. Clearly, specific problems arise in evaluating health promotion interventions, but these also occur in evaluating other public-sector programmes. Is difficulty a valid excuse for not attempting to overcome the problems? At the very least, a well conducted economic evaluation can list the effects that were quantified and those that were not.

One issue that needs to be addressed is the results for health promotion funding if no cost–effectiveness information is available. A hard fact of life is that decision-makers cannot fund all interventions. They must base their choices on the information available, and cost–effectiveness information is one of the criteria they may apply. If health promotion interventions are unable to demonstrate that the resources devoted to them have some outcomes – however these outcomes are measured – they will have difficulty securing funds. Economic evaluations are a means of making explicit the resource allocation decisions that may currently be based on a set of prejudices, often to the detriment of health promotion interventions. As suggested above, widening the definition of outcomes that should be used in such evaluations may help to ensure that broader notions of health are more widely adopted.

Economists recognize that economic evaluations are only one form of evaluation. Evaluations consume resources, so subjecting all interventions to economic evaluation is neither appropriate nor practicable. Further, a good economic evaluation cannot be based on a poor effectiveness study. A health promotion intervention can fail for many reasons, and other evaluation techniques are required to explore them.

Are economic evaluations ethical?

Some of the arguments that economic evaluations are unethical, especially the focus on financial cost, suggest a lack of understanding of the nature of such evaluations *(32)*. The reason for making full economic evaluations is that decisions should not be based on financial costs but on all resource use related to the outcomes achieved. Perhaps the lack of economic evaluations leads decision-makers to focus on cost alone. A similar lack of information may lead

166

health promotion practitioners to promise too much for the limited funds available. This may result in the perception that health promotion interventions are underachieving, while they are actually giving better value for money than many other services.

The principal criterion for economic evaluations is the maximization of outcomes, somehow defined, within a given budget. This criterion fails to take account of who receives the outcomes. For example, the most cost-effective intervention may be the one directed at currently well and well-off individuals. This may have the result of widening health inequalities. Clearly, most health promotion purchasers have other objectives. The effect of the intervention can be explored within an economic evaluation, and equity goals set alongside economic efficiency or value-for-money objectives.

A more specific but linked issue, which has an ethical component, is the value to put on life and indeed the comparison of worth over different individuals. Some methods have built-in weights. Obviously any measure based on expected earnings is biased towards people with higher earning capacity. In general, measures based on earning capacity, except when a population average is taken (as in Ginsberg & Silverberg *(17)*), are no longer widely used. Other measures, such as QALYs, have a built-in equity component. Without specific weighting, QALYs have the same worth, regardless of the characteristics of individuals. Especially in health promotion, however, any type of measure based on life expectancy may be considered biased against the old, who in general have fewer potential QALYs to gain. If considered a problem, the perceived bias could be corrected by the assumption that a QALY for an older person is worth more than a QALY for a younger one. This could be tested empirically by seeking general social values from the population.

Should health benefits be discounted?

Discounting future health benefits differentially affects young and old, and to some extent corrects the perceived agist bias of QALYs. In this instance, however, the assumption is that a QALY is of the same worth whatever the age of the person, but that QALYs gained in the future have less weight than those realized at present. Some think that life should be valued equally over time and that health should not be discounted. In reality, many current decisions may reflect implicit discounting, as health care funders invest in immediate life-saving interventions, rather than switching some resources to long-term prevention programmes. As suggested above, discounting may raise the cost per effect for health promotion interventions, but some interventions may well still compare very favourably with treatment options in value-for-money terms.

Does health promotion save money?

One of the arguments behind the phrase *prevention is better than cure* is that prevention should save costly health service interventions. In practice, demonstrating that health promotion saves money is difficult, possibly because they would only materialize over a long period. This is essentially an empirical question and will vary from intervention to intervention. In some cases, finding the individuals at risk can consume a lot of resources and only a proportion of those at risk may have gone on to incur large health service costs. The question should be, is the prevention programme achieving sufficient benefits for its costs? Simply comparing the costs of interventions with the potential health care cost savings and rejecting the intervention lacking savings would completely ignore any health gain.

More difficult is the question of whether any savings in specific health care expenditure should be adjusted by any future extra health service costs from all causes because people are living longer. A study in the United States, which resulted in published guidelines on undertaking and reporting economic evaluations, suggests that evaluation exclude these so-called unrelated costs *(27)*, but others argue that such adjustments should be made *(33)*. Estimates of care that may be projected to take place 20 or 30 years in the future are clearly subject to considerable uncertainty. Discounting may narrow the impact of different assumptions. As with many other aspects of economic evaluations, final judgement may need to be left to the user of the study. While some issues cannot always be resolved easily, economic evaluation at its best should seek to clarify and make explicit the impact of different decisions on such issues.

Concluding remarks

There is a large gap between the demand for and supply of cost–effectiveness information. Bridging it poses challenges for both economists and health promotion specialists. The most challenging task is finding rigorous but pragmatic evaluation designs for establishing effectiveness to which economic evaluations can be attached. Even with good designs, there are several specific measurement problems. In particular, the outcome measures designed must be practical, while capturing the full impact of health promotion interventions.

Economic evaluation should be used wisely, not widely or without the application of other evaluation methods. Less formal economic appraisals could be built into the planning process and there is certainly considerable scope for more partial evaluations. Even where economic evaluations are considered, simple broad calculations may indicate the dominance of some interventions over others.

Many of the criticisms of economic evaluation arise not from the method but its practice. Policy-makers need education on the dangers of using poorly designed evaluation results or focusing on cost information alone. The importance of guidelines has become increasingly apparent and the articles and books mentioned here can give more details about how to undertake or make a critical review of economic evaluations. Other problems remain, whose solution requires better communication between health promotion specialists, funding agencies, decision-makers and interested health economists.

References

1. DRUMMOND, M. ET AL. *Methods for the economic evaluation of health care programmes*, 2nd ed. Oxford, Oxford University Press, 1997.
2. ROSEN, M. & LINDHOLM, L. The neglected effects of lifestyle interventions in cost–effectiveness analysis. *Health promotion international*, **7**(3): 163–169 (1992).
3. SHIPLEY, R. ET AL. Community stop-smoking contests in the COMMIT trial: relationship of participation to costs. *Preventive medicine*, **24**: 286–292 (1995).
4. Ottawa Charter for Health Promotion. *Health promotion*, **1**(4): iii–v (1986).
5. WILLIAMS, A. Why measure the total burden of disease. *CHE news: research update*, **3**: 2–3 (1998).
6. LANGHAM, S. ET AL. Costs and cost effectiveness of health checks conducted by nurses in primary care: the Oxcheck study. *British medical journal*, **312**: 1265–1268 (1996).
7. FIELD, K. ET AL. Strategies for reducing coronary risk factors in primary care: which is most cost-effective? *British medical journal*, **310**: 1109–1112 (1995).
8. KAHN, J. The cost–effectiveness of HIV prevention targeting: how much more bang for the buck? *American journal of public health*, **86**(12): 1709–1712 (1996).
9. BUCK, D. ET AL. Reducing the burden of coronary heart disease: health promotion, its effectiveness and cost. *Health education research: theory and practice*, **11**(4): 487–499 (1996).
10. JOHANNESSON, M. ET AL. Outcome measure in economic evaluations. *Health economics*, **5**(4): 279–296 (1996).
11. MURRAY, C.J.L. & ACHARYA, A.K. Understanding DALYs. *Journal of health economics*, **16**(6): 703–730 (1997).
12. ANAND, S. & HANSON, K. Disability-adjusted life years: a critical review. *Journal of health economics*, **16**(6): 685–702 (1997).
13. CRIBB, A. & HAYCOX, A. Economic analysis in evaluation of health promotion. *Community medicine*, **11**(4): 299–305 (1989).
14. FISCELLA, M. & FRANKS, P. Cost–effectiveness of the transdermal nicotine patch as an adjunct to physicians' smoking cessation counselling. *Journal of the American Medical Association,* **275**: 1247–1251 (1996).
15. HOLTGRAVE, D. & KELLY, J. Preventing HIV/AIDS among high-risk urban women: the cost–effectiveness of a behavioural group intervention. *American journal of public health*, **86**: 1442–1445 (1996).
16. DRUMMOND, M. & STODDART, G. Assessment of health producing measures across different sectors. *Health policy*, **33**(3): 219–231 (1995).
17. GINSBERG, G. & SILVERBERG, D. A cost–benefit analysis of legislation for bicycle safety helmets in Israel. *American journal of public health*, **84**(4): 653–656 (1994).

18. DALVI, M. *The value of life and safety: a search for a consensus estimate.* London, Department of Transport, 1988.
19. COHEN, D. & HENDERSON, J. *Health, prevention and economics.* Oxford, Oxford Medical Publications, 1988.
20. TOLLEY, K. *Health promotion: how to measure cost–effectiveness.* London, Health Education Authority, 1992.
21. WILLIAMS, A. Economics of coronary artery bypass grafting. *British medical journal,* **291**: 326–329 (1985).
22. GRAHAM, J. & VAUPEL, J. Value of a life: what difference does it make? *Risk analysis,* **1**(1): 89–95 (1981).
23. DRUMMOND, M. ET AL. Cost–effectiveness league tables: more harm than good? *Social science and medicine,* **37**(1): 33–40 (1993).
24. KIND, P. ET AL. Variations in population health status: results from a United Kingdom national questionnaire survey. *British medical journal,* **316**: 736–741 (1998).
25. COHEN, D. Health promotion and cost–effectiveness. *Health promotion international,* **9**(4): 281–287 (1994).
26. SHIELL, A. & HAWE, O. Community development and the tyranny of individualism. *Health economics,* **5**(3): 241–247 (1996).
27. GOLD, M. ET AL., ED. *Cost–effectiveness in health and medicine.* New York, Oxford University Press, 1996.
28. PARSONAGE, M. & NEUBURGER, H. Discounting and health benefits. *Health economics,* **1**: 71–76 (1992).
29. DRUMMOND, M. & COYLE, D. Assessing the economic value of antihypertensive medicines, *Journal of human hypertension,* **6**: 495–501 (1992).
30. BMJ WORKING PARTY ON ECONOMIC EVALUATION. Guidelines for authors and peer reviewers of economic submissions to the BMJ. *British medical journal,* **313**: 275–283 (1996).
31. BURROWS, R. ET AL. The efficacy of health promotion, health economics and late modernism. *Health education research: theory and practice,* **10**: 241–249 (1995).
32. TOLLEY, K. ET AL. Health promotion and health economics. *Health education research: theory and practice,* **11**(3): 361–364 (1996).
33. LEU, R. & SCHAUB, T. More on the impact of smoking on medical care expenditures, *Social science and medicine,* **21**: 825–827 (1985).

8

Health promotion: towards a quality assurance framework

Richard Parish

Quality assurance is a phenomenon of the late twentieth century. It has become a driving force in recent years in both manufacturing and service industries. The health sector has been no exception, and the organizations responsible for delivering health care are now expected to have systems and procedures to measure and promote the quality of their services. Moreover, public expectations have increased over the past decade and this development, along with heightened consumer awareness about health matters in general, has encouraged health care providers to adopt a more customer-oriented approach to service delivery. Not surprisingly, the purchasers of products and services want to know what return they will see on their investments. This is as true for health promotion as for anything else.

Processes govern the relationship between inputs and outcomes, and the quality of these processes largely determines whether the desired outcomes are achieved. Quality assurance is therefore at least partially concerned with efficiency, effectiveness and client satisfaction. As quality assurance is at the heart of planning, evaluation and accountability, it is also central to the concepts and principles of health promotion.

Although health promotion is a relatively new field, many studies in the past two decades have evaluated its practice and effectiveness. Despite this wealth of literature, there are still demands to evaluate every health promotion programme, even when the research indicates that what is proposed would be widely regarded as good practice. In other disciplines, such as medicine, nursing or engineering, the conclusions drawn from research and evaluation become embedded in standards for practice. This prevents unnecessarily repetitive evaluation, with all its attendant costs. Quality standards are therefore at least partially derived from the work of previous evaluation studies. Translating evidence into everyday practice is at the heart of quality assurance.

Despite the growing interest in quality, relatively little work has been done to advance quality assurance practice in health promotion. Speller et al. *(1)* argue that no guidance existed in the United Kingdom until HEA funded a project in 1994 to provide a practical set of quality assurance methods for practitioners. The outcome was a manual that incorporates the characteristics of good practice in health promotion *(2)*. Despite these recent attempts to clarify the concepts, principles and practice of quality assurance, however, concerns remain. Speller et al. *(1)* identify three such concerns in the United Kingdom: pressures of organizational change, anxiety that quality assurance would restrict individual professional judgement and confusion over terminology. The last is particularly worrying. If terminology is a problem for native English-speakers, how much greater difficulty might it cause for people who do not have English as their mother tongue, but must use it in their work?

Despite the perceived problems, Speller at al. *(1)* also identify a number of potential advantages, including the value quality assurance could add to planning and internal communications, staff development, external relations and contract negotiations. All would benefit from the rigour imposed by a quality assurance framework.

The work undertaken thus far seems to show that quality assurance in health promotion is still at an embryonic stage. Nevertheless, support for its introduction and refinement appears to be growing, not least among health promotion practitioners. Indeed, the European Committee for Health Promotion Development, sponsored by the WHO Regional Office for Europe, designated the development of a framework for quality assurance as a priority in 1995. A paper submitted to the Committee *(3)* argues that quality assurance is a process of continuous improvement and thus the quality standards of today should rapidly become outdated. Nevertheless, initial success requires further clarification of the principles, practical application and terminology.

Background

J. Edward Deming is widely regarded as the father of contemporary quality assurance. Deming's introduction to quality thinking started in 1941, but he began to achieve international prominence nine years later. Following the Second World War, Deming was asked to play a major role in the reconstruction of Japan. At a meeting with the Japanese Union of Scientists and Engineers in 1950, he introduced what later became known as the Deming quality assurance cycle (planning, acting, doing and checking). Deming's philosophy is rooted in three main principles.

1. Client or consumer satisfaction is the most important aspect in the development of any product or service.
2. Quality is based on teamwork.
3. Quality assurance is a scientific process based on the collection, interpretation and application of data.

Quality assurance started to become formalized as part of national standards some 30 years later. The British Standards Institute (BSI) claims that, in 1979, it was the first organization in the world to publish "quality systems standards" *(4)*. These were later adopted by the International Organization for Standardization (ISO) and became known as the now familiar ISO 9000 group of quality standards. By the mid-1990s, more than 70 000 organizations worldwide had registered for ISO 9000. Registration involves reviewing, documenting and assessing an organization's procedures. This means:

- defining what the organization does
- describing the processes
- ensuring that the organization actually does what it says it does
- making sure that it does it effectively
- learning from the process so as to improve it in the future.

BSI suggests that the following benefits will derive from the adoption of a comprehensive approach to quality:

1. increased consumer satisfaction
2. improved efficiency
3. better value for money
4. less duplication of work
5. less waste
6. fewer errors
7. cost savings
8. better motivated employees
9. better use of time and resources
10. improved communication
11. improved customer confidence.

The experience of BSI suggests that the benefits of ISO 9000 registration can be seen in three distinct areas: management, people and finances *(4)*.

From a management perspective, the introduction of quality assurance results in a structured approach to quality, with greater emphasis on internal monitoring and review. It helps to promote leadership and direction for the organization, and helps to identify the areas in which the organization should change. The process defines the standards of performance necessary to achieve high-quality outcomes and thus introduces greater efficiency and effectiveness. Among the most significant benefits of an explicit approach to quality is that it results in the early identification of problems and encourages preventive measures. In this sense, quality assurance is a form of continuous monitoring and evaluation, and it facilitates the process of staff development.

Quality assurance has significant advantages for the people involved. A comprehensive approach to quality helps to empower employees and provides for a greater sense of ownership of the process. Their roles and responsibilities are more explicit, and this helps them to make more effective use of their time. Quality assurance results in more effective internal communication, and creates the context for staff development. In short, it benefits consumers, the organization and its staff.

Perhaps most important from a policy-maker's perspective, quality assurance identifies areas of waste and unnecessary bureaucracy. It can thus result in cost savings.

Quality assurance is by definition a monitoring and evaluation mechanism designed to ensure that an organization gets it right the first time, every time. This is a contrast to more traditional approaches to evaluation, which measure the final outcome against stated objectives, but do not consider the processes involved. In this sense, quality assurance has similarities with process evaluation, with the added advantage that it could be used from a health promotion perspective as a management tool, for example, constantly to realign the development of a community programme.

Deming's principles

Deming identified key principles for the management of any organization interested in delivering quality *(5)*:

1. ensuring that the organization is geared to constant improvement;
2. rejecting the belief that delays and mistakes are inevitable;
3. building quality into production processes and demanding statistical proof;
4. minimizing total cost, not merely initial cost, by considering meaningful measures of quality in addition to price in purchasing products or services, and reducing the number of suppliers by eliminating those who cannot produce evidence of quality;
5. constantly improving all aspects of planning and production, thereby enhancing overall quality and reducing total costs;
6. maximizing the potential of all employees by instituting continuous on-the-job training;
7. ensuring that the organization has clear leadership focused on helping people do a better job;
8. encouraging effective two-way communication between staff and management;
9. breaking down barriers between different departments and groups of people to encourage multifunction teamwork;
10. acknowledging that most impediments to productivity are inherent in the system, not the workforce;
11. eliminating arbitrary numerical work quotas and introducing monitoring systems that enable continual improvement to be measured;
12. encouraging self-improvement and introducing a comprehensive programme of continuing education; and
13. creating a top-management structure that will focus on continually improving quality.

174

The case for quality in health promotion

Health promotion has been a developing priority for many countries in recent years. This commitment has led to increasing investment in terms of both funding and policy development. The growing recognition of health promotion's potential to improve public health, however, has paralleled a burgeoning concern about the ever spiralling costs of health care. Health promotion has been caught up in the debate, because in most countries it is funded from the same budget as hospital and community health services. Justifiable demands have therefore been made that health promotion prove its worth.

As health care costs continue to escalate, policy-makers have increasingly demanded evidence of both efficiency and effectiveness in the use of resources. They want assurances that the significant financial investment in health care – whether through taxation, corporate provision or personal subscription – will result in the best possible health outcomes for the population concerned. Moreover, they rightly demand that all services be responsive to client needs, and be consistently and reliably delivered. In short, they demand quality.

The current debate about health care reform, along with the separation of health purchasers from health care providers in some countries, has given added momentum to the quality issue. Purchasers – either public bodies or medical insurance schemes – want evidence to demonstrate that funds are being used effectively and that consumer aspirations are being met. Contracts no longer specify only cost and volume but also quality standards.

What quality means

Despite the widespread use of the term *quality assurance*, confusion about its meaning remains. One definition used in health promotion is: "Quality assurance is a systematic process through which achievable and desirable levels of quality are described, the extent to which these levels are achieved is assessed, and action is taken to enable them to be reached" *(2)*. This definition implies the need to set standards, to develop tools to audit their achievement and to engage in organizational and/or professional development where performance falls short of the standard expected. Evans et al. *(2)* argue that quality assurance in effect describes an integrated series of activities that include:

- deciding to develop a quality assurance programme and identifying its key areas;
- setting standards and agreeing on criteria for measurement;
- measuring performance;
- taking action to improve quality; and
- making regular reviews.

Quality is clearly a multidimensional issue. From a health promotion perspective, quality assurance helps to ensure that all of the input to health promotion realizes its maximum potential in terms of outcome. Health promotion programmes have four types of component:

*   inputs, such as funding, personnel, legislation and policy change;
*   processes, such as policy analysis, public involvement, training, communication and evaluation;
*   outputs, such as improved access, better services and safer environments; and
*   outcomes, such as better health.

Although quality is ultimately assessed in terms of the final product or service, thinking about quality should pervade every aspect of health promotion. Quality assurance is by definition a planning and monitoring exercise; if applied appropriately, it will achieve the outcomes envisaged when resources were committed to the programme. It focuses on systems, procedures and processes, rather than the final product. The latter will realize its potential if the former are addressed as part of a comprehensive approach to quality.

The notion of quality assurance implies continuous evolution; constant review against set standards and the revision of the standards (once achieved) establish quality assurance as a dynamic enterprise. Quality is not so much achieved as enhanced at each stage of the cycle. By definition, quality assurance is therefore a developmental and incremental process.

The quality assurance cycle

Evans et al. *(2)* describe the cyclical nature of the quality assurance process and identify the factors that should be taken into consideration at each stage:

1. identifying and reviewing key areas
2. setting standards
3. selecting measurement criteria
4. constructing an audit tool
5. comparing practice with standards
6. identifying reasons for failing to meet standards
7. making an action plan
8. reviewing progress.

The Ottawa Charter for Health Promotion: the starting point for quality

The Ottawa Charter for Health Promotion *(6)* gave momentum to the increase in the importance of health promotion in many countries; it established a framework for health promotion policy development and programme implementation. Building on the concepts and principles already proposed by the WHO Regional Office for Europe *(7)*, the Charter argues strongly that action for health promotion means:

176

1. building healthy public policy
2. creating supportive environments
3. strengthening community action
4. developing personal skills
5. reorienting health services.

These principles are just as valid in planning for quality.

Stages of the quality assurance cycle

Planning must be the entry point for quality. Without clear plans, there is no context for the application of quality systems. As noted above, the first stage of the quality assurance cycle is to identify the key areas for application.

Identifying key areas

The process of identifying priorities in health promotion is more complex than it may first seem. Most policy-makers, for example, see health promotion in terms of specific health issues, such as coronary heart disease, cancer or HIV/AIDS. Governments frequently set health (or, perhaps more accurately, disease reduction) targets on this basis and allocate resources to specific programmes of this kind. Many health promotion professionals, however, would argue for priorities to be set according to the environments within which health promotion can take place, such as schools, workplaces or particular communities. In contrast, the intended beneficiaries of health promotion (the public) see themselves as belonging to groups within the community that share some common characteristics. Priorities would thus be, for example, health promotion for women, older people or particular ethnic minorities.

In practice, of course, these are merely three ways of looking at the same set of considerations. Almost every health promotion intervention addresses health issues, is aimed at identified groups within the community and is delivered through one or more designated settings. What often exists in reality is a three-dimensional matrix (of topics, target groups and settings), which can be a valuable aid to planning.

Different people – politicians, professionals and members of the public – thus view priorities in different ways. From a quality point of view this is irrelevant, because the processes involved in health promotion ultimately determine quality. In effect, the Ottawa Charter provides the framework for quality assurance.

Over and above the five interrelated action areas, the Ottawa Charter *(6)* also emphasizes the importance of advocacy, enabling and mediation. The Charter therefore defines a number of action areas and processes that should underpin all health promotion activity, irrespective of how priorities are determined. Quality will be achieved by setting standards related to these processes and by continuously measuring performance against them.

The concepts and principles of health promotion *(6, 7)* are accepted as universally applicable. This means that the framework for quality assurance can be applied in any country, irrespective of the health issues to be addressed or the socioeconomic context.

Setting standards

Standards describe the performance criteria to be achieved. Standard setting has two dimensions: specifying the level of performance in measurable terms and clearly indicating the extent to which the standard should be consistently met (for example, on 97% of occasions). One should probably start by establishing a modest level of performance that can be achieved consistently, rather than higher standards that will seldom be attained. Focusing on the achievable and progressively raising standards permit the demonstration of increasing levels of performance, and have the added benefit of giving policy-makers, professionals and the wider community the view that the health promotion initiative is achieving everything it set out to do.

Specifying measurement criteria

Criteria should be precisely specified, and must be achievable, measurable, observable, understandable and reasonable *(2)*. They should also be acceptable to the providers of the service or intervention, to the consumers or recipients and to those responsible for purchasing or funding the initiative.

Constructing an audit tool

Establishing criteria is of little value without an effective mechanism for measuring whether the standards have been achieved. An audit framework will therefore be necessary, and this usually consists of a number of both qualitative and quantitative probe questions for each specified performance criterion. According to Wessex Regional Health Authority *(8)* in the United Kingdom, the auditing method employed must:

- be appropriate to the environment of the audit;
- recognize that the person(s) carrying out the audit may make different professional or value judgements; and
- use weightings that are tailored to the subject of the study *(8)*.

Clearly, the significance of different aspects of the audit will be based on value judgements, and the exercise should be undertaken in conjunction with the people who funders and recipients of the health promotion initiative. At the end of the day, quality, like beauty, is in the eye of the beholder.

Comparing practice with standards

Who should conduct the audit is an important question (see also Chapter 4). For example, any or a combination of the following could undertake a quality assurance audit:

- providers of the health promotion programme (self-audit);
- managers, who have overall accountability but are not directly involved in operational matters;
- external reviewers from outside the organization;
- peer reviewers from within the same organization but involved in other areas of work;
- consumers or recipients of the programme; or
- purchasers (those who fund the initiative).

Whoever assumes responsibility must be skilled in auditing procedures. Indeed, the audit process should be subject to specified quality criteria, and this necessitates training in audit techniques.

Identifying reasons for failing to meet standards
Failure to meet specified standards can have many causes. One of the functions of quality assurance is to enable these to be identified so that the necessary action can take place. Possible reasons for apparently not achieving the required standards are:

- inappropriate standards (perhaps too ambitious)
- low level of resources
- inadequately trained personnel
- organizational constraints
- unclear objectives
- poor communication
- inaccurate audit methodology.

Making an action plan
Having identified the causes of any failure to achieve the stated standards, one should devise a clear plan for remedial action. It should identify the action to be taken, when and by whom.

Reviewing the situation
Conversely, it may be necessary to set more demanding quality standards if existing ones have been met in full. In any event, periodic review should be built into the quality assurance programme.

Planning for success
Planning in two areas – policy formulation and programme development – is essential to successful quality assurance.

Policy formulation
There is no substitute for comprehensive initial planning as the starting point for quality. A clear plan will define the parameters for setting standards. This

means that the nature of the policy decisions that gave rise to the health promotion initiative should be examined, before any consideration of the quality issues relating to programme development or service delivery. The following probe questions might be asked when health promotion policy is formulated.

1. Are there clear policy goals and objectives?
2. Has a range of policy instruments been considered, such as research, legislation, taxation, subsidy, education, organizational change and regulation?
3. Is there a clear strategy for research and evaluation?
4. Is a mechanism in place to measure the health impact of current policy?
5. Have the intended beneficiaries of the policy been consulted in the process of policy formulation?
6. Is organizational capacity adequate to ensure that the policy can be translated into practice?
7. Do the human resources have the necessary skills exist to develop policy and deliver programmes?
8. Does a clear focus of responsibility exist for intersectoral planning?
9. Has equity been a key consideration during the process of policy formulation?

This list is not intended to be definitive; it merely indicates some of the considerations in policy development.

These issues are crucial, because the evidence available suggests that the framework for health promotion adopted at Ottawa in 1986 may not be having the desired impact in practice. The Second International Conference on Health Promotion, held in 1988, commissioned a large number of case studies considered to be at the leading edge of health promotion policy development. An audit of these case studies, however, demonstrated that few had really grasped the concepts and principles set out by WHO (7) or had implemented the framework described in the Ottawa Charter (6). The audit tool employed reviewed each case study for:

1. content and scope of policy
2. potential impact
3. political context
4. accountability
5. planning and consultation process
6. use of research and information
7. degree of multisectorality
8. coordination mechanisms
9. approach to equity
10. health service reorientation.

The audit led to the conclusion that few of the principles of health promotion had been implemented in practice, even though the projects described in the case studies were regarded as models of good practice. Only a small minority had engaged in any form of extensive multisectoral action, and most had employed a limited range of policy measures, notably education and research. The situation may have changed since then, but only an audit of contemporary policy can determine this.

Programme development
Logical and systematic programme development will help define the dimensions for quality assurance. The literature describes many planning models for health promotion, but Fig. 8.1 indicates the issues that need to be considered.

The training manual produced by the University of Keele *(9)*, as part of its project on managing health improvement, shows the need to plan for quality at the outset. The manual highlights key dimensions to any quality check-list applied to health improvement work *(9)*:

1. appropriateness of the intervention to the health needs of the individual, group or community concerned;
2. effectiveness in terms of optimum improvement;
3. social justice to ensure that the intervention produces, as far as possible, health improvement for all recipients and does not benefit some at the expense of others;
4. dignity and choice to ensure that the intervention treats all groups with dignity and recognizes people's rights to choose how to live their lives;
5. an environment conducive to health, safety and wellbeing;
6. participant satisfaction to ensure that all key stakeholders find the intervention acceptable;
7. involvement to assist all key stakeholders, particularly those who should benefit from the initiative, to participate in planning, design and implementation; and
8. efficiency and value for money to ensure that resources are deployed to maximum effect.

Dilemmas, contradictions and ethical considerations
In addressing quality, people engaged in health promotion potentially face some difficult issues. First is the question of competing priorities. The various interested parties may well hold differing views on priorities, methods and quality standards. For example, policy-makers (who often control the resources) may take a diametrically opposite view to that of the communities they are supposed to serve. This may result in pressure to limit the extent of consultation. Moreover, either policy-makers or intended beneficiaries may support the use of methods that health promotion specialists may view as either unethical or ineffective. Such dilemmas will exercise the mediation skills of even the most competent health promotion practitioner.

Fig. 8.1. The starting point for quality in health promotion planning

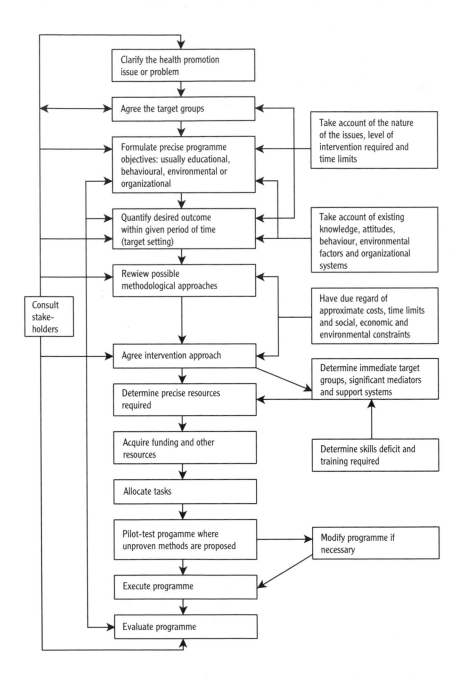

Second, multiple accountability is a related issue. Practitioners are accountable not only to funding agencies but also to the communities for which health promotion initiatives are designed, and to their own organizations and frequently their professional peers.

The third consideration concerns the nature of evaluation itself, and the question of who does what. Researchers customarily argue that outsiders should conduct the evaluation of any activity to ensure objectivity. By definition, however, quality assurance usually involves the people implementing an intervention in continuous monitoring and evaluation. This makes evaluation an everyday management tool, not merely a means of measuring final success or failure. This paradigm shift presents a challenge to the traditional view of scientific research.

In conclusion

Quality is at the forefront of the current debate on public expenditure in many countries, and health promotion must recognize this if it is to continue attracting investment. There is as yet no definitive quality assurance strategy for health promotion, although the issue now features as part of the work of the WHO Regional Office for Europe.

Quality is not an alternative to other forms of evaluation, but is central to other methodologies. Indeed, all areas of work, including the evaluation process, should be subject to the rigours of quality assurance and audit.

Quality assurance is by definition a process of continuous improvement. It is therefore a developmental exercise requiring constant revision. The speed with which today's quality standards become irrelevant to the delivery of health promotion tomorrow will be a key measure of success.

References

1. SPELLER, V. ET AL. Developing quality assurance standards for health promotion practice in the UK. *Health promotion international*, **12**(3): 215–224 (1997).
2. EVANS, D. ET AL. *Assuring quality in health promotion*. London, Health Education Authority, 1994, pp. 20–21.
3. PARISH, R. *Quality issues in health promotion*. Copenhagen, WHO Regional Office for Europe, 1995 (document).
4. *How to become registered to BS EN ISO 9000 with BSI Quality Assurance*. London, British Standards Institute, 1995.
5. NEAVE, H.R. *Managing into the 1990s: the Deming philosophy*. London, H.M. Stationery Office, 1989.
6. Ottawa Charter for Health Promotion. *Health promotion*, **1**(4): iii–v (1986).
7. *Discussion document on the concept and principles of health promotion*. Copenhagen, WHO Regional Office for Europe, 1984 (document).

8. WESSEX REGIONAL HEALTH AUTHORITY. *Using information in managing the nursing resource: quality.* Macclesfield, Greenhalgh and Co., 1991.

9. *Managing health improvement project – Managing for quality in health improvement work. Block 1. Unit 1.* Keele, University of Keele, 1994.

9

Investigating policy networks for health: theory and method in a larger organizational perspective

Evelyne de Leeuw[2]

Introduction

Policy development has traditionally been seen as a top-down, linear and planned endeavour. Even authors with the best intentions of strengthening community action for health have regarded policy-making as essentially one of the many roles of the health promotion professional *(1)*, who should act as a policy developer, advocate and analyst. This view of policy-making as an esoteric and elitist process does not necessarily lead to the shared involvement of all relevant stakeholders in policy development.

Many authors perceive the intricate relationship between certain preconditions and the process of policy development. Alamanos et al. *(2)*, for instance, recognize the value of reliable data for priority setting, as does Green *(3)*. Dean *(4)* adds that rigorous theory development is a quintessential element for the provision of such data. Crawley *(5)* emphasizes the mediating role that a health authority can play in broader health policy development. Hetzel *(6)* even gives a number of sequential steps in developing healthy public policy. Joffe & Sutcliffe *(7)* describe environmental impact assessment as a multidisciplinary instrument to clarify the range of health determinants and consequent policy domains.

Nevertheless, most authors who intend to add to the body of knowledge in health policy-making stop at the point at which policy-making actually begins. This chapter reviews this process, and describes how meaningful research can shed light on ways to modify or even steer it. Policy-making is an organizational endeavour in which individuals may play important roles. Research should be an intrinsic part of policy development, so the chapter describes the

---

[2]   I am very much indebted to Matthew Commers, Department of Health Promotion, University of Maastricht, the Netherlands, for his editorial assistance and eloquence in criticizing many of my assertions.

research process in methodological terms. In presenting three case studies, it illustrates how researchers' decisions determine the relevance of their work to policy development and its outcomes.

Policy studies

Policy is the expressed intent of an institution (government, corporation, volunteer group, etc.) to act strategically to attain specified goals. Policies do not necessarily identify intervention instruments, implementation strategies (including their required resources) or quantified or quantifiable objectives. All these must be operational and allocated, however, for an evaluation to take place. Policy evaluation focuses not merely on results but more importantly on the choices or processes that determine the allocation and use of resources and instruments.

For analytical purposes, policy is usually described as a sequential process with various phases: agenda building, policy theory development, instrumentation and resource allocation, implementation and termination, preferably through goal attainment. Hetzel (6) describes these steps as: situation analysis, communication to politicians, community and professionals, policy-making and planning, political decision-making, implementation and evaluation of the implementation process. Modern scientific insight, however, has revealed the policy process as dynamic, with a number of sometimes seemingly irrelevant feedback loops, and including actors who define their interests in the development of various stages of policy in different ways and participate at different times. Policy-making constellations continuously form and disintegrate, depending on perceptions of the issues at stake, which are hardly ever those determined by formal policy-makers.

For example, Goumans's investigation of ten Dutch and British cities participating in the WHO Healthy Cities project found it essential to describe the policy domains in which health issues are debated and prioritized (8). Health was found to be a container concept, depending on specific perceptions and values, and the often hidden agendas of individual actors and organizations involved. The health domain was therefore in constant flux. Some policy debates, for instance, deeply involved the education sector, while the actors in related debates did not consider education an issue. The instability of the health domain adds to the complexity and abstraction of the theoretical realm, yet does not preclude understanding the dynamics.

Even the participants may wish to limit the scope of their work; it is easier to work on single, quantifiable issues, rather than on the broader policy vision. As a result, policy debates often lead to the development of demonstration projects. The question is whether fixed-term projects can evolve into longer-term policies (9). Research has indicated that most health promotion endeavours suffer from "projectism" (8,9). No matter how well intended and effective most health promotion projects are or could be, they hardly constitute bases for sound public or private policies, because they remain projects, with fixed beginnings and endings, specified funding and prerequisite conditions that do not necessarily contribute to integration and institutionalization into broader policy frameworks, apart from government rhetoric that health promotion and disease prevention form parts of the national health policy package. Broad implementation (based on conscientious policy considerations) of interventions that have been proven effective and lasting remains rare *(10)*.

The Ottawa Charter for Health Promotion *(11)* calls for the development of healthy public policies. Although health education and health promotion professionals and academics often tend to pay lip service to policy development, their understanding of the intricacies of policy-making is generally naive, and does not take account of the wealth of theory development in the realm of political and policy science. Mullen et al. *(12)* provide an example of such naivety, insofar as they treat policy development as a mere phase in the health education planning process. Similarly, Green *(3)* regards both the public and the scientist as outsiders to the policy process. Even an issue of *Health education quarterly* devoted to policy advocacy *(13)* lacks any reference to the broad body of knowledge developed in the academic domain of political science.

A more compelling view of policy-making places it at the heart of community action. Communities may be regarded, in this respect, as organizational (although not always institutional) entities. In 1986, Milio *(14)* convincingly asserted that public policy sets and limits individuals', groups' and communities' options to lead a healthy life. A decade later, she continued this argument, clarifying the involvement of individuals, groups and communities in policy development *(15)* (see Chapter 16).

In general, one major question covers the difficult issues in policy development: who determines which policy will be made? The Healthy Cities project has recognized this question (see Chapter 14). Tsouros *(16)* asserted: "The WHO Healthy Cities project is a long-term international development project that seeks to put health on the agenda of decision-makers in the cities of Europe and to build a strong lobby for public health at the local level". This assumes that agenda status would lead to policy development and lasting political attention to health. Policy and political scientists now recognize that the process is more intricate, dynamic and iterative. Recent studies on policy agendas *(17,18)* and policy-making configurations *(18–22)* show a remarkable match with processes occurring in social-interactive and empowering community programmes (those in which products and outcomes are shaped by debate and consensus, rather than by power and expertise alone).

The public and official perception of the role of the state in policy formulation has been transformed. Various phrases have been coined to describe this new role; governments now talk of public–private partnerships or retreating government; philosophers take constructivist or neo-corporatist perspectives, while policy academics have started to talk of policy networks. No matter what role government has or how policy is debated, communities and institutions play a role in policy development. Apart from being potentially important political constituencies, they also constitute the quintessential domain for the formation of social agendas. The adoption of the Jakarta Declaration on Leading Health Promotion into the 21st Century *(23)* further emphasizes such a position. While the 1986 Ottawa Charter *(11)* may seem to put health professionals at the centre of networking for health, the 1997 Jakarta Declaration intensifies joint responsibilities and regards health as a crucial form of social capital. The policy-making perspective illustrated here underscores such perspectives.

Some metaphors might illustrate current insights into policy-making processes. While the network is a generally used image, a web metaphor – but not the traditional spider's web – is also useful. Here, the web represents the complex interactive set of relations in which policy is made; every actor feels the moves of all others within the web, and any move may ultimately change its structure. The image of an arena helps to convey the perspective that actors play their role while watched by others. Finally, the mosaic relates to a holistic perspective in which the whole is more than the sum of the parts. The pieces of a mosaic are just bits of colourful ceramic, but together they create a meaningful image.

Agenda building

Why are some issues defined as difficult, and others not? Why are some communities better able to structure policy agendas? Why are some policies easily formulated, while others materialize after years of debate? Policy scientists interested in agenda building (why some issues are considered difficult and thus to require policy solutions) address these questions.

Three perspectives can be distinguished: the romantic *(24)*, the cynical and power oriented *(18)*, and the pragmatic/social-interactionist *(17)*. Cobb & Elder *(24)* regard agenda building as essentially a democratic exercise in which public perceptions of problems and the expansion of these perceptions from smaller groups to larger ones determine access. The strategy they propose for issue expansion – moving an issue from the systemic (societal) to the institutional (political) agenda – is to present it as equivocal, with high social relevance, without historical precedents, relevant over a longer period and non-technocratic. One should remember that the difficulty of issues is always perceived; stakeholders construct and manipulate issues to mobilize other audiences. They use symbols and metaphors to help mobilize other stakeholders by changing their perceptions. Communities, depending on their degree of organization and capabilities to identify with difficult issues, play important roles in moving an issue onto an agenda and then making it the subject of policy.

Laumann & Knoke *(18)* take another starting point, seeing policy-making as largely a corporate endeavour. Their study of policy development in the energy and health domains in the United States found that the more corporate actors are able to monitor each others' and government's actions, the more able they are to influence the policy agenda to their advantage. Laumann & Knoke see hardly any relevance of community action to policy development, although their argument may have implications for power balances at the community level.

Kingdon *(17)* provides the most recent insight into agenda building. This perspective is the most realistic and yet the least tangible of the three. Kingdon identifies three more or less independent streams in each policy realm: problems, policies and politics. Each of these has all kinds of visible and less visible participants. Societies always have problems, he maintains, which can be tackled by solutions floating in the policy stream. Policies and attempts to produce them are in constant flux. Politics are determined by elective terms, and the community of political positions. The trick is to open a window of opportunity between the three; a small group of social entrepreneurs *(25)* links a preferred solution to a set of problems, policies and participants. The social entrepreneur can show the opportunistic advantages involved in effective agenda building. Goumans *(8)* has shown that this is why city administrations have joined the international Healthy Cities movement. The issue of health has rarely put Healthy Cities on the municipal agenda; social entrepreneurs have moved existing problems, policies and participants towards the Healthy Cities ideology as an opportunistic way of dealing with issues ranging from environment and employment to housing and community development.

Kingdon's perspective on the policy mosaic *(17)* is particularly relevant to research on the Healthy Cities paradigm, as the rhetorical and conceptual components of the former coincide very well with the latter. Participating cities aim to put health high on social and political agendas; social entrepreneurship is supposed to be key in this process, as is intersectoral collaboration. In Kingdon's terms, the policy, problem and politics streams determine social and political agendas; the social entrepreneur opens windows of opportunity by manipulating these processes (which are very much akin to those involved in establishing intersectoral collaboration) and their visible and invisible participants. The descriptions of cases 1 and 2 below, however, show that Kingdon's model alone cannot entirely explain Healthy Cities development processes.

Policy networks

Policy science has involved itself mainly with the why and what questions (above), rather than the issues of who answers them *(26)*. The reason for this limited view was the notion that government is a black box that directs policy-making in a unilateral and temporally linear way. Political scientists – and particularly local and national governments – saw making policy as a process of establishing goals and objectives, setting schedules and determining the instruments to use *(27)*. Of course, the primary actor was government bureaucracy. It was assumed that, through clever deployment of the regulatory, facilitative and communicative, control and steering instruments available, that government could make policies effective. More recently, however, the who question

189

has become much more prominent, as a result of better academic insights into the art of policy-making and the almost paradigmatic shifts in the perception of the role of government.

Kenis & Schneider *(28)* present the assumptions of the policy network approach:

> The mechanical view of the world established the idea of linear causality explaining social states and events as determined by external forces. The bio-organic perspective shaped the notion of functional causality in which societal subsystems contribute to prerequisites and needs of a global social organism. Both the mechanical and biological world pictures conceived ̶s̶ ̶e̶ ̶ ̶l̶e̶s̶s̶ ̶a̶n̶d̶ societal control as something beyond individual actors. Essentially, this perspective is changed in the network perspective of society. The core of this perspective is a decentralized concept of social organization and governance: society is no longer exclusively controlled by a central intelligence (e.g. the State); rather, controlling devices are dispersed and intelligence is distributed among a multiplicity of action (or "processing") units. The coordination of these action units is no longer the result of "central steering" or some kind of "prestabilized harmony" but emerges through the purposeful interactions of individual actors, who themselves are enabled for parallel action by exchanging information and other relevant resources.

Many local political administrations, however, have not yet recognized or have limited capacities to associate themselves with the networking perspective. While the traditional policy model clearly has fitted with deterministic and mechanical perspectives on society, networking modalities are not necessarily incompatible with more empowering and social-interactive models for community organization.

Ownership of public problems

Central to Gusfield's book on the culture of public problems *(29)* are the concepts of ownership and responsibility. Gusfield examines the fixing of responsibility for public problems. He discriminates between three aspects: ownership and two types of responsibility. One type is causal: who is held responsible for a problem? The other type, the political or policy concept of responsibility, has a wider scope. The politically responsible office or person is the one charged with solving the problem and open to reward for success or punishment for failure.

On the basis of values and beliefs, people develop ideas about causal (as opposed to final or problem solution) relationships, which they often mistake for fact. Causal relationships implicitly point out people or organizations as responsible. The adoption of these indications as facts has implications for the solutions sought to public problems; it assigns responsibility for action and an intervention type as a solution.

190

Gusfield *(29)* uses a concept of politics that extends beyond national or local government; the politically responsible organization or person is the one held liable for acting on the problem. Importantly, political responsibility does not necessarily involve causal responsibility. For instance, health care providers are not held causally responsible for cancer, but are held politically responsible for its cure.

Gusfield *(29)* uses the concept of ownership to illustrate that, in a debate about public problems, all actors (organizations or groups) do not have the same degree of power to define the facts of a problem. The degree of acceptance gained by an organization's concepts of causal responsibility and its proposed solutions is the degree of that organization's ownership of the problem. Further, the owner has the power to divide or share political responsibility. The owner thus has influence in defining the problem and its solutions, and thereby creates a symbolic order. Owners have authority; they can make claims and assertions. Others anxious for definitions of and solutions to the problem look and report to the owners. Even if opposed by other groups, owners can gain the public ear. Different groups and institutions have authority and influence for different problems at different times.

Gusfield's study *(29)* focuses on the relationship between the three aspects of structure: ownership, causation and political obligation. They may not reside with the same office or person. Those who own a problem often try to take political responsibility for its solution, and causal and political responsibility are sometimes related. The unique position of the state makes it a key figure in fixing responsibility. Government officials and agencies operate to define public issues, develop and organize demands upon themselves, and control and move public attitudes and explanations; for example, the Government of the Netherlands tried to influence public debate towards formulating a policy for health, rather than health care alone *(30)*. This is the subject of case 3 below.

Public problems comprise an arena in which a set of groups and institutions, often including government agencies, struggles over ownership, the acceptance of causal theories and the fixing of responsibility. Knowledge is a part of the process, providing a way of seeing the problems that is either congenial or contradictory to one or another way of assigning political responsibility. In other words, choices between theories of causation and loci of political responsibility are made in this arena. They may emerge from religious institutions, science or even folklore.

Constructing a theoretical mosaic

Policy studies in the field of health promotion *(31–34)* have demonstrated that analyses become more meaningful when several theories are combined; Kelly *(35)* asserts that such combination is among the challenges of health promotion research. Each theory sheds light on the same phenomenon from a different perspective. This approach produces case analyses that reflect the dynamics of the policy development process in a way that allows the dissection of its strengths

191

and weaknesses, and opportunities and obstacles in terms of power relations, stakeholder values, effective rhetoric, etc. Such case analyses are interesting both to academics and to participants in the development process. This theoretical mosaic enables the telling of stories that cover the following elements.

- Which actors feel they have a legitimate role in dealing with health policy (ownership and values)?
- How do they include or exclude others in the deliberations leading to priorities (networking, social entrepreneurship)?
- Why do only some issues acquire agenda status (agenda building, rhetoric)?
- How and to what tangible extent are policy objectives set (stakeholder values, ownership and responsibility)?
- Most important, how can a vision of health promotion be used to open windows of opportunity for health policy development among the visible and invisible participants in the policy arena?

The policy analyst usually enters late in the game, describing the processes to the stakeholders as they are ending. By that point, the policy-making process under study is irreversible, although a study may be instructive as future reference for participants in the policy game. From a truly social-interactive perspective, such studies therefore contribute only marginally to the quality of the processes that they describe, and do not enable social entrepreneurs for health to reconsider and re-evaluate their actions. This chapter suggests a methodology for these policy studies that makes them more useful in the processes that they examine.

Policy research methodology and policy development

In evaluation terms, only fourth-generation evaluation (4GE, pronounced "forge") methodologically challenges and maps the realistic view of the policy process *(36,37)*. It is a participatory, dialectic, post-modern scheme of reference ultimately leading to consensus on evaluation parameters, their use and expected outcomes. Methodology is the total body of methods, rules and postulates employed by a discipline. It thus guides the application of specific scientific methods; 4GE or participatory research would establish a methodological postulate on how to apply specific methods.

The 4GE methodology is not unique, extremely innovative or more advanced than others. Boutilier et al. *(38)* describe "community reflective action research" that incorporates stakeholder perspectives in policy development. Piette *(39)* demonstrates that polyarchic systems enhance effective community participation in policy-making. Delaney *(40)* relates intersectoral collaboration to making healthy public policy, and demonstrates that a networking perspective may be the only theoretical one relevant to the domain. Mutter *(41)* focuses on communication as an essential tool in policy building and agenda setting, and describes ways to analyse the communication process. Wyllie & Caswell *(52)* strategically analyse the political elements of that process. Even though none of these studies has employed a theory from the domain described above, they ask similar questions and have a methodological toolkit that is adequate for answering them.

As stated above, policy analyses routinely follow a *post hoc* case study design. Such studies establish a singular perspective; even though scientific quality assurance measures (validity, reliability, triangulation of data sources and data interpreters) may be in place, ultimately the case is relevant only for the specific conditions under which it was found. Such studies can provide pointers or proxies for further studies, and may validate certain theoretical perspectives. They also provide after-the-fact learning opportunities for the participants in the case.

A study sometimes aims for a collection of cases (the multiple case study). Such studies would provide more validated patterns of development, and may indicate pathways to success. Again, even though the collection of cases may reflect scientific rigour (traditional quality assurance measures), the findings are presented after the fact. Participants in new policy development processes may interpret these findings and translate them into action, but the average bureaucrat or social entrepreneur more often follows his or her gut feelings, rather than scientific case descriptions. Also, as each case is unique, rejecting its applicability to new cases seems easy.

In a time when randomized controlled trials and evidence-based practice have been established as dominant, funding agencies often dismiss or even ridicule case study designs, which are not perceived as producing hard evidence. Few mainstream health professionals and academics recognize that the quality of policy development is a proxy for the effectiveness and efficiency of interventions. The question thus becomes whether policy study protocols can be phrased in a way to meet the demands of mainstream research paradigms.

Policy studies almost never have traditional quasi-experimental designs, first and foremost because the methodological barriers to applying such methods to policy science seem insurmountable. For instance, one would have to find a number of parallel environments in which very similar policy developments were sought. One would have to develop protocolized interventions to enhance the policy development process in the experimental environments, and simply monitor the policy process in the control environments.

One would assume that a theoretical mosaic as proposed above, combined with the 4GE protocols, would establish a more or less standardized intervention package. 4GE assumes the following steps in the development process:

1. contracting;
2. organizing;
3. identifying stakeholders;
4. developing within-group joint constructions of the problem;

5. enlarging joint stakeholder constructions through new information or increased sophistication;
6. sorting out resolved claims, concerns and issues;
7. prioritizing unresolved items;
8. collecting information or adding sophistication;
9. preparing the agenda for negotiation;
10. carrying out the negotiation;
11. reporting; and
12. recycling.

Essentially, each step aims at the clarification of roles and stakes in a developmental process. This closely relates to the social entrepreneurial role in Kingdon's theory *(17)*, as well as to the issues of ownership and responsibility raised by Gusfield *(29)*. Bringing values and stakes to the surface may be assumed to strengthen the policy development process. It would facilitate Kingdon's preferred option specification process, which would enable the opening of windows of opportunity; it would also clarify the often hidden and power-related debates about interests and perceptions of causality. Ultimately, the approach would ease the conflict resolution that is at the core of policy debates. The approach presented here serves two purposes: satisfying the quasi-experimental preferences of funding agencies and providing hands-on and highly interactive consultancy to those involved in the policy development process.

Case 1. A quasi-experimental policy research design

The methodological perspective proposed would certainly be feasible in numerous situations, such as a project developed in the southern part of the province of Limburg, the Netherlands. Law in the Netherlands requires public health services to cover a service area with a substantial population, which often comprises more than one municipality. The law requires the municipalities jointly to maintain the services. The Public Health Service of Southern South Limburg covers five municipalities; the city of Maastricht (with a population around 120 000) and the rural municipalities of Valkenburg, Meerssen, Eijsden and Margraten (each with a population of around 30 000). In 1993, the five municipalities and their Public Health Service decided to initiate a community health development programme combined with a reorientation of health care services towards the monitoring of high-risk populations. Incidentally, the Mayor of Meerssen proved to be a strong social entrepreneur, as he was also a member of the Board of the Netherlands Heart Foundation. By 1997, the Foundation had decided to fund the larger part of an array of heart health interventions in Southern South Limburg under the name Heartbeat Limburg. The University of Maastricht Hospital and its Faculty of Health Sciences allocated further funds for evaluation. The project was officially launched in the autumn of 1998 *(43)*.

The programme was developed similarly to a previously validated approach in the Netherlands *(44)*. Southern South Limburg was the experimental setting, with a matched control region elsewhere in the country. Health promotion was delivered to all of the experimental region's population through so-called work books from which neighbourhoods (sometimes facilitated through focus group sessions) could choose interventions already validated as effective behavioural modification programmes or empowerment strategies. In the control region, services continued as usual. In addition, even after external funding ceased, local authorities were supposed to have integrated a number of the changes initiated by Heartbeat Limburg, to make health policy development a sustained part of health activities in the region.

The setting was ideal for the mosaic approach described above. Four equal-sized small municipalities established a common frame of reference, and would be exposed to virtually the same health interventions. They would vary only in the accountabilities and legitimacies shaping their policy development procedures. Two of these municipalities were selected as 4GE areas, and two others as controls.

Commentary

Even though the research design may seem rather standard, serious problems arose, especially during protocol development. Regular intervention studies in health promotion use a pre-determined intervention format (a description of who will do what, when, where, for what target group and area, and for what purpose) and evaluation parameters (the goals to be pursued, and the conditions under which the intervention may be declared a success). Clearly, 4GE aims to produce such objectives and parameters in the course of the intervention, under the assumption that those constructed through negotiation and consultation will more closely suit the interests and stakes of the varying participants.

The funders' protocol referees were very uncomfortable with this, however. An attempt was therefore made to phrase the evaluative process into more traditional terms, asking whether the municipalities in which 4GE was applied would show better results than the controls in:

1. extensive and unequivocal involvement of stakeholders in local health policy development;
2. the shape and substance of interorganizational collaborative activities (such as the quality concept in ISO 9000 norms);
3. efficient allocation of human and other resources;
4. the establishment of a sustainable health policy (with longer-term allocation of resources and clear procedures for decision-making and resource allocation) by the end of the implementation period; and
5. the explicit and unequivocal mention of health affairs in overall policy.

Another concern was the quality of intervention, which seemed to depend on the training, skills and capacities of the action researcher who was to be recruited for the process. As funding is usually made available only for a junior researcher (working for a doctorate), no guarantees could be made. As a solu-

195

tion, a monitoring team was established, composed of staff of the University of Maastricht Faculty of Health Sciences and of the local Public Health Service.

These methodological and contextual decisions meant that the research process was intricately linked with the quality of the policy development process. Indeed, the interrelation of both processes challenges more traditional research paradigms.

Everyday research challenges

In contrast to many other domains, who or what constitutes the research population is not immediately clear in policy studies. Theoretical insights may indicate the type of information the researcher seeks, but the provider of such information is less clear. Even more obscure is the answer to the question of the level at which to aggregate the raw data for analysis. Gusfield's distinction between different types of ownership and responsibility (29) indicates two methods of data gathering as appropriate: document analyses and contact with stakeholders.

Different types of document should be analysed. As the allocation of ownership and responsibility is, according to Gusfield, contested to a certain extent in the public realm, documentation from that realm would be a primary source for mapping the arena for the debate. An analysis of mass-media coverage of the issue under investigation would yield insights into the composition of the arena, and a list of stakeholders. Such an analysis would have to be time sensitive; Gusfield assumes that perceptions and attribution change. A reasonably accurate image of the issues and the stakeholders may be based on this analysis. Any invisible participants potentially influencing ownership and responsibility, however, must be identified. The usual means is snowball sampling, in which the stakeholders listed as a result of the media analysis are asked to add to or modify the list. Laumann & Knoke (18) used this method in establishing the scope and limits of the domains that they investigated. In a Delphi-like procedure (45), the list can be repeatedly returned to the growing collection of stakeholders until additions cease.

While a media analysis might give a superficial picture of the debate, coloured by the need to present news to specific target groups (readers, viewers, etc.), an analysis of stakeholders' documents would yield further insights into their motivations for perceiving or presenting reality to their own advantage. Naturally, such documentation is often hard to obtain. A distinction is usually made between so-called white literature (available in the public domain), grey literature (semi-official memoranda and policy papers) and black literature (internal memoranda, meeting briefings and personal notes). Such documentation can help to modify and refine the map initially traced by the media analysis.

Document analyses do not necessitate close or direct contact with stakeholders. Some disciplines (notably history, ethics and philosophy) once accepted so-called library research as yielding adequate findings, but now

196

recognize that contact with stakeholders often provides a more lively and process-oriented image. Researchers can use a questionnaire, as did Laumann & Knoke *(18)*, or conduct interviews, as did Kingdon *(17)* and Gusfield *(29)*; I prefer interviews. More recent advances show the value of focus groups.

Of course, the respondent to a questionnaire or subject of an interview is a human being. Should his or her responses reflect personal views or organizational perspectives? Laumann & Knoke *(18)* and Gusfield *(29)* typically find that organizations are the relevant units under investigation, while Kingdon *(17)* would regard individuals as the movers and shakers. Thus, the theoretical framework used will establish whether people or organizations are being questioned. Once this has been fixed, the researcher can brief the respondents accordingly. With questionnaires, ascertaining the validity of the chosen perspective is difficult. During interviews, investigators may want to check continually whether a respondent is speaking in organizational or personal terms. They should also request appropriate stakeholder documentation, as this would validate the representation.

The data compiled through document analysis and written or verbal interaction with stakeholders typically comprise lengthy text files. Researchers must choose the ways in which the raw material will be compiled and made available for analysis.

There are usually two options in document analyses. The first and less labour intensive is to make annotated bibliographic reviews of the material, emphasizing remarkable statements on both issues and stakeholders. The advent of scanners and software for optical character recognition has created another option: the transformation of documents into material that can be subjected to automated analysis.

Questionnaire and interview material must be handled differently. The use of questionnaires assumes the availability of a number of conceptual presuppositions. Thus, the questionnaire material can be structured along the lines of classes of information, or may even have a precoded format. Individual questions and subquestions are then related to parts of the conceptual or theoretical framework. This should enable researchers to classify the answers while typing up the response. Material represented in such a format can then be analysed further.

Interviews usually involve considerable labour, both to conduct the interaction and to transform the response into processable material. Researchers usually tape interviews (and should always ask respondents whether they permit recording), and use the tapes to create verbatim transcripts of everything that was said. In my experience, transcripts include a great deal of so-called noise: talk irrelevant to the topic. I have found it possible to write down the essence of the interview, using the recordings for fact checking while typing up the texts. This creates texts that exclude noise but still yield the information sought. Nevertheless, it is advisable to make verbatim transcripts of statements that characterize the respondents' views.

197

Case 2. Healthy Cities second-phase policy evaluation: theory and units of investigation

The WHO Healthy Cities project was established in 1986 to demonstrate the validity of the Ottawa Charter's principles at a local level. Putting health high on social and political agendas remains its main objective (see also Chapter 14). The project completed two five-year phases and began a third in 1998. Although the global popularity of the idea (over 3000 cities worldwide celebrated Healthy Cities principles on World Health Day 1997) is a strong indicator of its success, evaluations demonstrating substantial achievements have been few. Evaluations of the first phase (1986–1992) mainly focused on the description of models of good practice. Some of the outcomes have been widely used as a source of inspiration and Healthy Cities development; the most notable are a review of progress in 1987–1990 *(46)* and the *Twenty steps* booklet *(47)*.

The EU funded research that would evaluate the WHO project. After a pilot phase including all 38 WHO-designated European project cities, 10 were selected for further in-depth study. The goal of the second-phase evaluation was to show whether cities had included health promotion in their policies, and the factors leading to success or failure. As the project's objective was to develop policy, this was the central research issue. We in the WHO Collaborating Centre for Research on Healthy Cities, in the Department of Health Promotion of the University of Maastricht, formed the research team.

We took a two-tiered approach to the pilot phase. We sent all 38 coordinators of the projects in designated cities open-ended questionnaires, asking about the reasons cities wanted to be associated with the WHO project, the resources available to fulfil their obligations to the project, the problems that their Healthy Cities activities addressed and the role of coordinators and project offices. In addition, we interviewed coordinators and politicians, on the basis of the questionnaire findings, during one of the biannual business meetings during which city representatives meet with WHO staff and establish priorities. The main purpose of the interviews was checking facts, although we asked some preliminary pilot questions to test the applicability of the theoretical framework under construction.

The ten cities selected for further study were evenly distributed across the EU and reflected the diversity of project cities. The sample therefore included small towns and big cities, cities with a rich tradition in health promotion as well as novices to the urban health domain, and cities with clearly surveyable organization and those with highly complicated governance structures. The final stage of selection comprised cities' consent to participate.

The WHO Healthy Cities project office provided us with further documentation on all cities through an easily accessible database. On the basis of the conceptual framework, the pilot questionnaire, fact checking and an examination of individual city documentation, we invited each city to nominate the following interview partners:

1. a politician/councillor for health, social affairs, environment and/or finance, a representative of the city council committee for health and the director or deputy director of public health services;
2. a researcher from its own organization and one from an academic institution covering the city and in its service area;
3. the city project coordinator, other project team members, the coordinators of specific projects and any other counterpart desired by the coordinator; and
4. the mayor and other community leaders.

After visiting each city, we sent a confidential report to the project coordinator for comment on the findings. We then used the validated and edited reports for the final aggregate report.

Commentary

Surprisingly, the researchers' requests for interviews resulted in new dynamics in the selected cities. The research visits legitimized coordinators' efforts to bring together stakeholders who had not previously met in a formal Healthy Cities context. On a number of occasions, this was the first encounter with Healthy Cities aims and strengths for actors who should already have been part of the programme. This often created new accountabilities on the spot. The coordinators highly appreciated this unanticipated result of the research, even though the final report could not – for strategic or political reasons – incorporate formal statements on new commitments and accountabilities. For instance, in one city a working relationship was established during the interview session between the Healthy Cities project office and a quango responsible for carrying out municipal welfare policies in an intersectoral context with non-governmental organizations.

The decision to send confidential reports to city coordinators proved to be wise. The coordinators considered the reports very valuable, although not always pleasant. For example, one coordinator said that the report indicated changes needed in the city project, but hoped that these would not be drawn to a politician's attention. This feedback process was also very relevant for validation purposes.

The analytical process

Analysis is the step in the research process that transforms the raw data into surveyable and comparable pieces and then into meaningful information. Analysis starts with assigning unequivocal labels to specific bits of information. In quantitative approaches, these labels are usually numbers (for example, scaling techniques), and called codes. The numbers can then be ranked, represented in (frequency) tables and statistically manipulated. Assigning labels in qualitative research is more intricate, but has the same purpose. The range of labelling enables the researcher to say something about the degree to which data and information conform to the conceptual framework. The codes used may be words, as well as numbers.

Thus, codes need to be based to a large extent on a previously existing framework. Some qualitative research approaches (phenomenology, anthropology and grounded theory (48)), however, see the transformation of data into meaningful information as an emerging process of interpretation and reinterpretation. Nevertheless, when a conceptual or theoretical framework is available, as in the kind of policy research described here, a code book can be established beforehand; it translates concepts and theoretical presuppositions into the range of responses that would be expected. A code book is not necessarily static. Frequent anomalies in responses might encourage the adding of new codes to the list. In such a case, however, all data must be run through again to assess whether the new code applies to material not previously coded, or to codes that turned out to be container concepts, which could be further dissected.

A qualitative code book typically comprises both codes and an unequivocal definition or descriptor for each. In an ideal world, a team of coders (or observers) would be briefed on the code book and its definitions and descriptors. After coding, an inter-observer kappa could be calculated (49) to measure the consistency and coherence of the coders' work. An insufficient kappa value (about 0.7; a value of 0 is chance observation and 1, full agreement) would mean that the coded material could not be used for further analysis: the codes were too vague; observers did not stick to their briefing or the raw material was unsuitable for coding. In this world, however, time may be too short or the budget insufficient to recruit experienced observers, so the researcher must justify his or her analytical practices unequivocally in the final research report. One way of securing a valid and reliable analysis is to share analysis with respondents through, for example, the 4GE procedure, although a Delphi-like technique is also suitable (26,27).

The use of more observers and the calculation of kappas are sometimes irrelevant. This is often the case in explorative research (26,50). Such research aims to discover ranges of interests or perceptions. The principal aim is detecting the limits of these ranges. When the investigation also aim at establishing internal consistencies within research groups, however, multiple observer coding (and the kappa) would have to be initiated, as this is, again, a process of interpretation.

In the past, two practical ways of coding were prevalent: colour coding with coloured pencils or, more recently, felt-tipped pens, and cutting parts from the original records and pasting them together to make new documents, each containing similarly coded material. The researcher would then have to interpret either the coloured mosaic or the collection of texts. Computers have made both processes much easier; word processing can do both, and a more advanced step is now available. Fielding & Lee (51) describe the use of software packages in qualitative research: for instance, Ethnograph (for DOS and Windows) or HyperQual (Macintosh) facilitate the coding, structuring and interpretation of data. Neither, however, can overcome inter-observer coding problems.

The analysis is followed by interpretation, usually labelled as results or findings in the report.

Case 3. Policy research – a planned endeavour

In 1986, the Government of the Netherlands presented a memorandum to Parliament and its social partners with a radically new perspective on its health policies *(52)*. The memorandum proposed that policy focus on health, rather than health care delivery. The Government envisaged a three-year process of national debate, culminating in Parliament's acceptance of the new perspective. With strong support from the University of Maastricht and the health ministry, I investigated the feasibility of such an innovative approach, both in substance and process *(26)*. I structured the research process by means of a pre-planned set-up, and formulated specific research questions on the basis of Cobb & Elder's theory of agenda building *(24)*. As shown in Fig. 9.1, three domains were determined that could yield valuable information: stakeholders (left column), mass-media coverage (centre column), and the factual developmental chronology of the memorandum (right column). The ovals represent triangulation areas between different domains, theories and methodologies.

Fig. 9.1. Study of the national debate on health policy in the Netherlands, 1980s

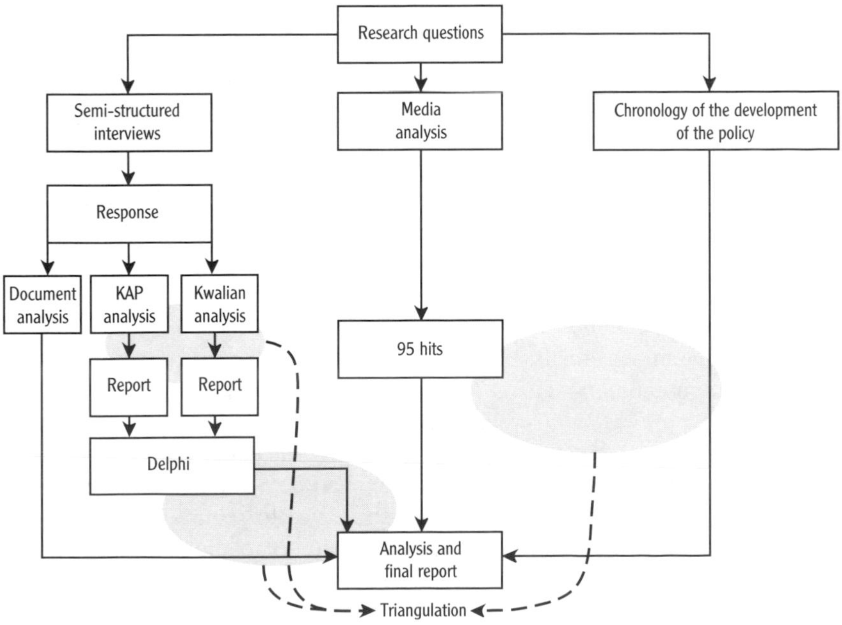

Snowball sampling determined the set of stakeholders: 56 organizations and actors. They were invited to participate in one-on-one interviews, whose contents were structured along the lines of elements of the theory. The response was 60%. Supporting documentation was requested and its content analysed. Interviews were analysed by means of an analysis of knowledge, attitudes and perceptions, and by using Kwalitan software. The former was intended to distinguish between factual knowledge of the policy, attitudes towards it and subjective perceptions. I produced a separate report for each analytical method and sent them back to the entire research population, not just respondents, for validation. This increased the response to 95%. Mass-media reports were also analysed for content. The chronology of policy development was based on access to grey and black literature at the health ministry. Separate reports were produced for each stream and their findings compared (data triangulation).

The policy's feasibility proved to be extremely limited. Direct financial and organizational threats in the care realm overtook its visionary stance *(26,27)*. Vision-based policy-making appeared to be feasible only in times of financial stability.

Commentary

Few problems arose in the course of the investigation. The triangulation procedures revealed that the various data sets were of high quality. The interpretation of the findings, however, was complicated. Application of the theory indicated that the initiators of the policy closely followed the ideal process of agenda building, and that most components of the theory were in place. This would indicate that the memorandum was likely to be implemented without substantial problems. By the time the data were analysed, however, the memorandum *(52)* had disappeared from the policy stage. What was wrong with the study? Were there faults in the data or their analysis and interpretation, or was the theory inappropriate?

I returned to the original data, scrutinized their analysis and interpretation once more and detected no faults or mistakes. This meant that either the theory or our interpretation of it was inappropriate. I compared my procedures with those of other studies using the same theory, and found them highly similar.

I therefore reviewed the theory and its presuppositions and discovered two problems. First, the theory overlooked the possibility that two issues could simultaneously compete for institutional agenda status in the same policy domain. The memorandum's vision of policy-making to create health had had to compete with a move towards market-driven resource considerations in health care. Because most stakeholders had perceived the latter as an immediate threat to their organizational survival, they had turned their attention from longer-term vision development towards strategies to secure short-term survival. Second, the theory did not recognize that power relations between stakeholders and audiences influence the expansion of issue perceptions from one group to the other. Powerful stakeholder organizations had voiced a benevolent scepticism about the memorandum, while those with less power but an allegiance to the memorandum's vision had failed to counter this by combining their efforts to identify the status quo as unacceptable and in need of remedy. These discoveries allowed me to formulate recommendations on theorizing about agenda building in general, and on the importance of monitoring competing agenda issues and power positions when visionary policy is proposed in particular.

Conclusion

This chapter has reviewed theories in policy development that share an interactive networking perspective. Such theories seem more appropriate in describing actual political processes than more traditional, linear, top-down lines of action. The discussion of methodological considerations and researchers' decision processes, however, shows that the application of such theories should go hand in hand with a compatible research attitude. Researchers should be aware of the epistemological and interactive dimensions of policy research. They cannot detach themselves from the organizational, tactical, strategic and contextual issues in the domain under investigation.

Policy research thus steps away from standard methodological approaches to challenge the capacities of both academics and policy-makers. The latter seem to appreciate the consequences of the approach described here more than they did traditional studies. In the end, the approach advocated here yields more immediate, pregnant and tangible results for the policy-making process. Such results are intimately related to the quality of policy outcomes under study.

References

1. McLEROY, K.R. ET AL. An ecological perspective on health promotion programs. *Health education quarterly*, **15**(4): 351–377 (1988).
2. ALAMANOS, Y. ET AL. Assessing the health status and service utilization in Athens: the implications for policy and planning. *Health promotion international*, **8**(4): 263–270 (1993).
3. GREEN, L.W. Three ways research influences policy and practice: the public's right to know and the scientist's responsibility to educate. *Health education*, **18**(4): 44–49 (1987).
4. DEAN, K. Using theory to guide policy relevant health promotion research. *Health promotion international*, **11**(1): 19–26 (1996).
5. CRAWLEY, H. Promoting health through public policy. *Health promotion international*, **2**(2): 213–216 (1987).
6. HETZEL, B.S. Healthy public policy and the Third World. *Health promotion international*, **4**(1): 57–62 (1989).
7. JOFFE, M. & SUTCLIFFE, J. Developing policies for a healthy environment. *Health promotion international*, **12**(2): 169–174 (1997).

8. GOUMANS, M. *Innovations in a fuzzy domain. Healthy Cities and (health) policy development in the Netherlands and the United Kingdom* [Thesis]. Maastricht, University of Maastricht, 1998.
9. GOUMANS, M. & SPRINGETT, J. From projects to policy: 'Healthy Cities' as a mechanism for policy change for health? *Health promotion international*, **12**(4): 311–322 (1997).
10. PAULUSSEN, T.G.W. *Adoption and implementation of AIDS education in Dutch secondary schools*. Utrecht, National Centre for Health Education and Promotion, 1994.
11. Ottawa Charter for Health Promotion. *Health promotion*, **1**(4): iii–v (1986).
12. MULLEN, P.D. ET AL. Settings as an important dimension in health education/promotion policy, programs, and research. *Health education quarterly*, **22**(3): 329–345 (1995).
13. SCHWARTZ, R. ET AL. Policy advocacy interventions for health promotion and education. *Health education quarterly*, **22**(4): 421–527 (1995).
14. MILIO, N. *Promoting health through public policy*. Ottawa, Canadian Public Health Association, 1986.
15. MILIO, N. *Engines of empowerment: using information technology to create healthy communities and challenge public policy*. Ann Arbor, Health Administration Press, 1996.
16. TSOUROS, A. *The WHO Healthy Cities project: state of the art and future plans*. Copenhagen, WHO Regional Office for Europe, 1994 (document).
17. KINGDON, J. *Agendas, alternatives and public policies*, 2nd ed. New York, Harper Collins College, 1995.
18. LAUMANN, E. & KNOKE, D. *The organizational state*. Madison, University of Wisconsin Press, 1987.
19. GOUMANS, M. An ecological perspective on the health of a city – The Healthy City project of the WHO. *In: Prospects for climate-oriented planning in European cities*. Berlin, European Academy of the Urban Environment, 1995, pp. 19–24.
20. GOUMANS, M. Putting concepts into (health) policy practice. *In*: Bruce, N. et al., ed. *Research and change in urban community health*. Avebury, Aldershot, 1995, pp. 327–338.
21. MARIN, B. & MAYNTZ, R., ED. *Policy networks. Empirical evidence and theoretical considerations*. Frankfurt, Campus and Boulder, Westview, 1991.
22. SCHARPF, F.W. *Games real actors could play: the problem of connectedness*. Cologne, Max-Planck-Institut für Gesellschaftsforschung, 1990 (MPIFG Discussion Paper 90/8).
23. *Jakarta Declaration: on leading health promotion into the 21st century. Déclaration de Jakarta sur la promotion de la santé au XXIe siécle* (http://www.who.int/hpr/docs/index.html). Geneva, World Health Or-

ganization, 1997 (document WHO/HPR/HEP/4ICHP/BR/97.4) (accessed on 22 November 2000).

24. COBB, R. & ELDER, C. *Participation in American politics: the dynamics of agenda building*. Baltimore, John Hopkins University Press, 1983.

25. DUHL, L. *The social entrepreneurship of change*. New York, Pace University Press, 1995.

26. DE LEEUW, E. Health policy, epidemiology and power: the interest web. *Health promotion international*, **8**(1): 49–52 (1993).

27. DE LEEUW, E. *Health policy: an exploratory inquiry into the development of policy for the new public health in the Netherlands*. Maastricht, Savannah Press, 1989.

28. KENIS, P & SCHNEIDER, V. Policy networks and policy analysis: scrutinizing a new analytical toolbox. *In*: Marin, B. & Mayntz, R., ed. *Policy networks. Empirical evidence and theoretical considerations*. Frankfurt, Campus and Boulder, Westview, 1991, pp. 25–59.

29. GUSFIELD, J. *The culture of public problems: drinking–driving and the symbolic order*. Chicago, University of Chicago Press, 1981.

30. DE LEEUW, E. & POLMAN, L. Health policy making: the Dutch experience. *Social science and medicine*, **40**(3): 331–338 (1995).

31. ABBEMA, E. *Twenty steps on North Shore: Healthy City development in New Zealand*. Maastricht, WHO Collaborating Centre for Research on Healthy Cities, University of Maastricht, 1997 (World Health Organization Collaborating Centre for Research on Healthy Cities Monograph Series, No. 14).

32. DANEN, S. *The World Health Organization Healthy Cities project second phase evaluation – Forging a process*. Maastricht, WHO Collaborating Centre for Research on Healthy Cities, University of Maastricht, 1998 (World Health Organization Collaborating Centre for Research on Healthy Cities Monograph Series No. 15).

33. LOGGHE, K. *Integratie: het beste gezondheidsbeleid? Een onderzoek naar uitgangspunten voor lokaal gezondheidsbeleid en de zorgverlening aan asielzoekers en vluchtelingen* [Integration: the best health policy? An inquiry into principles of local health policy and health care delivery for asylum seekers and refugees]. Maastricht, WHO Collaborating Centre for Research on Healthy Cities, University of Maastricht, 1996 (World Health Organization Collaborating Centre for Research on Healthy Cities Monograph Series No. 13) (in Dutch).

34. MILEWA, T. & DE LEEUW, E. Reason and protest in the new urban public health movement: an observation on the sociological analysis of political discourse in the 'healthy city'. *British journal of sociology*, **47**(4): 657–670 (1995).

35. KELLY, M.P. Some problems in health promotion research. *Health promotion international*, **4**(4): 317–330 (1989).

36. GUBA, E.G. & LINCOLN, Y.S. *Fourth generation evaluation*. Thousand Oaks, Sage, 1989.

37. GUBA, E.G. & LINCOLN, Y.S. *Naturalistic evaluation: improving the usefulness of evaluation results through responsive and naturalistic approaches.* San Francisco, Jossey-Bass, 1981.

38. BOUTILIER, M. ET AL. Community action and reflective practice in health promotion research. *Health promotion international,* **12**(1): 69–78 (1997).

39. PIETTE, D. Community participation in formal decision-making mechanisms. *Health promotion international,* **5**(3): 187–198 (1990).

40. DELANEY, F.G. Muddling through the middle ground: theoretical concerns in intersectoral collaboration and health promotion. *Health promotion international,* **9**(3): 217–226 (1994).

41. MUTTER, G. Using research results as a health promotion strategy: a five-year case-study in Canada. *Health promotion international,* **4**(3): 393–400 (1989).

42. WYLLIE, A. & CASSWELL, S. Formative evaluation of a policy-orientated print media campaign. *Health promotion international,* **7**(3): 155–162 (1992).

43. *Hartslag Limburg. Samen gezond! De achtergrond; de mensen; de actie* [Heartbeat Limburg. Healthy together! The background; the people; the action]. Maastricht, GGD Zuidelijk Zuid-Limburg, 1997 (in Dutch).

44. VAN ASSEMA, P. *The development, implementation and evaluation of a community health project* [Thesis]. Maastricht, University of Limburg, 1993.

45. LINSTONE, H.A. & TUROFF, M., ED. *The Delphi method – Techniques and applications.* Reading, Addison-Wesley, 1975.

46. TSOUROS, A.D., ED. *World Health Organization Healthy Cities project: a project becomes a movement: review of progress 1987 to 1990.* Milan, Sogess, 1991.

47. *Twenty steps for developing a Healthy Cities project.* Copenhagen, WHO Regional Office for Europe, 1992 (document ICP/HCC 644).

48. GLASER, B.G. & STRAUSS, A.L. *The discovery of grounded theory.* Chicago, Aldine, 1967.

49. LIGHT, R.J. Measures of response agreement for qualitative data: Some generalizations and alternatives. *Psychology bulletin,* **76** (1971).

50. FIELDING, N.G. & FIELDING, J.L. *Linking data.* Beverly Hills, Sage, 1986 (Qualitative Research Methods, Vol. 4).

51. FIELDING, N.G. & LEE, R.M. *Using computers in qualitative research.* Newbury Park, Sage, 1993.

52. *Nota 2000* [Health memorandum 2000]. The Hague, Ministry of Welfare, Health and Cultural Affairs, 1986 (in Dutch).

Part 3
Settings

Introduction

Michael Goodstadt

The concept of settings provides a natural and powerful methodological tool for health promotion; it suggests a framework for analysing and understanding the context within which health promotion occurs. The dynamics of health promotion vary as a function of the cultural, community and social settings within which health-related issues are embedded. Health behaviour, health status and health outcomes are the products of their unique environments.

The significance of settings in health promotion extends beyond an awareness of environmental influences on health. The settings concept is recognized to provide an efficient and effective framework for planning and implementing health promotion initiatives and ultimately assessing their impact. The power of this concept lies in its two dimensions. A setting is the context within which and through which health occurs. As much of society's formal and informal structure and government is based on the settings in which its citizens live and work, these settings provide both an efficient way to analyse, understand and influence the determinants of health and an extensive array of leverage points and incentives for effectively reaching and influencing individuals and communities.

Settings differ widely. The name covers large and sometimes poorly defined communities (such as municipalities), large well defined societal or community structures (such as health care systems), smaller discrete organizations (such as sports clubs), community-based entities (such as schools and hospitals) and life contexts (such as the family). Some settings (such as schools and the workplace) have particular relevance to different stages of life. Others are defined with reference to populations, such as the homeless (the streets), indigenous people (reservations) or religious or spiritual groups (places and communities of worship). Finally, many settings refer to the ways in which people spend their leisure time, such as sports venues, restaurants, bars and cafés.

Part 3 of this book examines a limited number of the large array of settings for health:

- cities and communities, the larger environments that influence the health of individuals and society;
- schools and workplaces, the contexts within which major clusters of individual behaviour occur; and
- hospitals, a part of the health care system with major influence on individual and community health.

209

The chapters included provide excellent examples of settings that are important for health promotion, and the evaluation of health promotion initiatives.

The chapters discuss a variety of issues related to the evaluation of health promotion when considered through the lens of settings. Many of the questions and challenges involved arise in every setting and have relevance to the evaluation of health promotion in general. Thus, Chapter 10 discusses five issues common to all evaluations, but especially those of community initiatives:

1. what the evaluation should be
2. what kind of design to use
3. what and how to measure
4. how to analyse the data
5. what relationship the evaluator should have to the programme.

Similarly, Chapter 11 provides a five-stage logic model for community evaluation that has general applicability to the evaluation of both community-wide and smaller initiatives:

1. collaborative planning
2. community implementation, action and change
3. community adaptation, institutionalization and capacity
4. more distal outcomes
5. dissemination.

Finally, Chapter 13 recommends a six-step framework developed for the evaluation of workplace programmes:

1. clarifying the aims and objectives of the proposed health promotion programme;
2. deciding what questions to ask;
3. deciding how to measure change;
4. collecting the data;
5. evaluating the results to determine the effectiveness of the programme; and
6. making recommendations.

Given the overlap in authorship, chapters 13 and 14, dealing with the evaluation of workplace and Healthy Cities initiatives, respectively, share some features. Both give special attention to the setting as a locus for change, the purposes of and questions addressed by evaluation, multimethod and interdisciplinary approaches and ownership, partnership and power issues. Chapter 14 is particularly helpful in distinguishing between foci of evaluation, which can include infrastructure, policies and programmes, environments and/or health status.

In addition to the valuable contributions made in identifying and clarifying conceptual and methodological issues, these chapters offer a wealth of recommendations that should assist the planning and implementation of health promotion initiatives in a variety of settings. Chapter 10, for example, provides extensive, scholarly but clearly stated guidelines and recommendations related to each of the five evaluation issues identified. Chapter 13 presents five principles for the evaluation of health promotion in the workplace:

1. starting the formative evaluation process with health needs assessment
2. including participation and feedback
3. ensuring clarity about the purpose of the evaluation
4. collecting data to produce useful information
5. paying attention to ethical issues.

In making recommendations for improving evaluation practice in the workplace, the authors highlight five challenges:

1. integrating evaluation with other workplace activity
2. choosing evaluation methodologies
3. bridging multisite workplaces
4. ensuring that evaluation indicators are relevant to the organization involved
5. bridging interfaces.

Chapter 11 concludes an extensive discussion of the evaluation of community initiatives with specific recommendations on how policy-makers and practitioners can promote and support the five stages comprising the authors' evaluation framework. Chapter 12 concludes its discussion of an extensive and systematic review of the literature on health promotion in schools with recommendations that are important to both policy-makers and practitioners. Finally, Chapter 14 presents three case studies that provide insightful examples of the evaluation of Healthy Cities initiatives at three different levels: the international level, urban policy and the community.

The authors hope that readers' appreciation will extend beyond the challenges faced in evaluating health promotion to include a more profound awareness of the contributions that a settings approach can make to the planning and evaluation of health promotion. The Ottawa Charter for Health Promotion explicitly emphasizes the importance of settings in its call for creating supportive environments and strengthening community action. The five chapters that follow reflect the Charter's values, principles and strategies.

10
Evaluating community health promotion programmes

Louise Potvin and Lucie Richard

For the last 30 years or so, practitioners have tried to develop and implement what many perceive to be a potent intervention strategy for health promotion: community programmes *(1)*. Noteworthy efforts were made in the fields of mental health *(2)*, heart health promotion *(3,4)*, substance abuse prevention *(5)*, breast cancer screening *(6)*, comprehensive multifactorial approaches *(7)* and single risk-factor (such as smoking) prevention *(8,9)*. The evaluation literature has discussed issues related to comprehensive community programmes since the 1970s *(10)*, but epidemiology, public health and health promotion journals started publishing papers debating the evaluation of community health promotion programmes only after interest was created by the three community heart health promotion programmes funded by the national Heart, Lung and Blood Institute in the United States and implemented in the 1980s *(11–13)*.

A student of this literature would find four categories of papers, presenting:

1. research designs implemented for the comprehensive evaluation of ongoing programmes;
2. intermediate results, often about programme processes or mid-term analyses;
3. the results of overall outcome evaluations; and
4. discussions of methodological issues arising from the first three types.

Papers from the first group are rare. They usually introduce interesting methodological ideas, but, because they are published while studies are under way, their value in terms of new knowledge is somewhat limited. The second group of papers contains most of what has been learned about community health promotion programmes. It provides a rich source of data documenting various aspects of community programming. The third group presents what is usually seen as the main results from outcome evaluation. These papers are often disappointing; few programmes can show an overall beneficial effect on risk factors *(14)*, so readers face the uncomfortable conclusion that community programmes are not effective. Finally, the fourth group of papers provides reflections, critiques and insights on the conduct of evaluation research. The authors are usually researchers involved in the evaluation of community programmes, and the issues debated reflect the state of the field.

This chapter aims to provide the reader with an introduction to the fourth category of papers, with some intrusions on the other three groups for illustrative purposes. Community programmes are complex interventions, involving many community actors from a variety of backgrounds with diversified interests. Of course, this complexity affects the evaluation components. As a result, many issues are raised about this type of study. Unfortunately, few have found widely agreed and easily implemented solutions. What characterizes the debate about the evaluation of community programmes is the impossibility of implementing methodological solutions that have been proven useful and rigorous in more controlled situations such as clinical research. Not surprisingly, no consensus can be realistically expected at present.

Planning the evaluation of a community health promotion programme requires the clarification of numerous difficult issues. Community programmes and settings are unique, and evaluators are well advised to tailor a combination of methodological solutions to suit the peculiarities of the programme, the characteristics of the community and the needs for information about the programme. Anyone who is planning the evaluation of a community health promotion programme should address the issues raised in this chapter. Intervention and evaluation teams should examine and discuss them before starting their work.

The unique characteristics of community programmes comprise a very specific approach to health promotion, and should not be confounded with other forms of intervention.

Characteristics of community programmes

If great effort has been put into defining the notions of community (15–17) and programme (18), the task remains to integrate the many elements characterizing community programmes into a clear definition. Green and his colleagues (18–20) have offered a first distinction between two complementary approaches to improving the health status of a community. First, community interventions or large-scale programmes have a community-wide scope; they seek small but pervasive changes for most or all of the population. Such an approach rests on numerous studies in public health that show that a slight reduction in risk in an entire population yields more health benefits than greater reductions in a small subset of at-risk individuals (21). This is in opposition to a second type of approach: interventions in the community. These microinterventions or small-scale programmes seek changes in a subpopulation, usually in a site such as schools, workplaces and health care facilities. The objectives are usually to attain intensive and profound changes in the risk behaviour of the targeted subset of the population. This chapter focuses on large-scale community programmes, which have five essential characteristics. They must be: large, complex, participatory, long lived, and flexible and adaptable.

First, given their objective of reaching the entire community, community programmes are large in scope and magnitude *(18,19)*. They usually require much planning and coordination, and large human and financial resources.

Second, community programmes differ qualitatively, as well as quantitatively, from small-scale programmes or interventions in the community. While the latter are often rather restricted in focus, community programmes embrace a multilevel, multistrategy vision of individual change. In line with social science research that identifies the important influence of various facets of the environment on individuals' behaviour *(22–24)*, community programmes not only target limited aspects of individual behaviour but also try to modify the whole social context assumed to influence health and health-related behaviour. Changes in social norms and local values, institutions and policies are thus the primary targets *(25–28)*. To succeed, community programmes involve many settings, organizations and partners *(18,29,30)*. Kubisch et al. *(22)* have expressed a similar idea with their notion of these programmes' complexity in horizontal (work across systems, sectors or settings) and vertical (interventions directed to many targets such as individuals, families and communities) terms. Such diversity of intervention strategies and the complex synergy resulting from them *(31)* are thought to be essential to reach "the community and everyone in it" *(18)*.

A third characteristic of community programmes refers to a critical element of any change process at both the individual and community levels: participation. As described by Green & Kreuter *(18)*, ethical, practical and scientific considerations call for the active integration of targeted individuals in any planned process of change. This is most necessary when large-scale change objectives are pursued in a community *(18,22,31–33)*.

In practice, community organization is often seen as the key strategy to mobilize citizens, organizations and communities for health action and to stimulate conditions for change *(25)*. Community organization not only ensures the local relevance of both the problem identified and the solution envisioned but also extends and helps raise scarce resources, maintains citizens' interest in programme activities and encourages the sustainability of interventions *(29,34)*. It also increases communities' problem-solving abilities and competence in addressing issues threatening the residents' health and wellbeing. By far its most important outcome, however, is the development of a sense of ownership of the programme in the community. For many authors, the only way to attain these goals is to favour high involvement of community actors in every aspect of programme planning, implementation and evaluation *(33)*, so that they can be considered senior partners in the process *(35)*, up to the point at which authority for the programme moves from external partners to neighbourhoods and communities *(22)*.

215

A fourth essential characteristic of community programmes – longevity – stems directly from the first three. Gaining community actors' confidence, encouraging their involvement and establishing a working agenda that satisfies all the partners involved in the programme comprise a time- and energy-consuming process. Moreover, targeting environmental aspects calls for numerous steps, the most crucial of which relate to educating the population about the need for and relevance of the proposed changes (4).

Last, because of their long life-span and particularly because of the complex and dynamic nature of the targets of intervention, community programmes must be flexible and adaptable to cope with changing realities (22,31) and to carry out a process involving many partners, among which neighbourhood and community organizations and citizens are considered senior.

Key issues in evaluating community health promotion programmes

How are the main characteristics of large-scale community programmes associated with issues raised by the evaluation of these programmes? The issues discussed here are grouped into five categories:

1. identifying the evaluation questions
2. deciding on the design
3. selecting and assessing outcome variables
4. analysing the data
5. choosing the role of the evaluator.

Issue 1. Identifying the evaluation questions
Defining the objectives of the evaluation raises two related questions. The first deals with the importance of specifying a model for the intervention, to facilitate the process of identifying an evaluation question. The use of such a model also helps clarify the second question, which deals with process and outcome evaluations.

Agreements/Disagreements
Defining the evaluation question should be high on the evaluator's list of priorities. Most often, the question pertains to the effects of the programme on individual risk factors or population health indicators. For example, the main evaluation questions of the Stanford Five-City and the Minnesota and Pawtucket heart health programmes (11,13,36) were whether the programmes contributed to the reduction of the prevalence of selected modifiable risk factors in the target communities. These outcome questions can be formulated with or without reference to the effective mechanisms that link the programme to an

216

observed effect. When these links are not specified, the study is often called a black-box evaluation *(37)*:

> This type of evaluation is characterised by a primary focus on the overall relationship between the inputs and the outputs for a programme without concern for the transformation processes in the middle. Such simple input/output or black box evaluations may provide a gross assessment of whether or not a programme fails but fail to identify the underlying causal mechanisms that generate the treatment effects.

Black-box evaluation works well when the programme is precisely defined and encapsulated into a series of operations that can be described with detail and accuracy. Because community health promotion programmes rest on citizens' participation, however, this kind of standardization is impractical for them (see also chapters 2 and 4).

In addition to these input/output questions, many evaluations have included questions aimed at discovering elements of the causal mechanisms in community programmes. These theory-driven evaluations *(37)* begin with a programme theory *(38)* describing how the programme should produce the expected outcome. Arguing for increasing the use of programme theory in the evaluation of community programmes, Weiss *(39)* states that founding evaluations on theories of the programme serves several purposes: focusing the evaluation on key issues, facilitating the aggregation of results from several studies into a comprehensive framework and helping both evaluators and practitioners make their assumptions explicit. Programme theory therefore helps coordinate evaluation with intervention strategies.

In the health promotion literature, the PRECEDE/PROCEED model *(18)* operates with a similar logic of linking input, process and outcome measures through the specification of a conceptual model. By establishing a series of intermediate objectives, the PRECEDE section of the model helps practitioners formulate the theory of the programme, while the PROCEED section uses these objectives as milestones for the evaluation.

Programme theory has been increasingly used to focus the evaluation of community health promotion programmes. For example, the Pawtucket Heart Health Program highlighted the role of voluntary organizations in community development *(40)*, while the Henry J. Kaiser Family Foundation's Community Health Promotion Grant Program developed a series of hypotheses on the importance of improving collaboration among organizations in a community to spur action on single or multiple health promotion issues *(41)*. Indeed, in a review of particularly important issues in the evaluation of community programmes, Koepsell et al. *(42)* insist on the necessity of formulating a programme's theory to build a model that shows how the programme should work. Researchers can use such a model to specify the key steps in programme implementation, set the evaluation design, measurement and data collection, and clarify the meaning of the findings.

A related issue is whether to do a process or an outcome evaluation. Authors often oppose them in a way that positions the former as easier and less costly and the latter as real science (29,43). The result is a more or less explicit prescription that, once outcome evaluations have used enormous resources to show a programme to be effective, the task for further evaluations is to show that the conditions for the effect to occur were in place. This position has been challenged on at least two grounds.

First, because community participation in the planning, implementation and evaluation phases of programming seems to be an essential ingredient for success (18,34,44), some have argued that conclusions on the outcomes of programmes not emerging from communities are hardly applicable (45). Thus, failure to show a significant positive effect on selected health indicators – as in the Minnesota (12) and Pawtucket heart health programmes (46) and the community trial for smoking cessation (COMMIT) (9) – could be attributable to the failure to involve the community as a senior partner at every stage (35).

Second, complex community programmes evolve following dynamics that remain mostly unknown (47). Each time a community programme is implemented, interaction in a unique context produces something different from what was previously designed or tested elsewhere (48). This is true even when programmes apply the same planning principles. Abandoning outcome evaluation because a programme has been proven effective in previous trials is weak logic, since the programme changes with its context (49).

Guidelines and recommendations

Many authors seem to agree that contributing to the understanding of how a programme works is much more important than merely determining whether it works (39,50,51). Altman (49) argues that evaluations of process, intermediate and ultimate effects, and social relevance all help to determine how programmes work. One should recognize that no single study can answer all relevant questions about a programme (52). Different evaluations of similar programmes should be coordinated to form comprehensive research agendas. Each study could thus contribute to the development and testing of the programme theory.

Within this perspective, the question is no longer whether to emphasize process or outcome evaluation. Ideally, evaluation and intervention teams should come together early in the planning stages of the programme and work out a treatment theory to build a model of the programme. Then, depending on the resources available, the questions raised by a literature review, the vested interests of the teams and other relevant factors, evaluators can use this model to formulate evaluation questions. They should remember, however, that process evaluation questions are aimed at producing local knowledge on what is delivered in the community. This information often serves as feedback that allows the intervention team to tailor the programme to the needs of the community, thus making it more likely to produce an outcome. As a counterpart, outcome evaluation questions produce both local and generalizable knowledge (53).

218

Locally, outcome results may be used to make funding decisions on a programme, although some have argued that evaluation results are just one among many factors influencing such decisions *(54,55)*. As generalizable knowledge, the results can be accumulated to foster understanding of health promotion mechanisms that are active at the community level. To gain validity, this knowledge should be replicated in a variety of evaluation studies using different methodologies *(56)*. As many evaluations as possible should therefore include some outcome questions in their objectives. Not all are required to implement sophisticated and complex methodological features, but every piece of knowledge produced should find its way to a scientific journal where it can be debated and added to the body of knowledge.

A related issue pertains to how evaluation questions are determined. This problem has no easy answer. Patton *(57)* argues that all programmes' stakeholders should take part in identifying relevant research questions. Although this represents the ideal situation, Pirie *(58)* warns that stakeholders differ in their information needs. There is tension between senior managers, who are interested in efficacy and effectiveness; practitioners, who want to learn about the process; and academic researchers, who want to produce information that has some degree of generalizability to contribute to the development of programme evaluation.

The implementation of some form of cooperative inquiry could help ease these tensions *(59)*. In the orthodoxy of participatory research, everyone involved in such a project has a role in setting the agenda, participating in data collection and analysis and controlling the use of outcomes *(60)*. Because it does not establish a clear distinction between the researcher and the object of inquiry, this type of methodology questions the foundations of positivist research (see Chapter 4). Participatory research is committed to research as a praxis that develops a change-enhancing, interactive and contextualized approach to knowledge building *(61)*. While implementing all principles of participatory research would not seem feasible to many academic researchers, this does not need to be the case. Green et al. *(62)* have shown that these principles have various levels of implementation, and offer guidelines to help address these questions.

Issue 2. Deciding on the design

The two main design issues are: assigning communities to either a control or an intervention group (and consequently determining the appropriateness of random assignments) and maintaining the integrity of one or several control communities as intervention free.

Agreements/Disagreements

In the experimental/quasi-experimental tradition of programme evaluation, the validity of the causal inference about programmes' outcomes depends on the researcher's ability to rule out plausible rival hypotheses other than the one stipulating that the programme produces the expected effect *(52)*. The use of a control group allows comparisons of units that are not exposed to the pro-gramme with those that are. Such comparisons are useful to rule out hypoth-eses pertaining to maturation or historical phenomena (63). For example, in North American countries, cigarette smoking has been declining for the last 25 years (64,65) so, to be judged effective, a programme would have to be asso-ciated with a decrease in cigarette smoking that is higher than the decrease expected from the secular trend. Assuming that the controlgroup has not been exposed to the programme, its use allows the monitoring of the secular trend under natural conditions. In addition, the random assignment of the units into either the programme or the control group provides a simple means of ruling out a great number of alternative explanations related to the equivalence of the groups to be compared before the programme's implementation (66).

Because community health promotion programmes are implemented in communities and individuals within a community cannot therefore be assigned to different groups, the assignment units must be communities (42). For ran-dom assignment to play its role in making the groups statistically equivalent, a great number of units would have to be assigned and enrolled in a single study. This is difficult, but the fact that half of them would not receive any treatment for the entire study period increases the difficulty. The recent literature has often debated the problem of randomizing communities.

Some authors argue that random assignment is as important to ensure valid results in studies about community programmes as in individual-based pro-grammes (51,67). The problem is simply having adequate funding to conduct a study on a sufficient number of communities. For example, COMMIT ran-domly assigned 22 communities to either a control or an experimental group (8). Other authors say that, although random assignment would improve the capacity to draw valid causal inferences from community studies, the number of communities available is likely to remain small. Randomization alone would therefore not ensure the statistical equivalence of groups (42,68), unless paired with other procedures, such as blocking or stratification.

Two characteristics of community programmes lead yet other authors to question the appropriateness of randomizing even a large number of commu-nities. First, community programmes follow their own dynamic and evolve differently in interaction with their specific contexts, so creating standard programmes for implementation in all experimental communities is almost impossible (47). Local variations, coming from a lack of control over the ex-perimental conditions, would undoubtedly have a differential effect on the observed outcomes in the different communities, resulting in a lack of power to detect existing effects (69,70). Second, the long lives of programmes and the long delay between exposure and potential outcomes lead to uncontrol-lable and uneven changes in the composition of the groups (47,71). The longer the delay, the more likely it is that external events, whether or not they are independent of the programme, will affect the observed outcomes. For example, the community health promotion environment may change, as well as the composition of the groups. Here again, the lack of control over the context in which the programme evolves would concur to lower the theoretical power of the study.

The greater the experimenter's control of the experimental situation, the more efficient is the randomized controlled trial to estimate effects that can be attributable to a treatment or a programme. Areas of control include the treatment itself, the context for its delivery and the subjects receiving it. In open and complex systems such as communities, none of these can be controlled. Interventions evolve in relationship to their implementation contexts; community populations are mobile, and many components of an intervention are available through other channels. Randomizing communities in community health promotion trials is therefore unlikely fully to isolate the relationship under scrutiny. Even when funding is sufficient to enrol a large number of communities to be randomly assigned to either a treatment or a control group, one is well advised to doubt the effectiveness of the technique in producing groups equivalent in all respects other than the treatment under study.

Independently of the feasibility of randomizing communities, the other important design issue is the maintenance of the integrity of the control group. Even when no health promotion efforts are deliberately invested into control communities, the level of health promotion activities has been observed to increase, parallel with the level of activities in communities exposed to health promotion programmes (51,72,73). Evaluators can do nothing to prevent such compensatory behaviour in control communities (74). All they can do is closely to monitor the level of health promotion activity in various control communities, using process data collected with methods that are as unobtrusive as possible. In an article based on the experience of major community heart health programmes, Pirie et al. (75) thoroughly discuss measures and methods to assess important issues for process evaluation.

Guidelines and recommendations

Evaluating community trials challenges the very notion of scientific rigour. Even if the feasibility of implementing methods effective in other settings were ensured, this could not guarantee the validity of the causal inference. Communities are complex systems, wide open to numerous external and internal influences. The traditional criteria for rigour, based on standardized, repeatable and formalized procedures (76), are not applicable in evaluations of community programmes. One must turn to other criteria, such as the transparency of the decision process (77) or the critical implementation of multiple methodological procedures (78).

Design issues in the evaluation of community interventions are critical. The appropriateness of using recognized methodological tools, such as random assignment and control groups, must be weighed each time an evaluation is planned. Their use does not guarantee the validity of the causal inference of programmes' effectiveness. Although the systematic manipulation of isolated elements has been the golden rule for scientific knowledge since John Stuart Mill (74), it is far from the only one. Campbell (79) proposes a post-positivist theory of science in which four principles, derived from modern epistemology, characterize the scientific process:

1. judgmental and discretionary decisions are unavoidable in science;
2. scientific activities take place within a broader paradigmatic environment that partly shapes every aspect of a study;
3. scientific activities are historically determined in the sense that they can only build on existing knowledge, which characterizes scientific activity as epistemologically, historically, culturally and paradigmatically relativist; and
4. science is a social process and the scientific method is a social system product.

These principles lead to the recognition that:

1. no universal methodological recipe works in all situations;
2. a plurality of critical perspectives and evidence is necessary to form scientific knowledge; and
3. transparency and accountability in decision-making about methodological issues are necessary ingredients of validity.

Observational methods in the evaluation of community health promotion programmes need rehabilitation. Profound and detailed knowledge gained from the systematic observation of the implementation of a programme, in tandem with the tracking of expected effects within various community subsystems, can prove useful for the understanding of whether and how community programmes are effective health promotion strategies. Evaluators of community programmes are thus invited to create new ways of answering their questions about programmes' processes, implementation or outcomes. Evaluators should, however:

1. document the justifications for their decisions, paying special attention to clarity about their own values;
2. try to implement multiple research strategies, acknowledging that none of them is bias free;
3. interpret critically their results, using existing knowledge and acknowledging that their conclusion is one among many other plausible ones; and
4. share their results with the scientific community to contribute to the augmentation of its common understanding of health promotion processes.

Recognizing the lack of a magic bullet for the evaluation of community trials is of primary importance. Evaluators should deal with design issues individually, and select procedures on the basis of a thorough examination of the characteristics of the communities involved and in relationship to the evaluation questions.

Issue 3. What should be measured and how?

The two measurement-related issues in community trials concern the types of indicators needed to assess the various components of the programme and the optimal survey design to assess intermediate and ultimate outcomes (the choice between following a cohort of citizens or conducting a series of independent cross-sectional surveys).

Agreements/Disagreements

The problem of community-level outcome indicators is closely linked to the development of the intervention model. Indeed, to the extent that the latter establishes effective mechanisms for the programme to trigger, it is much easier for an evaluator to include various types of indicators in the evaluation design. Best et al. *(80)* and Hollister & Hill *(81)* argue that the selection of outcome and process measures for health promotion programme evaluation should parallel the systems that are targeted by various programmes' activities. Limiting evaluation indicators to individual outcome indicators of health or health behaviour jeopardizes the evaluator's capacity to understand the effective route of the programme. Because community programmes are likely to modify environmental and community determinants of health, system-level indicators are important outcome and process variables.

Cheadle et al. *(82)* define community-level measures as all "approaches used to characterize the community as a whole as opposed to individuals within it". They divide community-level indicators into three categories: individual-disaggregated, individual-aggregated and environmental. The first category is derived from observations of individuals within geographic boundaries. The indicators were widely used in most evaluations of community health promotion programmes. In the second category, individual data cannot be retrieved; they are aggregated to form rates. The third category is based on the observation of community processes or environments. Authors have noted that, despite their potential usefulness for assessing important intermediate factors, system-level indicators badly lack attention from the scientific community *(42)*. Very few have been developed and fewer have been studied to assess their reliability and validity.

Some examples of system-level variables, however, are available. Reasoning that, to induce changes at the individual level, community programmes should first activate communities for health promotion and health issues, Wickiser et al. *(83)* and Cohen et al. *(84)* developed a measure of levels of community activation and health promotion activity based on key informants from various organizations in the participating communities. Cheadle et al. *(85)* developed an indicator of community fat consumption based on the survey of shelf space devoted to certain products, especially low-fat milk products, in supermarkets.

A second important issue related to measurement is the design of the surveys to assess the health-related and risk factor outcome variables. Independent of the problems related to control communities and the definition of the

223

outcome variables, one must decide whether to assemble a cohort at baseline and follow these subjects until the final post-test, or to conduct a series of independent cross-sectional surveys. Both designs have been used to evaluate community health programmes. Cross-sectional surveys were used on the North Karelia Project and the Stanford Three-Community and the Heartbeat Wales programmes (86–88). The Stanford Five-City and the Minnesota and Pawtucket heart health programmes used cohort and cross-sectional sampling designs (11,13,36).

The epidemiological literature suggests that a cohort design in which subjects are assessed both at baseline and later, using one or several post-tests, theoretically leads to lower standard errors of estimates of change than independent cross-sectional samples. Subjects in a cohort are their own controls, and thus the variability of the estimate of change can be calculated with greater precision. In addition, because differential attrition and subjects' loss to follow-up make cohort sampling designs much more vulnerable to a variety of biases, these designs often produce biased estimates.

Several authors have raised the issue of the best design to use in community trials. Koepsell et al. (42) note that self-selection at recruitment is a concern with cross-sectional and cohort designs, while cohort designs are more vulnerable to attrition, testing, maturation and history bias. Feldman & McKinlay (89) review several advantages and disadvantages of both designs. When the units of assignment (communities) are relatively small, cohorts are preferred because obtaining independent non-overlapping consecutive samples is difficult. When the population within the units of assignment is expected to remain relatively stable throughout the study period, one can assume that a cohort sample will remain representative; this is not the case when migration in and out is expected to be high. A short intervention span, for example, favours cohorts because assignment units are more likely to remain stable. Evaluators should prefer a cross-sectional design when measurement is expected to influence subsequent behaviour. Finally, controlling for the level of exposure is easier in a cohort sample.

This shows that the gain in precision from using a cohort design can entail the cost of greater susceptibility to a variety of biases. To keep the likelihood of these biases low, a cohort design requires two activities that are not required in cross-sectional studies: over-sampling at baseline to account for attrition, and an aggressive strategy to follow up cohort members. As noted by Feldman & McKinlay (89), the essential problem is therefore to identify the experimental conditions under which the cohort design is more cost-efficient than the cross-sectional design. They show that, even in the absence of any bias, three features of the study context work against the theoretical gain in relative efficiency associated with a cohort design. The gain in precision is substantial only when the auto-correlation of the dependent variable over time is very high. It decreases when the units of assignment (clusters) are large, and when the cluster and measurement variances are very large.

Using graphic illustrations and real data from their study, Diehr et al. *(90)* argue convincingly that, when the community population is not stable, a cohort sample assembled at baseline is not representative of the other segments of the population. These other segments are: the migrants out and in, and the so-called stayers (people who remained in the community) that were not part of the cohort. Their results, derived under simple assumptions, show that:

1. the cohort estimate of change has a higher bias than the cross-sectional estimate;
2. the bias seems to be equivalent in control and in experimental communities; and
3. in large samples obtained from large communities, the cross-sectional data become less variable while remaining bias free.

They suggest that cross-sectional samples should be used and the analysis performed on the sample sections that represent stayers only. This entails the elimination from the baseline data of the respondents that are no longer living in the community at the time of the post-test, and screening potential post-test respondents to ensure that they were living in the community at baseline.

Guidelines and recommendations

Guidelines for dealing with measurement issues must refer to the context of the study and the intervention model. Indicators should be selected to correspond to points of interest in the model, either because they will help the intervention team to better their understanding of their own programme and people's reactions to it, or because they can contribute new knowledge. Evaluators should not hesitate to use environmental process indicators in their studies. There are numerous determinants of health at various levels, and evaluations should use ecological models of health *(91)*. Evaluators will have to be creative, owing to the paucity of environmental indicators, particularly validated ones, in the literature. More developmental research is needed in this area.

The choice between a cohort or a cross-sectional sampling design should be based on a thorough analysis of the community context in relationship to the peculiarities of the evaluation questions and the characteristics of the programme. Evaluators can consider using both types of survey within a single evaluation, although they run the risk of ending up with non-convergent results. In the Minnesota Heart Health Program, for example, results from the cohort data do not correspond to the results from the cross-sectional data *(12)*, because sampling designs help to answer different research questions. A cohort design is useful for identifying individual and environmental variables associated with changes in the target behaviour. Valid conclusions can be reached on individual-level change processes, but generalization problems can be expected to the extent that survivors in a cohort are not representative of the entire population exposed to the programme. Cross-sectional designs, for their part, allow better control for secular trends.

Issue 4. Analysing the data

The important issue related to analysing data from community trials is the use of the appropriate level of analysis, given that communities, not individuals, comprise the intervention and control groups.

Agreements/Disagreements

One of the fundamental principles in experimental studies lies in this simple slogan: "Analyse them as you randomized them". In other words, the sampling units and the units of analysis should be the same. Cornfield *(92)* explained that assigning groups to different treatments, and then analysing individual-level data, without taking account of their origin in a smaller subset of clusters, leads to a bias in the standard error of estimate, unduly inflating the power of the analysis. It is well documented that clustered observations violate the assumption of independence of observation that underlies most analytical procedures based on the linear model. Briefly, the variance of the observations within the community is smaller than that between communities, because for various reasons people from the same cluster are more similar than those from different clusters *(93)*. This leads to an intraclass correlation between the observations that should be included in the standard error of estimate of the parameters under study *(94)*. The point estimate is unbiased, but the likelihood of falsely rejecting the null hypothesis is inflated. This inflation factor increases with the increase in the intraclass correlation within the clusters. To avoid this bias, Murray argues that, "community trials should be evaluated using standard errors computed at the level of the unit of assignment" *(95)*.

An appropriate analytical strategy for dealing with this problem has recently been developed under the general label of multilevel models of analysis *(96)*, with a special application called "hierarchical linear models" *(97)*. The strategy was used to evaluate the Henry J. Kaiser Family Foundation's Community Health Promotion Grant Program *(98)*. The models comprise regression equations that include different levels of variables, nested in a hierarchical manner, and involving as many stages of model specification as the model has levels. Typically, community trials have at least two levels of variables: individual-level variables covering individuals' risk factors or other characteristics, and community-level variables describing characteristics of the community as a whole. In their simplest form, the latter are indicators that differentiate communities *(99)*. At the first level, the regression equations define the outcome variables as a function of a series of individual-level predictors, resulting in a series of regression parameters for each cluster. At the second level, these regression parameters become outcome variables to be predicted by community-level variables. The two-level model allows all individual-level variables to be defined as a function of every community-level predictor and to have a component of random variation.

226

Donner et al. *(94)* discuss power and sample-size issues related to the analysis of community trials. These trials have at least two sampling units: communities and the individuals within them. Increasing the number of individuals sampled within each community has a very limited impact on the power of the analysis once a certain threshold is reached *(95)*. Indeed, the most important factors affecting power are the number of communities assigned to the different arms of the study and the magnitude of the intraclass correlations. The higher the correlations, the more important is the effect of the number of communities.

Guidelines and recommendations

As mentioned, community programmes are complex entities and their evaluation poses complex questions, most of which still await satisfactory answers. Despite their apparent complexity, however, the questions about analysis are probably the most thoroughly studied. The problems have been clearly identified; their effects on the results have been documented, and known statistical procedures and models can be used to solve them. The main difficulty is finding people with statistical knowledge sophisticated enough to carry out the appropriate analyses.

We strongly suggest that an evaluation involve such people right at the beginning of the planning phase of the programme. It is always easier to implement procedures that have been anticipated from the start. The early inclusion in an evaluation team of people educated in statistical theories offers two advantages. These people can both foresee analytical problems (and build solutions into the collection procedures) and learn the cost of good data by taking an active part in the data collection procedures. Dangers such as missing values, incomplete questionnaires, self-selected participants, unbalanced designs and abnormal distributions are all part of the evaluation of programmes, and particularly community programmes.

Issue 5. Choosing the role of the evaluator in relation to the programme

This chapter has provided ample evidence of the challenges of evaluating community programmes. The complexity and magnitude of these programmes force evaluators to redefine their criteria for rigour, to combine methodologies creatively, to develop new instruments and analytical approaches, and to take part in the elaboration of programme theory. In addition, evaluating community programmes is a practical endeavour, meaning that an evaluator must develop a relationship with the programme as it is developed and implemented. This relationship can take many forms, depending on the programme, the evaluator's skills and the programme staff's expectations. The nature and rules of this relationship should be clarified early in the process.

Agreements/Disagreements

Programme evaluations may be external or internal (see Chapter 4). External evaluations are carried out by someone outside the delivery of the programme, and are associated with summative or outcome evaluation. Internal evaluations are conducted by staff or other people involved with a project *(100)*. The association of outcome evaluation with an external evaluator – owing to the belief that external evaluations give more credible results – has been challenged. On the one hand, Campbell *(79)* claims that the trustworthiness of scientific reports does not come from the indifference of the researcher to the hypotheses under study; "competitive cross-validation", a process in which validation comes from the replication of results by other researchers, leads researchers to be critical of their own results. On the other hand, examining the actual practice of evaluation, Mathison *(101)* concludes that, although rarer than external outcome evaluations, internal outcome evaluations do not seem to lack credibility.

In addition, the health literature makes a distinction between internal and external evaluation, although formulating it differently. The double-blind standard for conducting clinical research *(102)* certainly calls for separating the evaluation resources as much as possible from the intervention. Surprisingly, the literature on community health promotion programmes says nothing about the coordinating features and relationships that should exist between programmes' intervention and the evaluation components. Mittelmark *(35)* comes closest to discussing these issues by describing the possible forms of relationships between citizens and academic researchers in community trials. As Mittelmark refers to the Minnesota Heart Health Program, in which academic researchers led both the intervention and the evaluation components, it is difficult to extrapolate his comments to evaluators' relationship with the intervention of a community programme.

The latest trend in the evaluation literature is towards encouraging evaluators to work as closely as possible with the various programme's stakeholders in general *(57)*, and even more closely with the intervention team *(103)*. Patton *(57)* calls for maximum collaboration between the intervention and the evaluation in four steps in the evaluation effort:

1. establishing the focus of the evaluation and formulating the questions
2. making decisions on the design and measurement options
3. reviewing the measurement instruments and data collection plan
4. interpreting the results of the analyses.

More recently, building on the principles of participatory research and on Cronbach's claim that "the evaluator is an educator; his [or her] success is to be judged by what others learn" *(104)*, Fawcett et al. *(105)* have presented the evaluation of community programmes as an empowerment initiative; academic evaluators act as a support team that assists a community in the different components of an evaluation through a series of "related enabling activities". In addition to providing programme information, empowerment evaluation is a capacity-building process that is collaborative (in that the support team responds to the needs of the community), interactive (in that the initial planning is allowed to evolve in reaction to the information the evaluation feeds back into the system) and iterative (in that success in completing one cycle of evaluation contributes to the launching of another).

Guidelines and recommendations

Evaluators can adopt a wide range of possible roles. Depending on their background and epistemological beliefs, evaluators will position themselves differently in relationship to programmes. Positivist evaluators tend to distance themselves as much as possible. They maintain minimal and instrumental contact with the intervention component. At the other end of the spectrum, constructivist and critical evaluators try to understand the programme from within. They maintain close and frequent contact with the intervention, often take part in modifying it and, like everybody else involved, are ready to be changed by their experience with the programme *(103)*. In principle, we agree that such a spectrum of relationships between the evaluators and the programmes can be found in programme evaluation. We contend, however, that the features of community programmes constrain the range of relationships an evaluator can maintain with the community, to produce valid evaluation results and to contribute to programmes' sustainability.

Brown *(31)* suggests that, in addition to the traditional methodological expertise, most of the new roles evaluators have taken when working with community programmes serve to bridge the gap between the evaluator and the activity. They develop strategies of engagement. She provides four reasons for adopting such an approach:

1. to demystify and democratize the knowledge development process;
2. to help position evaluation as an integral part of the programme;
3. to enhance community understanding, stakeholder commitment and use of the results; and
4. to provide the evaluator with contextual knowledge of the participants and thus increase the relevance of the results.

To these we add a fifth: to ensure the validity of the results. The evaluation of community programmes depends on the participation of many actors in the community, from programme staff to local organizations and individual survey participants. Wide participation is crucial to obtain valid results, and this participation cannot be secured unless everyone involved with the programme values the evaluation component.

Our discussion of the issues pertaining to the five domains of the evaluation of community programmes indicates that evaluators should offer methodological expertise, stimulate participation and lead negotiations for the identification of the evaluation questions, transfer part of their expertise (so that communities can use the information produced) and assist communities to develop their own agendas. According to Brown *(31)*, evaluators need to develop pedagogical and political skills and the ability to gain stakeholders' interest and trust. We add negotiation skills to the list. Reaching the goal of implementing a sustainable and effective community programme requires continuous and open negotiation involving the evaluation and intervention components and the community itself. The success of this process depends entirely on all parties' acknowledgement that everyone's contributions are essential. This can only happen when all members of the partnership are equal and take equal responsibility for the programme's success.

Redefining rigour

The evaluation of community health promotion programmes raises challenging issues for the scientific community. Although evaluations of community programmes have produced a wealth of data that have helped scientists understand the secular trends of major cardiovascular risk factors *(106)*, this kind of study still presents difficulties that exceed their ability to adapt their scientific creed to situations such as community trials. When researchers are able to show positive results, these are not convincing and usually fall within the range of random variation from the secular trends *(106)*. Maybe the problem lies in the creed. Reflecting on the lack of positive results from community trials using experimental or quasi-experimental methods, Susser *(14)* notes:

> trials may not provide the truest reflection of the questions researchers intend to pose and answer. Still, faith in the randomized controlled trial is so firm among epidemiologists, clinical scientists, and journals that it may justly be described as a shibboleth, if not a religion. Science, like freedom, dies of dogma; subversion is its lifeblood. We need a more rounded and complex perspective. ... Observational studies have a place as epidemiological armament no less necessary and valid than controlled trials; they take second place in a hierarchy of rigor, but not in praticability and generalizability. One can go further. Even when trials are possible, observational studies may yield more truth than randomized trials. In the population sciences, of which epidemiology is one, generalizability requires deep penetration of the world as it is, usually with an unavoidable loss of rigor.

Scientists should thus welcome any opportunity to increase their knowledge of "what kinds of community approaches have which kinds of effects" *(107)*. Because they represent unique opportunities for learning about health promotion processes, community programmes should always be coupled with some kind of evaluation effort. Variations in the scope and magnitude of these studies will be an indicator of the health and productivity of the health promotion field as a domain of scientific inquiry. Researchers should thus remember that no single study can provide a definitive answer to any scientific inquiry, so they should set more modest goals and realistic expectations for the significance of the results of their evaluation studies. Acknowledging also that a little knowledge is always better than none, researchers and public health practitioners should realize that even very small inquiries, using meagre resources, have the potential to contribute significant information.

Recommendations and conclusion

Defining rigour as the systematic, lucid and critical appraisal of the relationship between an observer and the empirical world, rather than the blind application of some kind of methodological recipe, we echo Susser in urging an increased use of observational methods for the evaluation of community programmes. The issues discussed in this chapter are useful for the planning of both observational and manipulative approaches to the evaluation of community programmes. We strongly believe that the level of skills and expertise necessary to conduct this kind of evaluation can vary according to the scope of the evaluation questions. What cannot vary, however, is the critical perspective that researchers need to adopt towards their results. The phenomenon under study is too complex to yield easy solutions, and creativity should be the highest priority. In the light of the discussion above, we offer five recommendations for the development of high-quality evaluations of community health promotion programmes.

First, evaluation efforts should be encouraged whenever community health promotion programmes are developed and implemented. They present invaluable opportunities for learning about complex health promotion processes. As no single study, regardless of its methodological strengths, can ever provide a definitive answer to a scientific inquiry, variability in the scope and magnitude of evaluation studies should be welcome.

Evaluation's contribution to both local and generalizable knowledge should be recognized. Most decisions about funding and continuing programmes are based on local knowledge generated by process and outcome evaluations. To provide such knowledge, evaluation must be part of the programme. A systematic information feedback mechanism allows practitioners and decision-makers to adjust interventions according to the reactions observed in the targeted communities. Evaluators must therefore maintain contact with programme staff and their information needs. In turn, programme staff should receive relevant information in a timely and regular fashion. We do not, however, find the monitoring role of evaluation incompatible with the production of more generalizable knowledge. Indeed, all empirical knowledge is primarily local (108). Local knowledge gains acceptance as scientific and generalizable through a process of critical replication (79).

Funding agencies should encourage evaluators to expand their research to produce more generalizable knowledge. Basing programmes and their evaluations on existing models and theories makes this process easier. Scientific journals should publish papers that elucidate the underlying mechanisms of programme effectiveness, even if such studies are not always able to rule out plausible rival hypotheses owing to methodological limitations. These results could then become a starting point for other programmes, and their generalizability could be tested.

Second, the insistence on randomization as the only process capable of ensuring valid knowledge about health promotion community interventions should be seriously questioned. In fact, even the more flexible quasi-experimental designs might not be the most appropriate forms of inquiry for community programmes. Twenty years of research have shown that experimental and quasi-experimental evaluations of community programmes are barely able to demonstrate positive results of state-of-the-art community programmes (4); even when positive results were detected, they were generally within the range of random variations from the secular trends (106). Perhaps community programmes cannot significantly add to the secular trends. Before accepting such a discouraging conclusion, however, one should first question the methods used to reach such a conclusion.

There is a gap between the conditions for which experimental and quasi-experimental methods were developed and those in which community programmes operate. These methods work best when the experimenter controls the treatment, its delivery and the context. This control is required to isolate the causal relationship under study. By definition, however, community programmes operate in complex and changing contexts. Using controls, as required by experimental and quasi-experimental methods, carries the cost of oversimplifying the programmes and their relationships to the contexts in which they operate. Owing to this important gap, one cannot rule out the hypothesis that community programmes are effective, despite scientists' inability to measure and to assess their effectiveness.

Ways of studying complex relationships in complex environments usually involve systematic observation, with or without modifications of some of the environmental conditions. We admit, however, that knowledge resulting from this kind of methodology is based on more circumstantial evidence than that of controlled experiment, and therefore that reasonably reliable scientific claims can be constructed only from the convergence of a greater amount of such evidence (14). Nevertheless, given the poor record of controlled experiments for evaluating community programmes, the use of alternative methodologies should be encouraged. The results of such studies should then be used to elaborate models that deepen understanding of the mechanisms of effective community programmes.

Third, funding agencies should invest in the development of community-level indicators of health promotion processes. By definition, direct contact with targeted individuals and educational processes are not the only means through which community programmes are thought to be effective. Recent papers on the ecological perspective on health and health promotion point to implementation of diverse and complementary approaches as an effective strategy to improve health and to increase individuals' and communities' control over their wellbeing and its determinants (24,109). Some of these approaches clearly have a direct impact only on the community and environmental features, and therefore reach individuals indirectly. To conduct fair evaluations of complex programmes whose interventions aim at various community, social and environmental features, evaluators must use indicators of health promotion processes occurring at these various levels. Our review shows the paucity of

232

such indicators. Most of those used in the evaluation of community programmes are individual-level indicators aggregated for a targeted population. There is an urgent need to develop better indicators to assess the processes that community programmes are believed to trigger.

Fourth, the role and the impact of community participation in the evaluation of community programmes need close examination. As such participation is a fundamental condition for the planning and implementation of effective community programmes, it should be present in most of them. Because of its empowering role, community participation is likely to influence and interact with the evaluation process in important ways. Advocates of participatory research even argue that such participation is necessary to ensure the validity of the results. How this confers validity, however, remains unclear; there is a dearth of empirical data on the impact of community participation on validity. In conclusion, funding agencies should consider researching the research process itself.

Our discussion of methodological issues related to the evaluation of community health promotion programmes aims at reflecting the issues and problems debated in the current literature. The fact that most of the literature focuses on issues related to outcome evaluation and its related statistical problems indicates that epidemiologists and statisticians have shown the most interest in the evaluation of community health promotion interventions. The debate should be broadened to include the practical issues raised by trying to conduct evaluations with minimal research capacity.

References

1. GREEN, L.W. & RAEBURN, J. Contemporary developments in health promotion: definitions and challenges. *In*: Bracht, N., ed. *Health promotion at the community level.* Thousand Oaks, Sage, 1990, pp. 29–44.
2. DERENZO, E.G. ET AL. Comprehensive community-based mental health outreach services for suburban seniors. *Gerontologist*, **31**(6): 836–840 (1991).
3. SHEA, S. & BASCH, C.E. A review of five major community-based cardiovascular disease prevention programs. Part II. Intervention strategies, evaluation methods and results. *American journal of health promotion*, **4**: 279–287 (1990).
4. GREEN, L.W. & RICHARD, L. The need to combine health education and health promotion: the case of cardiovascular disease prevention. *Promotion and education*, **11**: 11–17 (1993).
5. KAFTARIAN, S.J. & HANSEN, W.B.. Community Partnership Program Center for Substance Abuse Prevention. *In*: Kaftarian, S.J & Hansen, W.B., ed. *Journal of community psychology. CSAP Special issue*, pp. 3–5 (1994).
6. NCI BREAST CANCER SCREENING CONSORTIUM. Screening mammography: a missed clinical opportunity? Results of the NCI breast cancer

screening consortium and National Health Interview Survey Studies. *Journal of the American Medical Association*, **264**: 54–58 (1990).

7. WAGNER, E.H. ET AL. The evaluation of the Henry J. Kaiser Family Foundation's Community Health Promotion Grant Program: design. *Journal of clinical epidemiology*, **44**: 685–699 (1991).

8. COMMIT RESEARCH GROUP. Community intervention trial for smoking cessation (COMMIT). I. Cohort results from a four-year community intervention. *American journal of public health*, **85**: 183–192 (1995).

9. COMMIT RESEARCH GROUP. Community intervention trial for smoking cessation (COMMIT). II. Changes in adult cigarette smoking prevalence. *American journal of public health*, **85**: 193–200 (1995).

10. O'CONNOR, A. Evaluating comprehensive community initiatives: a view from history. *In*: Connell, J.P. et al., ed. *New approaches to evaluating community initiatives. Concepts, methods and contexts*. New York, Aspen Institute, 1995, pp. 23–69.

11. FARQUHAR, J.W. ET AL. The Stanford Five-City Project: design and method. *American journal of epidemiology*, **122**: 323–334 (1985).

12. LUEPKER, R.V. ET AL. Community education for cardiovascular disease prevention: risk factor changes in the Minnesota Heart Health Program. *American journal of public health*, **84**: 1383–1393 (1994).

13. CARLETON, R.A. ET AL. The Pawtucket Heart Health Program: an experiment in population-based disease prevention. *Rhode Island medical journal*, **70**: 533–538 (1987).

14. SUSSER, M. The tribulations of trials – Interventions in communities. *American journal of public health*, **85**: 156–158 (1995).

15. HELLER, K. The return to community. *American journal of community psychology*, **17**: 1–15 (1989).

16. MCMILLAN, D.W. & CHAVIS, D.M. Sense of community: a definition and theory. *Journal of Community Psychology*, **14**: 6–23 (1986).

17. HAWE, P. Capturing the meaning of "community" in community intervention evaluation: some contributions from community psychology. *Health promotion international*, **9**: 199–210 (1994).

18. GREEN, L.W. & KREUTER, M.M. *Health promotion planning: an educational and environmental approach*, 2nd ed. Mountain View, Mayfield, 1991.

19. GREEN, L.W. & MCALISTER, A.L. Macro-interventions to support health behaviour: some theoretical perspectives and practical reflections. *Health education quarterly*, **11**: 323–339 (1984).

20. FRANKISH, C.J. & GREEN, L.W. Organizational and community change as the social scientific basis for disease prevention and health promotion policy. *Advances in medical sociology*, **4**: 209–233 (1994).

21. ROSE, G. *The strategy of preventive medicine*. Oxford, Oxford University Press, 1992.

22. KUBISH, A.C. ET AL. Introduction. *In*: Connell, J.P. et al., ed. *New approaches to evaluating community initiatives. Concepts, methods and contexts*. New York, Aspen Institute, 1995, pp. 1–21.

23. STOKOLS, D. Establishing and maintaining healthy environments: toward a social ecology of health promotion. *American psychologist*, **47**: 6–22 (1992).

24. GREEN, L.W. ET AL. Ecological foundations of health promotion. *American journal of health promotion,* **10**: 270–281 (1996).

25. THOMPSON, B. & KINNE, S. Social change theory: applications to community health. *In*: Bracht, N., ed. *Health promotion at the community level*. Thousand Oaks, Sage, 1990, pp. 45–65.

26. BRESLOW, L. Foreword. *In*: Bracht, N., ed. *Health promotion at the community level*. Thousand Oaks, Sage, 1990, pp. 11–14.

27. ELDER, J.P. ET AL. Community heart health programs: components, rationale, and strategies for effective interventions. *Journal of public health policy*, **14**: 463–479 (1993).

28. SCHWARTZ, R. ET AL. Capacity building and resource needs of state health agencies to implement community-based cardiovascular disease programs. *Journal of public health policy*, **14**: 480–493 (1993).

29. MITTELMARK, M.B. ET AL. Realistic outcomes: lessons from community-based research and demonstration programs for the prevention of cardiovascular diseases. *Journal of public health policy*, **14**: 437–462 (1993).

30. FARQUHAR, J.W. ET AL. Community studies of cardiovascular disease prevention. *In*: Kaplan, N.M. & Stamler, G., ed. *Prevention of coronary heart disease: practical management of risk factors*. Philadelphia, Saunders, 1983.

31. BROWN, P. The role of the evaluator in comprehensive community initiatives. *In*: Connell, J.P. et al., ed. *New approaches to evaluating community initiatives. Concepts, methods and contexts*. New York, Aspen Institute, 1995, pp. 201–225.

32. BROWN, E.R. Community action for health promotion: a strategy to empower individuals and communities. *International journal of health services*, **21**: 441–456 (1991).

33. MINKLER, M. Improving health through community organization. *In*: Glanz, K. et al., ed. *Health behavior and health education: theory, research and practice*. San Francisco, Jossey-Bass, 1990.

34. BRACHT, N. & KINGBURY, L. Community organization principles in health promotion. A five-stage model. *In*: Bracht, N., ed. *Health promotion at the community level*. Thousand Oaks, Sage, 1990, pp. 66–88.

35. MITTELMARK, M.B. Balancing the requirements of research and the needs of communities. *In*: Bracht, N., ed. *Health promotion at the community level*. Thousand Oaks, Sage, 1990, pp. 125–139.

36. JACOBS, D.R. Community-wide prevention strategies: evaluation design of the Minnesota Heart Health Program. *Journal of chronic disease*, **39**: 775–788 (1986).

37. CHEN, H.T. *Theory-driven evaluation*. Thousand Oaks, Sage, 1990.

38. LIPSEY, M.W. Theory as method: small theories of treatments. *In*: Sechrest, L. et al., ed. *Research methodology: strengthening causal interpretations of nonexperimental data*. Washington, DC, US Department of Health and Human Services, 1990, pp. 33–51.

39. WEISS, C.H. Nothing as practical as good theory: exploring theory-based evaluation for comprehensive community initiatives for children and families. *In*: Connell, J.P. et al., ed. *New approaches to evaluating community initiatives: concepts, methods and contexts*. New York, Aspen Institute, 1995, pp. 65–92.

40. LEFEBVRE, R.C. ET AL. Theory and delivery of health programming in the community: the Pawtucket Heart Health Program. *Preventive medicine*, **16**: 80–95 (1987).

41. CHEADLE, A. ET AL. An empirical exploration of a conceptual model for community-based health promotion. *International quarterly of community health education*, **13**: 329–363 (1993).

42. KOEPSELL, T.D. ET AL. Selected methodological issues in evaluating community-based health promotion and disease prevention programs. *Annual review of public health*, **13**: 31–57 (1992).

43. NUTBEAM, D. ET AL. Evaluation in health education: a review of progress, possibilities, and problems. *Journal of epidemiology and community health*, **44**: 83–89 (1990).

44. SALONEN, J.T. ET AL. Analysis of community-based cardiovascular disease prevention studies – Evaluation issues in the North Karelia Project and the Minnesota Heart Health Program. *International journal of epidemiology*, **15**: 176–182 (1986).

45. POTVIN, L. ET AL. Le paradoxe de l'évaluation des programmes communautaires multiples de promotion de la santé. *Ruptures, revue transdisciplinaire en santé*, **1**: 45–57 (1994).

46. CARLETON, R.A. ET AL. The Pawtucket Heart Health Program: community changes in cardiovascular risk factors and projected disease risk. *American journal of public health*, **85**: 777–785 (1995).

47. KIM, S. ET AL. An innovative and unconventional approach to program evaluation in the field of substance abuse prevention: a threshold-gating approach using single system evaluation designs. *In*: Kaftarian, S.J & Hansen, W.B., ed. *Journal of community psychology. CSAP Special issue*, pp. 61–78 (1994).

48. POTVIN, L. Methodological challenges in evaluation of dissemination programs. *Canadian journal of public health*, **87**(Suppl. 2): S79–S83 (1996).

49. ALTMAN, D.G. A framework for evaluating community-based heart disease prevention programs. *Social science and medicine*, **22**: 479–487 (1986).

50. GOODMAN, R.M. & WANDERSMAN, A. FORECAST: a formative approach to evaluating community coalitions and community-based initiatives. *In*: Kaftarian, S.J & Hansen, W.B., ed. *Journal of community psychoogy. CSAP special issue*, pp. 6–25 (1994).

51. FORTMANN, S.P. ET AL. Community intervention trials: reflections on the Stanford Five-City Project experience. *American journal of epidemiology*, **142**: 576–586 (1995).

52. BRAVERMAN, M.T. & CAMPBELL, D.T. Facilitating the development of health promotion programs: recommendations for researchers and funders. *In*: Braverman, M.T., ed. *Evaluating health promotion programs*. San Francisco, Jossey-Bass, 1989 (New Directions for Program Evaluation, No. 43), pp. 5–18.

53. ROSSI, P.H. & FREEMAN, II.E. *Evaluation. a systematic approach*, 4th ed. Thousand Oaks, Sage, 1989.

54. WEISS, C.H. Evaluation for decisions. Is there anybody there? Does anybody care? *Evaluation practice*, **9**(1): 15 20 (1988).

55. WEISS, C.H. If program decisions hinged only on information: a response to Patton. *Evaluation practice*, **9**(3), 15–28 (1988).

56. CAMPBELL, D.T. Guidelines for monitoring the scientific competence of prevention intervention research centers. *Knowledge: creation, diffusion, utilization*, **8**: 389–430 (1987).

57. PATTON, M.Q. *Qualitative evaluation methods*. Beverly Hills, Sage, 1980.

58. PIRIE, P.L. Evaluating health promotion programs. Basic questions and approaches. *In*: Bracht, N., ed. *Health promotion at the community level*. Thousand Oaks, Sage, 1990, pp. 201–208.

59. REASON, P. Three approaches to participative inquiry. *In*: Denzin, N.K. & Lincoln, Y.S., ed. *Handbook of qualitative research*. Thousand Oaks, Sage, 1994, pp. 324–339.

60. McTAGGART, R. Principles of participatory action research. *Adult education quarterly*, **41**(3): 168–187 (1991).

61. LATHER, P. Research as praxis. *Harvard educational review*, **56**: 257–277 (1986).

62. GREEN, L.W. ET AL. *Study of participatory research in health promotion. Review and recommendations for the development of participatory research in health promotion in Canada*. Ottawa, Royal Society of Canada, 1995.

63. CAMPBELL, D.T. & STANLEY, J.C. *Experimental and quasi-experimental designs for research*. Chicago, Rand McNally, 1963.

64. MAO, Y. ET AL. The impact of the decreases prevalence of smoking in Canada. *Canadian journal of public health*, **83**: 413–416 (1992).

237

65. GIOVINO, G.A. ET AL. Surveillance for selected tobacco-use behaviors – United States, 1990–1994. *Mortality and morbidity weekly report*, **43**(3): 1–43 (1994).

66. RUBIN, D.B. Estimating causal effects of treatments in randomized and nonrandomized studies. *Journal of educational psychology*, **66**: 688–701 (1974).

67. GREEN, S.B. Interplay between design and analysis for behavioral intervention trials with community as the unit of randomization. *American journal of epidemiology*, **142**: 587–593 (1995).

68. KOEPSELL, T.D. ET AL. Invited commentary: symposium on community intervention trials. *American journal of epidemiology*, **142**: 594–599 (1995).

69. COOK, T.D. ET AL. Randomized and quasi-experimental designs in evaluation research. *In*: Rutman, L., ed. *Evaluation research methods*. Beverly Hills, Sage, 1977, pp. 103–135.

70. CRONBACH, L.J. Beyond the two disciplines of scientific psychology. *American psychologist*, **30**: 116–127 (1975).

71. JACKSON, C. ET AL. Evaluating community-level health promotion and disease prevention interventions. *In*: Braverman, M.T., ed. *Evaluating health promotion programs*. San Francisco, Jossey-Bass, 1989 (New Directions for Program Evaluation, No. 43), pp. 19–32.

72. NIKNIAN, M. ET AL. Are people more health conscious? A longitudinal study of one community. *American journal of public health*, **81**: 205–207 (1991).

73. NUTBEAM, D. ET AL. Maintaining evaluation designs in long term community based health promotion programmes: Heartbeat Wales case study. *Journal of epidemiology and community health*, **47**: 127–133 (1993).

74. COOK, T.D. & CAMPBELL, D.T. *Quasi-experimentation: design and analysis issues for field settings*. Chicago, Rand McNally, 1979.

75. PIRIE, P.L. ET AL. Program evaluation strategies for community-based health promotion programs: perspectives from the cardiovascular disease community research and demonstration studies. *Health education research*, **9**: 23–36 (1994).

76. SPRINGER, J.F & PHILLIPS, J.L. Policy learning and evaluation design: lessons from the Community Partnership Demonstration Program. *In*: Kaftarian, S.J & Hansen, W.B., ed. *Journal of community psychology. CSAP special issue*, pp. 117–139 (1994).

77. RATCLIFFE, J.W. & GONZALEZ-DEL-VALLE, A. Rigor in health-related research: toward an expanded conceptualization. *International journal of health services*, **18**: 361–392 (1988).

78. SHADISH, W.R. ET AL. Quasi-experimentation in a critical multiplist mode. *In*: Trochim, W.M.K., ed. *Advances in quasi-experimental design and analysis*. San Francisco, Jossey-Bass, 1986 (New Directions for Program Evaluation, No. 31), pp. 29–46.

79. CAMPBELL, D.T. Can we be scientific in applied social science? *In*: Connor, R.F. et al., ed. *Evaluation Studies Review Annual, Vol. 9*. Beverly Hills, Sage, 1984, pp. 26–48.

80. BEST, J.A. ET AL. Conceptualizing outcomes for health promotion programs. *In*: Braverman, M.T., ed. *Evaluating health promotion programs*. San Francisco, Jossey-Bass, 1989 (New Directions for Program Evaluation, No. 43), pp. 33–45.

81. HOLLISTER, R.G. & HILL, J. Problems in evaluating community-wide initiatives. *In*: Connell, J.P. et al., ed. *New approaches to evaluating community initiatives. Concepts, methods and contexts*. New York, Aspen Institute, 1995, pp.127–172.

82. CHEADLE, A. ET AL. Environmental indicators: a tool for evaluating community-based health-promotion programs. *American journal of preventive medicine*, **8**: 345–350 (1992).

83. WICKISER, T.M. ET AL. Activating communities for health promotion: a process evaluation method. *American journal of public health*, **83**: 561–567 (1993).

84. COHEN, R.Y. ET AL. Measuring community change in disease prevention and health promotion. *Preventive medicine*, **15**(4): 411–421 (1986).

85. CHEADLE, A. ET AL. Evaluating community-based nutrition programs: comparing grocery store and individual-level survey measures of program impact. *Preventive medicine*, **24**(1): 71–79 (1995).

86. FARQUHAR, J.W. ET AL. Community education for cardiovascular health. *Lancet*, **1**: 1192–1195 (1977).

87. PUSKA, P. ET AL. *The North Karelia Project. Community control of cardiovascular diseases. Evaluation of a comprehensive programme for control of cardiovascular diseases in North Karelia, Finland, 1972–1977*. Copenhagen, WHO Regional Office for Europe, 1981.

88. NUTBEAM, D. & CATFORD, J. The Welsh Heart Programme evaluation strategy: progress, plans and possibilities. *Health promotion international*, **2**: 5–18 (1987).

89. FELDMAN, H.A. & MCKINLAY, S.M. Cohort versus cross-sectional design in large fields trials: precision, sample size, and a unifying model. *Statistics in medicine*, **13**: 61–78 (1994).

90. DIEHR, P. ET AL. Optimal survey design for community-intervention evaluations: cohort or cross-sectional? *Journal of clinical epidemiology*, **48**: 1461–1472 (1995).

91. FRENK, J. ET AL. Elements for a theory of the health transition. *In*: Chen, L.C. et al., ed. *Health and social change in international perspective*. Boston, Harvard University Press, 1994, pp. 25–49.

92. CORNFIELD, J. Randomization by group: a formal analysis. *American journal of epidemiology*, **108**: 103–111 (1978).

93. DONNER, A. ET AL. A methodological review of non-therapeutic intervention trials employing cluster randomization, 1979–1989. *International journal of epidemiology*, **19**: 795–800 (1990).

239

94. DONNER, A. ET AL. Randomization by cluster: sample size requirements and analysis. *American Journal of Epidemiology*, **114**: 906–914 (1981).

95. MURRAY, D.M. Design and analysis of community trials: lessons from the Minnesota Heart Health Program. *American journal of epidemiology*, **142**: 569–575 (1995).

96. GOLDSTEIN, H. *Multilevel models in educational and social research.* London, Charles Griffin, 1987.

97. BRYK, A.S. & RAUDENBUSH, S.W. *Hierarchical linear models in social and behavioral research: applications and data analysis methods.* Newbury Park, Sage, 1992.

98. KOEPSELL, T.D. ET AL. Data analysis and sample size issued in evaluation of community-based health promotion and disease prevention programs: a mixed-model analysis of variance approach. *Journal of clinical epidemiology*, **44**: 701–713 (1991).

99. MURRAY, D.M. ET AL. Design and analysis issues in community trials. *Evaluation review*, **18**: 493–51418

100. SCRIVEN, M. *Evaluation thesaurus.* Inverness, Edgepress, 1980.

101. MATHISON, S. What do we know about internal evaluation? *Evaluation and program planning*, **14**: 159–165 (1991).

102. FRIEDMAN, L.M. ET AL. *Fundamentals of clinical trials*, 2nd ed. Littleton, PSG, 1985.

103. MATHISON, S. Rethinking the evaluator role: partnerships between organizations and evaluators. *Evaluation and program planning*, **17**: 299–304 (1994).

104. CRONBACH, L.J. Our ninety-five theses. *In*: Freeman, H.E. & Solomon, M.A., ed. *Evaluation studies review annual, Vol. 6.* Beverly Hills, Sage, 1981.

105. FAWCETT, S.B. ET AL. Empowering community health initiatives through evaluation. *In*: Fetterman, D.M. et al., ed. *Empowerment evaluation. Knowledge and tools for self-assessment and accountability.* Thousand Oaks, Sage, 1996, pp. 161–187.

106. WINKLEBY, M. The future of community-based cardiovascular disease intervention studies. *American journal of public health*, **84**: 1369–1372 (1994).

107. FISHER, E.B. The results of the COMMIT trial. *American journal of public health*, **85**: 159–160 (1995).

108. CAMPBELL, D.T. Relabelling internal and external validity for applied social scientists. *In*: Trochim, W.M.K., ed. *Advances in quasi-experimental design and analysis.* San Francisco, Jossey-Bass, 1986 (New Directions for Program Evaluation, No. 31), pp. 67–77.

109. RICHARD, L. ET AL. Assessment of the integration of the ecological approach in health promotion. *American journal of health promotion*, **10**: 318–328 (1996).

11

Evaluating community initiatives for health and development

Stephen B. Fawcett, Adrienne Paine-Andrews,
Vincent T. Francisco, Jerry Schultz, Kimber P. Richter,
Jannette Berkley-Patton, Jacqueline L. Fisher,
Rhonda K. Lewis, Christine M. Lopez, Stergios Russos,
Ella L. Williams, Kari J. Harris and Paul Evensen[3]

Introduction

Throughout the world, local people and organizations come together to address issues that matter to them. For example, community partnerships have formed to reduce substance abuse and violence *(1,2)*, to lower the risks of adolescent pregnancy, HIV/AIDS and cardiovascular diseases *(3–5)* and to prevent child abuse and neglect, domestic violence and injury *(6–8)*. Local collaborative efforts to promote health and development may be part of global trends in building democracy and decentralization *(9)*.

Community initiatives, such as those to reduce adolescent substance abuse or promote the wellbeing of older adults, attempt to improve health and development outcomes for all people who share a common place or experience *(10,11)*. Prevention efforts often use both universal approaches – for all those potentially affected – and targeted approaches – for those with multiple markers that put them at higher risk *(12,13)*. They aim to change the behaviour of large numbers of people, such as drug use or physical inactivity, and the conditions in which the behaviour occurs, such as the availability of drugs or lack of safe recreational areas *(14)*.

Community health promotion is a process of development: it "enables people to increase control over, and improve, their health" *(15,16)*. It uses multiple

[3] This chapter is based on work supported by grants to the Work Group on Health Promotion and Community Development at the University of Kansas from the Kansas Health Foundation (9407003D, 9206032B and 9206038B), the Ewing Kauffman Foundation (95-410), the Greater Kansas City Community Foundation, the Robert Wood Johnson Foundation and the John D. and Catherine T. MacArthur Foundation. We appreciate the support of Rachel Wydeven, of the Work Group on Health Promotion and Community Development at the University of Kansas, United States, in preparing this manuscript, and offer special thanks to colleagues from communities who continue to teach us about how better to understand and strengthen community initiatives for health and development.

strategies, such as providing information and modifying access, and operates at multiple levels, including families and organizations, and through a variety of community sectors, such as schools, businesses and religious organizations. It aims to make small but widespread changes in health by transforming the environments in which health-related behaviour occurs *(17)*. The goal is to promote healthy behaviour by making it easier to adopt and more likely to be reinforced. Models for promoting community health and development include the Healthy Cities/Healthy Communities model, the PRECEDE/PROCEED model, the Planned Approach to Community Health (PATCH) and others *(12,18–20)*. Community-based efforts to prevent cardiovascular diseases, for example, engage local people in changing the environment in which they make choices about diet, tobacco use and physical activity *(5)*. Although evidence of effectiveness is somewhat limited, these and other community approaches aim to increase opportunities for local people to work together to improve health and development outcomes and the quality of life.

The process of community development requires the fullest possible reliance on indigenous resources to identify and address local concerns *(21–24)*. In the Declaration of Alma-Ata, WHO embraced a community development approach to health promotion *(15,16)*. Such efforts support local participation in health promotion *(25)*. Although community-oriented approaches to public health are usually implemented in neighbourhoods, towns and cities, they may be encouraged and coordinated at the broader levels of provinces, regions or countries.

Community-based funding promotes community, not researcher, control of interventions *(12)*; funds are awarded to communities to address local concerns and often to researchers to support local efforts and help discover what is working. Information on the effectiveness of community-based initiatives is modest, however, since evaluation practice has yet fully to catch up with this innovation in community practice. Although models are available for studying community health efforts at the organizational and community levels *(26–28)*, the research methods used are often borrowed from clinical trials and other researcher-controlled models of inquiry *(12)*.

Several models and traditions inform the practice of community evaluation (see chapters 2, 4, 10 and 15). Action anthropology *(29)* refers to the use of research to facilitate empowerment in local communities. Qualitative research *(30)* highlights the value of the experience of those studied in understanding the meaning of the effort. Participatory action research *(31,32)* uses dialogue to produce knowledge and to inform action to help a group or community. Similarly, empowerment evaluation *(33,34)* aims to assess the merit of the effort while enhancing community capacity and self-determination. These and other varieties of action research *(35)* and action science *(36)* engage local people in designing and conducting the inquiry, and in interpreting the meaning of the results. The various approaches to community evaluation highlight different balances between the potentially competing ends of understanding and empowerment. They underscore the tension between experimenter and community control in the methods of community intervention and inquiry.

Evaluation can strengthen efforts to promote health and development at the community level *(33,37)*. First, descriptive data about process and outcome can contribute to the understanding of how community initiatives develop over time. Second, providing continuous feedback on progress can improve implementation and encourage adjustments in this open and adaptive system *(38,39)*. Third, engaging local people in the evaluation process may strengthen the capacity of marginalized groups to understand and improve local efforts. Finally, better documentation of community initiatives can help ensure the accountability of implementers to communities and funding agencies and of funding agencies to the communities that they serve. As communities receive more responsibility for addressing their health and development concerns, the demand for community evaluation increases.

This chapter presents models, methods and applications of community evaluation in understanding and improving community initiatives for health and development. We outline some challenges in evaluating community initiatives, describe a model of the community initiative as a catalyst for change, and discuss some principles, assumptions and values that guide community evaluation. Then we outline a logic model for system of community evaluation that we use in the Work Group for Health Promotion and Community Development at the University of Kansas, describe an example that draws on our field experience in the United States, outline key questions related to philosophical, conceptual, methodological, practical, political and ethical issues and offer specific recommendations on how practitioners and policy-makers can address these issues. Finally, the closing discussion examines broad issues and opportunities in evaluating health and development initiatives at the community level.

Challenges to community evaluation

Despite the potential benefits, evaluating community initiatives for health and development poses 12 serious challenges.

1. The determinants of many societal and public health problems, such as substance abuse or violence, are poorly understood, making it difficult to identify appropriate interventions and indicators of success.
2. Key constructs, such as community capacity or quality of life (see Chapter 6), are ambiguous, making the detection of changes in important processes and outcomes a formidable task *(33,40)*.
3. The complexity of community initiatives makes it daunting to describe the intervention in sufficient detail to the permit replication of effects *(33,41)*.
4. The lack of reliable and valid community-level measures of outcome for community concerns such as child abuse or domestic violence makes it difficult to assess the effects of an initiative *(42)*.

243

5. The ultimate outcomes of community efforts, such as those to reduce risk for cardiovascular diseases or HIV/AIDS, may be delayed for a decade or more, necessitating the identification of measures of intermediate outcome, such as changes in the community or system *(12,38,40)*.
6. Estimating the intensity of community-driven interventions may be impossible without more precise information on the type of component implemented, who was exposed to it and for how long.
7. Data aggregated for individuals may not permit analysis of impact at the community level *(43)*.
8. The absence of suitable experimental designs or appropriate comparisons may make it difficult to attribute observed effects to the community initiative, and not to some other variables *(44,45)*.
9. The evolving and adaptive nature of community initiatives, with resulting implications for the fidelity of implementation, may make it difficult to assess the general applicability of effects *(41,46,47)*.
10. Participatory evaluation must guard against potential confusion resulting from conflicting interpretations from multiple sources *(46,48,49)*.
11. Broader goals for the evaluation – contributing to both understanding and empowerment, and related increased responsibilities – may make it difficult to meet standards for feasibility *(33,50)*.
12. It may be difficult to reconcile the competing goals of evaluation – such as assessing merit and enhancing community control – in the same endeavour *(33,37,49)*.

Despite the challenges, some models and principles may help guide the practice of community evaluation.

The community initiative as a catalyst for change

Although the missions and specific interventions may vary, many community initiatives for health and development use a common model or framework: that of the initiative as a catalyst for change *(40)*. Such initiatives attempt to transform relevant sectors of the community: changing programmes, policies and practices to make healthy behaviour more likely for large numbers of people. Fig. 11.1 displays the several nonlinear and interrelated elements of this catalyst model, adapted from earlier models *(12,19)* and based on theories of empowerment *(40)*.

This model is nonlinear in that community partnerships engage in multiple and interrelated activities simultaneously. A new initiative to reduce the risk of violence in young people, for example, may refine its plans for action while pursuing highly visible and relatively easily achieved changes, such as posting billboards that describe the negative consequences of gang-related activity or arranging alternative activities that promote connections between young people and caring adults.

244

Fig. 11.1. The community initiative as a catalyst for change

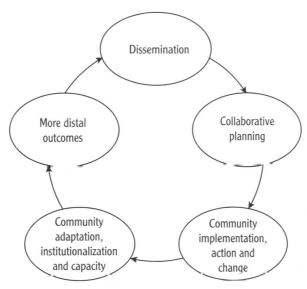

Source: adapted from Fawcett et al. *(26).*

The five components of the model are interrelated. Collaborative planning should identify specific model components and community changes to be sought, thereby guiding community action and change. Key components may be adapted to fit local conditions and sustained through policy change, publicly supported programmes or other means of institutionalization *(51)*. A pattern of successful change should increase the community's capacity to create additional changes related to the mission, which may in turn affect more distal health outcomes. Successful initiatives or components may be disseminated for adoption and adaptation by other communities addressing similar concerns *(47)*.

The goals and expectations of community initiatives vary. A community may attempt to address a single mission, such as increasing physical activity or improving diets, or multiple ends, such as reducing child abuse and domestic violence, that may share common risk and protective factors. Some communities have a relatively free hand in selecting locally appropriate interventions. Funding agencies may require other partnerships to replicate tried and true strategies or interventions based on research and development efforts *(52)*. Hybrid approaches may combine model replication and catalyst roles by implementing core components, such as sexuality education and peer support for preventing adolescent pregnancy, as well as developing new community or systems changes related to desired outcomes, such as increasing access to contraceptives *(53)*.

Components of community interventions should be expected to evolve and be reinvented by their users *(47)*. To deliver an intervention component of

245

supervised alternative activities for adolescents, for example, communities may use a variety of different programme elements, such as recreational opportunities, summer jobs or community gardens. Locally controlled adaptation may facilitate community ownership, help ensure that components are institutionalized and build capacity for self-determined change.

Consistent with the principles of social marketing *(54)* and diffusion *(47)*, key components of successful community programmes or the entire innovation may be disseminated in the later stages. For example, comprehensive interventions for reducing the risk of cardiovascular diseases or specific components, such as increasing access to low-fat foods, might be actively disseminated. Potential adopters need to know what works, what does not and what are the best conditions for implementation. This helps connect local efforts to the lessons learned from other community-based projects and the best or most promising practices suggested by experience and research.

Principles, assumptions and values of community evaluation

Some principles, assumptions and values underpin the process of evaluating community initiatives for health and development. They reflect the challenges of addressing seemingly contradictory aims in the same endeavour: contributing to the understanding and effectiveness of community initiatives while fostering community self-determination and capacity to address locally important concerns *(33,41)*. The following ten principles, assumptions and values help guide the work of community evaluation.

1. Community initiatives often function as catalysts for change in which local people and organizations work together to transform the environment for a common purpose *(40)*.
2. They are complex and evolving phenomena that must be analysed at multiple levels *(19)*.
3. They help launch multiple interventions that citizens plan and implement.
4. Community evaluation must understand and reflect the health or development issue addressed, and the context of the community and the initiative *(55)*.
5. Because local initiatives should be planned and implemented with maximum involvement of community members *(10,25)*, community evaluation is a participatory process involving collaboration and negotiation among multiple parties *(31,33,56,57)*.
6. Evaluation activities and resulting data should be linked to questions of importance to key stakeholders, such as community members and funding agencies *(10,58)*.
7. Community evaluation should strengthen local capacities for understanding, improved practice and self-determination.

8. Evaluation should begin early in the development process, offering continuing information and feedback to enhance understanding, improvement and self-determination *(12,33,59,60)*.
9. Evaluation results should help sustain the community initiative by enhancing its ability to secure resources, maintain efforts and celebrate accomplishments *(51,55)*. If the initiative has demonstrated promising outcomes, community evaluation data can be used to promote widespread adoption of the initiative or its components *(47)*.
10. Evaluation should be coupled with technical assistance to provide an integrated support system for increasing the effectiveness of the initiative *(40)*. The enabling activities of a support and evaluation team can assist a community initiative throughout its life-span.

Logic model

Fig. 11.2 depicts the logic model for the Work Group's community evaluation system *(33,61)*. Grounded in the catalyst model described earlier, this framework reflects an attempt to fulfil the ideals of community evaluation. Each phase has products and each product leads to the next.

Initiative phases and evaluation activities

Evaluation and support activities and related products are based on the five-stage, iterative model of the community initiative as a catalyst for change (Fig. 11.1).

Collaborative planning

Agenda setting, determining what issues and options are worthy of consideration, is a particularly powerful aspect of planning in democracies *(62)*. In community initiatives, agendas shape the choice of which issues should be addressed and which related strategies implemented. Assessment tools can be used to gather information about community concerns *(63)* and epidemiological information on health problems *(19)*. Media advocacy *(64)* may assist agenda-building efforts, enabling local people to articulate the health and development issues that matter to them.

Involving a diverse group of local people in collaborative planning is a hallmark of the community development process *(12,23)*. Key support activities include helping the initiative clarify its mission, objectives and strategies. A particularly critical factor in promoting change is developing action plans that identify the specific changes to be sought (and later documented) in all relevant sectors of the community *(65)*. Identifying local assets and resources *(66)* for addressing concerns complements the problem- or deficit-oriented planning activities.

Community implementation, action and change

Evaluation documents the implementation of key elements of community initiatives. It monitors local efforts and accomplishments, documenting changes

Fig. 11.2. Logic model for the documentation and evaluation system of the University of Kansas Work Group on Health Promotion and Community Development

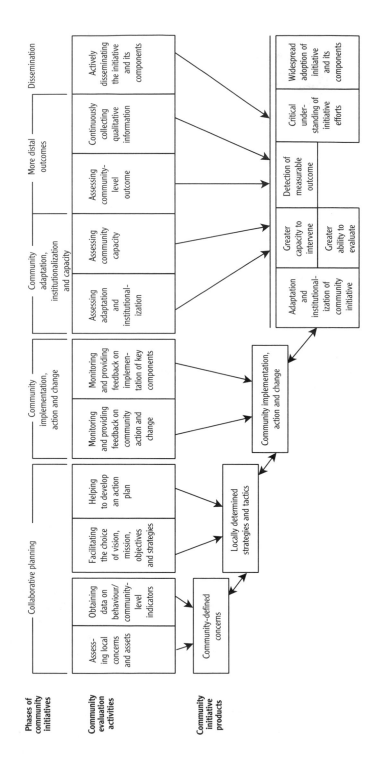

in programmes, policies and practices (community or systems changes) *(38)*. Evaluators provide feedback on process (how components of the intervention were implemented) and intermediate outcome (the number and distribution of community changes). They may also conduct intervention research *(52)* to examine more systematically the effects of particularly promising interventions, such as modifying school lunches to reduce fat and retain energy or providing school-based clinics to increase access to contraceptives.

Community adaptation, institutionalization and capacity

Community evaluators assess the adaptation or reinvention of key initiative components, examining whether adjustments to fit local conditions increase or preserve effectiveness. They also assess the effects of efforts to promote institutionalization through policy change, the adoption of key components by established agencies and other approaches *(51)*. Finally, evaluators help document community capacity: the ability of communities to facilitate important changes and outcomes over time and across concerns.

More distal outcomes

An ultimate goal of most community initiatives is to improve community-level indicators of health and development, such as the incidence of injuries or HIV/AIDS. To detect measurable outcome, community evaluators use quantitative methods such as behavioural surveys (of abstinence or unprotected sexual activity, for example) and records of outcomes (estimated rates of adolescent pregnancy, for example). They also use qualitative methods, such as interviews with key informants or participants, to better their understanding of the meaning and value of the work. When integrated, quantitative and qualitative information contributes to a critical understanding of the initiative's efforts *(67)*.

Community-level outcomes are often too delayed to be useful in fostering the continuous improvement of initiatives. Evaluation should document intermediate outcomes, such as community or systems change. Measuring such change helps detect and amplify information about new programmes, policies and practices that reflect the creation of a healthier environment *(38)*. Future research may help clarify the conditions under which patterns of community change are associated with more distal outcomes *(65)*.

Dissemination

Evaluators help community-based initiatives disseminate information about their effectiveness to relevant audiences, such as community boards and funding agencies. They provide data and interpretative reports about successes and failures, and the factors that may affect the wider adoption of initiatives *(11,47)*. Dissemination activities may include presentations, professional articles, workshops and training, handbooks and communications in the mass media *(68)*.

Products of evaluation, support and development activities

Evaluation and support activities enable local initiatives to produce products, such as community-identified concerns or community change, related to the phases in the process. According to the logic model of community evaluation (see Fig. 11.2), identified community-defined concerns may facilitate (and be influenced by) the development of locally determined strategies and tactics. These, in turn, may guide community implementation, action and change. Key components may be adapted and important community or systems changes may be institutionalized. This may enhance the community's capacity to intervene and to evaluate local efforts, and may result in measurable outcomes and critical understanding of the initiative. This may help promote the widespread adoption of the initiative or its more effective components. The products of evaluation activities may influence each other, as well as the future agenda of community-defined concerns.

Example: evaluating community health initiatives in Kansas

This section outlines a composite case study, drawing on several community health initiatives in the state of Kansas for which we in the Work Group had evaluation and support responsibilities. Their missions included preventing adolescent pregnancy and substance abuse, reducing risks of cardiovascular diseases and some cancers, and promoting health (as determined locally) in rural communities. All the initiatives aimed at building local capacity to address community health concerns.

Background

A variety of communities participated in these initiatives with grant support from the Kansas Health Foundation, a philanthropic organization working to improve health in the state. The communities included cities (such as Wichita, population: 350 000), communities with military bases (such as Geary County, population: 29 638) and prisons (such as Leavenworth County, population: 69 323) and rural communities (such as Dighton, population: 1342).

In one initiative, three Kansas communities responded to a request for proposals to use a model to prevent adolescent pregnancies: the school/community sexual risk reduction model, first used in South Carolina (3,69). Three other communities received grants to establish community coalitions to reduce the risk of adolescent substance use and abuse, using the Project Freedom coalition model (65,70). Another initiative attempted to reduce the risk of cardiovascular diseases and some cancers through a state-wide partnership (71,72) and related school-linked initiatives in several rural communities (73). In a rural health initiative, eight sparsely populated and relatively agrarian Kansas counties received grants to identify and address their health concerns. Each initiative attempted to serve as a catalyst for change by involving local people in dialogue about how best to change community programmes, policies and practices to address locally identified concerns *(26)*. Related task forces or action committees refined and implemented the action plan for each objective by specifying and pursuing the community changes to be sought.

Participants and stakeholders

The participants in these initiatives were community members, leaders and service providers. They included people affected by the programmes' concerns and the leaders of organizations able to facilitate change; various targets of change, such as young people or elected officials whose action or inaction contributed to the problem; and agents of change, such as religious leaders or peers, who could contribute to the solution. Other major stakeholders included members of the steering committees, directors and staff of the community health initiatives, programme officers representing the funding agency and evaluation and support staff of our Work Group at the University of Kansas.

Stakeholder interests in the evaluation included understanding whether the efforts were having an effect and using this information to improve the functioning of the initiative and its specific projects (see Chapter 9). Major stakeholders posed several key questions to be addressed by the community evaluation.

- Is the initiative making a difference?
- Is the initiative serving as a catalyst for change?
- How is the initiative distributing its efforts?
- What factors influence the functioning of the initiative?

The evaluation system used a variety of measurement instruments, such as a documentation or monitoring system, and community-level indicators to address these and other questions *(12,26,33,38,61)*.

Implementation of the model

The remainder of this section describes the application of the catalyst-for-change and community-evaluation logic models (see Fig. 11.1 and 11.2) to community health initiatives in Kansas.

Collaborative planning

Community initiatives often use technical assistance from public agencies or university-based centres to help them identify concerns, and gather and interpret epidemiological data. For example, in the rural health initiative, our Work Group used several means to gather information about local concerns. First, the concerns survey *(63,74)* enabled community members to rate the importance of various health issues and their satisfaction with how each of these issues was being addressed in their community. Data were summarized according to major strengths – issues of high importance and relatively high satisfaction – and relative problems – issues of high importance and relatively

251

low satisfaction. Locally determined rural health issues varied, including such concerns as promoting the health of older adults and preventing substance abuse and adolescent pregnancy.

Second, the Work Group helped local residents conduct informal listening sessions in which members of the community came together to define issues, identify barriers, articulate assets and resources, and brainstorm solutions. Third, we obtained epidemiological data to determine whether the archival records of public health and other relevant agencies substantiated perceived community problems.

Agenda setting involves artistry: local people achieving consensus on a modest set of goals in the face of multiple and diverse community issues and unavailable, inaccurate or insensitive community-level or epidemiological data. Conflicts may arise when the available hard data do not substantiate the importance of issues to the community. For example, although epidemiological data on causes of death may suggest the public health importance of addressing cardiovascular diseases, the legitimacy of other community concerns, such as child abuse or domestic violence, may be contested if supporting data are unavailable. These tensions test the commitment of funding agencies and evaluators to assessing merit and promoting accountability while nurturing community self-determination and capacity.

The Work Group supported action planning in communities. Staff helped each community initiative to form a vision, create a mission, set objectives and develop strategies and action plans. Local people and key leaders in each community sector, such as schools or religious organizations, were encouraged to participate so that a variety of important and feasible changes could be facilitated across all relevant sectors of the community. The Work Group developed practical guides to support action planning for a variety of community health issues, including substance abuse, pregnancy and violence in young people, chronic disease, child abuse and neglect, and health promotion for older adults *(75–80)*. Technical assistance from us enabled each community partnership to identify action plans: specific, locally determined changes in programmes, policies and practices consistent with its vision and mission.

Community implementation, action and change

We worked with programme staff and leaders to document the community changes (new or modified programmes, policies and practices) facilitated by each community partnership. Fig. 11.3 illustrates one key measure of intermediate outcome, the cumulative number of community changes, for a local partnership to prevent adolescent pregnancy. In a cumulative record, each new event (such as a new peer support group or policy change in schools to provide sexuality education) is added to all previous events; a flat line depicts no activity, and a steeper slope shows increased activity or accomplishment over time. Illustrative community changes represented by discrete data points for this initiative included each new programme (such as a mentoring programme), policy (such as increased hours of operation for a school-linked clinic) and practice (such as teachers attending graduate level training on sexuality) facil-itated by the initiative and related to its mission of preventing adolescent preg-nancy. Ratings by community members and outside experts helped inform programme leaders and the funding agency about the importance of such changes. Graphs and regular reports of accomplishments were used to inform stakeholders about the pattern of progress in this intermediate outcome. The Work Group created prototypes for communicating information about the ini-tiative's accomplishments to relevant audiences and provided information on how to incorporate such information in status reports and grant applications to potential funding sources.

Fig. 11.3. Community changes (intermediate outcomes) from work to prevent adolescent pregnancy in Geary County, Kansas, 1993–1996

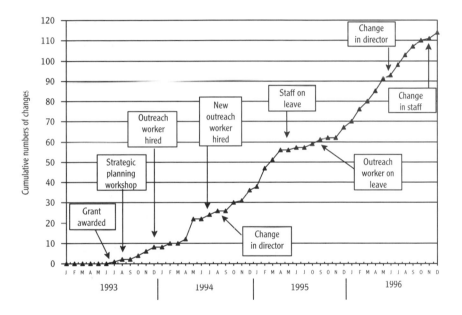

We also documented the implementation of initiatives. For example, we tracked the implementation of sexuality education (for preventing adolescent pregnancy) through teachers' reports and records *(53)*. The Group also col-laborated with initiatives in conducting intervention research studies to deter-mine if the changes caused by the initiatives were having the intended effects. For example, in intervention studies, Lewis et al. *(81)* found that citizen sur-veillance and feedback reduced sales of alcohol and tobacco to minors only when the intervention was fully implemented, and Harris et al. *(82)* found that changes to the school environment led to reduced fat content in school lunches and better eating habits and more physical activity in students.

Community adaptation, institutionalization and capacity

The Work Group used technical assistance and consultation to facilitate necessary adjustments in key components in the school/community model used by Kansas communities to prevent adolescent pregnancy *(53)*. To provide peer support and education, communities implemented a variety of different programme elements, including male-to-male support groups, abstinence clubs and social events for young people. The Work Group examined institutionalization by asking whether new programmes, policies and practices were still in place some months after their initial implementation. We studied community capacity by ascertaining the pattern of community change over time and, where possible, whether high rates of community change were generated for newly emerging health and development concerns.

More distal outcomes

The Work Group obtained data from behavioural surveys and archives to help assess whether changes in the environment were associated with corresponding changes in reported behaviour and community-level indicators. For example, the local initiatives for preventing adolescent substance abuse used school surveys to assess young people's reported use of alcohol, tobacco and drugs. The Work Group gathered data on community-level outcomes, such as rates of adolescent pregnancy, or single nighttime vehicle crashes for initiatives to prevent substance abuse. We examined possible relationships between rates of community change and changes in community-level indicators to help draw inferences about whether the initiative made a difference on more distal outcomes *(26,40,65)*.

Dissemination

The Work Group used local and national presentations, journal articles and book chapters to communicate the results of the work. We also prepared handbooks, such as those for guiding action planning *(40)* and community evaluation *(26,61)*. Staff conducted workshops and training sessions and collaborated with lay opinion leaders *(5)* to help disseminate core elements of the model for community evaluation and support. Finally, our team helped develop a free, Internet-based system, the Community Tool Box (http://ctb.lsi.ukans.edu, accessed 17 May 2000), to disseminate information about promising practices for bringing about community change. The Tool Box provides practical information on strategic planning, advocacy, community evaluation and other methods used by community initiatives for health and development.

Key issues of community evaluation

This section identifies a number of salient issues in evaluating community initiatives for health and development. Our experience and understanding of the literature lead us to organize them under three broad categories (philosophical

254

and conceptual, methodological and practical, and political and ethical) and to frame them as questions categorized according to the ten principles, assumptions and values of community evaluation. In addition, we have linked the questions to the recommendations that follow.

Philosophical and conceptual issues

The process of community health and development raises philosophical issues, such as the proper relationship between researchers and communities and the kinds of knowledge that can and should be obtained and by whom. Similarly, conceptual issues, such as how to define *community* and what theories of change to use, influence the process of understanding and improving community initiatives.

Catalysts for change

What is the theory of change (implicit or explicit) that guides the initiative, and is the evaluation consistent with it (see recommendations 1, 2, 4, 5, 16 and 19–21)?

Complex and evolving phenomena requiring analysis at multiple levels

Are targeted health and development concerns significant to the community? Are they clearly defined, and is the community aware of their level (see recommendations 1, 3 and 24)?

How well does current knowledge explain the determinants of the community issue(s)? What causes do community members and other stakeholders assign? What assumptions and values are implicit in the analysis of the problem, and does the evaluation acknowledge and reflect current knowledge about them (see recommendations 1–3)?

What does current knowledge suggest about how the intervention should balance universal with targeted interventions (see recommendations 1, 4 and 20)?

Multiple interventions planned and implemented by citizens

What is the role of local people as agents for or champions of change in facilitating community or systems change (see recommendations 4 and 10)?

Does the evaluation help document the type and intensity of the community intervention (see recommendations 5, 6, 10, 12 and 16)?

If an intervention model is being replicated, how faithful is the replica to the original? What intervention components are modified and how? Are monitoring systems in place to detect effectiveness over time, especially after adaptation (see recommendations 7, 8 and 16)?

Reflecting the issue and the context

How is *community* defined? How are differences within communities (within neighbourhoods or quadrants of neighbourhoods, for example) reflected in the data and their interpretation? In particular, how are differences among more and less powerful members of the community addressed (see recommendations 1, 3, 15 and 18)?

How is the experience of community members valued alongside the expert knowledge of researchers? When differences in perspective or interpretation arise, how are they reconciled (see recommendations 1, 3, 7, 8, 15 and 18)?

What is the relationship between the community initiative and its larger cultural, historical and community context? How does one account for interactions among context, methods, researchers and community members? How much of the context needs to be understood to design and conduct the intervention and evaluation, and to interpret the results (see recommendations 3, 4, 7, 8, 15 and 16)?

Collaborative and participatory process involving multiple parties

What are the interests and values of the stakeholders involved in the community evaluation? How are they involved in decision-making? What are the stakeholders' visions for the community and its health and development? How are differences in stakeholders' interests, values, purposes and visions reconciled (see recommendations 1, 3, 15, 16 and 18)?

What knowledge and resources (and limitations and barriers) do key stakeholders bring to the initiative (see recommendations 1, 3, 4, 10 and 16)?

What is the purpose of the evaluation: understanding, improvement, empowerment or accountability? Who decides what questions to address and how information will be collected and interpreted? By what process is the research agenda set? Who interprets the meaning of the findings (see recommendation 3)?

Methodological issues

The study of community initiatives for health and development lies at the applied end of the research continuum *(83)*. Basic research and clinical trials use powerful experimental designs (and extensive researcher control) to identify personal and environmental factors that either promote or limit health and development. Traditional methods of selecting participants, such as using random assignment and tight control of the intervention, cannot be used in community-controlled initiatives (see chapters 10 and 14). As collaborative partners, researchers assist in designing new interventions proposed by community members, advise on which interventions or practices to implement and assist in adapting, implementing and evaluating chosen interventions. When building community capacity to address issues of local importance is an aim of such partnerships, maximum researcher control is inapplicable and undesirable (see Chapter 4). The evaluation of community initiatives raises a number of methodological issues.

Complex and evolving phenomena requiring analysis at multiple levels

Do the evaluation measures reflect both personal and environmental contributors to the community concerns? Do evaluation measures reflect the behaviour of actors who are both upstream (such as elected officials) and downstream (such as people affected by the problem) of the causes of the concern (see recommendations 2, 4, 6, 11 and 14)?

What designs will be used to increase confidence in the reliability and generalizability of conclusions? What degree of experimental and researcher control does the design require? How and with whom is the experimental control negotiated (see recommendations 3, 5 and 14)?

Do the measures permit an evaluation at the community level of analysis? How are links established between measures of intermediate outcome (community changes) and of more distal community-level outcomes (see recommendations 6, 14 and 18)?

Multiple interventions planned and implemented by citizens
Does the evaluation help build understanding of the process of development? What aspects of continuity and change characterize the gradual unfolding of the community initiative (see recommendations 4, 8–12 and 16)?

How does the evaluation help determine the value added by the community initiative? Does it help determine what new things the initiative brings to the community? How does it assess the significance of the initiative's contribution to addressing community concerns (see recommendations 15 and 16)?

Information linked to questions important to stakeholders
Do the evaluation methods and resulting information correspond to the questions being asked, and to the interests of stakeholders (see recommendations 3, 5, 11, 15, 18 and 19)?

What quantitative and qualitative methods best address stakeholders' questions and interests? Are diverse evaluation methods used to address the variety of these questions and interests, and do they fit the culture and context? What measurement instruments provide more reliable and valid (accurate, consistent and sensitive) information (see recommendations 3, 4 and 16)?

Practical, political and ethical issues
Issues of practicality, politics and ethics circumscribe the process of promoting community health and development, and should be considered in the design and implementation of a community evaluation.

Collaborative and participatory process involving multiple parties
Who determines the criteria for success? Who sets the agenda for the evaluation? Who are the clients for the evaluation? Whose interests does it serve (see recommendations 1, 3 and 15)?

What is the evaluators' role in the initiative? To whom and for what are they accountable? Do evaluators work with, rather than on or for, communities (see recommendations 3, 5, 15 and 17)?

Information linked to questions important to stakeholders

What is the purpose of the evaluation: assessing the merit or worth of the initiative, contributing to its effectiveness, building capacity and/or promoting self-determination (see recommendations 1, 3 and 15)?

To whom and how often are the data reported? How, by whom and under what circumstances are they best communicated to ensure maximum impact (see recommendations 3, 11 and 18)?

Building local capacity

What decisions are to be informed by the evaluation (see recommendations 1, 3 and 15)?

How does the evaluation help assess and strengthen the community's readiness and ability to address its issues (see recommendations 5, 10, 11, 13 and 21)?

Who defines the problem or issue and acceptable solutions? Do evaluation methods contribute to shared responsibility within the community for defining the agenda and for selecting, adapting and sustaining interventions (see recommendations 1, 2, 4, 7–10, 13 and 20)?

Does the evaluation help make the initiative accountable to the community it is intended to serve (see recommendations 1, 5, 8 and 15)?

How does the evaluation contribute to and/or limit community control? How does it strengthen community capacity to understand and develop solutions for locally identified concerns? Does the evaluation help local people to solve problems and make decisions independently (see recommendations 1, 5 and 7–13)?

Continuing part of the development process

Does the evaluation start early enough to help the initiative improve and adapt, and last long enough to help people understand whether the initiative has more distal outcomes (see recommendations 14 and 18)?

Do the evaluators avoid doing harm (see recommendations 3 and 16)? For example, if the initiative addresses illegal or socially sanctioned behaviour (such as drug use or violence), what special considerations are taken to help ensure confidentiality?

Do the evaluators share relevant information with stakeholders often enough and at the right times to affect important decisions (see recommendation 3)?

Using positive results to promote initiatives

How does the evaluation contribute to the sustainability and institutionalization of the initiative and its core components (see recommendations 7, 10, 13 and 19)?

What criteria are used to decide whether the initiative merits continued support and whether the initiative or its components should be disseminated (see recommendations 1, 3 and 15–18)? Who should be involved in identifying the criteria? What happens if the results are not positive?

Integrated support system for community health and development

Is the evaluation useful? How well do its measures and feedback correspond to the initiative's desired results (see recommendations 3, 5 and 16)?

Is the evaluation feasible or a burden to the community initiative, reducing its capacity to affect identified concerns? Are the time, effort and monetary costs of the evaluation justified in light of the benefits (see recommendations 3, 5, 14 and 16)?

Recommendations for practitioners and policy-makers

We group the recommendations according to the five phases of the catalyst and logic models (see Fig. 11.1 and 11.2), and address them to practitioners (especially community researchers and implementers) and policy-makers (including elected and appointed officials and funding agencies).

Supporting collaborative planning

1. Policy-makers should support and practitioners assist community members in:

   - identifying community health and development concerns and collecting data that document locally defined problems and assets; and
   - strategic planning: identifying a vision, mission, objectives, strategies and action plans.

2. Practitioners and policy-makers should create opportunities for community members to participate in developing an evaluation plan for the initiative that reflects the interests of key stakeholders.

3. Practitioners should:

   - develop and communicate information on risk and protective factors for community concerns and the most promising practices for addressing them;
   - help elicit local explanations and knowledge and assist in the critical analysis and interpretation of available data;
   - develop a reciprocal relationship with community initiatives, providing technical assistance and resources, as well as making requests for information and data; and
   - develop and regularly review research plans, schedules, expected outcomes and data with community members and other stakeholders.

Supporting community implementation, action and change

4. Practitioners and policy-makers should:

   - create opportunities for community members to select interventions and prioritize desired community changes that reflect local and expert

259

knowledge of what is important and feasible (for example, by using a survey of goals); and

- encourage community initiatives to be a catalyst for change, focusing their efforts on transforming modifiable features of the environment (programmes, policies and practices), rather than individual behaviour only.

5. Practitioners should:

- highlight the products of planning, such as forming committees or completing action plans or grant applications, rather than the process;
- provide technical support and feedback in identifying, developing and implementing promising interventions and best practices;
- evaluate the effects of interventions or initiative components of particular interest to the stakeholders to assess their actual impact on behaviour, risk factors and outcomes; and
- assess and feed back information for process measures that are of importance to the initiative (such as the units of media coverage, number of community members and organizations participating, resources generated and services provided).

6. Policy-makers should request and practitioners provide a measure of community or systems changes (new or modified programmes, policies or practices) facilitated by the initiative to indicate how the environment is changing to support health and development.
7. Policy-makers should allow and practitioners support the adaptation of community models and interventions to fit local conditions.
8. Practitioners should collect data on process and outcome to determine whether locally implemented and adapted innovations are effective.
9. Policy-makers should encourage long-range planning for sustainability, and provide support (such as training and links to support networks) and gradually reduce long-term funding to promote the institutionalization of initiatives.
10. Practitioners should:

- conduct periodic (annual) assessments of the proportion of community or systems changes that are sustained (incorporated into policy, programmes or the budget of government agencies) as an indication of institutionalization;
- collect data on rates of community change over time and across concerns to provide an indication of community capacity; and
- collect data on the engagement of citizen agents of community or systems change to provide a measure of community capacity and social capital.

11. Policy-makers should request and practitioners should provide, regular (monthly or quarterly) feedback of process and outcome data to improve the functioning of the initiative.

12. Practitioners should provide feedback on the distribution of community change by risk factor, strategies used, goals sought and settings engaged to help understand and improve efforts to address community issues.
13. Policy-makers should provide funding that enhances the capacity of a diverse team of community leaders to implement the initiative (to provide training for requesting funding and to support community capacity to plan and carry out the mission, objectives and strategies).

Detecting and influencing more distal outcomes
14. Practitioners should:

* collect data on reported behaviour related to risk and protective factors (such as reported tobacco use or physical inactivity) and validated physiological measures (such as measures of fitness);
* use longitudinal environmental measures to assess the conduciveness of the environment to health and how it changes over time, which may include prospective case studies of rates of community or systems change and their relationship to changes in relevant community-level indicators of health and development; and
* develop practical and standardized methods for collecting data on relevant risk and protective behaviour and community-level indicators over the same time frame and geographic area, covering communities in which the intervention is implemented and appropriate comparison communities.

15. Policy-makers should encourage and practitioners support community members and outside experts in assessing the public health or social significance of initiative achievements (using an outcome survey to assess perceived importance to the mission, for example) to increase accountability to community members and other stakeholders.
16. Practitioners should use qualitative methods (such as interviews with key informants about critical events, barriers, resources and lessons learned) to increase critical understanding of the initiative's process and outcomes.
17. Policy-makers should provide funding mechanisms that help make outcome matter to communities. These could include annual renewal of multi-year grants based on evidence of high rates of community change, outcome dividends or bonuses for improvements in more distal outcomes.
18. Practitioners should:

* feed back data on health and development outcomes, behavioural risk and protective factors, and community change early and regularly to a broad cross-section of initiative participants, including staff, community members, board members and funding agencies; and
* collaborate with initiative leaders to develop meaningful ways to present evaluation data to stakeholders.

Supporting dissemination

19. Practitioners should present data, in collaboration with community members and initiative staff, at local, state, national and international venues to create a broader audience for local efforts.
20. Practitioners and policy-makers should spread information on programmes and components known to be effective, and encourage other communities to replicate them.
21. Policy-makers and practitioners should use all communication media to disseminate information about successful interventions, promising practices and lessons learned in doing the work.

Conclusion

Answering an overarching question may assess the merit of a community evaluation. How does the evaluation contribute to (or restrict):

- understanding of the community initiative; and
- the improvement of the community and its capacity to effect valued ends?

This perspective adds empowerment to the traditional purposes of assessing merit *(33)*. The traditional evaluation paradigm asks how to configure community conditions, participants and interventions to get an answer to a research question. In contrast, the paradigm of community evaluation asks how to structure the evaluation to understand better and to improve what is important to the community.

In community evaluation, community members, funding agencies and evaluators collaborate to choose evaluation strategies to fit the local context. The factors determining the mix of strategies comprise the health and development outcomes to be addressed, the stakeholders' interests and needs, the resources available and the types of intervention methods chosen. For example, an injury prevention initiative might collaborate with the local clinic to track the incidence of deaths and injuries related to violence, road accidents or other locally important contributors. Although a child welfare initiative might find direct observation of parent–child interactions too expensive, it could use archives to collect data on the number of children living below the poverty line and other indicators.

A situation analysis of the community is a crucial step in planning for health and development at the local level *(19)*. Community evaluation informs the development process in which a community gains knowledge about its situation and identifies locally important concerns. Optimally, community evaluation is an early and integral part of the support system, helping inform the choices of culturally sensitive goals and strategies, and later documenting the community's mobilization and progress with its identified concerns. Evaluation methods contribute to a knowledge base from which community leaders, researchers and funding agencies can better understand the social and cultural conditions and processes that support or inhibit community change.

Communities may have built-in mechanisms for change, such as financial resources or service networks, that enable them to accept responsibility for transforming local conditions *(84)*. Community evaluation can help communities recognize and act on their own abilities to change. In this endeavour, the community has a collaborative relationship with the evaluation team, as both work together to understand and improve the initiative. Communities identify and mobilize existing resources to initiate and help document changes that relate to community health improvement. By documenting such changes, community evaluation can prompt community members and leaders to discover where change does (and should) occur.

When communities do not facilitate change, however, the role of the community evaluation team may shift to promoting accountability. When intermediate and main outcomes remain minimal over extended periods, for example, local trustees and funding agencies can use community evaluation data to encourage leaders to make adjustments. In extreme cases, community initiatives may be encouraged to seek change in local leadership. To help make outcome matter to local implementers, funding agencies may structure funding so that annual renewal depends on evidence of progress.

Detecting community capacity is a particularly important challenge for community evaluation, but community change, as illustrated in the Kansas initiatives, is a promising measure. For example, a community initiative for preventing substance abuse that displays a sustained pattern of relevant community changes over time and related improvements in more distal outcomes (such as reported drug use) might be said to demonstrate greater community capacity than a counterpart with no sustained change. Evidence that members of the same initiative later effect community changes related to a new mission or concern, such as preventing violence by young people, provides further conviction of increased capacity. Further research may help reveal a variety of sensitive and reliable measures of community capacity *(85)* and the related constructs of community competence *(43)* and social capital *(86,87)*.

Successful community partnerships create, adopt and/or adapt the interventions and practices best suited to local conditions. How interventions are adapted and implemented becomes almost as important a research issue as what happened as a result *(47)*. Future research may refine the art of supporting and documenting the process of reinvention. Such knowledge should enhance the capacity to support contextually appropriate efforts to promote health and development.

Relationships between scientists and communities appear to be evolving in the context of community partnerships for health and development. This may reflect a minor revolution in traditional modes of science and practice *(88)*. In the late 1980s, community-based funding emerged as an innovation in funding practice: awarding grants to communities to address their concerns and not primarily to research scientists to design and implement interventions in or on communities. Traditional methods emphasized control over communities; they could not achieve the multiple goals of community initiatives: to increase understanding, improvement, capacity and self-determination. Widespread discontent with the inadequacies of traditional models of research and evaluation, and challenges to basic assumptions about their purposes created the conditions in which new community-oriented approaches to intervention and evaluation emerged.

A new paradigm offers changes in models, methods and applications *(88)*. For example, the community evaluation system described in this chapter outlines a conceptual framework for examining and improving community initiatives that act as catalysts for change. The methods include various support activities and instruments for documenting and feeding back information about process and intermediate and more distal outcomes *(12,26,38,47,61)*. The variety of problems tackled through community initiatives in both urban and rural areas suggests the generalizability of this approach.

To be adopted, candidate approaches to supporting and evaluating community initiatives must show their advantage over others *(47,88)*. New models and methods should solve problems not addressed well by others. For example, a community evaluation system might offer the capacity to collect and feed back information about community change, an intermediate outcome of community initiatives. The innovation must also preserve the strengths of earlier and competing methods; community evaluation approaches should draw from the strengths of models from public health *(19)*, applied research methods from behavioural science *(41)*, strategies from community development *(23)* and key constructs such as prevention *(13,89)* and empowerment *(90,91)*.

Finally, a candidate approach to community evaluation should leave a variety of unresolved issues and questions to be addressed by scientists and practitioners drawn to the new or adapted paradigm. The many issues highlighted here and the related recommendations offer multiple niches for contribution. Perhaps this and other approaches will help unlock the secrets and power of community initiatives. Such efforts may contribute to the capacity of communities and support systems to address locally valued and evolving health and development concerns, now and in future generations.

References

1. HAWKINS, J.D. & CATALANO, R.F. *Communities that care.* San Francisco, Jossey-Bass, 1992.
2. ROSENBURG, M.L. & FENLEY, M.A. *Violence in America: a public health approach.* New York, Oxford University Press, 1991.
3. KOO, H. ET AL. Reducing adolescent pregnancy through a school and community-based intervention: Denmark, South Carolina, revisited. *Family planning perspectives,* **26**(5): 206–211, 217 (1994).

4. ZIMMERMAN, M.A. & FREUDENBERG, N., ED. *AIDS prevention in the community: lessons from the first decade.* Washington, DC, American Public Health Association, 1995.

5. PUSKA, P. ET AL. *The North Karelia Project: 20 year results and experiences.* Helsinki, National Public Health Institute, 1995.

6. GABARINO, J. & KOSTLENY, K. Neighborhood-based programs. *In:* Melton, G.B. & Barry, F.D., ed. *Protecting children from abuse and neglect: foundations for a new strategy.* New York, Guilford Press, 1994.

7. FLETCHER, S. Fear on the farm: rural women take action against domestic violence. *Women & environments,* **38**: 27–29 (1996).

8. COMMITTEE ON TRAUMA RESEARCH, COMMISSION ON LIFE SCIENCES, NATIONAL RESEARCH COUNCIL AND INSTITUTE OF MEDICINE. *Injury in America: a continuing public health problem.* Washington, DC, National Academy Press, 1985.

9. ESTEVA, G. & PRAKASH, M.S. From global to local thinking. *The ecologist,* **24**(5): 162–163 (1994).

10. BRACHT, N., ED. *Health promotion at the community level.* Thousand Oaks, Sage, 1990.

11. SCHORR, L.B. *Common purpose: strengthening families and neighborhoods to rebuild America.* New York, Doubleday, 1997.

12. FAWCETT, S.B. ET AL. Promoting health through community development. *In:* Glenwick, D. & Jason, L.A., ed. *Promoting health and mental health: behavioral approaches to prevention.* New York, Haworth, 1993.

13. KELLAM, S.G. & REBOK, G.W. Building developmental and etiological theory through epidemiologically based preventive intervention trials. *In:* McCord, J. & Tremblay, R.E., ed. *Preventing antisocial behavior: intervention from birth through adolescence.* New York, Guilford Press, 1992.

14. FREUDENBERG, N. Shaping the future of health education: from behavior change to social change. *Health education monographs,* **6**(4): 372–377 (1978).

15. Ottawa Charter for Health Promotion. *Health promotion,* **1**(4): iii–v (1986).

16. GREEN, L.W. & RAEBURN, J.M. Health promotion: what is it? What will it become? *Health promotion,* **3**: 151–159 (1988).

17. EPP, J. *Achieving health for all: a framework for health promotion.* Ottawa, Health Canada, 1986.

18. ASHTON, J. ET AL. Healthy Cities: WHO's new public health initiative. *Health promotion,* **1**: 55–60 (1986).

19. GREEN, L.W. & KREUTER, M.M. *Health promotion planning: an educational and environmental approach,* 2nd ed. Mountain View, Mayfield, 1991.

20. US DEPARTMENT OF HEALTH AND HUMAN SERVICES. *Planned approach to community health: guide for the local coordinator.* Atlanta, US Department of Health and Human Services, Centers for Disease Control

and Prevention, National Center for Chronic Disease Prevention and Health Promotion, 1996.

21. DUNHAM, A. Some principles of community development. *International review of community development*, **11**: 141–151 (1963).

22. GOULET, D. *The cruel choice: a new concept in the theory of development*. New York, Atheneum, 1971.

23. ROTHMAN, J. & TROPMAN, J.E. Models of community organization and macro practice perspectives: their mixing and phasing. *In*: Cox, F.E., ed. *Strategies of community organization: macro practice*. Itasca, F.E. Peacock Publishers, 1987, pp. 3–26.

24. *Social progress through community development*. New York, United Nations, 1955.

25. GREEN, L.W. The theory of participation: a qualitative analysis of its expression in national and international health policies. *Advances in health education and promotion*, **1**: 211–236 (1986).

26. FAWCETT, S.B. ET AL. *Evaluating community efforts to prevent cardiovascular diseases*. Atlanta, Centers for Disease Control and Prevention, National Center for Chronic Disease Prevention and Health Promotion, 1995.

27. VOTH, D.E. Evaluation of community development. *In*: Christenson, J.A. & Robinson, J.W., ed. *Community development in perspective*. Ames, Iowa State University Press, 1989, pp. 219–252.

28. WINDSOR, R.A. ET AL. Evaluating program effectiveness. *Evaluation of health promotion and education programs*. Palo Alto, Mayfield, 1984, pp. 126–170.

29. STULL, D. & SCHENSUL, J. *Collaborative research and social change: applied anthropology in action*. Boulder, Westview, 1987.

30. DENZIN, N.K. & LINCOLN, Y.S., ed. *Handbook of qualitative research*. Thousand Oaks, Sage, 1994.

31. GREEN, L.W., ET AL. *Study of participatory research in health promotion. Review and recommendations for the development of participatory research in health promotion in Canada*. Ottawa, Royal Society of Canada, 1995.

32. WHYTE, W.F., ED. *Participatory action research*. Thousand Oaks, Sage, 1991.

33. FAWCETT, S.B. ET AL. Empowering community health initiatives through evaluation. *In*: Fetterman, D.M. et al., ed. *Empowerment evaluation: knowledge and tools for self-assessment and accountability*. Thousand Oaks, Sage, 1996, pp. 161–187.

34. FETTERMAN, D.M. ET AL., ED. *Empowerment evaluation: knowledge and tools for self-assessment and accountability*. Thousand Oaks, Sage, 1996.

35. LEWIN, K. Action research and minority problems. *Journal of social issues*, **2**(4): 34–46 (1946).

36. ARGYRIS, C. ET AL. (1985). *Action science*. San Francisco, Jossey-Bass.

37. *WHO-EURO Working Group on Health Promotion Evaluation: executive summary report of meeting, Atlanta, Georgia, USA, July 27–28, 1995.* Copenhagen, WHO Regional Office for Europe, 1995 (document).

38. FRANCISCO, V.T. ET AL. A methodology for monitoring and evaluating community health coalitions. *Health education research: theory and practice*, **8**: 403–416 (1993).

39. WHEATLEY, M.J. *Leadership and the new science.* San Francisco, Berrett-Koehler Publishers, 1992.

40. FAWCETT, S.B. ET AL. Using empowerment theory to support community initiatives for health and development. *American journal of community psychology*, **23**(5): 667–697 (1995).

41. FAWCETT, S.B. Some values guiding community research and action. *Journal of applied behavior analysis*, **24**: 621–636 (1991).

42. PUBLIC HEALTH SERVICE. *Healthy people 2000. National health promotion and disease prevention objectives. Conference edition.* Washington, DC, US Department of Health and Human Services, 1990.

43. ENG, E. & PARKER, E. Measuring community competence in the Mississippi Delta: the interface between program evaluation and empowerment. *Health education quarterly*, **21**(2): 199–220 (1994).

44. CAMPBELL, D.T. & STANLEY, J.C. *Experimental and quasi-experimental designs for research.* Boston, Houghton Mifflin, 1963.

45. KOEPSELL, T.D. ET AL. Selected methodological issues in evaluating community-based health promotion and disease prevention programs. *Annual review of public health*, **13**: 31–57 (1992).

46. GUBA, E.G. & LINCOLN, Y.S. *Fourth generation evaluation.* Thousand Oaks, Sage, 1989.

47. ROGERS, E.M. *Diffusion of innovations.* New York, Free Press, 1995.

48. PATTON, M.Q. *Qualitative evaluation methods.* Beverly Hills, Sage, 1980.

49. STUFFLEBEAM, D.L. Empowerment evaluation, objectivist evaluation, and evaluation standards: where the future of evaluation should not go and where it needs to go. *Evaluation practice*, **15**(3): 321–338 (1994).

50. SANDERS, J.R. & JOINT COMMITTEE ON STANDARDS FOR EDUCATIONAL EVALUATION. *Program evaluation standards: how to assess evaluations of educational programs.* Thousand Oaks, Sage, 1994.

51. STECKLER, A. & GOODMAN, R.M. How to institutionalize health promotion programs. *American journal of health promotion*, **3**(4): 34–44 (1994).

52. FAWCETT, S.B. ET AL. Conducting intervention research: the design and development process. *In*: Rothman, J. & Thomas, E.J., ed. *Intervention research: design and development for human service.* New York, Haworth, 1994, pp. 25–54.

53. PAINE-ANDREWS, A. ET AL. Replicating a community-based initiative for the prevention of adolescent pregnancy: from South Carolina to Kansas. *Family and community health*, **19**(1): 14–30 (1996).

267

54. ANDREASEN, A.R. *Marketing change: changing behavior to promote healthy social development and the environment.* San Francisco, Jossey-Bass, 1995.

55. KELLY, J.G. *A guide to conducting prevention research in the community.* New York, Haworth Press, 1988.

56. HIMMELMAN, A. *Communities working together for change.* Minneapolis, MN, 1992 (unpublished manuscript).

57. MITCHELL, R.E. ET AL. A typology of prevention activities: applications to community coalitions. *Journal of primary prevention,* **16**(4): 413–436 (1996).

58. BAUM, F. Researching public health: behind the qualitative–quantitative debate. *Social science and medicine,* **40**(4): 459–468 (1995).

59. CARLETON, R.A. ET AL. The Pawtucket Heart Health Program: community changes in cardiovascular risk factors and projected disease risk. *American journal of public health,* **85**: 777–785 (1995).

60. MITTELMARK, M.B. ET AL. Realistic outcomes: lessons from community-based research and demonstration programs for the prevention of cardiovascular diseases. *Journal of public health policy,* **14**: 437–462 (1993).

61. FAWCETT, S.B. ET AL. *Work Group evaluation handbook: evaluating and supporting community initiatives for health and development.* Lawrence, Work Group on Health Promotion and Community Development, University of Kansas, 1995.

62. COBB, R. & ELDER, C. *Participation in American politics: the dynamics of agenda building.* Baltimore, John Hopkins University Press, 1983.

63. PAINE-ANDREWS, A. ET AL. Assessing community health concerns and implementing a microgrant program for self-help initiatives. *American journal of public health,* **84**(2): 316–318 (1994).

64. WALLACK, L. ET AL. Doing media advocacy. Wallack, L. et al. *Media advocacy and public health.* Thousand Oaks, Sage, 1993.

65. FAWCETT, S.B. ET AL. Evaluating community coalitions for the prevention of substance abuse: the case of Project Freedom. *Health education and behavior,* **24**(6): 812–828 (1997).

66. MCKNIGHT, J.L. & KRETZMAN, J.P. *Building communities from the inside out: a path toward finding and mobilizing a community's assets.* Evanston, IL, Center for Urban Affairs and Policy Research, Neighborhood Innovations Network, 1993.

67. STECKLER, A. ET AL. Toward integrating qualitative and quantitative methods: an introduction. *Health education quarterly,* **19**: 1–8 (1992).

68. PARCEL, G.S. ET AL. Beyond demonstration: diffusion of health promotion innovations. *In:* Bracht, N., ed. *Health promotion at the community level.* Thousand Oaks, Sage, 1990.

69. VINCENT, M.L. ET AL. Reducing adolescent pregnancy through school and community-based education. *Journal of the American Medical Association,* **257**(24): 3382–3386 (1987).

70. PAINE-ANDREWS, A. ET AL. Community coalitions to prevent adolescent substance abuse: the case of the *Project Freedom* replication initiative. *Journal of prevention and intervention in the community*, **14**(1/2): 81–99 (1996).

71. JOHNSTON, J. ET AL. Kansas LEAN: an effective coalition for nutrition education and dietary change. *Journal of nutrition education*, **28**(2): 115–118 (1996).

72. PAINE-ANDREWS, A. ET AL. Evaluating a statewide partnership for reducing risks for chronic diseases. *Journal of community health*, **22**(5): 343–359 (1997).

73. RICHTER, K.P. ET AL. Measuring the health environment: a review of the literature and applications for community initiatives. *Preventive medicine*, **31**(2): 98–111 (2000).

74. FAWCETT, S.B. ET AL. The concerns report method: involving consumers in setting local improvement agendas. *Social policy*, **13**(4): 36–41 (1982).

75. FAWCETT, S.B. ET AL. *Preventing adolescent substance abuse: an action planning guide for community-based initiatives*. Lawrence, Work Group on Health Promotion and Community Development, University of Kansas, 1994.

76. FAWCETT, S.B. ET AL. *Preventing adolescent pregnancy: an action planning guide for community-based initiatives*. Lawrence, Work Group on Health Promotion and Community Development, University of Kansas, 1994.

77. FAWCETT, S.B. ET AL. *Preventing youth violence: an action planning guide for community-based initiatives*. Lawrence, Work Group on Health Promotion and Community Development, University of Kansas, 1994.

78. FAWCETT, S.B. ET AL. *Reducing risk for chronic disease: an action planning guide for community-based initiatives*. Lawrence, Work Group on Health Promotion and Community Development, University of Kansas, 1995.

79. FAWCETT, S.B. ET AL. *Preventing child abuse and neglect: an action planning guide for building a caring community*. Lawrence, Work Group on Health Promotion and Community Development, University of Kansas, 1996.

80. RICHTER, K.P. ET AL. *Promoting health and wellness among older adults: an action planning guide for community-based initiatives*. Lawrence, Work Group on Health Promotion and Community Development, University of Kansas, 1998.

81. LEWIS, R.K. ET AL. Evaluating the effects of a community coalition's efforts to reduce illegal sales of alcohol and tobacco products to minors. *Journal of community health*, **21**(6): 429–436 (1997).

82. HARRIS, K.J. ET AL. Reducing elementary school children's risks for chronic diseases through school lunch modifications, nutrition education,

and physical activity interventions. *Journal of nutrition education*, **29**(4): 196–202 (1997).

83. TEUTSCH, S.M. A framework for assessing the effectiveness of disease and injury prevention. *Morbidity and mortality weekly report*, **41**(RR-3): 1–12 (1992).

84. HOMAN, M.S. *Promoting community change*. Pacific Grove, Brooks/ Cole, 1994.

85. GOODMAN, R.M. ET AL. An initial attempt at identifying and defining the dimensions of community capacity to provide a basis for measurement. *Health education and behavior*, **25**(3): 258–278 (1998).

86. KREUTER, M.W. ET AL. *Social capital: evaluation implications for community health promotion*. Copenhagen, WHO Regional Office for Europe, 1997 (document).

87. PUTNAM, R.D. Bowling alone: America's declining social capital. *Journal of democracy*, **6**(1): 64–78 (1995).

88. KUHN, T. *The structure of scientific revolutions*. Chicago, University of Chicago Press, 1970.

89. PRICE, R.H. ET AL., ED. *14 ounces of prevention: a casebook for practitioners*. Washington, DC, American Psychological Association, 1988.

90. RAPPAPORT, J. Terms of empowerment/exemplars of prevention: toward a theory for community psychology. *American journal of community psychology*, **9**: 1–25 (1987).

91. WALLERSTEIN, N. & BERNSTEIN, E. Introduction to community empowerment, participatory education and health. *Health education quarterly*, **21**: 141–148 (1994).

12
Evaluating health promotion in schools: reflections

Sarah Stewart-Brown[4]

This chapter draws on the experience gained from a series of reviews of health promotion in schools, some of which are still under way *(1–6)*. It describes some of the strengths and difficulties of experimental research and systematic reviews in school health promotion. It raises issues in the development and evaluation of school health programmes; some are specific to the school setting and some relate to programmes in a variety of settings. The chapter concludes with recommendations for the future development and evaluation of school health promotion programmes.

Schools as a setting for health promotion

For more than a century, schools have proved a popular setting for initiatives designed to promote health and prevent disease. This has happened for a number of reasons, both theoretical and practical. Policy-makers in both health and education recognize the interdependence of health and learning; children need health to benefit fully from schooling, and learning is important for the maintenance of health. In countries where education is compulsory, schools provide direct access to the whole population of children, independent of their parents. Schools can reach children at an early age, before they have embarked on health-damaging behaviour. Schools thus provide an infrastructure for programme delivery, which is at least in part free to health promotion practitioners.

In some countries, schools have been the setting for the entire range of health promotion and disease prevention initiatives, from screening and im-

---

[4] The systematic reviews described in this chapter were undertaken in conjunction with Sarah Chapman, John Fletcher, Jane Barlow and Jane Wells at the Health Services Research Unit (HSRU) at the University of Oxford, and Deborah Lister-Sharpe and Amanda Sowden from the Centre for Reviews and Dissemination at the University of York, United Kingdom. I have very much enjoyed working with them; without their work this chapter could not have been written. HSRU is supported by the United Kingdom National Health Service Executive (Anglia and Oxford), as were several of the HSRU reviews undertaken. The United Kingdom Health Technology Assessment Programme funded the continuing review of reviews of health promotion in schools.

munization programmes and the provision of clinics, through classroom health education programmes to community outreach initiatives trying to ensure that schools' physical and social environments are conducive to health (through smoking policies and the provision of healthy school meals and recreation facilities, for example) *(7,8)*. The former are generally regarded as disease prevention initiatives and the latter as health promotion, but distinguishing between them is not always easy. The most widely accepted definition of health promotion includes the concept of empowerment *(9)*. If health promotion is a process of enabling children to increase control over their health, improving access to preventive services by offering them in schools can promote health. The distinction may depend less on the content and aim of the service than on its provision: whether, for example, the service involves coercion or offers young people a genuine choice.

The study and development of health promotion initiatives, in schools and other settings, have led to the recognition that different approaches to health promotion may be synergistic and that effective programmes may require a multifaceted approach *(7)*. In school health promotion, this has meant involving parents and the community, as well as all the school staff, so that pupils perceive congruent messages. The European Network of Health Promoting Schools (ENHPS) takes this multifaceted approach *(8)*. Developed by the WHO Regional Office for Europe in partnership with the European Commission and the Council of Europe, the initiative requires participating schools to work in three domains: developing a school ethos and environment that support health, working with families and communities and working with pupils through health education in the school curriculum *(10)*. It is built on the understanding that self-esteem is important for health and that changes in health-related behaviour need to be achieved through empowerment, not coercion. Multifaceted initiatives are complex, and their evaluation presents many challenges. The 1995 WHO evaluation of ENHPS proposed a framework for the evaluation of health promoting schools *(11)*. This defines three types of evaluation, focusing on the process of the initiative and its impact on both intermediate factors and health or wellbeing.

The role of experimental studies

In many instances, formal evaluation is not necessarily essential for research and development. People can develop successful programmes by trial and error, and learn whether they work by observation. This process can be very effective if programme developers are keen observers, who resist the influence of personal bias. Formal evaluation is useful, however, because it enables others to learn from the experience of those who develop programmes.

Evaluation can be observational or experimental. Observational studies aim to document events, perceptions or changes and experimental studies, to describe what happens when an intervention is made, usually comparing the results with those of making no intervention or another intervention. Experi-

272

mental studies are useful to demonstrate that the observations made during the course of studies were not biased. Because bias is very common, experimental studies have come to be viewed as the methodology of choice. Many of the limitations of theses studies, however, are pertinent to school health promotion research. Control of both the design and data collection by outsiders hinders either the research staff or those involved in the experiment in making pertinent observations of both expected and unexpected effects. Participatory research enables researchers to base their conclusions on the observations of a much larger number of people, including the targets of the intervention, and is therefore more likely to discover answers. Participation is difficult to achieve in experiments over which the participants feel that they have no control. Chapters 1–4 discuss these issues in more detail.

The randomized controlled trial is often recommended as the optimum experimental design *(12)*. The random allocation of individual children causes unacceptable disruption to school timetables. Classes or schools can be randomly assigned to experimental and control groups, but this causes another problem in the evaluation of programmes intended to provide knowledge, as almost all school health promotion programmes do: contamination between the control and programme groups. Useful knowledge spreads from person to person. Randomly allocating schools reduces this problem, but does not eliminate it. Randomly allocating cities or communities reduces it still further. Allocating individuals to groups on the basis of their class, school or city, however, introduces complications to statistical analysis based on independent observation. Children in the same class share and are influenced by their classroom teacher. Children in the same school are exposed to a common school ethos, and are likely to have more similar socioeconomic backgrounds than a random sample of the general population. Overcoming these complications requires both sample-size calculations and analyses of results to take account of intraclass correlations *(13)*. This process tends to increase very significantly the sample size and thus the cost of evaluation studies. In addition, interclass correlations theoretically affect the analysis of the results of controlled trials, as opposed to randomized controlled trials. Controlled trials are subject to the additional criticism that investigators may have been biased in deciding which schools got the interventions.

Both controlled and randomized controlled study designs tend to be based on the assumption that delivering a standardized intervention, which can be faithfully reproduced in different schools, is possible and desirable. In ENHPS *(10)* and some studies covered by our review of reviews *(3)*, schools were encouraged to customize the programme under evaluation to increase their participation and ownership, but most studies examined standardized interventions. The requirement for standardized interventions creates problems for health promotion evaluation in all settings. The randomized controlled trial requires a passivity in participants that is the antithesis of health promotion, in which active participation is central to success and empowerment a desirable goal in its own right. Health promotion programmes aim to enable participants to do a potentially difficult thing for themselves. Enabling people to help themselves is more difficult than doing something for them. Help tailored to the participants' needs may be more effective than offering a standard package.

The process of delivery may be particularly important in the school setting. Children, especially primary school children, are more accepting and less critical than adults: less likely to identify misinformation incorporated into health promotion programmes and more susceptible to manipulation. For example, saying that illegal drugs are more harmful than they actually are could achieve short-term improvements in attitudes, but only at the cost of reducing children's ability to trust teachers and other experts in the future. Such approaches disregard children's right to make informed choices. The assessment of these aspects of the delivery process can be built into experimental studies (14), but the qualitative methodologies sensitive to their measurement are time consuming and expensive.

Finally, some element of coercion is regarded as positively desirable in schools. This means that health promotion programmes can be implemented in schools that could not be implemented elsewhere. Children can be required to take part in physical education sessions to ensure that they are physically fit, and to participate in classes in which sexual health is discussed. Changing children's lunch-time nutritional intake is relatively easy in a school that provides meals and in which no other food is available. Experimental studies can show the short-term effectiveness of programmes such as these in changing risk factor prevalence (15,16). Such programmes may develop a taste for healthy foods and exercise in children who might not otherwise have had the opportunity to discover them. Programmes that require children to submit to activities in which they do not want to take part, however, model coercion rather than respect. Respect for others is an important part of a healthy society, so coercive programmes are unlikely to promote health in the long term. Reports of experimental studies seldom discuss such possible adverse effects of school health promotion programmes.

The role of systematic reviews and reviews of reviews

Systematic reviews were developed to ensure that the results of sound medical experiments were incorporated into professional practice as soon possible (17). Systematic searching guards against reviewer bias in the selection of studies. Critical appraisal, using specified criteria, is intended to ensure that conclusions are based on the most robust studies. Combining the results from several studies that have used the same outcomes provides the statistical power to decide whether small differences between intervention and control groups could have occurred by chance. Reviews of reviews therefore present a unique opportunity to comment on what has and has not been evaluated, and to identify effective and ineffective interventions and areas in need of further research.

Systematic reviews also have certain important limitations, and some of these are particularly pertinent to reviews of studies of health promotion initiatives. Systematic searching and critical appraisal do not need to be confined to experimental studies, but they usually are. As a result, systematic reviews are less likely to take account of what other methodological approaches have revealed. Driven by the quality standards established by the Cochrane Collaboration (18), most recent systematic reviews have aimed to search for both published and unpublished studies, but published studies are much easier to identify. The views of journal editors and reviewers about what constitutes good research may therefore bias these reviews. Similarly, the conclusions are subject to potential bias in the types of initiatives that are favoured by funding organizations and therefore studied. Using information only from completed studies, systematic reviews may fail to make use of the experiential knowledge of practitioners or to take account of the most recent methodological advances. In addition, their search strategies are a source of potential bias; reviewers who are unaware of a specific body of research or unfamiliar with specialist terminology may fail to find important studies.

Finally, systematic reviews are rarely complete. Our systematic reviews of reviews (3) found multiple reviews on all the topic areas, but only 10% of the studies appeared in more than one review. There were reasons for this; reviews may have varied in focus or covered studies published in different periods. Nevertheless, even thorough reviews are unlikely to be complete and, even within this group, we noted inexplicable discrepancies between reviews reporting on the same study.

Experimental studies of health promotion in schools

Systematically reviewing systematic reviews enables one to develop an overview of the very large number and wide range of studies of health promotion in schools, and to build on the work of previous reviewers. The latest of our systematic reviews of reviews (3) identified over 200 reviews of health promotion in schools, a measure of the volume of research in this field. Systematic reviews ask focused research questions, and ours focused on population approaches to primary prevention. It therefore excluded programmes targeted at high-risk groups (such as obese children or teenage mothers) and those delivered to individuals rather than groups (such as those for screening and immunization). Perhaps most important, by excluding reviews that did not include some controlled or randomized controlled studies, it focused on experimental studies. Reviewing reviews, rather than primary studies, meant that the project was limited by the focus of the original reviews and by the process of data extraction carried out by the reviewers. We included only the reviews that met certain quality criteria: those that showed evidence of a systematic search strategy, gave key information about the studies reviewed and included some controlled trials. The reviews finally included covered over 400 studies of health promotion in schools. With these important caveats, the project thus provided the opportunity to make some useful observations on experimental studies of health promotion in schools.

The systematic reviews that were identified and met the inclusion criteria focused on one or two specific topics: usually health-related behaviour. The greatest number covered studies of substance abuse: illegal drugs, alcohol and tobacco, either alone or in combination. The next most common were reviews of studies of nutrition and/or exercise. Multiple reviews of sex or family life education, accident and injury prevention, personal safety, oral health and mental health were less numerous. The reviews included did not cover school health promotion programmes in general, the effectiveness of different approaches (for example, multifaceted programmes) regardless of the topic, or the ENHPS approach. This is not surprising, given the lead-time required for the evaluation and publication of results of studies of a new approach. No reviews focusing on studies of holistic approaches to health promotion (such as empowerment or self-esteem development) were suitable for inclusion.

The number of studies reviewed in each topic area correlated with the number of reviews. Much the greatest number focused on substance abuse. If, as seems likely, the number of high-quality reviews reflects the volume of research and development, investment in research on substance abuse programmes appears to have been disproportionate. The most pressing health needs of school-age children are injury prevention and mental health promotion (1). Drug and alcohol abuse are related to both of these, and the disproportionate investment might be justifiable on these grounds. On the other hand, the emphasis on substance abuse programmes may reflect societies' concern with the antisocial behaviour that frequently accompanies abuse, rather than the health of young people.

Aims and content of programmes

Most of the reviews had been commissioned to evaluate the impact of school health promotion programmes on health-related behaviour, and focused on improvements in health-related behaviour specific to a group of diseases (such as cardiovascular diseases) or health problems (such as injuries and drug abuse). Among reviews concentrating on aspects of health, rather than behaviour, the aim of reducing the prevalence of particular diseases was more common than that of improving aspects of wellbeing. Although some of the reviewed programmes on the prevention of substance abuse and on sex or family life education aimed to improve wellbeing, either by increasing self-esteem or by reducing stress, the latter aim appeared to be common only in mental health promotion programmes.

Almost all the initiatives covered in these reviews aimed to increase pupils' knowledge of the relevant health issues and included a classroom component, but the intensity and delivery of classroom programmes varied significantly. The amount of curriculum time tended to range from, for example, one fifty-minute session to weekly sessions over two years. Programmes were delivered by teachers (with or without special training), other professionals, peers, community volunteers and students in higher education. Most evaluated programmes used interventions developed and standardized outside the school. Thus schools involved in the research would not usually have participated in intervention design and development.

The classroom components extended beyond the development of knowledge, covering the range of components described by Hansen in his review of substance abuse programmes *(19)*. These may be grouped into four broad areas: skill development, promotion of wellbeing, support and other approaches. Examples of programmes on all topics aimed to increase children's skills, but the types of skills promoted varied. In substance abuse and sex and family life education programmes, these tended to be generic skills in making decisions, solving problems, assertiveness and resistance, communication and listening, coping and building social networks. Programmes for accident and injury prevention and, to a lesser extent, nutrition and exercise promoted more specific skills in road crossing and cycling, food preparation and physical education. Programmes aiming to develop skills used a variety of techniques, from information and discussion through video modelling to role playing, simulated experience and supervised cooking or physical education instruction. Most of the programmes on substance abuse and sex and family life and some of those on nutrition and exercise also used one or more of the following approaches: learning about social norms, clarifying values, identifying alternatives, setting personal goals or giving pledges and assistance.

This classification has weaknesses. Goal setting, alternatives and pledge programmes could all strengthen children's powers of resistance and enable them to be more assertive. Some of the programmes trying to help children learn individual skills (in, for example, assertiveness, coping, communication and family life) have the potential to affect emotional wellbeing. While the reviews focused on health-related behaviour and extracted data only on these outcomes, some of these programmes might have had the explicit or implicit aim of improving wellbeing.

Programmes on different topics appeared to differ in the frequency with which they included interventions aimed at developing the school ethos or environment. Nutrition and exercise and accident and injury programmes – working for nutritional improvements to school lunches, advertising in school, staffed road crossings and helmet discount schemes, for example – most frequently reported such interventions. A few examples were reported in reviews of environmental initiatives in sex and family life programmes (transport to community clinics) and substance abuse programmes (school policy development). None of the reviews reporting mental health or personal safety programmes appeared to include these approaches. Reviews of nutrition and exercise and accident and injury prevention programmes concluded that school health promotion programmes could affect the environment.

Nutrition and exercise reviews most frequently reported a programme aim of influencing the family and community where it appeared to increase programme effectiveness; interventions included activities after school that allowed parents to experience some of the approaches used in the classroom. Accident and injury prevention reviews commonly reported programmes' aim of influencing the community; activities included engineering measures, mass-media campaigns, raising community awareness and police enforcement. Family and community approaches formed part of a few of the reviewed sex and family life programmes: homework to promote communication with parents, links to clinics, family sessions with values clarification, life skills training, initiatives through voluntary agencies and churches, and media campaigns. Approaches involving parents and the community appeared relatively rare in substance abuse, personal safety and mental health programmes.

On the basis of the programmes included in the reviews, nutrition and exercise programmes appear to be the most comprehensive, in terms of the number of domains covered, but are less likely to be based on cognizance of the potential importance of general wellbeing for health-related behaviour. These programmes differ from substance abuse programmes and sexual health programmes in that they permit evaluation of the impact of programmes on behaviour in primary school children. At this age, what children eat and the amount of exercise they take is very largely controlled by the adults who care for them at home and at school.

Accident and injury prevention programmes also appear to be based on an understanding that what happens in the community affects schoolchildren. These programmes focused their community activity on the physical environment. This is in line with accident and injury prevention programmes outside schools, which regard engineering and design measures as very effective. The accident and injury programmes covered in the reviews did not appear to be based on explicit psychological or social models, and approaches such as resistance skills training and assertiveness and self-esteem development seem to have played no part in them. As wearing a cycle helmet, in the face of peer pressure against it, may require the same level of self-confidence as refusing cigarettes or drugs, however, these approaches might be worth trying. Substance abuse and sexual health programmes appeared more likely to be based on a theoretical model, and to take account of psychological research on why teenagers begin to use alcohol and illegal drugs and to have unprotected sex, in the face of warning of the potential hazards by adults. The programmes, however, appeared less likely to cover all three domains of health promotion, particularly family and community approaches.

Study designs
Because the inclusion criteria required reviews to include at least one controlled trial, the systematic review of reviews does not cover the full range of health promotion research, but some interesting observations can still be made. Overall, the most common study design was the randomized controlled trial, in which either schools or classes had been randomly allocated to programme or control group. Many of the reviewed trials, however, covered fewer than ten schools or classes. At this level, the design retains its ability to prevent inves-

tigator bias in deciding which school gets the intervention, but loses much of its power to distribute confounding factors equally between programme and control groups. Many reviewers failed to take account of the statistical implications of the cluster-randomized design of these studies in their assessment of results.

Randomized controlled trials were the most common type of design reported in reviews of substance abuse and sexual health programmes, and the least common type in reviews of accident and injury prevention evaluations. In the few examples of the latter, the unit of randomization was the city or community as often as the class or school. Observational studies with measurements before and after the intervention, but no control group, were rare in substance abuse and sex and family life education reviews, and more common in nutrition and exercise and accident and injury prevention reviews. The preponderance of randomized controlled trials in the former may either reflect a larger number of evaluations in total, offering reviewers more choice of studies to include, or indicate genuine differences in the type of design selected in different topic areas. Accident and injury prevention programmes were more likely to cover all three domains: classroom activities, school environment and family and community approaches. These are necessarily very complex interventions, and the most complex interventions may be least suited to the randomized controlled trial.

Outcome measures

The range of outcome measures reported reflected the aims of the reviews. Additional outcomes may have been reported in the individual studies, but not in the reviews, because they were not seen as central to these aims. Measures fell into six groups: knowledge and attitudes, skills and behaviour, changes to the environment, physiological measurements, measurements of wellbeing and event rates. The first three are intermediate outcomes in terms of the classification used in evaluating ENHPS *(11)*. The second three are health status measures. Most of those reported were disease-specific measures (accident rates or blood pressure) rather than measures of health or wellbeing. The reviews rarely reported measures of the process of programme implementation. This gap makes it impossible to establish whether lack of impact on the other types of outcome were attributable to inadequate implementation or to an ineffective programme, and difficult to establish whether the programmes were delivered in a health-enhancing way: that is, that they were developed and implemented with schools' participation and were neither coercive or manipulative.

Changes in knowledge and attitudes were mostly assessed in questionnaires. The reviews rarely provided information about the aspects of knowledge assessed or the extent to which the questionnaires had been pilot-tested or validated. Changes in health-related behaviour were measured mostly by self-report and sometimes by reports from parents or teachers, using a range of instruments, some of which were well validated. Telephone interviews were also used to gather this type of data. Some studies used direct observation of behaviour, such as cycle-helmet use and choice of meals in school canteens or shops. Some used observation in role playing, such as resisting abduction. This approach is clearly less practical for some topics, such as sex and drugs education. The reviews did not always indicate the means by which skills were assessed, but role playing has been used to assess generic skills (such as decision-making, resistance and assertiveness) and direct observation in real life or simulated settings to assess specific skills (such as crossing roads). The reviews did not always make clear the extent to which either reviewers or investigators had critically appraised the validity and reliability of the outcome measures. Lack of comment may indicate that this was not considered of great importance.

Changes to the environment (such as the nutritional content of school meals and availability of cycle helmets in the community) were most commonly reported in reviews of nutrition and exercise and accident and injury programmes. Impact on parents' behaviour (as shown by the contents of children's lunch boxes) was reported in nutrition and exercise studies. Reviews of nutrition and exercise programmes reported on a broad range of physiological measures: body fat, blood lipids, fitness, endurance and blood pressure. With the exception of salivary cotinine measurements in smoking prevention programmes, physiological measurements tended not to be used to evaluate other types of programme.

Accident and injury and sex and family life education reviews used event rates to evaluate the impact of programmes: accident or pregnancy rates or changes to the environment. Measures of wellbeing included self-esteem, self-concept, self-efficacy, empathy, locus of control, peer and family relationships, stress and anxiety, depression, hopelessness, loneliness and suicide intention. Reviews of mental health promotion programmes and some substance abuse and sex and family life programmes reported these most frequently. Such measures would in theory be valuable in detecting unexpected adverse outcomes in other topic areas, but, from the results reported in reviews, this did not appear to have happened

Efficacy

Most of the reviews concluded that school health promotion programmes improved knowledge and attitudes. Since knowledge is essential for health, these programmes could all be said to be successful. Some of the reviews were also able to show an impact on health-related skills. Reviews of nutrition and exercise and accident and injury programmes were able to show changes to the environment.

Although studies in all topic areas reported a positive impact on health-related behaviour, no reviews reported a consistent impact. If the goal was to improve health-related behaviour, no programmes were reliably successful. Nevertheless, the number of studies demonstrating an adverse effect on behaviour was very much smaller than the number showing a beneficial impact. Thus, although the impact may be small, on balance school health promotion programmes do more good than harm in the experimental setting. The results of these studies, combined with those of experimental studies in other settings and those of non-experimental studies using other methodologies, support the conclusion that health-related behaviour change is very difficult to achieve.

Reviews of nutrition and exercise reported studies that showed an impact on physiological measures. Some of the programmes reviewed in studies of mental health promotion were able to show improved wellbeing. Few adverse outcomes were reported, but the identification of adverse outcomes in our project depended on both the inclusion of appropriate outcome measures in the studies and the extraction of these measures into the reviews.

In general, reviewers seem to have assumed that improvements in behaviour are synonymous with improvements in health or wellbeing. Although biomedical-model research shows that health-related behaviour has an unequivocal impact on the incidence of specific diseases, the relationship between behaviour and health in its broadest sense (defined by WHO as "a state of complete physical, mental and social well-being" *(20)*) is much less clear cut. The argument is easier to support when applied to physical wellbeing than to emotional, mental and social wellbeing. The latter components of health are more likely to be damaged by health promotion initiatives. Most medical services and many public health services still concentrate on physical wellbeing. For a number reasons, one may suppose that further improvements in health may require the inclusion of emotional, mental and social wellbeing *(21)*. These aspects have been considered difficult to tackle, but several of the studies included in the two reviews of mental health promotion suggest that school-based programmes can affect emotional wellbeing. The concept of the health promoting school *(8)* was developed in part to allow a more holistic approach to health promotion. The development of self-esteem in and good relationships between staff and pupils are central to ENHPS, which encourages schools to develop programmes that cover the range of health-related lifestyles. Outcome measures that encompass emotional, mental and social wellbeing, as well as physical wellbeing, may need to be developed to evaluate these programmes.

Interestingly, reviewers of health promotion programmes seem not to have yet made the connection between emotional literacy programmes, social competence programmes and the promotion of mental health *(5)*. By enabling pupils better to understand their own and other people's emotions and behaviour, these programmes have the potential to improve both mental health and social wellbeing.

The development of valid and reliable measures of emotional, mental and social wellbeing would make an important contribution to the evaluation of school health promotion programmes. The use of such measures, in addition to measures of physical health, would enable evaluators to distinguish the programmes that improve behaviour only from those that improve health in its broadest sense, and perhaps to identify the occasional programme that improves behaviour at the expense of health. The use of outcome measures incorporating wellbeing also would begin the process of identifying programmes in which the process of delivery is respectful and honest, and guards against the potential abuse of children's greater vulnerability to coercion, misinformation and manipulation.

Conclusions and recommendations for policy-makers

Further development of health promotion in schools may depend on changing the goals of programmes. If the goal is to improve health, programmes should be designed, implemented and evaluated in a socially healthy way, and evaluated using outcome measures encompassing health in its broadest sense. Concentration on the promotion of physical wellbeing to the exclusion of emotional, mental and social wellbeing may have detracted from the effectiveness of school-based programmes.

Different types of health promotion programme could learn from each other. Focusing on a narrow range of disease-based outcome measures may have contributed to the apparent failure of, for example, accident prevention programmes to make use of the knowledge that informs substance abuse programmes and vice versa. Many of these suggestions have already been incorporated in the health promoting school initiative.

Concentration on experimental methodologies, particularly the randomized controlled trial, is likely to be misleading in school health promotion research. Evaluations of school health promotion programmes need to take account of the nature of the intervention. Researchers should recognize the limitations of the experimental model in programmes that require the active engagement of participants, and that experimental evaluation is rarely able to take account of the process of delivery, which is critically important in the development of health. Evaluation of delivery requires observational methodologies, particularly qualitative research. Research and development that take equal account of the contribution made by different research methodologies are more likely to be successful in the long run.

References

1. STEWART-BROWN, S.L. New approaches to school health. *Progress in community child health*, **2**: 137–158 (1998).
2. FLETCHER, J. ET AL. *Systematic review of reviews of health promotion in schools*. Oxford, Health Services Research Unit, University of Oxford, 1997.
3. LISTER-SHARP, D. ET AL. *Health promoting schools and health promotion in schools: two systematic reviews*. Alton, Core Research, 1999 (Health Technology Assessment, Vol. 3, No. 22).
4. BARLOW, J. & STEWART-BROWN, S.L. Systematic review of the school entry medical examination. *Archives of disease of childhood*, **78**: 301–311 (1998).

5.   WELLS, J. A systematic review of mental health promotion in schools. *In*: Buchanan, A. & Hudson, B., ed. *Promoting children's emotional well-being*. Oxford, Oxford University Press, 2000.
6.   CHAPMAN, S. & STEWART-BROWN, S.L. *The school entry health check: the literature*. Oxford, Health Services Research Unit, University of Oxford, 1998.
7.   *Promoting health through schools*: report of a WHO Expert Committee on Comprehensive School Health Education and Promotion. Geneva, World Health Organization, 1997 (WHO Technical Report Series, No. 870).
8.   PARSONS, C. ET AL. The health promoting school in Europe: conceptualising and evaluating the change. *Health education journal*, **55**: 311–321 (1996).
9.   Ottawa Charter for Health Promotion. *Health promotion*, **1**(4): iii–v (1986).
10. HICKMAN, M. & HEALY, C. The European Network of Health Promoting Schools: development and evaluation in England. *Health education journal*, **55**: 456–470 (1996).
11. PIETTE, D. ET AL. *Towards an evaluation of the European network of health promoting schools*. Brussels, Commission of European Communities, WHO Regional Office for Europe, Council of Europe, 1995.
12. STEPHENSON, J. & IMRIE, J. Why do we need randomised controlled trials to assess behavioural interventions? *British medical journal*, **316**: 611–613 (1998).
13. HSIEH, F.Y. Sample size formulae for intervention studies with the cluster as unit of randomization. *Statistics in medicine*, **8**: 1195–1201 (1988).
14. HAMILTON, K. & SAUNDERS, L. *The health promoting school: a summary of the ENHPS evaluation project in England*. London, Health Education Authority, 1997.
15. ROE, L. ET AL. *Health promotion interventions to promote healthy eating in the general population: a review*. London, Health Education Authority, 1997.
16. KEAYS, J. *The effects of regular (moderate to vigorous) physical activity in the school setting on students' health, fitness, cognition, psychological development, academic performance and classroom behaviour*. York, Ontario, North York Community Health Promotion Research Unit, 1993.
17. ANTMAN, E.M. ET AL. A comparison of results of meta-analyses of randomized control trials and recomendations of clinical experts. Treatments for myocardial infarction. *Journal of the American Medical Association*, **268**: 240–248 (1992).
18. CHALMERS, I. ET AL. *Systematic reviews*. London, BMJ Publishing Group, 1995.
19. HANSEN, W. School based substance abuse prevention: a review of the state of the art in the curriculum 1980–1990. *Health education research*, **7**: 403–430 (1992).

20. Constitution of the World Health Organization. *In*: *Basic documents*, 42nd ed. Geneva, World Health Organization, 1999.
21. STEWART-BROWN, S.L. Emotional wellbeing and its relation to health. *British medical journal*, **317**: 1608–1609 (1998).

13
Evaluating health promotion programmes in the workplace

Lindsey Dugdill and Jane Springett

Introduction

Workplace health promotion has become a focus of increasing activity in recent years, particularly in countries where employers have an economic interest in the reduction of health care costs and worker compensation benefits through health insurance schemes *(1,2)*. While the incentive for employers is reduction in costs and absenteeism, government agencies see the work setting as "the single most important channel to systematically reach the adult population through health information and health promotion programmes" *(3)*.

Health promotion programmes were first introduced in the workplace in the 1960s as part of occupational health schemes, largely for safety and product quality reasons, but have since evolved into a wide range of approaches to improve employees' health *(4)*. The early programmes focused on one illness or risk factor, such as coronary heart disease or smoking. As an example of subsequent development, the wellness programmes in the United States offered a more complex range of intervention, featuring a variety of risk and behavioural factors. Currently, the most comprehensive types of intervention are corporate health care strategies, which have taken a multilevel approach; examples include the Du Pont health promotion programme *(5)* and programmes undertaken by a number of companies in Germany *(4)*.

Although workplace health programmes within large companies tend to be more comprehensive than those adopted in the past, they still focus mainly on the health of the individual worker, rather than the health needs of the organization. They rarely consider the relationship of the organization to the broader community, but making changes that promote workplace health requires an organizational understanding of health that reaches beyond individual responsibility *(6)*. Recognition of this has led to a call for what Goldbeck *(7)* has called fourth-generation programmes, which consider all activities, policies and decisions within an organization related to the health of employees, their families and the communities in which they live, as well as the companies' consumers. Different models have been put forward to suggest the form such a comprehensive approach should take *(8–10)*. All advocate the use of a multilevel approach designed to integrate individual, organizational and community-level strategies in a manner similar to that advocated in the framework of the business sector's response to the AIDS crisis in the United States (11).

Integrated approaches to health in organizational settings have implications for how worksite evaluation strategies are undertaken (12–14). While the literature contains studies that evaluate the individual components of such strategies, few have examined comprehensive strategies as a whole, owing to the difficulties of separating out the effects of different components of these complex interventions. In addition, little evidence in the literature compares organizational interventions with those focusing on individuals and/or restricted to specific lifestyle issues such as alcohol consumption or exercise participation. Since many of these interventions are short term (12 months), there is little research evidence on the crucial issue of the sustainability of health change. The available evidence on interventions to promote behavioural changes suggests a limited population effect over time (15). Further, the issue of process evaluation is often inadequately addressed. An extensive review of workplace research in the United States concluded that many evaluation studies were of limited breadth, despite the widespread adoption of health promotion programmes in enterprises (11). One reason for this is the lack of incentive for employers to document outcomes, and the lack of integration of evaluation into the design and implementation of workplace health programmes.

Moreover, most health promotion activity takes place in organizations with over 500 employees. Large organizations have traditionally had occupational health services. Most people work in small and medium-sized enterprises, particularly those with fewer than 100 employees, however, and the problems of delivering occupational health care to these enterprises are well attested (16). Persuading smaller businesses to accept the advantages of integrating health promoting activities into their working practices, in addition to statutory health and safety requirements, is a difficult challenge: one that the appropriate evaluation of health interventions in small workplaces, currently rare, may help to achieve.

Recent literature suggests that evaluation within the workplace setting is receiving higher priority, as it is now seen as a vital mechanism for planning appropriate health activities and empowering workers to make decisions about their health needs. WHO (4) has identified five main reasons for undertaking worksite evaluation:

- promoting the systematic planning and implementation of workplace health activities;
- making health and business successes more visible, which in turn can act as a public relations vehicle for the company/organization;
- providing a convincing argument for having a long-term company health policy;
- helping to identify changes that need to be made in a worksite health promotion plan or policy; and

286

- providing substantial information on the social nature of the employees within the organization, which can be used in planning future facilities or staff development programmes.

This chapter provides an overview of the main types of evaluation undertaken, the main findings on the effectiveness of workplace interventions, the methodologies used and their appropriateness both to the workplace as a setting and to evaluating comprehensive approaches. We then suggest a way forward in addressing these issues, including ways of encouraging health promotion planning and implementation that incorporate an evaluation component.

Types of evaluations undertaken

Broadly, evaluations of workplace interventions have fallen into two categories:

- those focusing on single interventions and seeing health promotion as acting within the work environment; and
- those examining comprehensive approaches and wider organizational issues, and evaluating activities that help to create healthy organizations as a setting.

The following review considers these two approaches within the following categories: studies using control groups, process evaluations and studies aiming to measure cost–benefit, cost–effectiveness or both.

Studies using control groups

The dominant methodological approach for single interventions has been the use of either a control group or a retrospective case study. The latter has been used largely in studies comparing firms. Some experimental studies have been carried out, particularly looking at mental and physical fatigue and psychological stress (drawing on a long tradition of occupational psychological research) and, more recently, exercise, nutrition, weight control and smoking programmes. Among a great number of research studies, however, it is hard to find examples of evaluations of full-scale changes in the working environment or of health action programmes of meaningful scope. Case-study research has been more successful in identifying the impact of more comprehensive strategies, but comparison has been difficult, as programme designs are so complex and vary between organizations and between countries.

In quasi-experimental studies, difficulties have arisen where control groups have been used. Finding appropriate control groups has proved very difficult, because they need to consist of workers who are employed in a workplace comparable to the experimental setting. Very often, working with organizations within a geographical area creates a ripple effect: as other organizations hear about what is going on in one business, they may be eager to try to implement health-related interventions for themselves. This can reduce the number of potential control workplaces. In addition, many studies report self-selection and attrition as methodological problems.

Often, too, the evaluation takes place over a limited time (12 months on average): too short to measure the long-term benefits of programmes or assess the sustainability of changes. Moreover, as mentioned, many evaluations focus only on outcomes; few have measured the extent to which different strands of an intervention programme contribute to the reported benefits. The Norwegian Work Research Institute made a study of restaurant workers, analysing the work environment in holistic terms. It demonstrated that factors in the work environment were rather insignificant when examined separately, but had a synergistic impact on health when considered together *(17)*.

Evaluations of workplace health promotion activity that use control groups have focused mainly on measuring changes in health behaviour *(15)*. Such studies usually take pre- and post-intervention measurements of one or more of the following: physical activity levels, smoking behaviour, alcohol consumption, stress levels and diet. They assess effectiveness by looking for significant positive changes in behaviour, such as smoking cessation *(18–20)*. The best designed studies of this type have included both physical and behavioural measures.

Current research shows that one-off fitness or screening programmes, which tend to be self-selecting towards the healthier members of the workforce, have a limited effect that is not sustained over time. Erfurt et al. *(21)* evaluated the effectiveness of intervention designs in controlling various lifestyle factors (blood pressure, obesity and smoking) in manufacturing plants. The programme designs (which included counselling, a menu of intervention types and assessment of the social organization of the plant) were more successful in reducing risk factors than programmes that featured screening alone or a more restricted intervention choice. This study emphasizes the importance of using personal outreach to at-risk groups, giving workers a choice of intervention type and using counselling to enable people to make sustainable health decisions. While comprehensive support systems within the workplace, such as peer support through self-help, are probably one of the most important factors in sustaining behaviour change over time, evaluation studies often ignore such psychosocial variables.

Larger studies often report attempts to measure changes in absenteeism; for example, Bertera *(22)* studied absenteeism among full-time employees in a large, multilocation, diversified industrial population. Over two years, absenteeism declined 14% in blue-collar employees participating in a comprehensive health promotion intervention and 5.8% in control groups. Reduced absenteeism offset programme costs within the first year.

Process evaluation

Some recent studies have looked at the process: how workplace health programmes and policies have been implemented and the implications of this for success. Process evaluation should take account of the cultural context in which the intervention is implemented; some now consider it an essential part of rigorous evaluation design *(23)*; hence it is a fundamental requirement for the efficient and effective planning of health activity in any workplace. Although most workplace evaluation studies describe programme effectiveness in quantitative terms (such as increased productivity or reduced sick-leave), an increasing number focuses on qualitative issues as well, since many of the positive benefits of health promotion (such as better staff morale) cannot immediately be measured in monetary terms.

Oakley et al. *(24)* identify the necessity for including process measures into evaluation studies; of the few reported studies that do so, most are from the United States and nearly all tend to focus on lifestyle issues, rather than more comprehensive health processes that involve organizational structure and policy. Gottlieb & Nelson *(25)* carried out one such study, and describe the implementation of a policy restricting smoking in decentralized worksites. Their evaluation framework included elements that explored concept, context, process and outcomes, and was used to identify characteristics that influenced implementation: the degree of policy restrictiveness, job characteristics, perceived level of worker participation in formulation and implementation, and support of supervisors responsible for day-to-day enforcement. Low levels of participation underlay many of the problems experienced during implementation.

A limited number of high-quality evaluations gives equal weight to process, impact and outcome measures. Such holistic evaluation frameworks, however, are more likely to provide data useful in exploring a programme's progress towards its goals. In turn, a broad portfolio of relevant, appropriate evaluation data can best inform the future development of sustainable health interventions.

Cost–benefit and cost–effectiveness

Some authors argue strongly that the future of both intervention programmes and their evaluation lies in the use of behavioural science models, integrated with financial models of programme evaluation *(15,26)*. For example, Katzman & Smith *(27)* have developed a methodology to determine the effectiveness of occupational health promotion programmes from a cost–benefit perspective. In the past, formal cost–benefit or cost–effectiveness analyses were rare even in the largest companies, and tended to focus first on occupational health activities, such as medical screening, and second on the immediate impact of an intervention. Pelletier's extensive review of over 76 studies of cost–effectiveness *(1)* indicates a growing body of evidence demonstrating cost–effectiveness outcomes from health promotion programmes. The evaluation periods of these studies ranged from six months to seven years. The findings showed that any evaluation study of cost–effectiveness should consider the differential impact on different at-risk groups. In some cases, the failure to target high-risk groups diluted the cost–effectiveness of the intervention.

Assessment of intervention efficiency (whether the end result of the programme could have been achieved at lower cost) has been rare, probably because measuring costs and benefits is very difficult. These difficulties arise for many reasons; for instance, measuring many health benefits requires the use of subjective measures that are not quantifiable. No single cost–benefit analysis process is widely accepted anyway. Nash et al. *(28)* remark: "... there can be no uniquely 'proper' way to do cost–benefit analysis; it is to be expected (and in our view welcome) that the studies will be done in many different ways ... each technique must reflect one or more value judgements".

Some authors advocate carrying out cost–benefit analysis by one consistent method, whose value judgements are agreed on professional grounds by economists. Lichfield *(29)* argued that, as it is more useful to accept the variety of schools of economic thought, it is wiser to take account of the relevant values of stakeholders and decision-makers when developing cost–benefit models. This view is in keeping with the philosophy of empowerment at the core of health promotion (see Chapter 1). Considering the complexity of the analysis process, it is not surprising that comprehensive cost–benefit analysis of workplace health programmes is in its infancy.

Ergonomic issues and work design are often the key factors in cost–benefit evaluation in Scandinavian studies. Spilling et al. *(30)* made a retrospective analysis of work at Standard Telefon og Kabelfabrik (STK) in Kongsvinger, Norway. The mainly female workforce assembled parts for telephone exchanges. Average sick-leave for musculoskeletal problems in the seven years before the ergonomic redesign of workstations was equivalent to 5.3% of total production time, but peaked at 10% in the final year before ergonomic changes were introduced. In the seven years following the changes, the sick-leave figure remained relatively steady: an average of about 3.1%. Labour turnover fell from 30.1% per year in the period preceding the changes to 7.6% in the period following. The financial implications were that – taking account of the cost of changes and reductions in recruitment, training and sickness benefit – an investment of about 340 000 Norwegian *kroner* (NKr) had saved STK more than NKr 3.2 million in operating costs over a twelve-year period.

This example illustrates the type of indicators that predominates in evaluations. It reflects the priorities of the chief stakeholders: company shareholders. Cultural differences play an important role here. The type of approach adopted reflects who initiates the health promotion programme and why, along with dominant management style. Weinstein *(31)* argues that North American and European programmes differ markedly. The former are usually initiated by senior management and focus on beneficial changes in personal health behaviour, and hence reduction in associated medical care costs, while European programmes, as exemplified by Scandinavian work, aim at legislative and structural change *(32)*. In Europe, trade unions usually initiate the activity and it focuses on psychosocial and environmental issues and job redesign.

Issues in the development of effective evaluation

This section identifies the issues that we believe are vital to the development of effective evaluation strategies for health activities in the workplace setting. Fundamental to that development is the acknowledgement that the process used to develop an evaluation strategy is as important as the final decision on what measurements are actually made.

Workplace and organizational issues

Some have argued that workplace health promotion should ideally be holistic, with interventions that focus on both the environment and the individual and that use multiple strategies. Considering the number of companies and organizations that have introduced some form of health promotion programme, however, rigorous evaluations have been rare (11,12). Reasons for this arise from the nature of occupational health practice, the current inadequacies of health promotion practice and the nature of businesses.

The traditions of occupational health practice, to which most workplace activity has been confined, evolved within the context of health and safety legislation and are divorced from wider public health issues. Thus, occupational health has tended to focus on screening and the assessment and control of threats to workplace health that arise from the chemical, physical and biological environments. It has failed to take account of newly recognized threats to health, particularly those due to the psychosocial environment (32). Most occupational health professionals are from single-discipline backgrounds and may be unfamiliar with the multidisciplinary, participatory approach that health promotion demands and that could challenge current professional practice. As a result, many have resisted a broader approach. Trade unions, too, are more likely to engage in traditional health and safety activities than to encourage health promotion. Indeed, a European survey of health-related activity at work indicated a low level of awareness of what constitutes comprehensive workplace health promotion. While action for safety is often quickly integrated into work practice, health is often seen as a medical issue quite separate from working conditions, and medical audit is rarely considered (33).

To date, much health promotion practice in the workplace has lacked rigour, with many activities taking place in isolation and adopting a largely unsophisticated approach. Rarely is such activity part of a coordinated strategy with an integrated approach to problem analysis (needs assessment) and programme planning, implementation and evaluation procedures. Moreover, many workplace interventions are relatively short; they do not address the challenges of long-term maintenance or self-selection (whereby the employees most likely to benefit from, for example, lifestyle changes are not targeted). We believe that a rigorous evaluation study uses a variety of tools and methods to collect portfolios of data. These data should be highly relevant to the aims and objectives of the programme being evaluated and to the priorities of the target groups, and should be useful in directing change processes. If appropriate and useful data can be collected and relevant stakeholders engaged in the process, the evaluation is much more likely to bring about change.

Another issue in the development of effective evaluation is the field of operation of workplace health promotion, which potentially extends beyond the workplace. The settings approach provides a captive group of people, who are engaged in a setting for a significant portion of their time, and apparently have ability to control and therefore influence the factors that affect their health. While work indisputably influences general wellbeing, however, health promotion activities in the workplace artificially separate work from other aspects of people's lives, particularly for women. Women in paid employment report fewer symptoms of ill health and greater life satisfaction, but suffer increasing stress from the demands of multiple roles, including caring for children and elderly relatives, for example. Dean's quantitative study of Danish women *(34)* concluded that conditions of employment and family support services are needed to facilitate health promoting everyday routines. The prospects for this do not seem promising, given current pressure in western countries to work longer hours to maintain job security. We believe that health interventions and their concomitant evaluation strategies need to take account of and cross the interfaces between home and work domains, if they are to be truly effective.

This lack of attention to different groups' specific needs is reflected in the way needs assessment is undertaken. Making a health needs assessment before determining the nature of the intervention is now seen as good health promotion practice. This can also be seen as formative evaluation. Conventional approaches to health needs assessment, however, tend to reinforce existing practice. For example, questions are often chosen for questionnaires without reference to the population from whom the data will be collected. Thus, the agenda is already set, and the needs assessment tends to reflect the dominant employer view that health is about individual lifestyle. This results in the implementation of inappropriate interventions. Moreover, because workforce issues are neglected, response to questionnaires is poor and staff lack commitment, leading to poor data and compliance. It also means that activity tends to be targeted at the healthier staff. An effective process of development for health promotion activity should aim to overcome these problems.

If workers' realities differ from those of managers and even of health promotion practitioners, mechanisms need to be in place to allow these different experiences to be articulated and incorporated in the agenda for change. Participatory action research strategies are often seen as a way to overcome some of the problems of conventional approaches. Further, using qualitative techniques *(13)* such as focus groups can do much to break down the divide between the public and the private in health knowledge. Action research allows the lay perspective to be articulated.

The diversity and complexity of workplaces make them challenging settings for evaluation. Their multifaceted nature creates difficulties for conventional evaluation designs attempting to isolate intervention effects from other variables. Workplaces vary in organizational structure, as well as size, and much depends on their level of development, economic stability and culture, including management style. Other considerations include:

- the type of company: for example, whether the workplace is a branch of a larger company;
- employment conditions, such as staff's access to facilities, the nature of staff contracts and conditions, and the presence or absence of an active workers' union;
- the age, gender, ethnicity and skill mix of the workforce; and
- local socioeconomic conditions.

Measuring the success of a programme without reference to the conditions in which employees live would not give due weight to small-scale achievements in areas of poor living conditions, and might be a disincentive to any form of evaluation.

All these different dimensions are multiplied if the organization is a large, multisite operation. Many organizations have multiple sites (such as National Health Service (NHS) hospital trusts in the United Kingdom) and these pose particular challenges for health promotion practitioners trying to meet the health needs of workers at different sites. Sites might vary in combinations of job type and culture, as well as location. Moreover, companies increasingly use contractors who work from home. Organizations such as the NHS often have many staff who are not directly employed but work either freelance or as part of a contracted-in service. Workplace health programmes are not always explicitly extended to such workers, so they may have no workplace health support. Such complexities raise the issue of what constitutes the object of evaluation when defining the workplace and defining the boundary of the object of research in any evaluation.

Finally, a major barrier to effective evaluation is lack of resources: money, staff and time. This is a problem for small and medium-sized enterprises in particular but also for larger organizations, except those with strong traditions and philosophies of human resource management, well developed health policies and specific health budgets. Many employers fail, for example, to keep accessible sickness records that would provide the basis of a simple monitoring of progress. The difficulties of working with small and medium-sized organizations are even greater. Cash flow and the ever-present problem of survival create fluid environments and business practices that keep health low on the agenda.

Methodological issues

Decisions on evaluation methodology, mechanisms of employee participation, and evaluation measures and indicators should take account of many of the factors highlighted above. Validation approaches to methodological design,

293

such as the randomized controlled trial, are difficult to implement and do not integrate well into an environment where change is the norm. Reliance on highly structured, intensive and expensive interventions delivered by highly trained research staff creates a set of conditions difficult to replicate *(1,35)*, but the use of randomized control groups remains the gold standard for good evaluation, and this is reflected in the criteria used to assess the quality of research in this area. For example, the review of workplace health promotion and education interventions by Oakley et al. *(24)* highlighted eight criteria for rigorous evaluation:

- clear definition of aims;
- a detailed description of the intervention that would allow replication;
- a randomly allocated control group to increase the confidence with which observed differences in outcomes can be attributed to the intervention;
- the provision of data on numbers of participants involved in intervention or control groups;
- the provision of pre-intervention data;
- the provision of post-intervention data;
- attrition rates from intervention types; and
- reported findings from all outcome measures.

A literature review in the *American journal of health promotion* advocated comprehensive approaches to health promotion in the workplace and drew attention to the methodological difficulties casting doubt on the results of some of experimental and quasi-experimental studies. The authors gave three stars to evaluations without comparison groups and five stars to "properly conducted studies with randomized control groups", but also said that these ratings did not reflect the richness of individual studies and that "readers should venture past the overall ratings and judge each study on its merits, taking into consideration the study's unique objectives, methods and constraints" *(11)*.

We argue that these criteria reflect a particular paradigmatic perspective that requires a level of experimental control that is impossible to reach in the real world of the workplace. Moreover, they are too concerned with intervention, change and outcome, paying insufficient attention to the value of process measurement to enhance understanding of how and why an intervention works. The fluid nature of the workplace setting requires a holistic and innovative evaluation approach, drawing on a paradigm that places change at the centre of research design. Such an approach comes from the field of action-oriented methodologies, which fully engage the participants (in this case, the workers and managers of an organization) in the process. They are well known in business research and management science. Such approaches generate different criteria for high-quality evaluations, including those relevant to organizations. This is important if organizations are to be persuaded to implement and assess workplace health promotion.

In the public sector, for example, expenditure cuts and the tightening of budgetary control have increased the emphasis on performance, accountability and effectiveness. Carter et al. *(36)* have argued that, "good performance indicators should measure performance that is 'owned' by the organization and not dependent on external actors ... performance indicators should be relevant to the needs and objectives of the organization".

Similarly, discussions of effectiveness and efficiency in health promotion programmes need to be combined with issues of quality assurance. Workplace evaluations should aim to include some measures of quality, such as workers' self-reported opinions about the benefits of an intervention. Such measures have tended to be criticized for their lack of objectivity, and hence are often neglected in the development of an evaluation protocol. Qualitative data, however, can provide valuable information for the organization to use, for example, in public relations. To enhance the validity of such qualitative data, a variety of research methodologies can be used throughout the entire evaluation process, in a triangulation technique. Triangulation allows layers of quantitative and qualitative data to be built up in a way that cross-validates the information *(23,37)*. An action research approach to the evaluation would allow participants to develop a set of indicators as the evaluation process proceeds. These would both be appropriate and reflect existing concerns as they change.

Finally, methodologies should be developed to cross the interfaces between different settings. As mentioned, people live in a variety of different settings that affect their health, such as the home, school and workplace. While these settings have unique characteristics, people constantly move between them. Thus, considering people's health from a broad perspective requires taking account of their health needs within the variety of settings in which they interact from day to day. For the working population, this means taking account of factors that affect their health at home and in the wider community, and developing intervention and evaluation strategies that bridge this gap, as well as that between research and action.

Action research approaches to evaluation

Although most workplace evaluation studies have adopted a positivist approach, a growing number of studies has recently taken an action research and, potentially, a more holistic approach, enabling both environmental and individual issues to be addressed (see Chapter 4). Action research engages the participants as part of the evaluation process, thus enabling the managers and workers jointly to make fundamental decisions about the evaluation process and the measurements to be made.

This type of approach allows the rather complex nature of the workplace to be evaluated alongside continuing organizational changes and intervention planning. Since action research is an accepted approach in management practice and education, the workplace is a natural setting for its use. It has the added advantage of allowing the business agenda of the organization to play its part in generating relevant indicators of change. In addition, the evaluation of health promotion programmes can link with developments within the organizational setting, for example, through quality assurance programmes. Of course, firms vary widely in values and priorities, and between cultures and countries *(38)*, as well as sectors.

Hugentobler et al. *(37)* used an action research approach in a project conducted in a medium-sized plant manufacturing components, in Michigan. They argue that the use of multiple types of data provided a broad-based, cross-validated identification and in-depth understanding of the problems and needs in the worksite, and guided the development of interventions that were appropriate to the setting. Making evaluation an integral part of the programme also contributes to the integration of health promotion into the workplace culture.

Moreover, participatory intervention and evaluation themselves help to improve health, as demonstrated by much of the research work coming out of northern European countries. Glasgow et al. *(39)* show that smoking cessation programmes work more effectively if they are developed with strong input from employee steering committees. The authors also highlight how continuing programme modification, using knowledge of the implementation process, can continuously improve programme action.

One of the most comprehensive studies to date, which assessed effectiveness from a psychosocial and organizational-design point of view, is a longitudinal action research project conducted in a manufacturing plant in Scandinavia *(40)*. It looked particularly at social support and participation in and control over decision-making. Using both qualitative and quantitative data, it asked to what extent:

- varying degrees of exposure to the intervention resulted in different effects;
- changes in social support, participation, stress and behavioural and health outcomes could be attributed to the intervention; and
- changes in social support and participation resulted in changes in stress and behavioural and health outcomes.

The researchers made an initial needs assessment to provide baseline data on personal resources (such as self-esteem, mastery of work-related tasks, interpersonal relationships, participation in and influence over decision-making, and coping behaviour) and a basis for action. Interventions included the creation of a newsletter, information display boards and participation programmes, and modification of the performance appraisal system. This study was exceptional in its approach and scope because the firm, situated in an area where labour was scarce, was keen to retain the labour force. As Eklund *(41)* has demonstrated from an analysis of work organization in assembly plants, the nature of the labour market usually determines an organization's interest in the quality of working life.

Guidelines for the evaluation of health promotion programmes in the workplace

How, then, can employers be encouraged to adopt effective health promotion practices and, more important, to evaluate them? The guidelines for the United Kingdom Workplace Task Force report *(42)* were developed with these issues in mind. The Task Force was a multidisciplinary group of professionals, including representatives from businesses, who were brought together as part of the Government's strategic response to the improvement of health in the workplace setting, highlighted in *The health of the nation (43)*. Its main aims were to review and assess past and current activity on health promotion in the workplace. The development work focused on two areas:

- more effectively evaluating such activity
- marketing health promotion, particularly among small and medium-sized enterprises.

The review found very little evaluative work being implemented, particularly in the United Kingdom, so the Task Force commissioned us to write guidelines for the evaluation of workplace health activities. We developed the guidelines to enable health promotion and health care practitioners to create and use more effective evaluation strategies. As mentioned above, we strongly emphasize evaluation as a process of rigorous good practice, using a portfolio of tools and measures appropriate to a particular workplace and health promotion situation. Thus, each evaluation strategy would be unique, but the process used to develop it would be transferable between different workplace settings.

Table 13.1 shows the original guidelines. They outline a series of steps that an evaluation process should follow, and a set of principles to ensure that the evaluation is worth the effort spent on it. The process is iterative, the steps being followed in sequence, and describes an ideal at which to aim. In practice, the steps may need to be revisited; this changes the sequential progression into a series of dynamic cycles in which evaluators back-track to pick up vital information or to involve new groups of workers in the process. This chapter builds on the original guidelines and represents progress in thinking since they were produced.

The principles are derived from a tradition of evaluation developed by Patton *(23)*, based on social science methodology and grounded in the techniques of education and sociological inquiry. They also draw on the techniques of action research commonly used in management science for elucidating complex problems in industrial relations and contributing to decision-making on the management of change. Thus, the approach is particularly applicable to the workplace and has been used in Canada, the Netherlands, Sweden and the United States for workplace health promotion.

The basic premise was that the purpose of evaluation is to provide useful information in the most practical way possible. At its best, evaluation is a

Table 13.1. Participatory evaluation of a health promotion programme: main actions, associated actions and comments

Main actions	Associated actions	Comments
Step 1. Clarify the aims and objectives of the proposed programme.	Get the participants on board. Set up an evaluation group. Determine what the real health problem is. Establish baseline information.	The importance of spending time on this groundwork cannot be over-emphasized. Involvement of the right people will ensure commitment to the use of the information generated and a good response to any questionnaires. The evaluation group (at least three people) should reflect the range of interests. Proper clarification makes the evaluation straightforward.
Step 2. Design the framework for evaluation and what questions to ask.	Decide the purpose of the evaluation and who will use the information. Decide what questions are useful to ask in relation to achieving aims and objectives. Decide from whom to collect information. Decide whether process as well as outcome information is needed.	Take this action before deciding what measures to use. If the objectives have been stated clearly, this should be relatively easy. Be clear about the aims of the evaluation; this affects what questions are asked. The main aim is to see whether the activities in the programme resulted in achieving the stated objectives. Try to look at process as well as outcome.
Step 3. Design the framework for evaluation and decide how to measure change.	Decide what to measure and which methods to use. Decide on sample size and target population. Decide when to collect the information.	Good measurement depends on being clear about the issues. Methods should be appropriate to the questions and need not be numerical. Be realistic and honest about limitations of time and money.
Step 4. Collect the data.	Make sure data collection is unobtrusive and does not add to participants' workload or, if it does, they can see the value of doing it. Make sure participants are still on board. Keep participants informed by regular feedback. Remember that data are not information.	There will be problems of confidentiality and bias. Bias is most common in self-reported behaviour. Problems are smaller if all stakeholders have been involved. Participation is a key.

Main actions	Associated actions	Comments
Step 5. Evaluate the results to determine the effectiveness of the programme.	Interpret data in association with the evaluation group, comparing what actually happened with what was expected. Remember that numbers are only indicators of what the world is like.	Data are not information until they have been interpreted. This is best done as a collaborative process, so the participants understand how the results were obtained. Remember the value of so-called soft information, and that some health changes take time to be revealed.
Step 6. Make recommendations.	Clarify what is useful. Cover practical changes for immediate implementation. Include the costs and benefits of not implementing as well as implementing the recommendations. Challenge existing beliefs. Look for longer-term changes that may not yet be visible.	If the participants have been involved in the process, they will already be committed to acting on the findings and be receptive to results

Source: Workplace Task Force report. London, Department of Health, 1993.

299

learning process that is an integral part of action for change in the workplace. It therefore should not take place in isolation, but form part of an integrated approach to analysis, planning and implementation. The approach adopted emphasizes everyone's involvement in the process, so that the consumers or users of health promotion drive the process at their own pace. This increases the likelihood that the results of the evaluation process will be used. The guidelines developed do not offer a definitive answer to all evaluation problems, but describe the process by which an evaluation can best be conducted, so that the tools most appropriate for the situation can be selected to generate the information needed. Following the stages in the guidelines should ensure that all the participants understand the pay-offs and the reliability and validity of the information gathered. The framework was to be used for evaluating both small and specific programmes, such as fitness testing and smoking cessation classes, and the health impact of particular work practices or organizational and managerial changes, such as restructuring.

Most crucial of all, the original report *(42)* highlighted the importance of spending most of the evaluation time on the first steps in the process. Research has shown that companies that are most successful in implementing change spent 90% of their time on developing the strategy and getting people on board, and 10% on implementation *(44)*.

Principles for the evaluation of health promotion in the workplace

These principles add to and expand on those set down in the original guidelines. Both the guidelines and this chapter argue that, no matter what resources are available or the size of the company or programme, five basic principles need to be followed to achieve effective evaluation.

Starting the formative evaluation process with health needs assessment

First, a well planned needs assessment is a key precursor to the entire process. The needs assessment should be user driven, so that formative evaluation and intervention planning become one integral process, enhancing, not disrupting, current work practice. This is more likely to result in interventions tailored to particular settings. The precise intervention developed may not be transferable to other settings, but the principles used to generate ideas about the intervention and evaluation design are applicable everywhere. Hawe et al. *(45)* state:

> In the first instance it is better to direct people to a careful description and understanding of the problem and how it is being experienced and postpone argument about what might be the answer to the problem, as this may lead to the problem itself being obscured. The purpose of needs assessment is to do just this. After the problems have been understood, and one has been chosen as the first priority, a range of possible solutions might be put forward.

300

Recent health promotion literature includes numerous models of health needs assessment. For instance, Harvey *(46)* describes a community diagnosis model, using a wide range of quantitative and qualitative data, some of which already exist (epidemiological data) and some that have to be collected (community perceptions). In the workplace, existing data sources may include budget sheets, sickness/absence data, medical records from the occupational health department and workplace surveys. After reviewing the existing data, the participants can decide whether further data collection during the health needs assessment process is necessary and, if so, the types of additional data that need to be collected. Ideally, a working group comprising members of all different sectors of the workforce will make these decisions.

Participation and feedback

As indicated above, the evaluation process should be participatory. There are two reasons for this. First, an evaluation should show the views and perspectives of different interest groups, especially the less powerful in both management and workforce. People have different perceptions of what an evaluation should entail, and their views will vary according to the context, depending on priorities and organizational structures. Second, the participants should know what is happening.

Good feedback is crucial to success in any data collection exercise. If key managers are involved, the knowledge gained from evaluation is more likely to be used. Involving workers strengthens their psychological health and encourages their adherence to intervention strategies. Workplaces and groups within them have different cultural values. For example, groups of workers in Liverpool City Council's housing department reported varying levels of associated job stress, according to levels of contact with the general public *(47)*. Previously, management had not perceived this as a priority health issue for workers, but focused on lifestyle changes and the physical working environment. A wide cross-section of workers should ideally be involved in the needs assessment to identify relevant health issues.

Clarity about the purpose of evaluation

Evaluation varies in time-scale. Process evaluation examines what happens during programme planning and implementation. The Liverpool housing department, for example, developed different strategies to change work practice as solutions to problems associated with stress, such as reducing individual contact time with the general public. Impact evaluation measures the immediate effects of a programme, such as improved reported health status. Outcome evaluation measures longer-term effects, such as reductions in sickness absenteeism over a five-year period.

Ideally, a balance of process, impact and outcome indicators is required to assess progress towards planned health goals and to understand what health activities are successful and why. Thus, the programme's goal should have a rational fit with its activities, if it is to be evaluated effectively. For example, if the aim is to reduce stress, introducing a no-smoking policy is no good without some support to help people to find other coping strategies.

Moreover, decisions about evaluation should be made at the same time as workplace health activities are being planned, to ensure that relevant data are collected for the duration of the activity. Examples of basic information might include numbers and reasons for sickness absenteeism, what workers describe as their work health problems, numbers of smokers, means of transport to work, use of showers, knowledge of health issues, levels of perceived stress and self-esteem, and coping behaviour.

Producing useful information

The types of data collected should produce useful information, and will depend on who the evaluation is for and what information is required. The stakeholders will probably be a combination of the following: a chief executive, line managers, trade union representatives, health and safety personnel and workers. Data can be collected at different levels. For example, at the individual level, regular fitness testing (using physiological measures) provides workers with some feedback on how well they are doing while participating in an activity, and this encourages further participation in the programme. At the group level, a questionnaire will provide information on changes in attitudes, beliefs and behaviour before, during and after a programme. At the company level, data on absenteeism rates will provide information on how well the programme is doing and whether continued investment is worth while.

The timing of data collection is crucial for measuring effectiveness. Workplace programmes focusing on individuals, for example, should take account of the degree of adherence over time. Experience suggests that measurements should be taken twice after the programme ends: at 6 and 12 months at least. In contrast, organizational change usually lags behind individual change. The true impact may appear years later, and evaluation should ideally allow for follow-up at this later date, to enable full benefits to be monitored.

Attention to ethical issues

The collection of information raises sensitive ethical issues around confidentiality, involvement and feedback. Useful data may already be collected as part of existing records, such as personnel and budgetary information. The nature of their accessibility requires careful consideration and full agreement by all involved. If workers perceive that the information will be used to their detriment (for example, to decide who will be made redundant) their cooperation is likely to be limited and the data unreliable (47). Also, information about employees not participating in a health programme may need to be used for comparison, and this could be considered an infringement of their rights. Similarly, the evaluation should respect people's right to choose not to be involved in a participatory process. Using non-intrusive and appropriate forms of feedback, not relying on written reports alone, is also crucial.

302

Evaluation practice as a process in the workplace

Action research approaches could be criticized for a failure to address issues of generalizability. The wide differences between companies, however, may make the ability to generalize across companies an illusory goal. More important is the development of a culture of quality assurance for health promotion programmes. Thinking should shift towards models of good evaluation practice, so that a framework of effective principles to work towards during the process replaces a set menu of suggested action. Using a validated tool in the workplace setting is sensible if the resultant data can inform progression towards the intervention goals. If its use results in the expensive collection of much inappropriate data that lack utility, however, it is an expensive mistake. If the evaluation process follows an action-oriented model, evaluators have time within the process to develop a relevant and appropriate set of indicators that truly reflects the meaning, values, aspirations and motivations of the people involved *(48)*.

If the process is set up correctly, it becomes a natural and automatic review activity, integral to the whole programme of health activity and tasks. The effectiveness of an evaluation depends on how it is undertaken. If the process is carried out in the way suggested, the choice of the design, methodology and tools used will depend on the context in which the evaluation is done, and the purpose of the evaluation will be clear. When described in an equally logical form, the process will become available for scrutiny by others.

Evaluation is about measuring change, and ultimately the value of an evaluation depends on its usefulness. Basic research is still required to help develop standards, and training is needed to improve the quality of evaluation and make learning and reflection about health part of organizational culture. The approach outlined here will encourage a commitment to process, better information and effective action based on that information. This approach reflects the best practice in the management of change *(49)*.

Recommendations for improving evaluation practice in the workplace

This section highlights the main challenges that evaluators face in improving practice.

Integration of evaluation with other workplace activity

Mechanisms of evaluation – from the understanding of health priorities (health needs assessment) to the development of workplace health interventions and the assessment of their impact – should be integrated into the normal planning cycles of organizations, such as budgetary and human resources planning. This will enable processes, impact and outcomes to be measured continuously, rather than as an afterthought, and consequently is more likely to result in funding being set aside for evaluation activities. Greater emphasis should be placed on evaluating the processes of programme implementation at the individual, organizational and community levels.

Choice of methodology

Evaluation methods should be participatory, so that the questions asked are relevant and valid to all sectors, not just management. Managing the conflict that arises during participation processes is one of the skills required by the workplace evaluator. Relevant questions are likely to engage workers in the continuation of the research process. Participatory methods allow workers to influence and control the planning of health activities in the workplace. This enhances individuals' sense of self-efficacy (self-esteem and confidence in their ability to achieve certain targets). Dooner (50) discusses the role of self-efficacy and its contribution to individual workers' health and consequently the collective health of the organization.

Bridging multiple sites

As mentioned, the sophistication of evaluation design will have to take account of the changing face of the workplace, especially within large organizations, such as universities, municipal authorities and multinational enterprises. The health needs of workers within such organizations vary depending on job type and the geographical location and culture of the site. Evaluation design should become increasingly diverse, to match multisite requirements, and to take account of trends towards home-based work.

Relevant evaluation indicators

Ideally, a range of indicators should be used to measure the effectiveness of intervention: these should include both health and business indicators. Including measures of quality, such as expressed satisfaction with job or working conditions, should be a priority. To provide meaningful data and to engage the organization in continuing dialogue, the evaluation must take account of the organization's business agenda. Evaluation indicators should focus not only on individual health issues (such as behavioural change) but also on organizational factors that can affect health (such as the psychosocial environment). Inevitably, the needs of business will take equal priority with the aims of health promotion.

Crossing interfaces

Both workplace health activities and their integral evaluation should attempt to cross the interfaces between work, home life, and the community, to give coherence, continuity and sustainability to the intervention and its development. Such interventions are more likely to take account of some of the problems faced by women, who must often juggle the multiple roles of carer and worker.

Conclusion

In summary, workplace health promotion and its evaluation are in a state of dynamic change. The literature reflects the increasing awareness that approaches should become more action oriented, use participatory techniques and take the business agenda on board when designing tools for measuring change. We hope that this chapter provides a practical framework for those working towards these aims and contributes towards creating healthy organizations. This approach uses methodologies that are found in abundance in the literature on change management. Ways of measuring the processes and outcomes of health promotion programmes are in their infancy, but much can be learned from evaluations undertaken in non-health areas with similar complex issues, such as education and management science. The development of appropriate tools demands a more innovative approach, taking on board evaluation methods from other disciplines and, where necessary, developing the skills to be able to design new tools for measuring change.

References

1. PELLETIER, K.R. A review and analysis of the health and cost–effectiveness outcome studies of comprehensive health promotion and disease prevention programmes at the worksite. *American journal of health promotion*, **10**(5): 380–388 (1996).
2. GOETZELET, R.Z. ET AL. An evaluation of Duke University's Live for Life Health Promotion Program and its impact on employee health. *American journal of health promotion*, **10**(5): 340–342 (1996).
3. LEWIS, C.E. Disease prevention and health promotion practices of primary care physicians in the United States. *American journal of preventive medicine*, **4**(Suppl. 4): 9–16 (1988).
4. DEMMER, H. *Worksite health promotion: how to go about it*. Copenhagen, WHO Regional Office for Europe, 1995 (European Health Promotion Series, No. 4).
5. BERTERA, R. The effects of behavioural risks on absenteeism and healthcare costs in the workplace. *Journal of occupational medicine*, **33**: 1119–1124 (1991).
6. COOPER, C.L. & WILLIAMS, S., ED. *Creating healthy work organizations*. New York, Wiley, 1994.
7. GOLDBECK, W. Preface. *In*: O'Donnell, M. & Ainsworth, T., ed. *Health promotion in the workplace*. New York, John Wiley, 1984.
8. O'DONNELL, M. Preface. *In*: O'Donnell, M. & Harris, J. *Health promotion in the workplace*. Albany, Delmar, 1994.
9. DEJOY, D.M. ET AL. Health behaviour change in the workplace. *In*: Dejoy, D.M. & Wilson, M.G., ed. *Critical issues in worksite health promotion*. Boston, Allyn and Bacon, 1995.

10. DEJOY, D.M. & SOUTHERN, D.J. An integrative perspective on worksite health promotion. *Journal of occupational medicine*, **35**: 1221–1230 (1993).

11. WILSON, M.G. ET AL. A comprehensive review of the effects of worksite health promotion on health-related outcomes. *American journal of health promotion*, **10**(6): 429–435 (1996).

12. SPRINGETT, J. & DUGDILL, L. Workplace health promotion programmes: towards a framework for evaluation. *Health education journal*, **54**: 88–98 (1995).

13. DUGDILL, L. *NHS staff needs assessment: a practical guide.* London, Health Education Authority, 1996.

14. DUGDILL, L & SPRINGETT, J. Evaluation of workplace health promotion: a review. *Health education journal*, **53**: 337–347 (1994).

15. SHEPHARD, P. Worksite fitness and exercise programs: a review of methodology and health impact. *American journal of health promotion*, **10**(6): 436–452 (1996).

16. WYNNE, R. & CLARKIN, N. *Under construction: building for health in the EC workplace.* Dublin, European Foundation for the Improvement of Living and Working Conditions, 1992.

17. GUSTAVEN, B. Democratising occupational health: the Scandinavian experience of work reform. *International journal of health services*, **12**(4): 675–688 (1988).

18. SHERMAN, J.B. ET AL. Evaluation of a worksite wellness programme: impact on exercise, weight, smoking and stress. *Public health nursing*, **6**(3): 114–119 (1988).

19. TUXWORTH, W. ET AL. Health, fitness, physical activity and morbidity of middle-aged male factory workers I. *British journal of industrial medicine*, **43**: 733–753 (1986).

20. WILSON, M.G. ET AL. A comprehensive review of the effects of worksite health promotion on health-related outcomes. *American journal of health promotion*, **10**(6): 433 (1996).

21. ERFURT, J.C. ET AL. Worksite wellness programmes: incremental comparison of screening and referral alone, health education, follow-up counselling, and plant organization. *American journal of health promotion*, **5**(6): 438–448 (1991).

22. BERTERA, R.L. The effects of workplace health promotion on absenteeism and employment costs in a large industrial population. *American journal of public health*, **80**(9): 1101–1105. (1990)

23. PATTON, M.Q. *Practical evaluation.* London, Sage, 1982.

24. OAKLEY, A. ET AL. *Workplace interventions – Does health promotion work?* London, Health Education Authority, 1994.

25. GOTTLIEB, N.H. & NELSON, A. A systematic effort to reduce smoking at the worksite. *Health education quarterly*, **17**(1): 99–118 (1990).

26. EVERLY, G.S. ET AL. Evaluating health promotion in the workplace: behavioural models versus financial models. *Health education research*, **2**: 61–67 (1987).
27. KATZMAN, M.S. & SMITH, K.J. Occupational health promotion programmes: evaluation efforts and measured cost savings. *Health values: achieving high level wellness*, **13**(2): 3–10 (1989).
28. NASH, C. ET AL. An evaluation of cost–benefit analysis criteria. *Scottish journal of political economy*, **22**(21): 121–134 (1975).
29. LICHFIELD, N. *Community impact evaluation*. London, UCL Press, 1996.
30. SPILLING, S. ET AL. Cost–benefit analysis of work environment investment at STK's telephone plant at Kongsvinger. *In*: Corlctt, E.N. et al., ed. *The ergonomics of working postures*. London, Taylor and Francis, 1986, pp. 380–397.
31. WEINSTEIN, M. Lifestyle, stress and work: strategies for health promotion. *Health promotion international*, **1**(3): 363–371 (1986).
32. KARASEK, R. & THEORELL, T. *Healthy work: stress, productivity and the reconstruction of working life*. New York, Basic Books, 1990.
33. WYNNE, R. *Action for health at work: the next steps*. Dublin, European Foundation for the Improvement of Living and Working Conditions, 1993.
34. DEAN, K. Double burdens of work: the female work and health paradox. *Health promotion international*, **7**(1): 17–25 (1992).
35. PELLETIER, K.R. A review and analysis of the health and cost-effective outcome studies of comprehensive health promotion and disease prevention programmes at the worksite: 1991–1993 update. *American journal of health promotion*, **8**: 50–62 (1993).
36. CARTER, N. ET AL. *How organisations measure success: The use of performance indicators in government*. London, Routledge, 1992.
37. HUGENTOBLER, M.K. ET AL. An action research approach to workplace health: integrating methods. *Health education quarterly*, **19**(1): 55–76 (1992).
38. HOFSTEDE, G. *Cultures and organizations. Software of the mind*. New York, McGraw-Hill, 1989.
39. GLASGOW, R.E. ET AL. Implementing a year-long, worksite-based incentive programme for smoking cessation. *American journal of health promotion*, **5**(3): 192–199 (1991).
40. ISRAEL, B. ET AL. Action research on occupational stress: involving researchers. *International journal of health services*, **19**(1): 135–155 (1989).
41. EKLUND, J.A.E. Organisation of assembly work: recent Swedish examples. *In*: Megaw, E.D., ed. *Contemporary ergonomics*. London, Taylor and Francis, 1988, pp. 351–356.
42. *Workplace Task Force report*. London, Department of Health, 1993.
43. SECRETARY OF STATE FOR HEALTH. *The health of the nation*. London, H.M. Stationery Office, 1992.

44. BURNES, B. *Managing change.* Belmont, Pitman, 1992.
45. HAWE, P. ET AL. *Evaluating health promotion: a health workers' guide.* Sydney, McLennan and Petty, 1990.
46. HARVEY, J. Promoting mental health: whose priorities? *In*: Trent, D.R., ed. *Promotion of mental health.* Aldershot, Avebury, 1991, vol. 1.
47. BRODIE, D.A. & DUGDILL, L. Health promotion in the workplace. *Journal of the Royal Society of Medicine*, **86**: 694–696 (1993).
48. DE LEEUW, E. *Health policy: an exploratory enquiry into the development of policy for the new public health in the Netherlands.* Maastricht, Savannah, 1989.
49. WILSON, D.C. *A strategy of change.* London, Routledge, 1993.
50. DOONER, B. Achieving a healthier workplace: organisational action for individual health. *Health promotion*, Winter edition, pp. 2–6, (1990).

14
Evaluation in urban settings: the challenge of Healthy Cities

Lisa Curtice, Jane Springett and Aine Kennedy

Introduction

The Healthy Cities movement focuses on changing municipal policies to create health-enhancing environments. The original idea comes from a model developed in the 1980s by Hancock and Perkins, which emphasized interrelationships in what they called the mandala of health. Here, the urban environment is a place where a number of levels of influence could be brought into harmony *(1)*. More recently, Labonté has developed the model, characterizing a healthy city as one that balances health, the environment and the economy in a viable, equitable and, most importantly, sustainable way *(2)*; this recalls the objectives of local Agenda 21 *(3,4)*. Underlying the Healthy Cities concept is a commitment to equity and social justice and a recognition that, just as powerlessness is a risk factor for disease, empowerment is important for health *(5)*. This necessitates the involvement of both the community and other non-health sectors in decision-making on health, particularly municipal authorities, who have a key role in creating health *(6)* through their decisions on resource allocation, education, housing, water and air pollution and poverty. Healthy Cities is intended as a practical experiment in healthy public policy. It rejects limited, sectoral, ineffective and short-term policy responses to the complex, interdependent and multisectoral determinants of health, and looks for ways to involve people actively and collaboratively in producing health-enhancing and equitable environments *(7)*. Most Healthy Cities health promotion programmes therefore support a holistic and socioecological view of health and its promotion, as opposed to a behavioural model *(8)*.

The international Healthy Cities initiative started as a small project of the WHO Regional Office for Europe to encourage the implementation of the WHO health for all strategy at the local level and in a specific setting – the city – and to support development and learning by creating a European network of participating cities *(9)*. The project has had a major influence on developing the settings approach to health policy and health programmes, and has taken root world-wide as a social movement in a variety of forms. It has spawned a wide range of community-based projects and health promotion work, from small-scale undertakings to the development of healthy public policy at a city-wide level *(10)*. Some see the Healthy Cities concept as aiming to raise people's sights above everyday reality to bring about broad-based change. From this perspective, it has some of the characteristics of a social movement, albeit with bureaucratic tendencies *(11,12)*. Others see Healthy Cities as health promotion with a community focus *(10)*. At its most developed, it can be about coordinated planning and healthy public policy *(13,14)*. A healthy city is defined in terms of process and outcome: a healthy city is conscious of health and striving to improve, not one that has achieved a particular level of health. A city's participation in the movement depends on its commitment to health and having a structure and process to achieve it *(15)*, not current health status.

This chapter identifies some of the key issues in evaluating a Healthy Cities initiative and illustrates how cities and communities have tackled them. We argue that answers to fundamental questions, such as identifying key evaluation questions to ask and the data to collect, depend on the level of the evaluation (local project, city or national or international network) and the focus of the work (whether comprehensive policy or a programme). More fundamentally, any evaluation of a Healthy Cities initiative should be undertaken in manner consistent with the movement's principles and should, at minimum, include the core aims of community participation, intersectoral collaboration and equity, not just in impact and process indicators but in the evaluation process itself. While the tools are yet to be developed actively to capture the synergistic impact and outcome of a wide range of initiatives implicit in an ecological approach to health promotion at a city level, they are likely to emerge as those involved grapple with evaluation issues at the local level.

Characteristics of Healthy Cities that present a challenge for evaluation

Three characteristics of Healthy Cities have important implications for evaluation. The first is the place of the city as a unit within a wider system of connections, upwards to the national and international levels and downwards to the neighbourhood or community. Focusing on the urban context for clarity, we nevertheless recognize that a parallel argument about interdependence could be made for rural communities and that Healthy Cities/Healthy Communities has developed as both an urban and a rural movement. Next we consider Healthy Cities in the context of post-modernism, and highlight different ways in which the concept of community is being revived. Finally, we discuss research and theory on the process of policy-making, because this is what Healthy Cities primarily seeks to influence.

The city as part of a larger system

The urban setting is complex and comprises many communities and systems in ever changing interaction. Many underlying factors that influence urban change are beyond local control. Analysis of the city as a setting and, by extension, of initiatives in the city, cannot be confined to the city level, but must en-

310

compass the social and political policies and processes that contribute to both the opportunities for and the constraints on effecting change.

Examples from the United Kingdom – of evaluation of community development approaches to urban problems in the 1960s and 1970s and of urban regeneration initiatives in the 1980s and 1990s – provide useful lessons. Participants in the Home Office National Community Development Project in the early 1970s came to reject their given role as providing a local technical testing ground for innovative national programmes. They pointed out the need for their critical engagement with the wider social policies that constrained the development processes with which they were involved (16). Small-scale and under-resourced urban initiatives, set up to tackle major issues of social policy such as powerlessness or poverty, have a limited likelihood of making large-scale change in the short term (17). In addition, one can easily underestimate the difficulties of translating the results of community development initiatives into organizational or policy change (18).

Urban programmes in the United Kingdom since the 1970s have acknowledged that economic growth alone is not a sufficient response to problems of urban deprivation; what is needed is "to consider new forms of public action" (19). Successive evaluation of national urban regeneration initiatives has demonstrated the importance of considering the conflicts and limitations that raise barriers to the implementation of such policies. The evaluation of Action for Cities, the urban development grant programme for inner cities, used impact assessment to address not only performance in achieving objectives but also the factors that affected variations in effectiveness between the different sites (20). Thus, social capital in cities can be neither promoted nor analysed in isolation from national policy; implementation is an interaction, not a simple manifestation of local conditions versus regional, national or international goals.

The city in a post-modern society

Transforming the city environment as a means of tackling major social problems is a recurrent policy concern. Communities within cities have often been the site where political theories have located the possibility of active political engagement and participation. In small neighbourhoods, runs the argument, informal relations between people are more important; interdependence is more apparent and there are opportunities for action on individuals' concerns, collective action and political debate in some kind of public and common space.

The contradictions in a romanticized view of community have been well rehearsed. Localities cannot be assumed to contain communities with shared interests. A community contains a range of interests structured by power relations involving dimensions such as class, race, gender and disability, and these interests may conflict. Communities in the post-modern city may be defined not only in spatial but also in other terms. Some localities, on the other hand, lack either a sense of community or the social capital to counter fragmentation and the divisive effects of poverty *(21)*. Communities are not necessarily inclusive or open; they may also be founded on self-interest and seek to exclude those whom they perceive to be marginal. Different communities may have competing priorities; solutions that benefit one, such as the building of a factory, may well create health problems, such as traffic pollution, for another. The initiatives taken to improve the urban environment, such as regeneration funding, may increase this competition by inevitably creating winners and losers in the struggle for funding *(22)*.

Acknowledging that the concept of the cohesive community contradicts much of the experience and reality of contemporary urban living, debates about how to counter fragmentation and social exclusion continue to return to the relationships between individual agency and empowerment, social cohesion at the local level and management of the boundary between local structures and wider political and economic forces. Local social structures are clearly interdependent with, not independent of, wider social relations, but this does not necessarily mean that the individual must be disempowered; collective coherence in support of human agency is also an option *(23)*. Four goals, of direct relevance to Healthy Cities, underlie these reinventions of community as part of a wider coalition of action for social justice: local democracy, improved quality of life and of the urban environment, the development of social solidarity and the overcoming of social exclusion.

Writers on governance have sought to establish how local political action can be transformed into new forms of community government that represent a genuine form of local participation, rather than merely the delegation of central government's administrative powers to the local level *(24)*, and to encourage the actions of a range of stakeholders in what Duhl calls "the governance of diversity" *(25)*. Atkinson *(26)*, for example, argues for an "urban renaissance" through a combination of bottom-up local planning (involving partnerships between local people and community-oriented planners) with a redirection of educational and training resources to develop the community's capital, and a stronger political organization at neighbourhood level, supported by a reorganization of local government structure, from a hierarchical and vertical functional model to a wheel design, which would be integrated at the centre but would also link outwards to neighbourhood representatives.

The challenge of developing local partnerships to promote the quality of life is a current policy theme. Seed & Lloyd *(27)* identify a range of values for the promotion of quality of life, arguing that common values should first form the basis of defining a quality-of-life agenda (independent of the resources commanded by different social groups) and then provide a common base for new standards. Quality-of-life values, they claim, are a product of environments characterized by their counter-values such as oppression and social exclusion. Benevelo *(28)* considers that European cities still offer scope for the creation of harmonious and integrated physical environments, as idealized by Aristotle, to provide a physical setting appropriate for modern social needs.

312

As thinking on community increasingly focuses on shared concerns, not merely locations, the relationship of solidarity and community is being more clearly articulated. The case for a connection between a sense of a common identity, tolerance of difference and equitable distribution is gaining strength. Cattell *(29)* applies this thinking to the question of healthy communities, arguing that inequalities deprive communities of cohesion: "unhealthy communities are ... divided communities in divided societies". The positive, synergistic community needs linkages at all levels: in the neighbourhood to foster a sense of local community, through membership of a group in which shared interests can be developed and alliances formed and in democratic structures that make links outwards. Only open structures and values in communities, however, will contribute to the growth of social cohesion and recognition of the case for redistribution.

Although much contemporary social analysis still employs nineteenth-century language to blame the victims of social exclusion by locating them in the forgotten parts of the city, liberal and social democratic analysts have countered with an image of the city as soil for the organic growth and nurture of community responsibility and sustainable environments to meet diverse human needs. Critics calling this concept romanticized stress the conflicts within and between communities and the limitations imposed on local solidarity by impoverished economic and social infrastructures. We have suggested that one resolution of this problem lies in acknowledging the interdependence of the city with wider political, social and economic forces and the policies that seek to address them. In particular, identifying the qualities that cities must possess to promote equity and a sustainable quality of life leads to a more discriminating and action-oriented approach that focuses on the values, conditions and processes needed to make cities active agents in a democratic and inclusive society. This is at the heart of Healthy Cities thinking about the city.

The nature of the policy-making process

Theorization of the policy-making process is key to understanding the challenges of evaluating the Healthy Cities process. Policy development is an iterative and dynamic process involving a range of actors linked together through a network of activities, decisions and motivations *(30,31)*. Policy is not a specific decision or intervention *(32,33)*, but is produced through negotiation between participants. Thus in practice there is often no distinction between policy development and implementation; policy is developed during implementation *(34)*. Changing public policy is notoriously difficult *(35)*; policy maintenance is more the norm *(36)*. When policy changes occur, however, they are usually incremental, especially at the local level *(37)*.

How policy actually develops therefore depends on local context, so evaluation of its quality and effectiveness will depend on local priorities and constraints, and the views and interests of stakeholders. Both are parallel and emergent learning processes for those concerned. Political context and personal preferences, moreover, affect the direction and utilization of the evaluation process *(38)*. The theory that underlies any policy affects what can be evaluated and how, and what action is taken in response *(39,40)*. For example, data interpretation and the action chosen differ according to whether policy-makers assume that ill health is more closely related to individuals' lifestyles (victim blaming) or to factors outside individual control (such as poverty). Additional influences on the policy and evaluation processes are the stories behind the policies: power struggles, personality conflicts and feelings of mutual distrust.

Further, the selection of evaluation criteria depends on whether a top-down or bottom-up perspective on policy is adopted, as shown by the example of joint work or intersectoral collaboration. A planner taking a top-down perspective may assess the process in terms of a good administration structure, perfect coordination and measurable performance *(41)*, seeing them within the context of impact of the local political and economic situation and national government policy on the opportunities for effective joint work. Typically, such an assessment would emphasize setting compatible and consistent goals for joint work.

People taking a bottom-up perspective see joint work as a process of negotiation in which the people involved exchange their beliefs and values. From this point of view, a focus on clear goals and adequate control neglects the analysis of the underlying processes that influence effective joint work *(41)*. HEA took the latter perspective in developing a set of indicators for planning, evaluating and developing healthier alliances *(42)*. HEA based the resulting simplified tool *(43)* on a pack describing five process indicators (commitment, community participation, communication, joint work and accountability) and six categories of output indicators (policy change, service provision and environment change, skills development, publicity, contact, and knowledge, attitude and behaviour change). The choice of indicators reflected the knowledge and perceptions of the participants in the workshops that created them, most of whom were health for all coordinators *(44,45)*.

People have greater confidence in the information gained in assessing effectiveness when they understand and own the results, and their involvement in the process of evaluation strengthens ownership *(38)*. Public participation is therefore as important as the involvement of policy-makers. The people who are affected by a policy initiative know intimately the problem and how to act upon it. In practice, however, involving city inhabitants in evaluation has proved as difficult as involving them in political decision-making. People will participate only when they see a glimmer of a solution or feel empowered. Ensuring participation is probably the greatest challenge to the Healthy Cities movement in policy development. Conventional bureaucratic structures do not lend themselves easily to democratic involvement.

Consensus and controversies in evaluation

This section links specific issues in Healthy Cities evaluation with more general controversies in evaluation. We identify six areas for discussion: the purpose of the evaluation, the principles and values underlying the process being evaluated and the evaluation itself, and the process, methods, indicators of success and audiences of evaluation. We argue that the purpose of evaluation partly determines the focus of activity. Moreover, the relationship between Healthy Cities values and those of the evaluation must be clear. The evaluation process needs to be considered in the light of its potential to help develop knowledge. We give the reason for disillusionment with purely positivist methodologies, highlight the political nature of indicator selection and again underline the need for locally sensitive approaches.

Focus and purpose

The Healthy Cities movement has spawned many expectations for evaluation. Some have exhorted it to demonstrate the effectiveness of new public health approaches at the local level (46). The biomedical science community has sought systematic analysis of an intervention and its impact on disease prevention (47). Social scientists have wanted to use a more critical analytic stance to understand and contextualize the phenomenon itself (for example, as social movement or bureaucratic intervention), and practitioners have called for practical guidance on putting the approach into effect (48). The evaluation questions are therefore embedded in the theoretical and conceptual perspective of those involved. These models change as conceptual development changes.

The diversity of views about the direction that evaluation should take (whether to emphasize why or how-to questions, for example) probably arises from the number of different audiences for Healthy Cities evaluation, as well as differing opinions about strategy. Is the priority to clarify the Healthy Cities concept and to understand its role in bringing about change, to give practical guidance to those wishing to undertake similar activities or to demonstrate the effectiveness of Healthy Cities action to decision-makers and funding agencies? Each has different implications for evaluation strategy. The first leads to an emphasis on how the model is understood and implemented in different settings; the second, to analysis of process and outputs; and the third, to attempts to define outcomes and appropriate ways to measure them.

Consensus has probably been reached: the most important evaluation task is to clarify the models underlying Healthy Cities approaches and to understand more about what determines whether they are effective and sustainable and which approach or combination of approaches is most likely to lead to systems-level change. A key proxy indicator would be evidence that the determinants of health are changing, since a growing body of research literature supports some key connections, for example, between ill health and levels of unemployment or relative inequality (49).

Principles and values

The key principles of Healthy Cities are collaboration and participation. Some difficulties beset the evaluation of such processes. First, the members of an alliance may differ widely in their understanding of its common aims. The outcomes of collaborative work may be dispersed, and determining whether certain outcomes are attributable to the Healthy Cities initiative may be difficult because it aims to encourage action by others. Finally, participative and collaborative models may prove a difficult test bed for particular approaches because the process inevitably changes the model being implemented. These are common problems in the evaluation of community development approaches (50). A pluralist model of evaluation, which actively teases out the criteria for success held by different stakeholders and seeks evaluative data from a wide range of sources, is a well established methodology for dealing with some of these problems (51).

A particular feature of the evaluation of initiatives such as Healthy Cities is the need to spell out the principles and values of participants in order to interpret developments. The theories on health that underpin a health-related policy may drive the processes of implementation and evaluation (39). Whether evaluators of social movements need to share the value base of the movements they are evaluating is under debate. Within the Healthy Cities movement, people have debated the desired balance between different evaluation stances (observer/critic, participant or ally); these positions are sometimes characterized as evaluation of, with or for Healthy Cities, respectively.

An evaluation wholly based on the principles of participants and/or conducted by participants (internal evaluation) may be accused of being insufficiently critical or objective. Kennedy (52) has argued that principle-led, internal evaluation can result in evaluation questions and methods that are appropriate to practice, particularly when a participatory approach is adopted. Poland (53) has argued for combining, within Healthy Cities evaluation, the direct use of principles derived from participants with a critical stance. Building on the work of Springett et al. (54), he demonstrates how a participatory action research method can best capture the experiential and practical knowledge of participants, while adhering to the key principles of the health for all movement. He recommends building into the evaluation a process that encourages critical reflection on, for example, issues of power and contradictions between theory and practice.

Process

From early in the development of the WHO Healthy Cities project, it was recognized that evaluation should ideally be multidisciplinary, not least because of the number of sectors potentially involved in project work. This has proved elusive in practice. Another challenge is to develop cross-national research processes. Both these aims might ultimately lead to the development of a more holistic evaluation framework within which models of practice and their components could be clarified and identified. Without such a framework, evaluation may appear simplistic or superficial as soon as it is applied to any substantive area (the environment, for example) or may not reflect the various cultural perspectives contained in the Healthy Cities movement.

Given the complexity, developmental nature and political dimension of Healthy Cities, the evaluation process and methodology must be flexible enough to take account of change. Healthy Cities is as much about a way of working as a particular setting. In common with other community health interventions, the specific aims and objectives of any participating city and the subsequent activities and outcomes depend on local priorities, political structures and capacities *(55)*. Each project therefore needs to be judged against its own aims and objectives, so that measures of quality and effectiveness are developed that are useful in knowledge development *(53)*. A participatory evaluation model enables the derivation of a locally relevant evaluation framework that can be modified and revised as an initiative develops.

Policy-makers often lack first-hand knowledge of the problems they are called upon to solve, but the implementers who have such knowledge lack the power to adjust and improve the policy. Similarly, the beneficiaries of the policy may hold key information and be a resource in finding solutions, as well as a vital element in assessing policy effectiveness *(56)*. Without continual feedback between evaluation, planning and activity, quality is unlikely to improve, because those involved need to own the information and the process. This is particularly important where a multilevel process aiming for long-term change is under evaluation *(57)*. Unrealistic demands for short-term outcome measurement are likely to be moderated only by taking people through the decision-making process, and determining what questions to ask and how they can effectively be answered. Knowledge development is a key feature of the process, as is opening channels of communication within the policy process *(58–60)*.

Methods

Healthy Cities evaluation is most appropriately approached as a form of policy evaluation. In many other sectors, policy evaluation is moving away from a reliance on rigid scientific methodologies to more interpretative, process-oriented methods with an emphasis on learning *(61,62)*. In the United States, for example, disillusionment with positivist approaches to the evaluation of urban policy has increased. Many of the evaluative studies undertaken in the 1970s and early 1980s have had little impact on policy or practice. This resulted in a retreat from quantitative studies to qualitative assessments, use of an eclectic mix of evaluative methods and concern for developing learning networks, as well as the active involvement of stakeholders *(63)*.

This disillusionment reflects in part the consequences of a positivist approach to data collection, whereby data are collected without changing the situation of the people involved or giving them something in return *(64)*. The aim is to examine a hypothesis that is often unknown to those studied. To avoid bias, evaluators keep them in the dark about the purpose of the evaluation. This is both disempowering and unlikely to lead to change. Rigorously designed evaluations will not influence the policy process because they are scientific, objective or valid. Rist *(65)* denies that such a linear relation of evaluation to

317

action exists. In the real world, policy-making and implementation often throw up conditions that resist positivist methods, since policy systems are complex structures for political learning that comprise many subcultures and values *(66,67)*. One should consider the unquantifiable values, aspirations and motivations of the people involved *(68,69)*. A flexible, negotiated and process-oriented approach to the evaluation of urban healthy public policy, more in keeping with the nature of the policy process, is required. This does not mean abandoning outcome measures, qualitative or quantitative, but encouraging all the participants in the process to discuss what is appropriate and what is possible; this encourages reflection on existing perspectives and ideologies.

Combined with theory development, quantitative methodologies may have a role in elucidating the relationships between processes and outcomes in Healthy Cities. The approach is essentially multilevel and seeks to produce synergistic change. The complexities of the models involved and the number of sources of variation and interaction suggest that statistical modelling may be valuable. Also, the key importance of time-scale in assessing the level of expected change points to the need for a quantitative dimension to data collection and analysis. A note of caution is nevertheless appropriate. The kind of changes one can realistically expect in political processes, organizational structures and so forth may be not only long term but also invisible in statistical terms, unless a large number of measures is available over time.

Indicators

Health promotion research as a whole has not yet reached consensus on what comprises sufficient evidence of change resulting from community interventions. Can evaluators use intermediate or proxy indicators of impact, such as the development of community competence, or must they demonstrate modification of risk factors *(70–72)*? As Healthy Cities is not primarily concerned with changing individual lifestyles, it may escape the worst of this controversy, although tension remains between those who seek proof of effectiveness in direct measures of health status and those who accept intermediate indicators. Recent work conducted for Northern Ireland has attempted to provide a framework for evaluating initiatives at the community level. It proposes sets of proxy indicators that reflect the criteria for different aspects of a community in which quality of life is promoted, such as safety and sustainability *(73,74)*.

Some have wished for indicators of a city's status across a range of political, health and environmental dimensions that could be based on routine data and would enable comparisons of the relative impact of Healthy Cities initiatives. Given the wide variation in experience and in political, social and cultural context, the lack of agreement on concepts and the variable availability of data, this is likely to be wishing for the moon. One real value of an indicator is often its capacity to indicate change over time, but this presupposes continuity in both definition and data collection *(75)*. Experience in Canada demonstrated that there is no magic list of reliable and universally useful indicators. Indicators have proved most useful where they have been developed locally and used to collect baseline formative information to raise issues with local policy-makers.

Participatory action research integrates action and change with knowledge development and learning. Its adoption for evaluation has implications for the development of indicators. This implies that individual cities must develop their own sets of indicators to meet their particular needs as permitted by their resources. Indicators cannot be developed in isolation from the political and philosophical basis or the aims and objectives of a particular health-related policy. Indicators will vary according to who requests them, who pays for their selection, who uses them and what their agendas are (76). The process of developing and using indicators to evaluate healthy public policy in cities is thus more a political problem than a technical one, dependent on world views and power structures, including the ability to impose certain views on others (77). While one can draw on the wide range of indicators already available to measure almost any dimension of health-related policy concepts (78), indicators cannot be developed outside the wider processes of knowledge and policy development.

The issue of indicators may have obscured debate about the development of outcome standards. Knowledge development approaches can be used to develop consensus on goals and the criteria or standards to apply to judge the extent of their achievement. Such negotiated criteria for success might encourage dialogue between city projects and protect city initiatives from unrealistic assessment criteria. Many of the key Healthy Cities processes provide intermediate outcome measures of progress. Thus, for example, the extent of joint work between key sectors and agencies on health-related policies and practices, compared with a previous baseline, may be a measure of project effectiveness. City administrations want to know whether investment in Healthy Cities approaches gives better value for money than other options. This is a difficult question to tackle, given the role of Healthy Cities projects as catalytic or enabling mechanisms and the diversity of their functions.

The identification of outcome measures for Healthy Cities activities is complex. The effects may be measurable as environmental improvements or visible success in either developing health promoting opportunities or preventing health-damaging activities. A city in eastern Europe, for example, might use the absence of tobacco advertising on public transport to demonstrate success in mobilizing resources to prevent the exploitation of its citizens on economic, health and cultural grounds. The expression of some intermediate outcome measures as visual evidence can complement more formal statistical approaches in an effective way.

Audiences

Overall, two sets of people have a stake in Healthy Cities evaluation. The first comprises those outside the movement, such as funding agencies at the municipal and network level, who are interested in value for their investment money, and those interested in the new public health, who seek to learn from the Healthy Cities experience. The second group includes those inside the movement, who are keen to develop self-evaluation to avoid the risk that inappropriate evaluation criteria and methods will be imposed.

As suggested above, these two groups may have conflicting priorities for evaluation. Given the limited resources available, some priorities will influence the choices of the evaluation methods employed, privileging a value-for-money approach in some contexts and an in-depth case-study approach in others. This eclecticism carries the risk of obscuring the big picture, so that observers wonder whether they see the tip of an iceberg or all that exists of the ice-field *(78)*. A creative way out of this dilemma is to ensure that the process of knowledge development is not confined to the city level. Reflection and feedback are required at all levels in the Healthy Cities movement, so that emergent understandings and new responses are based on a variety of experiences.

Conclusion

So far, this chapter has considered Healthy Cities evaluation from the perspective of the challenges posed by aspects of the movement, and reviewed the debate on how it should be evaluated. We have attempted to show how differences in underlying assumptions and goals affect choices about evaluation strategies. A unifying theme is the centrality to Healthy Cities of the wish to change policy. From this flow many evaluation needs; if evaluation is to be useful and compatible with this wish, it must contribute to knowledge development by adopting an action-oriented approach, by involving participants at all stages of the evaluation process and by ensuring that the criteria for evaluation are meaningful in terms of local principles and priorities.

We have highlighted some of the creative tensions that the Healthy Cities movement poses for evaluation goals and processes. Healthy Cities initiatives aim to foster the development of coherent, health-enhancing local policies. As such, they must involve a wide range of stakeholders whose priorities and underlying assumptions may differ. Healthy Cities initiatives seek to act within a setting characterized by interdependence at all levels and to affect a policy process that is developmental. We have proposed locally developed evaluation frameworks that can be sensitive to local priorities, structures and processes as the mechanism most likely to deliver effective and appropriate evaluation strategies. It is essential, however, that links to enable learning be made between those engaged with Healthy Cities at the network, city and neighbourhood levels to elucidate the full implications of different models of work and their effects.

Evaluation at city level

This part of the chapter discusses the evaluation of the Healthy Cities policy process at the city level. It continues to explore the issues raised earlier, and examines the relationship of city evaluation to that at the international network level. We conclude with a description of participatory evaluation of a community project to show the need for Healthy Cities evaluations to reflect the importance of neighbourhood action and its relationship with a city-wide strategy.

An example of Healthy Cities evaluation: Liverpool

Liverpool is a city in the United Kingdom with about 477 000 inhabitants. For the last 20 years, it been dealing with the consequences of an economic recession due to the decline of its port and associated industries. Liverpool has been involved in the WHO Healthy Cities project since its inception in 1987 *(79)*. In the first five years of the project, in common with many other cities, it failed to move beyond the small-scale development associated with a model project to more fundamental healthy public policy, although the groundwork was laid for more effective coalition work in the second phase *(80)*. Changes of personnel and a commitment from the local and health authorities to work together more closely heralded a new phase of development in 1993. A Joint Public Health Team was established to direct action on the main health concerns in Liverpool; it is accountable to the Joint Consultative Committee, a political body consisting of district health authority and local municipal authority members. In addition, a Healthy City Unit provides administration and support for joint work between the agencies in the city and the community. The central plank of this new phase was the development of a city health plan or strategy. This was a key requirement of the membership of the second phase of the WHO project.

Using a framework developed as part of a European research project on health-related policies in cities *(81)*, this section documents the experience of grappling with evaluation issues at the urban policy level by outlining how Liverpool tackled the evaluation of its city health plan. The plan *(82)* is the health authority's five-year strategy and a corporate priority of the Liverpool City Council. The discussion of the evaluation process uses Rist's policy cycle as an organizing framework *(65)*, and describes three phases of the policy process: formulation, implementation and outcome.

Policy formulation

To formulate and write the strategies for the plan, four task groups were set up to address key areas (heart disease, cancer, sexual health and accidents) of the Government's *The health of the nation (83)*, along with a task group on housing for health. The parties concerned already shared a similar theory of health and its promotion firmly grounded in a socioecological model of change that built strongly on theories of the relationship between health and unemployment. This model, along with existing priorities, drove the original development of the plan, but circumstance obliged the participants to follow a much narrower model. The membership of the task groups comprised purchasers and consumers of services, but a total of 160 people worked on the production of the city health plan. The approach contrasts with that adopted in Sheffield, which started with needs assessment at the grass roots *(84)*. The explanation for this lies partly in the schedule set to produce the plan and partly in the bureaucratic tradition in Liverpool.

In this preliminary phase, evaluation largely involved understanding and defining the key health issues, and data collection was based on intuitive understanding and experience and collective knowledge, as well as existing research (85). In addition, existing policies and programmes were reviewed, highlighting where coordination was required between policies. As a result, aims and objectives were modified. The draft city health plan was launched in January 1995; then followed a five-month consultation process and revision of the plan, leading to its release in 1996 (82).

Participation in decision-making on plan development largely involved the task groups and the consultation process. Both processes were evaluated externally, using resources from the two local universities (86,87). The consultation process began with a public launch in January 1995, followed by encouragement to comment through newspaper inserts, posters, radio broadcasts and mailing of an abridged version of the plan to every household in Liverpool. As the main method, however, 53 trained facilitators from the statutory and voluntary sectors were available to hold group meetings, using a video as support. The evaluation of the consultation process did not consider whether the final plan met the concerns of the community members who participated.

This failure to look at evaluation systematically, to identify what should be evaluated and how it could be fed into the process was a key feature of the early phase. Information on the joint work was immediately fed back into the process and led to a review of joint care planning, but no specific action. The consultation review was only available some time afterwards; specific process changes are difficult to identify, although reference is made to reports on meetings. The lack of involvement of the key stakeholders in defining the questions for evaluation may account for the lack of ownership of the results.

The final plan resulted partly from the information gained during its formulation, but also reflected certain stakeholders' dominance in the decision-making process. In its broadest terms, the plan aims to influence, coordinate and integrate purchasing, service and business planning in Liverpool. It makes strong links with other city-wide initiatives for economic and social regeneration. It explicitly tackles the underlying causes of ill health: the environment, the economy (including poverty and unemployment), housing education, crime and transport (84). Specific action is aimed at smoking, nutrition and physical activity, and particular population groups: children and young people, ethnic minority groups and older people. It also has targets in the national health strategy areas of heart disease, cancer, mental health, sexual health and accidents (85). The final plan returned to the underlying determinants of ill health because, in their planning, the task groups had proposed overlapping solutions to the problems they identified. The outcomes of the consultation process reinforced this view; further information gained led to revamping the plan, moving the issue of the environment up the agenda. The environment had been a priority, not for the main authorities, but for the community (84).

Policy implementation

The second phase of the policy cycle focuses on the "day-to-day realities of bringing a new policy into existence" *(66)*. Intersectoral policies are notorious for failing to be implemented *(88)*. The evaluation of key aspects of this phase can act as an early warning and actively encourage the process of change.

After producing the plan, the task groups disbanded. Implementation was now the remit of existing organizations and their departmental managers. The Joint Public Health Team retained an overview of developments and monitoring and evaluation. The Healthy City Unit's role was to support the Team in that process and facilitate implementation. The key strategic stakeholders actively addressed the failure to engage in systematic evaluation only in the year following the launch of the plan; this failure is still under debate. For a time, the Team became very task driven, and its strategic role was unclear. The issue of evaluation was raised with the Team a number of times, and it was suggested that the evaluation process be used to extend participation in both decision-making and implementation to middle mangers, who had not been involved in developing the plan and yet were expected to deliver its contents. To move the debate forward, a series of workshops on priorities, indicators and community participation took place. Eventually a framework emerged that now drives the evaluation and monitoring process. A significant achievement is the placing of health issues on the agendas of the evaluation of the partnership areas. The Healthy City Unit has been a key player in making this happen. In 1997, the need for a more systematic approach to evaluation was finally accepted, and a plan was evolving to replace ad hoc evaluation with a process that has clear aims and objectives.

Policy outcome

Another reason that the issue of a broad and systematic approach to evaluation was slow to be addressed was the overriding concern of key stakeholders to measure policy outcome. "How will we know we have made a difference?" was the key question emerging from early workshops for the Joint Public Health Team. As a result, considerable time, energy and funds were spent on finding and developing key quantifiable indicators. As with other attempts to find high-quality, resource-efficient quantifiable indicators, the results were disappointing.

This outcome challenged assumptions about what should make good indicators. This led to:

1. a decision to balance quantifiable indicators with qualitative ones;
2. a recognition of the difficulty of developing indicators that truly reflect the web of causality that the city health plan tried to address;
3. an acknowledgement of the factors beyond local control that might actually reduce the chances of achieving the aims and objectives of the plan;
4. a search for new approaches to notions of health gain and health impact;

5. an increasing acceptance that the measurement of progress could not rely on indicators that bear little resemblance to the aims and objectives of the plan;
6. an acknowledgement of the need to look at process, as well as outcome; and
7. an acceptance of the key role of the Joint Public Health Team in making connections and evaluating and monitoring the implementation process.

The Team needed to go through the learning process; as a result, achieving a systematic approach to evaluation took 18 months after the launch of the plan.

The example of the evaluation process of the Liverpool city health plan shows that pragmatism and patience may be needed to build support for systematic evaluation. Knowledge of the policy process was not enough; participants had to discover for themselves the need for evaluation to inform their work. In Liverpool there were well supported efforts at consultation, but only a relatively informal attempt to feed local experience into policy development. Is it realistic to expect that bottom-up and participatory processes at the local level can be more fully developed? Analysis of 49 case studies of action for health, drawn from the first phase of the WHO Healthy Cities project across Europe, found that added value and quality in local activities were best expressed in terms of the collaboration and participation introduced into the way action was implemented *(89)*. A comprehensive survey of community/neighbourhood projects in Canada, the Netherlands and the United States by Ten Dam has revealed the wide variety of such projects' strategies and goals, but could not identify information on the extent of the achievement of stated goals *(90)*. He concluded that the separate evaluations were insufficiently comparable to generate any definite conclusions on effectiveness. From the empirical data collected, he developed a framework that he used to analyse 11 neighbourhood health projects in Amsterdam, Rotterdam and The Hague, the Netherlands. The results revealed positive scores for all areas within the framework except public participation and the ultimate goal of health promotion; that is, health, as measured by standard data, did not improve during the short life of the project.

Experience from elsewhere illustrates the principles and methods that can be applied to empower people taking part in community-based initiatives to play a central role in their evaluation.

Evaluating Healthy Cities initiatives at the community level: Drumchapel

Building on the evaluation of the Drumchapel Healthy Cities project in Glasgow, United Kingdom, Kennedy *(52)* developed a participatory model for evaluation at the community level. The Drumchapel project was established to test the relevance of the principles of community participation, empowerment and collaboration in a multiply deprived community on the outskirts of Glasgow. It aimed to catalyse new ways of working among member agencies of Healthy Cities in Glasgow, and to pilot-test innovative approaches to the empowerment and participation of local people through the training, recruitment and deployment of community health volunteers. The project's organizational structure and management style were designed to maximize participation, empowerment and collaboration.

The evaluation came at the end of the two-year pilot period and was driven largely by participants' concern to pilot-test an evaluation method capable of reflecting the project's principles and ensuring that the evaluation process did so, too. Participants felt that testing the evaluation was as important as testing the practice. They wanted the evaluation to contribute to the project and not the other way around. They hoped to gain from the evaluation new skills, a better informed perspective on the project, a stronger sense of direction, more commitment to a shared vision and knowledge on how things could be improved. They also wanted to record and reflect on the project's approach and achievements, with a view to disseminating the practice, so that they themselves and others could learn from it. At the outset of the exercise, however, many participants felt very fearful and doubtful about evaluation and associated it with being judged, scrutinized from afar by outside experts.

In this evaluation, the participants' agenda took priority. The aims of the evaluation were:

- to explore a variety of approaches to the evaluation of the Drumchapel Healthy Cities project;
- to seek the views of a range of participants on indicators of the project's success; and
- to assess the feasibility of reflecting the principles of participation, empowerment and collaboration in the evaluation process.

The evaluation process took place over about a year, between November of 1991 and 1992. It tried a variety of approaches to data collection to ensure that a range of voices was heard and to give participants experience with the different methods. Project participants filled out a questionnaire to provide baseline data on their attitudes to evaluation. They participated in training workshops to explore evaluation issues and be introduced to some qualitative methods. A series of group meetings on evaluation was held over three months. These meetings were the main vehicles for participation in the process and for key decision-making on what should be evaluated and how. Participants appreciated the opportunity that the meetings offered to gain an overview of the project, to exchange views with other groups and to reflect in this setting on the project's progress. This illustrates the use of evaluation to develop skills, participation and collaboration, not merely to collect data. Group interviews were held over a six-month period with representatives of various groups within the project, complemented by individual interviews with a selection of participants. To enable community health volunteers to tell their own stories, case studies were prepared with them throughout May and June 1992.

Participants employed a range of creative methods to share the lessons of the evaluation experience. These included a report and video recording the experience of undertaking a participatory approach to community health needs assessment, in which some of the people who subsequently became community health volunteers in the project had participated. A group art project designed a tree symbol for the Drumchapel project. The symbol became the cornerstone of an exhibition on the project that was widely used in teaching and presentations. It has since taken permanent form in a tile mosaic in the area's new health centre, where the project is now based. Drama was another vehicle that expressed participants' experiences. A volunteer wrote a play about her experience, which was performed by a group of volunteers at open days and other community events. To look at one aspect of the project's outreach, community health volunteers, with support from project staff, carried out a publicity survey to investigate the profile of the project in the community. Finally, a follow-up questionnaire was administered among project participants to ascertain their level of participation in evaluation and any changes in their attitudes and skills that they could identify as a result of the experience.

The most popular methods of evaluation were creative, informal and non-threatening, and allowed different groups within the project to exchange views. The group meetings and exercises such as the creation of the tree symbol were excellent ways of helping participants to see and appreciate the project as a whole, rather than just from their own vantage points. For evaluation to be a participative activity, a range of approaches should be adopted to maximize the chance of appealing to as many project participants as possible. Videos, exhibitions and drama are imaginative and attractive alternatives to the written word for both the participants in and the ultimate consumers of evaluation. Further, putting together a video or performing a play tends to be a collective activity in a way that writing or reading a report is not.

The evaluators decided as little as possible in advance, so that the evaluation process was free to evolve in negotiation with participants. This process helped the participants to develop new insights into the project, to clarify and refine its organizational structure and direction, and to identify weaknesses and strategies to rectify them. The questionnaires administered before and after the evaluation demonstrated a significant shift in attitudes, with the original fear disappearing almost completely and all categories of participants placing a very high value on evaluation. The only, repeatedly expressed concern was that time not be spent on evaluation to the detriment of sustaining practice. Capacity building for evaluation was a key feature of the process and has allowed a more outcome-focused approach to the next stage. Project participants no longer fear evaluation and have the skills and confidence to ensure its integration with practice.

Conclusion

These examples of Healthy Cities evaluation have illustrated the city-wide policy process and participant involvement in the community level. While the examples come from different cities, the two levels are connected. While the city policy process in Liverpool had not yet established very open channels of communication with communities, policy implementation was to depend partly on partnerships in local areas. The Drumchapel project aimed both to benefit local residents and to model participatory and collaborative work to agencies throughout the city to influence the wider structures and processes that affected health in Drumchapel.

In addition, both these evaluation accounts are connected to the development of Healthy Cities as an international network and to the expectations for evaluation within it. The city health plan was a requirement for participation in the international project. Because of their relationships to the wider health for all movement, the evaluators in both Liverpool and Glasgow were concerned to find appropriate ways to evaluate collaborative and participatory work and to test methods for feeding the results of evaluation into knowledge development for policy and practice.

Conclusions
Overview
The evaluation of Healthy Cities initiatives is under development, as is the implementation of the Healthy Cities concept. Only recently has the whole issue of evaluation been addressed; in the past, evaluation has often been after the fact, rather than integral to the process. The third phase of the WHO project includes evaluation in its conditions for involvement, and for the first time seeks consensus on the evaluation questions before the start of the phase. Experience in Canada and the United States demonstrates that a knowledge development approach is consistent with both the movement's ideals and the process of innovation diffusion. What is required now is general acceptance throughout the movement of the value of evaluation in influencing change, so that sufficient resources can be devoted to ensure it takes place in an effective, efficient and imaginative way. New methodologies need to be developed to identify the synergistic effect of different processes leading to key outcomes.

Guideline and recommendations
Any attempt at evaluating Healthy Cities is likely to demand lots of time and other resources. The first nostrum to emerge from this chapter is that those involved need to have confidence in applying core Healthy Cities principles to evaluation activities, as even large-scale evaluations can prove ineffective if they are not appropriate to the kinds of changes sought by Healthy Cities. The evaluation of Healthy Cities, like the movement itself, cannot be addressed by one set of stakeholders alone, for the resultant framework (and results) will inevitably be too narrow. Given the wide diversity of projects in resources, form, style and activity, there seems no alternative to a negotiated form of evaluation in which cities themselves identify appropriate subjects of inquiry and evaluation, and common links are then formed between cities and research resources, topics, methods and questions across the agenda so formulated. Any approach must be collaborative, entailing cooperation not only across disci-

plines but with researchers and project participants in different countries, who can share literature, adapt common research instruments and tools, and facilitate cooperation in their countries.

Project cities cannot afford to prove everything, or they risk demonstrating nothing. Evaluation should concentrate on evaluating what Healthy Cities is about. This may mean choosing to focus on the goals a particular city has set itself; this will facilitate the identification of appropriate questions, approaches and resources to support the evaluation. This does not mean that evaluations should focus only on areas where impact can be demonstrated. On the contrary, within a learning framework, stories and explanations of setbacks and failures may prove at least as important as accounts of success. Further, this approach does not imply that evaluating what is common to Healthy Cities initiatives is impossible. Rather, an understanding of which approaches may be more widely applicable is more likely to emerge from detailed accounts that take account of the context of local opportunities and obstacles than from summaries that are too general to be sensitive to local differences.

This chapter has urged extreme caution in using apparently scientific (but often actually technological) means to answer the complex questions posed by Healthy Cities evaluation. As illustrated by the search for indicators, attempts to achieve robust measurement tools may prove disappointing and fail to capture the processes actually at work. The developmental phase in Healthy Cities evaluation is the most important. If evaluators try to make the setting of aims a collaborative and participative process, involving all the appropriate stakeholders, then the subsequent work is much more likely to be true to the nature of the project and to be supported and sustained. Who makes the decisions about evaluation is ultimately more important than which methods are adopted. The justification for evaluation in Healthy Cities is that it should contribute to knowledge and policy development in an iterative and continuing way. For this to happen, the people who make and are affected by decisions about Healthy Cities developments need to be involved at all stages of the process.

The evaluation process can contribute to goal clarification, capacity building, collaboration and skills sharing. This requires that evaluators pay attention to the impact of approaches used on those involved in the evaluation process. Question formulation and information can be integrated with patterns of meetings, group work or other activities with which people are already familiar. Imaginative new approaches, such as those involving art or drama, can provide opportunities to demystify the process and to use and develop skills among those involved. Feedback is an essential and non-negotiable responsibility of those engaging in Healthy Cities evaluation. Without it, participation and commitment will soon dwindle, and the process of knowledge development will be aborted. This in turn implies that the resources needed to support an evaluation process be adequately analysed, to ensure that evaluation repays those who have given their time and skills. The potential tensions for Healthy Cities initiatives that can result from conflicting evaluation agendas and those who espouse the philosophies underlying different evaluation approaches cannot be understated. Participants need to understand the political implications of selecting an outcome-focused or a more process-oriented approach, for example.

Scientific methodologies do not necessarily hold the key to clarifying cause-and-effect relationships in the messy worlds of policy development and city politics. Despite the complexity of the issues, therefore, evaluation offers real scope for supporting Healthy Cities participants to elucidate the theory behind their actions, the lessons of their experience and the stories that illuminate the consequences of attempts to improve the urban environment. Such accounts, particularly if focused on key urban problems, may be more effective in starting dialogue with other sectors and showing the possibilities for collaboration than academic discourses have proved to be. This is not to reject the value of sophisticated analytic skills for supporting the evaluation process, but to urge that these resources be devoted to exploring models that participants recognize as salient and accurate representations of their concerns. We recommend that the people evaluating Healthy Cities initiatives listen to and reflect on the theorizing of community action and participation, follow principles that are likely to lead to open processes of learning and use these principles to seek negotiated decisions on process and method.

References

1. HANCOCK, T. The healthy city from concept to application: implications for research. *In*: Kelly, M. & Davies, J., ed. *Healthy Cities: research and practice*. London, Routledge, 1994.
2. LABONTÉ, R. Health promotion and empowerment: reflections on professional practice. *Health education quarterly*, **21**(2): 253–268 (1994).
3. HAUGHTON, G. & HUNTER, C. *Sustainable cities*. London, Jessica Kingsley, 1994.
4. MAESSEN, M. *Sustainable development/environmental health policy in cities: indicators*. Maastricht, WHO Collaborating Centre for Research on Healthy Cities, University of Maastricht, 1995 (World Health Organization Collaborating Centre for Research on Healthy Cities Monograph Series, No. 9).
5. WALLERSTEIN, N. Powerlessness, empowerment and health: implications for health promotion programs. *American journal of health promotion*, **6**: 197–205 (1992).
6. BLACKMAN, T. *Urban policy in practice*. London, Routledge, 1995.
7. MULLEN, K. & CURTICE, L. The disadvantaged – Their health needs and public health initiatives. *In*: Detels, R. et al., ed. *Oxford textbook of public health. Volume 3. The practice of public health*, 3rd ed. New York, Oxford University Press, 1997.
8. BRUCE, N. ET AL., ED. *Research and change in urban community health*. Avebury, Aldershot, 1995.

9. CURTICE, L. & MCQUEEN, D. *The WHO Healthy Cities project: an analysis of progress.* Edinburgh, Research Unit in Health and Behavioural Change, 1990.

10. POLAND, B. Knowledge development in, of and for Healthy Community initiatives. Part I: guiding principles. *Health promotion international,* **11**: 237–247 (1996).

11. STEVENSON, H. & BURKE, M. Bureaucratic logic in new social movement clothing: the limits of health promotion. *Health promotion international,* **6**: 281–91 (1991).

12. BAUM, F. Healthy cities and change: social movement or bureaucratic tool? *Health promotion international,* **8**: 31–40 (1993).

13. GOUMANS, M. *Innovations in a fuzzy domain. Healthy Cities and (health) policy development in the Netherlands and the United Kingdom* [Thesis]. Maastricht, University of Maastricht, 1998.

14. GOUMANS, M. & SPRINGETT, J. From projects to policy: 'Healthy Cities' as a mechanism for policy change for health? *Health promotion international,* **12**(4): 311–322 (1997).

15. TSOUROS, A.D., ED. *World Health Organization Healthy Cities project: a project becomes a movement: review of progress 1987 to 1990.* Milan, Sogess, 1991.

16. LEES, R. & SMITH, G. *Action research in community development.* London, Routledge and Kegan Paul, 1975.

17. POLLIT, C. *An evaluation of the community health projects at Walker, North Kenton and Riverside.* Newcastle, Riverside Child Health Project, 1984.

18. SMITHIES, J. & ADAMS, L. Walking the tightrope: issues in evaluation and community participation for health for all. *In:* Kelly, M. & Davies, J., ed. *Healthy Cities: research and practice.* London, Routledge, 1994, pp. 55–70.

19. MACGREGOR, S. & PIMLOTT, B. *Tackling the inner cities: the 1980s reviewed, prospects for the 1990s.* Oxford, Clarendon Press, 1990.

20. PUBLIC SECTOR MANAGEMENT RESEARCH UNIT AND DEPARTMENT OF ENVIRONMENT INNER CITIES DIRECTORATE. *An evaluation of the urban development grant programme, Action for Cities.* London, H.M. Stationery Office, 1988.

21. JACOBS, J. *Edge of empire: postcolonialism and the city.* London, Routledge, 1996.

22. DE GROOT, L. City Challenge: competing in the urban regeneration game. *Local economy,* **7**: 196–209 (1992).

23. COX, K. & MAIR, A. From localised social structures to localities as agents. *Environment and planning,* **A23**: 197–213 (1991).

24. STOKER, G. *From local action to community government.* London, Fabian Society, 1988 (Fabian Research Series, No. 351).

25. DUHL, L. *The social entrepreneurship of change.* New York, Pace University Press, 1990.

26. ATKINSON, D. *Radical urban solutions: urban renaissance for city, schools and communities.* London, Cassell, 1994.
27. SEED, P. & LLOYD, G. *Quality of life.* London, Jessica Kingsley, 1997.
28. BENEVELO, L. *The European city.* Oxford, Blackwell, 1993.
29. CATTELL, V. Community, equality and health: positive communities for positive health and well being? *Contested Cities: Social Processes and Spatial Form, British Sociological Association, University of Leicester, 10–13 April 1995.*
30. KLIJN, E. *Policy communities, subsystems and networks. an examination and reformulation of some concepts for analyzing complex policy processes.* Rotterdam, Department of Political Science, Erasmus University, Rotterdam, Leiden, University of Leiden, 1992 (Research Programme: 'Policy and Governance in Complex Networks' Working Paper No. 4).
31. CONSIDINE, M. *Public policy, a critical approach.* London, Macmillan, 1995.
32. ALLISON, G. *The essence of decision: explaining the Cuban missile crisis.* Boston, Little, Brown and Company, 1971.
33. HOGWOOD, B. & GUNN, L. *Policy analysis for the real world.* Oxford, Oxford University Press, 1984.
34. LIPSKY, M. *Street-level bureaucracy: dilemmas of the individual in public services.* New York, Russell Sage Foundation, 1980.
35. SILER-WELLS, G. An implementation model for health system reform. *Social science and medicine,* **24**(10): 821–832 (1987).
36. PETTIGREW, A. ET AL. *Shaping strategic change.* London, Sage, 1992.
37. NOCON, A. Making a reality of joint planning. *Local government studies,* **16**(2): 55–67 (1990).
38. PATTON, M.Q. *Practical evaluation.* London, Sage, 1982.
39. CHEN, H.T. *Theory-driven evaluation.* Thousand Oaks, Sage, 1990.
40. DOWNIE, R.S. ET AL. *Health promotion, models and values.* Oxford, Oxford University Press, 1990.
41. SANDERSON, I. *Effective intersectoral collaboration: the theoretical issues.* Leeds, Health Education Unit, Leeds Metropolitan University, 1990.
42. SPELLER, V. ET AL. Multisectoral collaboration for health: evaluative project. *In:* Bruce, N. et al., ed. *Research and change in urban community health.* Avebury, Aldershot, 1995.
43. FUNNELL, R. ET AL. *Towards healthier alliances: a tool for planning, evaluating and developing healthier alliances.* London, Health Education Authority, 1995.
44. FRIEND, J. ET AL. *Public planning: the intercorporate dimension.* London, Tavistock, 1974.
45. HANF, K. & O'TOOLE, L. Revisiting old friends: networks, implementation structures and the management of organisational relations. *European journal of political research,* **2**: 163–180 (1992).

46. MILIO, N. *Promoting health through public policy.* Ottawa, Canadian Public Health Association, 1986.

47. *Report of the Evaluation Advisory Committee of the WHO Healthy Cities project.* Copenhagen, WHO Regional Office for Europe, 1997

48. *Twenty steps for developing a Healthy Cities project.* Copenhagen, WHO Regional Office for Europe, 1992 (document ICP/HCC 644).

49. WILKINSON, R. *Unhealthy societies: the afflictions of inequality.* New York, Routledge, 1996.

50. CRUICKSHANK, J. The consequences of our actions: a value issue in community development. *Community development journal,* **29**(1): 75–79 (1994).

51. GUBA, E.G. & LINCOLN, Y.S. *Fourth generation evaluation.* Thousand Oaks, Sage, 1989.

52. KENNEDY, A. Measuring health for all – A feasibility study in a local community. *In*: Bruce, N. et al., ed. *Research and change in urban community health.* Avebury, Aldershot, 1995, pp. 199–217.

53. POLAND, B. Knowledge development and evaluation in, of and for Healthy Community initiatives. Part II: potential content foci. *Health promotion international,* **11**: 341–349 (1996).

54. SPRINGETT, J. ET AL. Towards a framework for evaluation in health promotion: the importance of the process. *Journal of contemporary health,* **2**: 61–65 (1995).

55. FAWCETT, S.B. ET AL. *Evaluation handbook for the Project Freedom replication initiative.* Lawrence, Work Group on Health Promotion and Community Development, University of Kansas, 1993.

56. DE KONIG, K. & MARTIN, M. *Participatory research in health.* London, Zen Books, 1996.

57. GOODMAN, R. ET AL. An ecological assessment of community-based interventions for prevention and health promotion – Approaches to measuring community coalitions. *American journal of community psychology,* **24**: 33–61 (1996).

58. SARRI, R.C. & SARRI, C.M. Organsiational and community change through participatory action. *Administration in social work,* **16**(3–4): 99–122 (1992).

59. COUSINS, J. ET AL. The case for participatory evaluation. *Educational evaluation and policy analysis,* **14**(4): 397–418 (1992).

60. WINJE, G. & HEWELL, H. Influencing public health policy through action research. *Journal of drug issues,* **22**: 169–178 (1992).

61. FETTERMAN, D.M. ET AL., ED. *Empowerment evaluation: knowledge and tools for self-assessment & accountability.* Thousand Oaks, Sage, 1996.

62. BARNEKOV, T. ET AL. *US experience in evaluating urban regeneration.* London, H.M. Stationery Office, 1990.

63. HART, D. US urban policy evaluation in the 1980s: lessons from practice. *Regional studies,* **25**: 255–265 (1992).

64. REASON, P. Three approaches to participative inquiry. *In*: Denzin, N.K. & Lincoln, Y.S., ed. *Handbook of qualitative research*. Thousand Oaks, Sage, 1994, pp. 324–339.

65. RIST, R.C. Influencing the policy process with qualitative research. *In*: Denzin, N.K. & Lincoln, Y.S., ed. *Handbook of qualitative research*. Thousand Oaks, Sage, 1994.

66. CONSIDINE, M. *Public policy: a critical approach*. Melbourne, Macmillan, 1994.

67. WEISS, C.H. Evaluation for decisions. Is there anybody there? Does anybody care? *Education practice*, **9**: 15–20 (1988).

68. DE LEEUW, E. *Health policy: an exploratory inquiry into the development of policy for the new public health in the Netherlands*. Maastricht, Savannah Press, 1989.

69. ZIGLIO, E. Indicators of health promotion policy: directions for research. *In*: Badura, B. & Kickbusch, I., ed. *Health promotion research: towards a new social epidemiology*. Copenhagen, WHO Regional Office for Europe, 1991 (WHO Regional Publications, European Series, No. 37).

70. HIGGINS, J.W. & GREEN, L.W. The ALPHA criteria for development of health promotion programs applied to four Healthy Community projects in British Colombia. *Health promotion international*, **9**: 311–320 (1994).

71. DEFRIESE, G.H. & CROSSLAND, C.L. Strategies, guidelines, policies and standards: the search for direction in community health promotion. *Health promotion international*, **10**: 69–74 (1995).

72. GREEN, L.W. & HIGGINS, J.W. Rejoinder by Green and Higgins. *Health promotion international*, **10**: 75–76 (1995).

73. BARR, A. ET AL. *Monitoring and evaluation of community development in Northern Ireland*. Belfast, Voluntary Activity Unit, Department of Health and Social Services (Northern Ireland), 1997.

74. BARR, A. ET AL. *Measuring community development in Northern Ireland: a handbook for practitioners*. Belfast, Voluntary Activity Unit, Department of Health and Social Services (Northern Ireland), 1997.

75. *Urban environmental indicators*. Paris, Organisation for Economic Co-operation and Development, 1978.

76. O'NEILL, M. Building bridges between knowledge and action: the Canadian process of healthy communities indicators. *In*: Kelly, M. & Davies, J., ed. *Healthy Cities: research and practice*. London, Routledge, 1994.

77. BAUM, F. Research and policy to promote health: what's the relationship? *In*: Bruce, N. et al., ed. *Research and change in urban community health*. Aldershot, Avebury, 1995, pp. 11–31.

78. *Action for health in cities*. Copenhagen, WHO Regional Office for Europe, 1994 (document EUR/ICP/HSC 669).

79. ASHTON, J. & SEYMOUR, H. *The new public health: the Liverpool experience*. Milton Keynes, Open University, 1988.

80. GOUMANS, M. & SPRINGETT, J. From projects to policy: 'Healthy Cities' as a mechanism for policy change for health? *Health promotion international*, **12**(4): 311–322 (1997).

81. COSTONGS, C. & SPRINGETT, J.A. *Conceptual evaluation framework for health related policies in the urban context.* Liverpool, Institute for Health, Liverpool John Moores University, 1995 (Occasional Paper 2).

82. *Liverpool health plan.* Liverpool, Liverpool Healthy City 2000, 1996.

83. SECRETARY OF STATE FOR HEALTH. *The health of the nation.* London, H.M. Stationery Office, 1992.

84. HALLIDAY, M. *Our city our health: ideas for improving public health in Sheffield.* Sheffield, Healthy Sheffield Planning Team, 1992.

85. TAYLOR, J. *Progress report to the Joint Public Health Team on the Liverpool city health plan.* Liverpool, Healthy City Liverpool, 1997.

86. COSTONGS, C. & SPRINGETT, J.A. *City health plan: the effectiveness of joint working.* Liverpool, Institute for Health, Liverpool John Moores University, 1995.

87. STROBL, J. & BRUCE, N. *Report on the evaluation of the consultation phase of Liverpool's draft city health plan.* Liverpool, Urban Health Research and Resource Unit, Liverpool University, 1997.

88. HUDSON, B. Collaboration in social welfare: a framework for analysis. *Policy and politics*, **15**: 175–182 (1987).

89. *National Healthy Cities networks in Europe.* Copenhagen, WHO Regional Office for Europe, 1994 (document EUR/ICP/HSC 644).

90. TEN DAM, J. *Gezonde stadsgezichten.* [Healthy Cities vistas – Thesis]. Amsterdam, University of Amsterdam, 1998 (in Dutch).

Part 4
Policies and systems

Introduction

David V. McQueen and Jane Springett

This part of the book emphasizes and reinforces one of the central characteristics of health promotion – complexity. Researchers in this field must remember that health promotion is multidisciplinary and intersectoral, presents difficult challenges for evaluation and seeks a sound theoretical base. Attempts to understand and evaluate policies and systems illustrate all of these features particularly well. Thus, we are not surprised that evaluation and its underpinning concepts at this system level are less well understood or at least less well established than evaluation of interventions on behaviour within fairly confined settings. In this field of action, policies and systems, the nature of evidence becomes even more complicated; the randomized controlled trial and the experimental approach appear even more distant from the needs of evaluation. The chapters in Part 4 reflect the complexity of evaluation of policies and systems, while presenting innovative and imaginative efforts to understand how evaluation can be relevant.

Health, as the Ottawa Charter for Health Promotion says, is created in everyday life. It is also created and promoted through interaction between many different factors at a number of levels. Thus, although much can be learned from demonstration projects, where there is some degree of control over the environment in which a health promotion intervention is delivered, most health promotion activity is embedded in complex, dynamic systems. Success, no matter how defined, therefore depends on the synergy between multiple interventions at different levels. While a setting is just a system whose boundaries have been artificially delimited for the purpose of an intervention, most people operate in systems that are open and vary considerably in size and context. All the chapters in Part 4 show that methodologies to evaluate complex interacting systems are very much in their infancy. Equally clear is the frustration of all the authors with the constraints imposed by the dominant paradigm of the health sciences, whose methodologies are inadequate for assessing anything more than single interventions in controlled environments. This has resulted in both too narrow a focus on outcomes at the expense of process (so people often are left with no clear understanding of what worked and why) and a failure to appreciate the importance of context and relationships.

Rütten's chapter on evaluating healthy public policies in a region of Germany clearly shows an appreciation of context. Chapter 15 puts forward a comprehensive schema for assessing how a policy built around the notion of investment in health can be implemented in a community and a region. The particularly noteworthy feature of the development of this project is the role

337

for evaluation throughout the initiative. The project is concerned with the impact, measurement and assessment of a model of investment developed and outlined by the WHO Regional Office for Europe and detailed in Chapter 22. Further, the evaluation of the planning process for the project takes seriously an evaluation approach that is both process oriented and participatory, thus presenting a model for evaluation in this type of work that meets many of the design problems posed throughout this book.

In Chapter 16, Milio provides an overview of the kind of issues that must be considered in the evaluation of health promotion policies. A prominent researcher in this field, she uses the eye of experience to identify the key questions an evaluator should ask. She notes that policy evaluation takes place in a political environment and thus by implication is a political process. This raises issues concerning the nature of the relationship between the evaluators and the various stakeholders and the extent to which this can be made explicit. The dynamic dimension of health promotion policy and the inherent complexities of an evaluation strategy for policy may help to explain why this area of health promotion evaluation is less developed than others.

In Chapter 17, Warren et al. illustrate the need to adopt a participatory approach to the development of an evaluation framework and indicators with an example from Canada. They show that stakeholders' involvement in making key decisions is as necessary for large-scale, multilevel programmes as for community projects. They document the experience of evaluating the Canadian federal health promotion programme, started in 1978, and the experience gained. They also examine the more structured approach to evaluation of the Ontario Tobacco Strategy, which has adopted a user-driven monitoring approach that is neither bottom up nor top down. In particular, the authors stress the need to generate consensus-based judgements on programme efficacy, rather than relying totally on expert assessment, and actively to involve participants in the dissemination of information through feedback. This creates commitment to continuing improvement. They emphasize the value of the logic model in defining the goals of a programme, the links between the different elements and the goals of the evaluation. Two key themes emerge. First, the dynamic context for evaluation means that programmes, policies and interventions change, so that evaluation is effectively the tracking of a moving target. Second, evaluation should have an array of information sets and use a range of methods from management science and systems analysis, as well as conventional evaluation research concepts, methods and techniques. In Chapter 18, for example, Frankish et al. discuss health impact assessment as one means of measuring the impact of systems and policies on health.

In Chapter 19, Kreuter et al. point to the importance of social and political context for the success of community-based health promotion interventions. They see *social capital* as a relational term, not an object. Individualistic societies largely ignore social capital because the benefits accruing to each individual are small; for the common good, however, the whole is greater than the sum of the parts. Kreuter et al. define social capital in terms of four key constructs: trust, civic involvement, social engagement and reciprocity. They explore the various potential ways of measuring them, emphasizing the need for measurement at both the community and individual levels. They then outline a project that has analysed social capital as an independent variable in the United States. They mention the problem of cultural specificity in defining and measuring these concepts, and their potential for identifying the extent to which health promotion can create social capital. (Chapter 11 provides another discussion of this capacity-building aspect of health promotion evaluation.)

Although health is created largely outside the health sector, health care systems see health promotion or, more specifically, disease prevention as within their domain. Most interventions in the health sector, however, tend to be based on individual transactions between a health care professional and a client. While the clinical approach to evaluation may be appropriate in such a context, interventions with comprehensive approaches and multiple outcomes require a very different approach. Literature on the evaluation of such programmes, however, is scarce. In Chapter 20, Stachenko contributes to making good this shortfall by describing the evaluation of the Canadian Heart Health Initiative, which is a good example of a well researched, well planned initiative working at multiple levels to build capacity for the prevention of coronary heart disease. The evaluation strategy included reflective and qualitative elements and established tracking systems at each of the levels, but left sufficient scope for an appropriate mix of different components. The process and outcome indicators were developed over two years in a participatory manner. The evaluation focused on the acquisition of practical knowledge to implement integrated approaches to health promotion and disease prevention, but also identified gaps in existing methodologies.

Communication is a key relational component of a human system, and Freimuth et al. focus on health communication campaigns in Chapter 21. Such campaigns are a traditional feature of health promotion intervention at the national level. They use multilevel strategies with multiple messages and multiple channels in trying to inform individual and community decisions in order to change behaviour. Campaigns have evolved well defined and well developed frameworks for evaluation. Ideally, formative evaluation – to identify the best mix for a given audience and the audience segmentation and profile – should underpin such campaigns. As well as traditional summative evaluation, process evaluation should be carried out to provide information on how to act. As in the other chapters, the authors argue that an explicit understanding of the underlying theory of action should inform the evaluation framework, and they echo some of key concerns running through the whole book, such as the inappropriate use of certain qualitative and quantitative methods and the failure to use a range of different qualitative approaches. In general, Freimuth et al. feel the constraining environment of health science research has led to a failure to employ a range of methods from other fields, particularly advertising, that health science has rejected as unscientific. This has reduced the potential for real understanding of what is effective.

Ziglio et al. discuss the WHO Regional Office for Europe's approach to health promotion as an investment for health. Rather than putting forward an evaluation strategy, Chapter 22 suggests elements of an evaluation that focuses on examining the impact of a range of public policies on social and economic development for health. The authors argue that evaluation must employ multi-faceted appraisal. They also argue that, because the investment for health approach is so new, it requires a profound rethinking of evaluation in terms of both the theory underpinning health promotion and the evaluation strategy or approach itself. The evaluation strategy must await the development of the investment-for-health strategy.

The chapters on policies and systems bring readers full circle in the debates over evaluation. Ways to evaluate in health promotion seem innumerable. Even some strategies in health promotion, such as investment in health, become their own evaluation strategies. We are left to conclude that initiatives at all levels, but especially at the macro levels, reveal the complexity and dynamism of health promotion. Evaluation that does not take account of these characteristics, despite the pitfalls and uncertainties, will always leave unanswered questions.

15
Evaluating healthy public policies in community and regional contexts

Alfred Rütten

Key issues in evaluating healthy public policies

Evaluation approaches must suit the field to which they are applied. Owing to both the complexity and specificity of health promotion and especially the making of healthy public policy, traditional evaluation concepts and methods, based on rather simple and generalized input–output models, are increasingly recognized to be inappropriate for this field (see chapters 1 and 22). Saying so, however, seems much easier than defining and putting in practice a comprehensive model of the complex phenomena under investigation *(1)*. In particular, gaps in knowledge for evaluating the impact of healthy public policies need to be addressed *(2–5)*. To specify an evaluation framework for healthy public policies, this chapter discusses five key questions.

1. What is meant by healthy public policies in the context of health promotion?
2. What generic contextual factors should be taken into account?
3. How can a strategy for healthy public policies work?
4. What is the impact of healthy public policies?
5. How can their impact be measured?

Defining healthy public policies

The Ottawa Charter for Health Promotion *(6)* specifies building healthy public policies as a core strategy of health promotion action. It aims to put health on the agenda of policy-makers in all sectors and at all levels. It emphasizes the combination of multiple approaches with coordinated joint action that contributes to healthier goods, services and environments, and fosters equity. It also considers the requirement to identify obstacles to the adoption of healthy public policies in non-health sectors, and ways of removing them.

In line with this general concept, this chapter focuses mainly on making healthy public policies outside the health sector, and intersectoral policy-making processes in particular. It demonstrates diverse but complementary methods of building alliances to promote healthy public policies, and outlines both concrete structural constraints and strategies to deal with them. Nevertheless, it begins and ends with the premise that scientific investigation of healthy public policies should move beyond the Ottawa Charter. Such investigations need a more specific focus on policy analysis and must be informed by theory on the structure and dynamic of the policy-making process. For the evaluation of healthy public policies, theory-driven approaches are needed that can guide research in very complex circumstances (7–10).

This chapter uses such an approach to the logic of policy-making (1,11) as a conceptual frame of reference. This approach helps to investigate the limited chances for success of healthy public policy initiatives. Such initiatives must not only struggle with the "bounded rationality" (12) of policy-makers, who usually prefer to stay with what has worked in the past (12–14), but also face the selective perceptions of established policy-issue networks and advocacy coalitions, which strongly adhere to their core concepts (15–17). Moreover, they must deal with policy arenas and other institutional arrangements that foster competition instead of cooperation, or hinder new players or new policies from entering the arena (18,19). Even if a healthy public policy initiative is included in a public policy agenda (20) and survives all further steps in the policy-making process, in the end it may vanish in a labyrinth of bureaucracy within the administrative structure (21–23). Thus, healthy public policy initiatives often need both a complex perspective and a multidimensional intervention strategy to overcome the multilevel obstacles of established policy environments. This is precisely the reason for developing a multidimensional concept of policy evaluation.

Generic contextual factors

Although the Ottawa Charter (6) has outlined a general concept of healthy public policy, making such policy faces certain generic challenges in developed countries. Countries that are developing or in transition, such as the countries of central and eastern Europe and the newly independent states of the former USSR, may face different challenges and structures. Policy-making must take account of particular cultural and political contexts (24,25) and contextual factors at the local level that differ from those at the national or international level. For example, the issue of community participation seems especially important at the local level, where citizens' knowledge and perspectives are crucial for shaping healthy public policies.

Thus, on the one hand, evaluations of healthy public policies must be highly aware of context (26). On the other hand, to develop theory in health promotion and to elaborate theory-driven evaluation in this field, they should search for generalizable contextual features and for programme success stories that might be adopted in similar contexts (27). This chapter deals primarily with the context and specific problems related to the transition in eastern Germany. Within this setting, I focus on implementing and evaluating healthy public policies at the local and regional levels, but discuss the interrelationship between the contexts of healthy regional development and public policies on other levels, as well as the generalizability of an example.

Making a strategy for healthy public policies work

To achieve real policy impact, health promotion approaches must develop a "responsibility for implementation" *(28)*. This chapter deals with implementation as a core concept. It raises a crucial issue for both the implementation and the evaluation of health promotion approaches: how to define and structure the implementation process. For example, interventions may be organized from the top down or the bottom up, at a multiplicity of intervention levels, by various agencies and with distinct measures applied to different issues.

The example outlined in this chapter demonstrates different ways of implementing healthy public policies. At the local level, a cooperative planning approach served as an intersectoral and participatory method of building healthy public policies. Here, a regional research centre took the primary responsibility for implementation. Further, a group of key stakeholders from different sectors and communities was formed to develop new alliances and partnerships to create health and to secure sustainable investment. An international group of experts, a project team from the WHO Regional Office for Europe, played a crucial role as facilitator.

Defining impact

The implementation process in health promotion is related to basic elements at the policy-making level and the population level *(1,11)*. Assessing the impact of healthy public policies means carefully investigating these elements. Basic elements at the policy-making level are the specific institutional arrangements and events that form a particular policy arena, as well as the political interactions and administrative processes related to it. Variables on this level are constitutional rules, formal legislative and administrative procedures, policy issue networks, advocacy coalitions and forms of bureaucratic procedures and organization (see also Chapter 22). Basic elements at the population level are related to specific lifestyle patterns that reflect behaviour, social networks and resources. Variables on this level are health behaviour and attitudes, personal capacities and obligations, and social, economic and physical living conditions. This chapter gives some examples of healthy public policies' impact, focusing on how such policies may influence policy-making processes at the local and other levels.

Of course, the input of health promotion implementation is rather diverse and has to be clarified for evaluation purposes. On the one hand, *health promotion* is used as an umbrella term for a wide variety of strategies and issues, including in some countries screening for disease, preventing risk factors, promoting healthy lifestyles and protecting the environment. On the other hand, the Ottawa Charter *(6)* has defined health promotion as a strategic concept to overcome the insufficiencies of previous approaches, particularly those focusing merely on individual health status and behaviour, and thus emphasizes building healthy public policies and creating healthy environments.

The expected outcomes of health promotion initiatives are as diverse as the meanings of health promotion. While the traditional public health perspective still tends to focus on reducing mortality and morbidity rates or controlling health care costs, the new public health expects improvements in the quality of life and the convergence of healthy public policy, socioeconomic development and population health. The example below definitely favoured the latter approach.

Measuring impact

Research in health promotion must be particularly careful to avoid ideological prejudice *(29)*. One way of dealing with the research problems caused by the hidden values of methodologies, methods and measurement is to be explicit about these values *(30–32)*. The approaches to evaluation measures described in this chapter are heavily based on participatory action research methods *(33–40)* (see Chapter 4). In particular, they emphasize the participation of science in building healthy public policies and of key stakeholders in evaluating them. Thus, the processes of knowledge construction and use are strongly interrelated.

The value of traditional survey methods must not be underestimated, but they are not an end in themselves. The present approach uses various survey methods at a series of intervention levels for collecting additional data to inform the evaluation processes and the different stakeholders involved in these processes.

Options for responding to the evaluation issues: example

To show concrete options for responding to the evaluation issues outlined above, I concentrate on the WHO demonstration project on investment for health in West Saxony (a region of the Free State of Saxony, a German *Land*), first sketching the policy environment and major contextual factors, then outlining the logic and concrete strategies of the demonstration project to influence current policies, and finally describing the evaluation processes, design and measures.

Policy environment

The generalizability of the West Saxony example discussed in this chapter may appear debatable. One could argue that the major financial investment in eastern Germany created an artificial environment that is not likely to be replicated elsewhere. This investment, however, not only did good but also created a number of problems, including health problems, that seem to be typical for other societies in transition, such as:

- increasing sectoral divergence caused by investment policies that concentrate on narrow-scope, market-oriented economic development and show rather low awareness of the social and cultural concerns of the population;
- increasing inequalities in society, with important evidence of negative public health impact *(41)*;

- high and rising unemployment, decreasing social support, a decreasing sense of coherence and increasing uncertainty and psychosocial stress; and
- recent changes in traditional public health indicators such as life expectancy and morbidity and mortality rates *(42)*.

The changes in indicators in eastern Germany seem to resemble those in other European countries in transition. For example, recent analysis of the "mortality crisis" in eastern Germany shows evidence of negative health and mortality effects that can "now be claimed to be causally related to the transition" *(43)*.

The divergence within the policy environment in West Saxony, primarily caused by rapid and unsustainable economic investment strategies, was observable within sectors, between sectors and between levels. For example, major investment in the development of commercial areas outside cities contradicted policies to revitalize the inner cities. Economic development policies to support the development of new small and medium-sized businesses contradicted unemployment policies that encouraged new businesses based on a state-funded second labour market. In addition, public and private investment policies that favoured competition among communities led to increasing regional discrepancies between winner and loser communities, and counteracted policies to support regional adjustment and overcome structural inequalities. The unintended consequences of this policy environment were crucial:

- in economic terms, wasting resources and working ineffectively and inefficiently;
- in social terms, possibly sowing the seeds of social and political disorder; and
- in health terms, providing a good example of an unhealthy policy environment needing to be tackled by policy-oriented health promotion strategy.

Logic of intervention for healthy public policy

In 1994, the Technical University of Chemnitz initiated a project to use WHO thinking about investment for health (see Chapter 22) to create an intersectoral strategy for regional development. The project, which continued into 2000, was intended to support changes in the policies of public institutions and communities, as well as private businesses and nongovernmental organizations (NGOs), to make them more conducive to the health of the population. In particular, the project supported the development of policies that could improve living and working conditions and empower the local community. Two kinds of benefit were expected from such policies: direct health gains for the population and help in overcoming the current divergence in policies, with its negative health impact, with indirect benefits to the health of the population.

As a first step, a network was developed that included communities, private enterprises, unions, several social, cultural and ecological institutions, and various scientific disciplines. In 1995, local projects were planned and discussed at a conference. In February 1996, the Research Centre for Regional Health

345

Promotion was founded in West Saxony to support the implementation of the projects.

Based on the actual problems of the region, the projects addressed, for example, town development, new management of industrial wasteland and the development of sustainable tourism in rural areas. While the projects varied in objectives, all worked for health gain and shared the same planning and implementation approach, based on intersectoral collaboration.

For each local project a cooperative planning group was founded that integrated the perspectives of the citizens affected, policy-makers, scientists and expert professionals. The groups integrated specific knowledge from each, and the mutual learning process supported the development of shared values and common understanding. The planning groups tackled three interrelated challenges:

- applied science: bridging the gap between science and public policy
- policy orientation: a particular focus on implementation
- empowerment: ensuring participation by and acceptability to the citizens affected.

The planning and implementation approach integrated top-down and bottom-up interventions, provided for organizational development, and created intersectoral networking and a sustainable infrastructure for the implementation of health promotion.

The Research Centre was responsible for organizing the planning processes. It employed, trained and supervised teams to organize and evaluate cooperative planning, provided external knowledge and expertise and links with other partners, such as external political structures and financing sources, and was responsible for public relations.

As a second step, the West Saxony region adopted the WHO Regional Office for Europe strategy for investment for health *(3)* as an appropriate vehicle for looking at the local projects in a unified manner. With the cooperation of the region, the WHO project team focused on interproject dynamics, communication and synergy; it helped to bridge the gap between policy-makers and project managers, and to identify the health implications of the various projects, so that health could become an investment resource for the social and economic development of the region. WHO also provided the opportunity to increase the visibility of the demonstration project.

Central to cooperation at the regional level was the formation and work of the Umbrella Group. It included one or two people responsible for the design and management of each of the local projects, and representatives of the different stakeholder groups involved. A major task of the Umbrella Group was to unite the projects into a cohesive programme to put health at the centre of regional development. This gave strength in negotiating with other interests. The prime purpose of the WHO project team was to support the Umbrella Group. The Research Centre ensured day-to-day coordination within the region.

Evaluating healthy public policies at the local level

I use one of the local projects of the WHO demonstration project on investment for health in West Saxony – Space Pro Motion, for the development of an integrated infrastructure for recreation and sport in Limbach-Oberfrohna – to illustrate options for evaluating healthy public policies at the local level. This section defines the basic elements of the implementation model, describes their use in the project and discusses methods of measuring and evaluating the different processes and outcomes.

Health promotion issues

As outlined in Fig. 15.1 (box 1), the WHO demonstration project on investment for health in West Saxony aimed to implement four health promotion principles: creating health, community engagement, building alliances and securing investment.

Fig. 15.1. Key elements of an implementation structure for healthy public policies at the local level

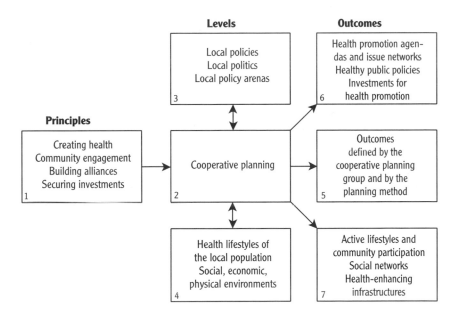

Socioeconomic development and health promotion are interdependent. For example, creating health through supportive environments means investing in both the quality of life and socioeconomic factors. Moreover, it supports the convergences of the different sectors (3). In the Space Pro Motion project, action on this issue worked to improve the city's infrastructure for recreation and physical activity.

Second, the specific knowledge and support of the community needs to be integrated in the development of healthy public policies. Within the local project, this meant empowering the community to take responsibility for the recreational infrastructure of their city, and, of course, preventing policy-makers from discouraging the community from doing so.

Third, building alliances means intersectoral collaboration in the community and the local policy-making processes, among different levels of public policy (regional, state, national and international) and between the public and private sectors. In the Space Pro Motion project, building alliances was related to the cooperation of public health and other sectors (such as sport and recreation, and city planning) and to negotiation between the providers and users of sports and recreation facilities and programmes. Further, building alliances among different communities at the regional level was important for the development of a health-enhancing recreational infrastructure.

Securing investment is closely related to the other three issues and building alliances seems to be a crucial prerequisite. Of course, a major focus is the allocation of funds from public budgets at the national or state level. To secure sustainable development, however, programmes should consider seeking investment from the private and voluntary sectors, as well as communities. Building or rebuilding facilities for health-enhancing physical activity may need financial support from the public sector, a private investor or a voluntary organization.

Implementation process

As shown in Fig. 15.1 (box 2), cooperative planning is a key intervention strategy to address health promotion issues. In the Space Pro Motion project, the cooperative planning group included: community stakeholders and representatives of sports organizations, local policy-makers (legislative, executive level), sports and health scientists and city planners and architects. The planning process started with a brainstorming session, continued with setting priorities and ended with a concrete list of measures to be implemented. In the second phase, the planning group supervised the step-by-step implementation of the measures.

Policy-making level

A key issue pertaining to the implementation process was how the work of the cooperative planning group interacted with the corresponding policy-making processes at the local level. As shown in Fig. 15.1 (box 3), the planning group had to pay attention to the decisions, programmes and measures developed by local authorities or private organizations. Moreover, the group had to be sensitive to the composition of local policy arenas. Was there a parliamentary committee responsible for sports and recreation? To what extent did the policy agenda consider health-enhancing physical activities? What stakeholder groups had the most powerful influence? What role did the mass media play?

While setting up an implementation infrastructure, the planning group might be influenced by the strategies of local political parties, interest groups and policy networks. Beyond this, policies at other levels have major influences on both local policy-making and the implementation process. For example, local actors can use state policies or private approaches to promote health-enhancing physical activities to build new alliances and secure investment.

Population level

One important part of creating health is to improve the health of the population and supporting the development of healthier lifestyles is a major way to reach this goal (see Fig. 15.1, box 4). Sedentary lifestyles are related to a number of health risks and diseases that the promotion of physical activity may help to prevent. The local environment may be conducive to physical activity because the population has access to a nearby sports and recreational infrastructure and a variety of programmes. In another case, the facilities available might be limited to competitive events or expensive private fitness centres. The environment also refers to the community. Who is allowed or able to use the facilities? Who is affected by the activities, both positively and negatively (by, for example, the noise of sporting events)?

Thus, a crucial part of the implementation process in the Space Pro Motion project was the improvement of the local population's opportunities to participate in health-enhancing physical activities (see Fig. 15.1, box 4).

Health promotion outcomes

According to the three levels of the implementation structure (cooperative planning, policy-making and the population), the local project was expected to have three kinds of health promotion outcome (see Fig. 15.1, boxes 5–7). One was related to the cooperative planning process and implied the implementation of concrete measures defined by the cooperative planning group (to create health and secure investment) and action towards the basic goals of the planning method (to build alliances and improve community participation in the planning group). At the policy-making level, outcomes were related to the structural issues and processes mentioned above, such as new policy agendas focusing on the development of an integrated infrastructure for physical activity and recreation, or new policy-issue networks that support this development. On the population level, outcomes were related to patterns of behaviour (such as more health-enhancing physical activity), social networks and community participation (such as more social contact and events facilitated by new opportunities for and forms of physical activity) and health-enhancing infrastructures (such as family-friendly sports facilities).

Evaluation design

The evaluation design of the local projects followed the implementation model as outlined in Fig. 15.1. In particular, the evaluation process (Fig. 15.2) focused on the implementation structure, referring to the internal cooperative planning process and to the external elements, structures and actors, at the policy-making and the population levels, that were related to the planning process.

Fig. 15.2. Design for an evaluation of healthy public policies at the local level

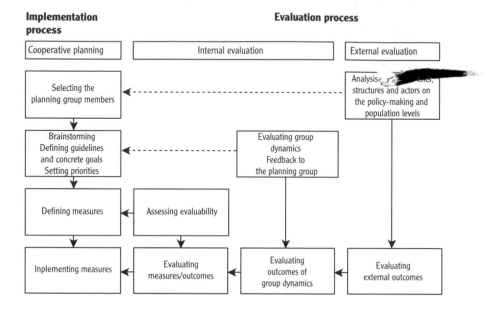

In evaluating cooperative planning, the form and content of the process are important. On the one hand, the evaluation team observes, for example, how members participate in the planning group's discussions, deal with the principles of the planning process (such as equity) and communicate with each other. On the other hand, the evaluation investigates the steps taken in developing the measures to be implemented. In both cases, the evaluation approach was process oriented and participatory. The evaluation team feeds back its observations to the organization team and the planning group. The team and group discuss how to optimize the group dynamics and improve their capacity for self-regulation (for example, by self-evaluation). In addition, the evaluation team interacts with the planning group by assessing the evaluability of the measures defined by the group. For example, the team and group jointly define both indicators for implementation and outcome measures. Thus, the final outcome evaluation was related to the measures and outcomes defined by the cooperative planning group. Beyond this, an outcome analysis of group dynamics (such as new alliances built during the planning process) helped to evaluate the effectiveness of the cooperative planning method.

The stakeholders who became members of the cooperative planning group comprised one source of information for evaluating external structures and changes in both local public policies and lifestyles (Fig. 15.2). Another source was surveys, such as those conducted by the Research Centre. The planning group also interacted with target groups or the whole local population by organizing group discussions and social events and using the mass media. These data were collected, not as an end in themselves, but for use in a process-oriented and participatory way *(44)*. In addition, the cooperative planning process was linked to evaluating policy and lifestyle dynamics. For example, planning group discussions could deliver information for discussion by focus groups at the policy-making and population levels.

Use of quantitative data

Following an action research approach, communication is crucial for measuring the impact of healthy public policies. Methods and data sources can differ significantly, but must be accepted as valid and reliable by both researchers and stakeholders.

In the Space Pro Motion project, survey data from the Research Centre on the health behaviour and physical activity patterns of the population in Saxony were used to inform both the cooperative planning group and focus group discussions at the local level. Questions raised by local stakeholders had already been integrated in the development of this survey. In a similar way, data derived from analyses of policy processes at the local and other levels were used to inform the planning and decision-making processes within the local project and the WHO demonstration project as a whole.

At the end of the first phase of the cooperative planning process, a major outcome evaluation took place in each local project, to determine what had been achieved so far. All members of the planning group were interviewed. Questions focused particularly on how they assessed the impact of the work on policy, society and health. For example, the perceived involvement of local policy-makers and success in securing public resources were used as indicators for policy impact; the development of new partnerships and the impact on other social contexts (style of communication with neighbours, co-workers and business partners) were indicators of social impact, and different measures of psychosocial wellbeing were indicators of health impact. The results of the outcome evaluation were fed back into planning group discussions and stimulated decisions on the specification of goals and measures for the subsequent implementation process in particular communities (including concrete indicators of impact) and of those that need concrete support from all participating communities to be implemented. As outlined below, the latter provided crucial information for the work of the Umbrella Group.

Evaluating healthy public policies outside the local level

To demonstrate options for evaluating healthy public policies outside the local level, the following deals with the WHO demonstration project on investment for health in West Saxony as a whole. This section concentrates on the constraints on implementing the key health promotion principles of the project in West Saxony, the strategies for healthy public policy developed to deal with these constraints and the evaluation designs developed to assess the impact of these strategies.

Implementation process

Identifying obstacles to the development of healthy public policies and ways of removing them is still a basic requirement of health promotion implementation. As the West Saxony example shows, this is especially important for societies in transition. For example, the President of Saxony and the State Cabinet were informed about the WHO demonstration project at an early stage, and their first reactions were quite positive. Because of the sectoral organization of state ministries and funding programmes (Fig. 15.3), however, getting any financial support from the state government proved very difficult. Similarly, the regional administration (Regierungspräsidium), although designed as an intermediary institution with specific tasks in intersectoral coordination, actually increased bureaucratic control to some degree.

Fig. 15.3. Current policy implementation structure

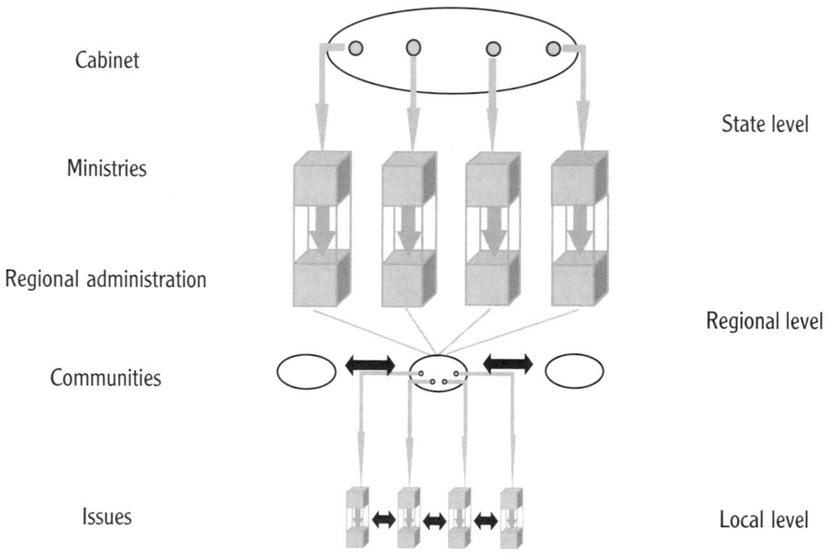

As outlined in Fig. 15.3, the policy implementation structure was not conducive to the growth of healthy public policies. Decision-making and resource allocation at the state, regional and local levels mainly followed a top-down model. This structure tended to discourage community engagement, alliance building and sustainable investment (45,46). It had already led to divergence among different sectors, regions and communities, and nurtured competition and distrust among various stakeholders. Thus, a crucial challenge to the WHO demonstration project was to try to modify this implementation structure.

The new interorganizational structure proposed by the project (Fig. 15.4) had three interrelated fora of intersectoral collaboration. As already noted, local cooperative planning groups ensured community involvement and the growth of new alliances to overcome the sectoral top-down approaches that had previously dominated policy-making at the community level. At the regional level, the Umbrella Group helped to overcome the intercommunity rivalries of the past, linked private and public partners and strengthened the corporate identity of the region. In addition, the project tried to establish an Audit Group at the state level, both to monitor the health impact of current state policies and to increase the capacity of the state government to develop healthy public policies.

Fig. 15.4. Desired implementation structure for healthy public policies

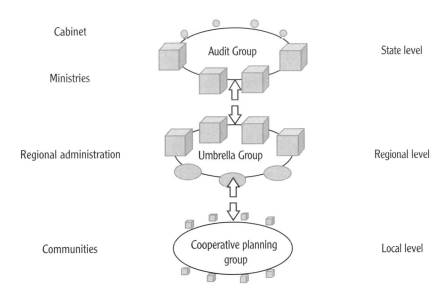

Of course, any organizational development remains a utopian idea, if it is not built on the strong commitment of key stakeholders to changing the current situation. The desire of key local decision-makers (who already had experienced the negative effects of increasing sectoral divergence) to develop a more integrated strategy for their communities was crucial to the successful development of the local projects. Similarly, community representatives' and business leaders' conviction that improving regional cooperation would serve their own interests was fundamental for the constitution of the Umbrella Group.

353

Further, the development of an Audit Group at the state level could be linked to current efforts of the State Cabinet to overcome sectoral divergence among ministries, especially in funding programmes, and to encourage the mutual adjustment of development strategies within the regions.

Nevertheless, turning wishes or duties into action requires appropriate opportunities, as well as capacity and knowledge. In this context, intermediaries that functioned as facilitators were crucial for the development of healthy public policies. Within the WHO demonstration project, the Technical University of Chemnitz and its Research Centre for Regional Health Promotion initially served in this capacity with increasing support from regional and international partners, especially from the WHO project team. Their major challenge was not just to facilitate cooperative learning within the different groups but to mediate between the local, regional, state and international levels.

Evaluation design

The demonstration project developed its own strategies for evaluating healthy public policies at the local and other levels. They were a major instrument of organizational learning within the Umbrella Group.

Phase 1. Case–consultancy approach

The regional Umbrella Group worked on the interface of the private and public sectors. Decision-makers and stakeholders from various sectors were involved. In particular, key representatives of different communities of the region had to cooperate in this context. In the first working phase of the Umbrella Group, a case–consultancy approach was applied to organize an intersectoral evaluation and learning process, to develop the corporate identity of the demonstration project and to reap the maximum benefit from WHO involvement.

As shown in Fig. 15.5, the case–consultancy approach applied the available experience and expertise to generic problems identified from one of the local projects. This included local expertise, that of the Umbrella Group and the WHO project team, and that derived from WHO case work and networks.

The case–consultancy approach is especially appropriate in evaluating healthy public policies within the context of action research, because it combines evaluation and action learning processes in mixed groups of stakeholders and experts. Focusing on one local project as a case study, the Umbrella Group worked collaboratively on the problems faced by individual projects, not only helping to solve them but also developing secondary problem-solving skills, as everyone involved carried the solution back home and applied it to their problems. This approach is an especially powerful learning device for senior managers and policy-makers. Working on real problems improves the individual learning process, facilitates joint work and encourages the development of integrated strategy.

Action learning via case–consultancy closely relates knowledge construction to knowledge use within the evaluation process. This has an especially

354

Fig. 15.5. Intersectoral evaluation and learning process: case–consultancy approach

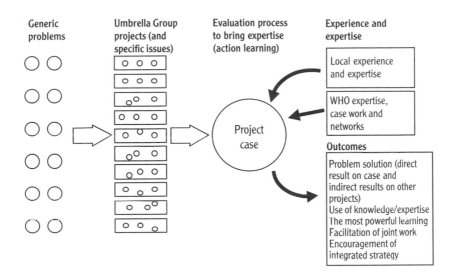

important impact on external policy-making. A "utility test" plays a crucial role in policy-makers' evaluation of alternative strategies, such as those for healthy public policy *(47)*. Thus, the key stakeholders involved in the Umbrella Group wanted to find out whether the lessons learned in their work could be applied to the real problems that faced them. In addition, as studies on the use of new concepts and insights in policy-making show *(48,49)*, these lessons had to be compatible with policy-makers' existing stock of knowledge and attitudes.

In some organizational or political contexts, single stakeholders and policy-makers may not find it rational immediately to transform new options into action. Especially in bureaucracies, where actors have developed a precise balance of power in a firmly established frame of institutional rules, innovation is often experienced as a threat *(22,23)*. The learning processes of individual stakeholders were closely related to issues of organizational capacity and development.

Phase 2. Measuring the impact of alliance building

Evaluating the impact of healthy public policies implies the assessment of both intra- and interorganizational processes. New networks, alliances and partnerships, as well as new institutional links among organizations, are important indicators of change in organizational structures. In particular, such intersectoral organizational adjustments and joint coordinated actions may help to overcome the negative impact of sectoral divergence and bureaucratic organization *(50–53)*.

After the first year of collaboration at multiple levels, the Umbrella Group, WHO project team and Research Centre reviewed their work. They decided:

- to emphasize implementation and concentrate on securing investment for health through alliance building;
- to strengthen existing relationships through further organizational development; and
- further to elaborate the principles under which the demonstration project operated to strengthen corporate identity and to identify specific criteria for both the review of existing local projects and the selection of new projects.

Moreover, to evaluate the impact of alliance building on securing sustainable investment for healthy regional development, the WHO project team and the Research Centre helped to establish cooperation between the demonstration project and The Prince of Wales Business Leaders Forum in the United Kingdom. One of the results was the inclusion of the demonstration project in the Forum's action research programme on measuring impact *(54,55)*.

In the second working phase of the Umbrella Group, the evaluation process included three major steps. First, following the first outcome evaluation of the local projects, the Umbrella Group dealt with the lists of local goals and measures (formulated by the cooperative planning groups) that required concrete support from all participating communities for implementation. The Group used these lists as input for formulating its own programme, and defined how to measure concrete progress by this programme. This built-in assessment of evaluability was crucial. For example, getting a private company to invest in a particular local project or getting public funding for another project could be used as an indicator of impact; other indicators might reflect concrete influences on regional and state policies (such as becoming part of a specific regional development plan that allocates funding from the state budget). The same procedure of defining concrete goals and measures and assessing their evaluability applied to further conceptual and organizational development.

Second, a process evaluation accompanied this phase of the Umbrella Group's work. In this context, the participatory evaluation measures to optimize the learning process (see Fig. 15.2 and 15.5) were completed by a reciprocal evaluation by local and regional agencies. Once the Umbrella Group decided on its programme, it fed back the overall list of goals and measures to the cooperative planning groups. After their review, the cycle began again. Thus, cooperation and particularly mutual monitoring between local and regional agencies became much more intensive.

Third, an outcome evaluation at the end of the second working phase of the Umbrella Group built on the evaluability assessment. Measures applied to the outcome evaluation of the first working phase could be reapplied to determine what had been accomplished thus far and to orient further work. Finally, as a crucial part of WHO work within the project, the WHO project team, along with the Research Centre, planned to help to identify the health outcomes of the new policy impacts reached by the Umbrella Group. In conclusion, these evaluations can demonstrate that alliance building is an important investment strategy.

Use of quantitative data

Within the demonstration project, the Research Centre and the WHO project team used quantitative data primarily to inform group discussions at different levels. For policy-making processes outside the local level, the "collective monitoring" (44) of various data sets by the regional Umbrella Group was of major importance. These data sets included important information about conditions for the population in West Saxony. For example, data on and analysis of the "mortality crisis" in eastern Germany (43) are used to discuss the context for economic, social and health development.

Other quantitative data were directly related to the work of the Umbrella Group. First, the members of the Umbrella Group were interviewed at the beginning of phase 1, to identify the core elements and problems of the various local projects. The results of this initial survey were used to define and evaluate the core principles of the demonstration project, and provided crucial input for the concrete design of the case–consultancy approach. Second, data were collected as part of a specific outcome evaluation. As with the evaluation of the local projects, questions focused on how the members of the Umbrella Group evaluated the impact on policy, society and health of the work done thus far. The results of the outcome evaluation, fed back into the group discussions, helped to stimulate decisions and to specify the goals and concrete measures of further work.

Audit of health impact of state public policies

The evaluation of intersectoral learning processes outside the local level has been related to the internal alliance building of the Umbrella Group and the development of a new partnership between the region and the Free State of Saxony. An additional assessment of the health impact of current state policies could complete the overall puzzle of an intra- and interlevel structure of interrelated policy elements (see Fig. 15.4). Participatory evaluation at this level could help to involve state representatives and other stakeholders from outside the region more actively in the WHO demonstration project.

Although one should be aware of the differences between evaluation and audit (56), auditing may be an appropriate strategy for evaluating public policies (see Chapter 8). The WHO Regional Office for Europe has developed an audit approach focusing on public policies, and applied it to two countries in transition: Hungary and Slovenia (57). Each used WHO expertise to assess its resources for health promotion and infrastructures supporting policy, the efficacy of intersectoral collaboration and the options for decision-making. Parliament, rather than any particular sector, proved to be an appropriate counterpart. Plans were made to apply this audit approach to West Saxony.

Again, an action research approach emphasizing cooperation appeared to be an appropriate framework within which to organize learning processes. For example, an audit group, including key stakeholders from different sectors and both government organizations and NGOs could give stakeholders an opportunity to provide input, increase their understanding of the audit's purpose and thus increase support. Representatives of the Umbrella Group could participate in the audit group to ensure communication among the key implementation agencies at the local level. In linking these agencies, the demonstration project could contribute synergistically to building capacity for healthy public policies at the local, regional and state levels in Saxony.

Conclusion: towards a framework for evaluating healthy public policy

Of the crucial terms used in the WHO demonstration project on investment for health in West Saxony – *health promotion, evaluation* and *policy* – the last appears to be least well defined and remains rather unclear. For example, in a recent attempt to define these key terms, Rootman *(44)* refers to a definition of policies as "broad plans of action which set the direction for detailed planning"; while this definition can be applicable to "any level, from international to the day-to-day work of a health promoter", it does not appropriately respond to the need for developing theory-driven approaches to policy analysis and evaluation in health promotion. Of course, other books and articles, particularly in the policy sciences, give more specific and sophisticated definitions of policy *(12,58–61)*. Nevertheless, each research agenda must specify the framework for its particular topic.

The WHO demonstration project in West Saxony showed how the concept of healthy public policy could be implemented. At the local level, cooperative planning groups developed and implemented joint coordinated actions, using multiple approaches to put health investment on the agenda of local policy-making processes. An intersectoral Umbrella Group performed this task in even more comprehensive policy settings. The West Saxony example also showed how to define relevant issues in healthy public policy, key elements at the policy-making and the population levels and relevant policy outcomes. It demonstrated how to assess changes at the different intervention levels and how to use quantitative data in these contexts. As a general feature, the policy evaluation concept strongly emphasized process and participatory evaluation. It showed how evaluative assessment could be integrated into cooperative learning processes and how survey data could be used for collaborative monitoring. The results also provided some evidence for a complementary use of qualitative and quantitative methods *(51,62,63)*.

For both further research and the development of policy evaluation methodology, one can debate whether evaluation approaches can keep pace with the increasing complexity of health promotion interventions. An alternative strategy might be to concentrate on a single, clearly defined healthy public policy and evaluate its impact. This is doubtless a complex endeavour, even when the implementation and evaluation frameworks discussed above are used. For example, a policy for sustainable development formulated by a ministry may focus especially on empowering local communities, and so act on a core aim of health promotion: enabling people to increase control over conditions that influence their health. This policy may particularly stress the need for community participation in the implementation process. An evaluation of the impact of such a policy in the context of health promotion research should take account of at least three levels of investigation.

First, the local policy environment can build a crucial intervening implementation structure. Important contextual factors at this level include the commitment of top local policy-makers and other stakeholders, the structure of relevant policy arenas, supportive issue networks and advocacy coalitions, and local political culture, history and administrative infrastructures.

Second, if the local policy environment is truly supportive in implementing a participatory policy, the next level of investigation is related to the receptiveness and sensitivity of the community. Here, further clarification will be needed on what participation actually means and how to measure it. For example, is it more closely related to involving community representatives or the whole local population?

Third, the health outcomes of the implemented policy must be investigated. In seeking health gain, the investigation could focus on psychosocial indicators, such as self-esteem, sense of control and a feeling of affiliation with the community, which are directly related to the health and wellbeing of the population.

Concentration on a single healthy public policy does not preclude a general, process-oriented, participatory design for the evaluation approach. On the contrary, a narrower focus and reduced complexity may help participating policy-makers and other stakeholders to follow the evaluation process. Nevertheless, health promotion practice, particularly when it is related to intersectoral alliance building, often transcends the focus of single policies, so appropriate evaluation must widen its focus, too. Policy evaluation within the health promotion context must avoid both becoming lost in the forest and missing the forest for the trees.

Finally, the need for elaborating policy analysis frameworks has a strategic dimension. Policy evaluation is neither a "neutral management tool" *(23)* nor a "referee within the political games that give life to public policies" *(64)*. In a political context, evaluation inevitably becomes part of the game *(65)*. Thus, policy evaluators should have in-depth knowledge about the rules of the game, the teams that are playing and their strategies and tactics in order to investigate at least the role that they and their work are expected to play. Moreover, "contra-intuitive effects" *(65)* are quite common in complex organizational and political contexts. Public policies designed to improve joint action and intersectoral networking may end by strengthening sectoral bureaucracies; in the same way, approaches using evaluation as a core instrument of policy development may contribute in the end to the fragmentation of evaluation as a discipline *(64)*. A careful recognition of the reciprocity of policy evaluation will help evaluators at least to understand these processes and avoid this danger.

References

1. RÜTTEN, A. The implementation of health promotion. A new structural perspective. *Social science and medicine*, **41**: 1627–1637 (1995).
2. GOUMANS, M. & SPRINGETT, J. From projects to policy: 'Healthy Cities' as a mechanism for policy change for health? *Health promotion international*, **12**(4): 311–322 (1997).
3. LEVIN, L.S. & ZIGLIO, E. Health promotion as an investment strategy: consideration on theory and practice. *Health promotion international*, **11**(1): 33–40 (1996)
4. MILIO, N. *Promoting health through public policy*. Philadephia, Davis, 1981.
5. WHITEHEAD, M. *The effectiveness of healthy public policies*. Toronto, Centre for Health Promotion, University of Toronto, 1996.
6. Ottawa Charter for Health Promotion. *Health promotion*, **1**(4): iii–v (1986).
7. CHEN, H.T. *Theory-driven evaluation*. Thousand Oaks, Sage, 1990.
8. DEAN, K. Using theory to guide policy relevant health promotion research. *Health promotion international*, **11**(1): 19–26 (1996).
9. MCQUEEN, D.V. The search for theory in health behaviour and health promotion. *Health promotion international*, **11**: 27–32 (1996).
10. WEISS, C.H. Nothing as practical as good theory: exploring theory-based evaluation for comprehensive community initiatives for children and families. *In*: Connell, J.P. et al., ed. *New approaches to evaluating community initiatives: concepts, methods and contexts*. New York, Aspen Institute, 1995, pp. 65–92.
11. RÜTTEN. A. et al. *Health promotion policy in Europe: rationality, impact and evaluation*. Munich, Oldenbourg Verlag, 2000.
12. LINDBLOM, C.E. *The policy-making process*. Englewood Cliffs, Prentice-Hall, 1968.
13. WILDAVSKY, A. *Speaking truth to power. The art and craft of policy analysis*. Boston, Little, Brown, 1979.
14. ZEY, M., ed. *Decision-making. Alternatives to rational choice models*. Newbury Park, Sage, 1992.

15.   HECLO, H. *Issue networks and the executive establishment. In:* King, A. *The new American political system.* Washington, DC, American Enterprise Institute for Public Policy Research, 1978.

16.   SABATIER, P.A. Towards better theories of the policy process. *PS – Political science & politics,* **24**(2):144–156 (1991).

17.   SABATIER, P.A. & Jenkins-Smith, H.C. *Policy change and learning. An advocacy coalition approach.* Boulder, Westview Press, 1993.

18.   LOWI, T.J. American business, public policy, case-studies and political theory. *World politics,* **16**(4):677–715 (1964).

19.   KISER, L.L. & OSTROM, E. The three worlds of action: a metatheoretical synthesis of institutional approaches. *In:* Ostrom, E., ed. *Strategies of political inquiry.* Beverly Hills, Sage, 1982, pp. 179–222.

20.   ROCHEFORT, D.A. & COBB, R.W. Problem definition, agenda access, and policy choice. *Policy studies journal,* **21**(1): 56–71 (1993).

21.   CAPLAN, N. Social science and public policy at the national level. *In:* Kallen, D.B.P. et al., ed. *Social science research and public policy-making: reappraisal.* Windsor, NFER-Nelson, 1982, pp. 32–48.

22.   CROZIER, M. *Le phénoméne bureaucratique.* Paris, Editions du Seuil, 1964.

23.   CROZIER, M. Comparing structures and comparing games. *In:* Hofstede, G. & Kassem, M., ed. *European contributions to organizational theory.* Assem, Van Gorcum, 1975, pp. 193–207.

24.   EDWARDS, R. *Building healthy public policies.* Toronto, Centre for Health Promotion, University of Toronto, 1996.

25.   MCQUEEN, D.V. Gesundheitsförderung und die neue Public Health Bewegung im internationalen Vergleich. *In:* Rütten, A. & Rausch, L., ed. *Gesunde Regionen in internationaler Partnerschaft.* Stuttgart, Naglschmid, 1996, pp. 5–12.

26.   GUBA, E.G. & LINCOLN, Y.S. *Fourth generation evaluation.* Thousand Oaks, Sage, 1989.

27.   WEISS, C.H. *Evaluation. Methods for studying programs and policies.* Englewood Cliffs, Prentice-Hall. 1998.

28.   KICKBUSCH, I. *Targets for health. Experiences and directions.* Geneva, World Health Organization, 1996 (document).

29.   MCQUEEN, D.V. Thoughts on the ideological origins of health promotion. *Health promotion,* **4**: 339–342 (1989).

30.   MYRDAL, G. *Value in social theory.* London, Routledge & Kegan Paul, 1958.

31.   PALFREY, C. & THOMAS, P. Ethical issues in policy evaluation. *Policy and politics,* **24**: 277–285 (1995).

32.   SHADISH, W.R. ET AL. *Foundations of program evaluation.* Thousand Oaks, Sage, 1991.

33.   CORNWALL, A. & JEWKES, R. What is participatory research? *Social science and medicine,* **41**(12): 1667–1676 (1995).

34. GREEN, L.W. ET AL. *Study of participatory research in health promotion. Review and recommendations for the development of participatory research in health promotion in Canada.* Ottawa, Royal Society of Canada, 1995.

35. KELLY, K. & VAN VLAENDEREN, H. Evaluating participation processes in community develoment. *Evaluation and program planning,* **18**: 371–383 (1995).

36. PAPINEAU, D. & KIELY, M.C. Participatory evaluation in a community organization: fostering stakeholder empowerment and evaluation. *Evaluation and program planning,* **19**: 79–93 (1996).

37. POLAND, B. Knowledge development in, of and for Healthy Community initiatives. Part I: guiding principles. *Health promotion international,* **11**: 237–247 (1996).

38. POLAND, B. Knowledge development in, of and for Healthy Community initiatives. Part II: potential content foci. *Health promotion international,* **11**: 341–350 (1996).

39. WHYTE, W.F. *Social theory for action. How individuals and organizations learn to change.* Newbury Park, Sage, 1991.

40. WHYTE, W.F., ED. *Participatory action research.* London, Sage, 1991.

41. WILKINSON, R. *Unhealthy societies: the afflictions of inequality.* New York, Routledge, 1996.

42. COCKERHAM, W.C. The social determinants of the decline of life expectancy in Russia and eastern Europe: a lifestyle explanation. *Journal of health and social behavior,* **38**: 117–130 (1997).

43. RIPHAHN, R. & ZIMMERMANN, K. *The mortality crisis in east Germany.* Helsinki, Uited Nations University World Institute for Development Economics Research, 1997 (document).

44. ROOTMAN, I. *Evaluating policies: new approaches consistent with health promotion.* Toronto, University of Toronto, 1997 (document).

45. KICKBUSCH, I. Think health: what makes the difference? *Health promotion international,* **12**: 265–272 (1997).

46. PUTLAND, C. ET AL. How can health bureaucracies consult effectively about their policies and practices? Some lessons from an Australian study. *Health promotion international,* **12**: 299–309 (1997).

47. WEISS, C.H. & BUCUVALAS, M.J. Truth tests and utility tests: decision-makers' frame of reference for social science research. *American sociological review,* **45**: 302–313 (1980).

48. CAPLAN, N. ET AL. *The use of social science knowledge in policy decisions at the national level. Report.* Ann Arbor, Institute for Social Research, University of Michigan, 1975.

49. WEISS, C.H. Congressional committee staffs (do, do not) use analysis. *In:* Bulmer, M., ed. *Social science research and government.* Cambridge, Cambridge University Press, 1987, pp. 94–112.

50. FRANCISCO, V.T. ET AL. A methodology for monitoring and evaluating community health coalitions. *Health education research*, **8**: 403–416 (1993).

51. GOODMAN, R.M. Principles and tools for evaluating community-based prevention and health promotion programs. *Journal of public health management practice*, **4**: 37–47 (1998).

52. HAWE, P. ET AL. Multiplying health gains: the critical role of capacity-building within health promotion programs. *Health policy*, **39**: 29–42 (1997).

53. MCLEROY, K.R. ET AL. Community coalitions for health promotion: summary and further reflections. *Health education research*, **9**(1): 1–11 (1994).

54. TENNYSON, R. *Managing partnerships: tools for mobilising the public sector, business and civil society as partners in development.* Aldershot, The Prince of Wales Business Leaders Forum, 1998.

55. *Measuring impact. an action research programme for international partnership practioners.* Aldershot, The Prince of Wales Business Leaders Forum, 1997.

56. SIMNETT, I. *Managing health promotion. Developing healthy organizations and communities.* Chichester, John Wiley & Sons, 1995.

57. *Investment for health in Slovenia. Report of a team from WHO Regional Office for Europe and the European Committee for Health Promotion Development.* Copenhagen, WHO Regional Office for Europe, 1996 (document).

58. DUNN, W.N. *Public policy analysis. An introduction.* Englewood Cliffs, Prentice-Hall, 1994.

59. HEIDENHEIMER, A.J. Politics, policy and policey as concepts in English and continental languages: an attempt to explain divergences. *Review of politics*, **48**: 3–30 (1986).

60. ROSSI, P.H. & FREEMAN, H.E. *Evaluation: a systematic approach*, 5th ed. Thousand Oaks, Sage, 1993.

61. VEDUNG, E. *Public policy and program evaluation.* New Brunswick, Transaction, 1997.

62. NUTBEAM, D. Evaluating health promotion – progress, problems and solutions. *Health promotion international*, **13**(1), 27–44 (1998).

63. SMITH, A. & SPENLEHAUER, V. Policy evaluation meets harsh reality: instrument of integration or preserver of disintegration. *Evaluation and program planning*, **17**: 277–287 (1994).

64. PALUMBO, D.J., ED. *The politics of program evaluation.* Newbury Park, Sage, 1987.

65. CROZIER, M. & FRIEDBERG, E. *L'acteur et le système.* Paris, Editions du Seuil, 1977.

16
Evaluation of health promotion policies: tracking a moving target

Nancy Milio

Introduction

An essential aspect of health promotion is public policy to foster conditions under which people can be healthy: healthful places and ways to live, work, learn, play and participate in community and public life *(1,2)*. The long-term health benefits and cost–effectiveness of policies that create healthier environments and lifestyle options have been demonstrated *(3–8)*.

Most health policy analyses focus on the substance of a policy: its costs, potential efficacy and effectiveness. For example, will higher tobacco taxes prevent cigarette smoking in young people? These studies are important in the repertoire of health promotion practitioners, although health promotion researchers rarely conduct them. A literature review of school health promotion studies illustrates the emphasis of evaluations *(9)*; of more than 500 studies conducted in the 1980s and 1990s, 85 involved interventions, of which 4 dealt with organization-based policy changes. These evaluations focused on descriptions of the policies and on clients' behavioural outcomes. The review suggests both the paucity of policy-oriented health promotion efforts and the limited types of evaluation assessing them.

Even when policy analyses show health benefits, many crucial questions remain for both the practitioner and the analyst. For example, if raising tobacco taxes benefits health, how might a tax policy be initiated, adopted and fully implemented locally or nationally? These are strategic questions that are as amenable to analysis and evaluation in a real-world setting as are the health effects and costs of policies. Because a policy is shaped by the processes that form and maintain it, strategic analyses of policy-making are needed *(10)*. They can tell practitioners what is the process in the empirical world, who affects it and how, how to teach and use such hands-on knowledge and how to measure all of these.

This chapter focuses on such strategic questions as the development and use of policy evaluation to support health policy action by health promotion advocates. The first section models policy-making processes to denote important variables and demonstrate how one might plan to evaluate an instance of policy development, illustrated with the case of tobacco-control policy. Then follows a discussion on general issues in policy evaluation.

Policy evaluation

Policy evaluation studies seek to assess the gaps between what is and what ought to be in policy objectives and results: gaps between goals and population effects or outcomes, action plans and actual progress, and means and ends *(11)*. This is a multidisciplinary and applied field intended to address real-world issues in timely ways. It is a pragmatic exercise, and must be user friendly and available in the short term to be most useful. Its audiences include an array of non-science groups, such as policy-makers in legislatures and administrative bodies, advocacy groups and organizations' governing bodies *(12)*.

Some basic questions
Process
An evaluation focus on policy-making suggests some of the specific questions that might be asked.

* How is the policy problem defined?
* What alternative goals and means are explored?
* Why and how were particular ones chosen?
* What kinds and amounts of resources were provided for implementation, monitoring and enforcement?
* What kind of strategic management unit, if any, was involved?

This approach explores the interplay of stakeholder organizations while analysing their interests (who gains and who loses), the strategic activities of groups attempting to influence the final policy, and the compromise reached through bargaining between groups throughout the policy-making process.

Effects
Questions can be asked about any part of the policy-making process: initiation (before a policy is formally placed on the agenda of the relevant legislative or executive authority), adoption, implementation, monitoring and enforcement, evaluation and disposition (revision, retrenchment or repeal). Questions might address some of the effects of a policy: positive and negative, direct and indirect, intended and unintended effects (favourable or not). They may affect organizations (for example, in fiscal and programme structure) and populations (for example, health and social characteristics). Finally, the potential sustainability of a policy may be assessed through analysis of the plans of and resource changes in the implementing organizations or policy authorities: organizational change. Such issues, of course, are relevant to local, national or organizational policy development.

Knowledge obtained from this kind of evaluation can then be used to inform policy actions in organizations, and to guide change in the original public policy. Its purpose is therefore strategic. Gleanings from policy evaluation should help health promotion proponents undertake the task of influencing policy-making. Understanding the ingredients in successes and failures in policy development can guide strategic planning to influence policy in favour of healthier populations: to select and use means that can increase the odds for reaching health-supporting policy goals.

A framework for health promotion policy-making
Evaluation: concept, problem and purpose

An evaluation model is a pair of glasses, a conceptual framework to guide the collection of data, develop indicators of change, analyse information and draw useful implications to inform future activity. An explicit framework is outlined below. It has been used previously and was developed to support strategic uses (13–16).

The basic purpose of evaluation is to address whether and how health promotion practitioners can affect any or all phases of policy development to bring about healthful changes in the real world. Evaluation focuses on the sentinel policy, the changes it undergoes during development processes and the influences that mould it. A policy is, in effect, a moving, evolving target, propelled by the actions of interested parties through formal and informal processes. The aim of evaluators is to track it empirically, attempting to account for each progressive movement, detour or reverse. The interested parties, as organized entities, are also objects of analysis to learn their purposes, resource base and strategies in pursuit of their interests in promoting, deterring or modifying the targeted policy.

Overview of the framework
Public policy: purpose and environment

Public policy is a guide to government action to alter what would otherwise occur. It guides coherent activity across public and private institutional systems. A policy has no clear beginning or end; its creation is continuous and non-linear, sometimes recursive. It never merely happens, but is determined by organized groups in and outside of government. Thus, policy-making can be monitored, measured and understood well enough to support health-supporting policy efforts. Organization policy is that of a single (for example, health department) or type of organization (for example, public schools), either public or private (for example, churches, childcare centres and corporations) and is closely tied to changes in government policy.

The purpose of policy-making is to shape the course and pace of change in a preferred direction by modifying current patterns of action. It is not to change the behaviour of every individual, each of whom is free to follow a policy or not, albeit with possible personal consequences. Rather, policy-making aims to change the decisions of organizations about their use of resources. This, in turn, will change the activities of managers and staff, clients and customers from former patterns towards new patterns in various settings, such as government agencies, nonprofit and commercial organizations, regulatory agencies, schools, clinics, construction firms or eating places.

Fig. 16.1. Health organizations and policy-making

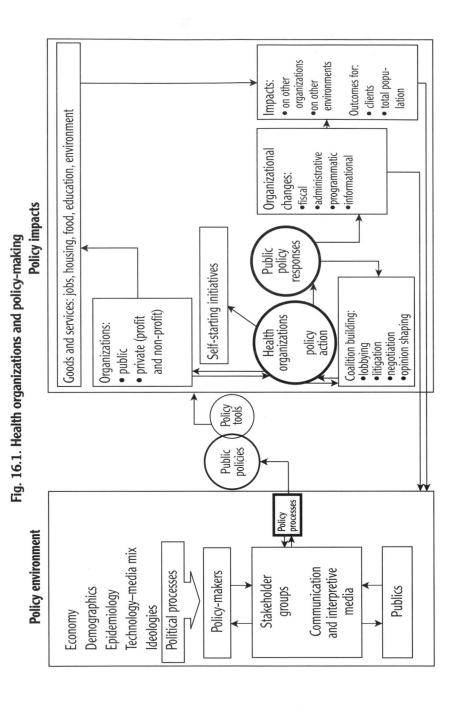

368

As indicated in Fig. 16.1, the policy environment or context includes the demographic and epidemiological characteristics of the population, the socio-economic and ethnic makeup of communities, the economy and technology, distribution of resources, political parties' agendas, organizational hierarchies and sudden disasters). All affect whether and how policy-making proceeds, regardless of the type of policy in question; the players, and therefore policy analysts, must take them into account to some extent. In addition, organized activity surrounding any specific policy is embedded in a historical context deriving from experience with similar issues and societal assumptions about the role of government. Evaluation of this environment indicates whether the social context, the climate, at a particular time enables or restricts the development of a sentinel policy (17).

Actors

Policies develop through the actions of the players and their relationships as they shape decisions about who pays and who gets how much of the determinants of health, such as housing, jobs and health care. The players or stakeholders are the organized groups whose interests are affected by current and prospective policies. They include political parties, the mass media, bureaucracies, voluntary and commercial organizations, and public interest groups (Fig. 16.2).

Fig. 16.2. Media and policy-making processes

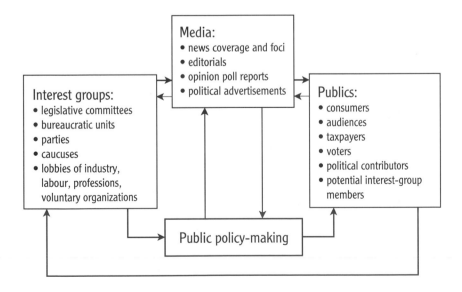

Organizations are social inventions for processing resources obtained from the environment, and turning them into services, products and information that

369

feed back into the environment. Whether governmental or private, organizations are both the makers and targets of policies and always potential active participants in policy-making processes. Private commercial or non-profit organizations make policy covering their own resources. Their policies, however, are subordinate to and often made in response to public (government) policies, which are made by legislative, executive or regulatory organizations (Fig. 16.1).

The media hold a unique position among organizations. They are conduits of information, but also create and shape issues (2). As large profit-making corporations, they seek to attract audiences and advertisers. Other players in the policy arena actively attempt to use the media for strategic purposes. Organized interest groups indirectly reach policy-makers and the public through heavy use of the media (18,19) (Fig. 16.2).

The public, in this framework, comprises several populations affected by policy-makers' decisions. Policy choices set the parameters for health in the form of prices, taxes and access to services, products, processes and information. Most members of the public are not active members of interest groups. The continuing outcomes of policy-making, among other things, shape the conditions for the health of populations, particularly disadvantaged subgroups.

Types of policies

For comparative purposes in evaluation, health promotion policies may be categorized according to their main intervention strategy (that is, informational/educational, behavioural or clinical regulatory and environmental policies) and the primary focus or target of the intervention (that is, individual or organizational change), as shown in Table 16.1.

Table 16.1. Strategies for disease prevention and health promotion

Intervention strategy	Focus
Individual-directed, information-mediated change	Homes and communities Organization settings
Organization-directed change	Policy bodies: • legislatural bodies • independent regulatory agencies • government administration Specific organizations: • government bodies • other organizations

The typical approach focuses on individual change through some form of information or education delivered in homes (through print or computers) and communities (through, for example, media campaigns and health fairs) or in health facilities, schools or workplaces (through, for example, counselling and small-group work with consumers, students or practitioners). A second ap-

370

proach involves policies directed at the organizations that affect the determinants of health (such as primary care systems, environmental polluters and commercial, educational and housing entities). The groups targeted by policy activity may be policy-making organizations themselves (such as state legislatures or regulatory authorities) or specific types of organizations in the public and private sectors (such as health departments, local schools or systems, health maintenance organizations and supermarkets or other firms).

A case in point: tobacco-control legislation

This section applies this model to a recent policy-making situation further to define and illustrate how a policy may be evaluated, dealing with the evaluation issues often encountered and noting how strategic guidance for future advocacy efforts may be derived and disseminated from the findings. The example involves the development of antismoking policy in several of the United States in the 1980s, based primarily on a recent descriptive report and related literature *(8,20)*. Studies compared states where strong laws were passed with those that enacted weaker legislation. Differences in policy-making effectiveness involved legislative leadership, coalition strength and support by top public health and public administration officials.

The kinds of data sources that can be used for addressing evaluation questions include the scientific literature, public secondary data, public reports, media coverage, opinion polls, internal documents of the players and the perceptions of players as proponents and opponents, competitors and collaborators, obtained through semi-structured interviews or surveys.

Environmental context: why there and then?

The basic evaluation question about context is, why there and then? What impelled tobacco-control initiatives at a particular time, or what environmental conditions enabled policy action?

Which components of the social ecology were more important to the outcome of the process? Relevant contextual data in the anti-tobacco case in the United States, for example, are the decline in the tobacco market and increase in costly legal challenges to the tobacco industry. This impelled manufacturers to seek overseas markets, facilitated by freer world trade policies. The offshore shift divided interests and weakened the oncefirm alliance between cigarette manufacturers and tobacco growers who, because of policy-supported farm consolidations, represent a shrinking political constituency. Taken together, these and other components of the environment make the industry increasingly vulnerable and present an opening for action by health promotion advocates.

From the viewpoint of health promotion, times of rapid environmental change may induce policy-makers to explore new approaches. The resulting turbulence impels organizations to re-examine what they do and revise their objectives in ways that help ensure their future. Alternatively, change and uncertainty could result in retrenchment, freezing new action. Successful policy-making activity is sensitive to the times; proposals must fit the circumstances of the day *(21)*. This implies that health proponents must be aware of current circumstances.

Policy frame and setting: how and where was the policy issue defined and legitimized?

How an issue or problem is framed affects whether it is regarded as a legitimate issue for government action, its priority on the public agenda and the kinds of policy solutions to be considered *(21)*. Several questions could be asked.

- How was the issue defined: as, for example, an individual, behavioural problem of young smokers or an organization-level problem related to tobacco production and marketing?
- What solutions were proposed (for example, youth education or market control)?
- Was the issue framed in the health interests of the public: as, for example, an environmental and child health issue or one of smokers' right to take personal risks in using a legal product?
- How did players resolve these early issues, if at all?

Many policy initiatives, of course, come to an end at their initiation. Stronger tobacco-control policies came about from framing the issues as a broad public concern about health, the market and young people's future.

The forum

Public fora can affect public opinion about the nature of the problem and enhance support for change.

Where did discussion occur, under whose sponsorship and initiative? How public was the debate?

Were the venues and communication channels favourable to proponents or the opposition? Tobacco-control advocates were more successful when they used the open arenas of legislatures or the public referendum process, and sought news media coverage to amplify their position, in contrast to the highly paid, behind-the-scenes activities and television advertising of the industry.

At what level of government did the policy action begin? For some anti-tobacco campaigns, local ordinances may be more readily enacted than state law, in spite of the narrower public health impact at local levels. Sufficient community-level action can be a learning laboratory and create political conditions for stronger statewide policy action.

Design, instruments and financing: what were the policy goals, tools and resources?

In addition to a policy's goals, its design usually includes the means to reach the goals. Goals as measurable objectives and the strength (or absence) of means significantly affect a policy's potential to benefit health. Without measurable objectives, progress towards health goals becomes contentious; without sound means and resources, little programme action is likely to occur, even though a weak policy is often more readily adopted.

Policy instruments

The means to achieve policy goals involve a limited list of instruments that are used by most governments and can be useful to evaluators for case comparisons. The instruments include economic incentives (such as tax breaks and subsidies) for businesses, governments and taxpayers; mandates and regulation; and the development and provision of information, education, training and services. Others are modelling, creating exemplars (for example, by forbidding smoking in government facilities) and market power and market management *(22)*.

Inflation-adjusted tobacco taxes are an example of an economic disincentive to smoking, especially for young people on limited incomes. Prohibition of smoking in public places is an example of a low-cost and effective use of regulation. Market management and market power are used when, for example, government offices redesign their vending machine policies around health promotion goals, such as prohibiting cigarettes and requiring healthy food items. Such changes require commercial suppliers to establish new practices and seek healthier products, which may in turn affect other buyers in the market.

Economic and regulatory instruments are more effective on a population basis than information and education *(10)*. The more effective means, however, tend to be the most difficult to put in place because they have a higher political cost; that is, offending tobacco interests by using economic instruments is riskier than simply informing the public of health risks through warning labels on cigarettes. The following, then, are important evaluation questions.

- What instruments were chosen?
- What groups advocated which instruments?
- What trade-offs among competing groups were made?
- What financing, if any, was attached to the instruments of choice?

Some of the states that passed weak anti-tobacco laws used less politically costly policy tools: narrow regulation and information/education to encourage compliance, with only minor penalties for infractions. The states with strong laws chose wide-reaching regulation with heavy penalties, along with information/education, as policy instruments.

Organizations: who were the players?
Interests

A policy issue draws the attention of public and private groups (stakeholders) that view a policy change as important to their interests. Stakeholders' inter-

373

ests include finances, facilities, staff, authority, control, status, legitimacy and image. These resources affect a group's bargaining power. Thus, stakeholders include elected or other officials as heads of committees, parties and bureaux; and commercial, scientific, medical and non-profit entities, including public interest groups *(23,24)*.

When organizations believe their interests are at stake, they attempt to influence the direction of change to strengthen them. They usually make an initial situation assessment, determining the importance of the issue (new tobacco-control policy) for the organization, and whether it is a legitimate one for action. More specifically, elected and other officials weigh political risk; they want assurances of political support. Voluntary organizations must please their boards and donors; commercial groups seek safe and expanding markets; advocacy groups must satisfy their current and potential supporters: boards, funding sources and members *(12,25,26)*.

Bottom-line judgments

The involvement of major health-related organizations in tobacco policy illustrates these calculations and accounts for their peripheral role. State health departments, public health associations, medical societies and large voluntary organizations did nothing more than lend their names to the anti-tobacco coalitions. Each of these mainline organizations had competing priorities (such as fears of budget cuts from opposition lawmakers, and lack of staff or legal restrictions in some local health departments). The medical societies chose to use their political capital to seek better clinical payment rates, and the large non-profit groups feared a backlash from some donors. These organizational decisions about public health advocacy were strategic choices that took account of trade-offs in resources for each group and its purposes. Similar risk protection was required before a state chapter of the American Cancer Society agreed to lead a tobacco taxation campaign.

Identifying stakeholders

Major players in a policy-making situation can usually be identified from relevant public legislative and administrative documents, the press, advocacy groups and voluntary societies. Communication with these organizations can yield additional group names in a kind of snowball sampling.

Organization indicators

After the major stakeholders are identified, each group can be characterized by indicators that denote its interests as the policy in question affects them: most usefully, its resource base. The size and sources of an organization's financing and its network of organizations in and outside of government are major indicators of its potential policy influence. Its funding sources also help identify its constituency: the groups that it must satisfy to retain their support. The most important constituents are usually the organization's governing body, such as a board of directors, or, in the case of a government agency, a higher administrative authority or legislative oversight committee. Another resource-related indicator of a group's policy influence is its allocation of staff and/or funds to the effort.

The question of values

An organization's values, always difficult to define, are not a useful variable for accounting for action. They are not measurable and can only be denoted by statements on mission or purpose. They are effective in practice only to the extent that resources are invested in functions that the organization attributes to them. One may well identify a group's values in practice by determining what activities, populations and localities receive larger shares of its resources. Basic questions to evaluate the impact of each stakeholder's participation in the policy-making process include the following.

- Why and to what extent did it seek participation in the process?
- What interests were at stake?
- What resources did it commit to the activities?

Interorganizational relations: how were players interlinked?

The interplay among organized entities – groups, coalitions, committees, companies and bureaux – determines whether, to what extent and in what form each stakeholder advances its agenda. To pursue their interests, organizations may link to each other in a variety of ways to influence policy development in any policy-making phase, including implementation.

Joint efforts

Alliances are more reliable when they are secured by written agreements, agreed rules or intense resource exchange (2). Collaboration can be distinguished from cooperation by the exchange of tangible assets in the former, in contrast with cursory and verbal support in the latter. Looser ties augur a shorter-term or less effective relationship. To be capable of influencing decision-makers in competition with well financed large-scale commercial interests, as in tobacco control, effective health policy work requires strategic planning and management and joint efforts, in spite of the difficulties of coalition formation (8,27).

Definitions of coalitions in the health promotion lexicon seem to reflect differences concerning individual versus organizational strategies. One definition views coalitions as organizations of individuals representing different organizations, while a polar view defines them as organizations of diverse interest groups (2). The latter concept is the one most suited to the evaluation framework used here, where organizational indicators are used instead of the member characteristics used in the individual concept.

Issues to explore

Relevant intergroup issues for evaluation are whether and how organizations with similar goals engaged in joint action, their previous relations, the resource base for joint efforts and policy success.

Organizations' strategies: what action did players take?
Types of strategic action
The most effective policy-making activities in the United States, demanding the most resources, include lobbying legislative or bureaucratic policy-makers directly or through their constituents, ensuring the election or appointment of supportive political leaders and engaging in litigation. Less effective means, often used by small groups, involve developing publicity through the media and organizing demonstrations, conferences and public education programmes *(28)*. To assess the adequacy of policy activity, one can explore the type, timing, cost and success of each strategy for single groups or alliances.

Bargaining
The central strategic activity for influencing policies and moving them through the phases of policy-making is negotiation, which always involves compromise. Effective bargaining requires taking account of the interests of governments and other stakeholders and being willing and able to trade away some valued interests to gain others in the foreseeable future (see Chapter 22).

As often occurs with the tobacco industry, opponents may offer sham compromise proposals to confuse and diffuse the issue for the public. These require public clarification and rebuttal from health proponents.

To give sound endorsement, elected and bureaucratic officials must have assurances of external support based on credible evidence. This involves developing information on group support for proponents' policy preferences from option polls, written endorsements by important groups or the promise of future support for a policy-maker's agenda.

In tobacco-control policy, the aim is not to win a scientific battle; this has long been done. Victory in the social, economic and political battle remains to be achieved. This effort has involved persuasion by reinterpreting available health, economic and political data for important political, community and professional constituencies. Such information, tailored to these groups' interests, can lower the political costs of their support if it can show how they will not lose, and may gain, status or resources. Group mobilization issues were illustrated in the anti-tobacco case by some organizations' reluctance to be actively and publicly involved. Before it would take the lead public role, the board of one large anti-cancer organization demanded evidence of external support from a special public poll, the approval of its local units and the formation of a coalition with adequate financial resources to support a policy campaign.

Basic evaluation questions about intergroup bargaining concern types and uses of information: rationales, counterarguments and evidence. These can be assessed and compared for contending stakeholders in relation to their policy success.

Information in policy-making: what types of information were used and how?

Regardless of the strategies used by policy participants, information is the medium of exchange. Even in the dubious instances when gifts are traded, information about such inducements is critical in policy negotiations. Information may be used passively, to monitor, analyse, evaluate, report or critique an issue, or more actively, to inform, educate, persuade, mediate, activate or mobilize others to act *(29)*.

The strategic problem for proponents of health-supporting policy is to use selected types of information to convince target groups that their policy position is economically feasible (to its supporters and users), politically acceptable (to the more powerful groups affected by it), socially doable within the milieu in which it is to operate and administratively and technologically possible *(30)*. Over recent decades, tobacco-control advocates have increasingly actively used ever more complex information in terse, timely and targeted ways.

Designing policy

For evaluation of policy-making, one can think of information as having two types, each having two purposes. Science-based information is mainly used for substantive policy purposes: for example, identifying problems and solutions, including the efficacy, effectiveness, and economic costs and benefits of a policy, as in defining strong or weak anti-tobacco policies. The primary and traditional purpose is to educate policy constituencies and inform the early design of a policy.

Other, less systematically verifiable information, from stakeholders' informed judgments and personal experience, often influences substantive policy issues. For example, tobacco-control proponents may call an emphysema patient as witness in a legislative hearing. The main purpose is to persuade, to promote the public legitimacy of an issue and to justify a place for it on the policy agenda *(21)*.

Enacting policy

Both types of information, properly translated, also have potential strategic uses: to promote proponents' policy choices and to persuade potential allied groups, policy-makers, the public and the press to support enactment. Policy-makers may use selected scientific findings to justify choices that have been made on a political, negotiated basis with major stakeholders *(11)*. Knowledge gained from policy evaluations that explore the forms, formats, information and channels for reaching and persuading policy-makers can be applied proactively to promote health-sustaining policies.

Media information and influence: how were media involved?

Information is conveyed directly or through various channels, interpersonal and technological. All such conduits select and shape the information they pass on according to their own priorities. The new media mix includes net-

377

work, cable and satellite television, videotapes, CD-ROMs, film and the print media, all merging on the Internet. This rapidly sprouting web has implications for both policy development activities and traditional health information/ education.

Effects on policy-making

The electronic world has vastly widened the political arena, raising new issues, proposing solutions and establishing the legitimacy of individuals and groups, and is influencing political choices (31). This offers the possibility of reframing public issues – such as smokers' rights versus others' right to breathe clean air – in health promoting ways. Issues, however, can be too simply defined, solutions made too superficial and legitimacy conferred only on groups selected by the media because of market criteria (19,32).

People necessarily use what they directly experience and what they learn through other routes to view and form opinions about reality. The media as businesses depend on advertisers, and select content and target audiences in the interests of sponsors (33). News, programming and advertising can amplify or minimize public issues and help shape interpretations in public fora, opinion polls and the political risk assessments made by policy-makers (34). In tobacco-control campaigns, short-term changes in public opinion on local policy proposals have tended to follow the amount of media advertising money spent by contending groups. The ultimate effectiveness of the campaigns depends on the balance and intensity of local groups' and policy-makers' leadership on the issue.

Useful queries

Questions about the interplay between information and the media in policy-making arenas are virtually essential for evaluations that can guide health advocates.

- Did public opinion change over time?
- What sorts of information (substantive or strategic) were conveyed to the public, by whom, through which channels and at what cost?
- Did changes in opinion, if any, affect policy-making?
- What was media opinion, as reflected in news coverage of the issue, editorials and opinion columns?

Implementation: did policy become reality?

The central question in policy implementation is: so what? Any health-supporting policy, successfully guided to adoption, can have no health impact unless it is also implemented in effective and sustainable ways. Most health promotion evaluations of this phase focus on individual health outcomes. Yet individual or population health benefits cannot be extensive if, as in the case of tobacco control, restrictions on smoking in public places are not put into practice, enforced or, as in one state, properly funded (8).

378

Implementation means changes in the workplaces and public spaces that organizations control. It requires reallocation of their resources. There are two relevant questions.

- What changes in fiscal, administrative, programme staff or training support, if any, were made in the accountable organizations?
- How were these changes managed?

Comparisons between organizations in a given situation can then suggest the conditions that promoted implementation to bring the policy into full effect (or not), and thereby assist health promotion practitioners in the future. The bigger the fund of understanding that evaluations of policy-making can build of generic policy processes – seen as the interplay of interested parties to gain in the allocation and reallocation of resources as they chart the course of change – the more effectively health advocates can engage in and influence these processes.

Policy evaluation issues
The environment of policy evaluation

Policy evaluation takes place in a political environment that may be less comfortable for researchers than that of traditional academic studies *(35)*. Groups with diverse interests often have stakes in the findings of a policy evaluation. Opponents may charge that findings are tenuous on methodological grounds, and may challenge interpretations as biased or based on insufficient evidence. In addition, during rapid and continuing policy changes, the moving target of a specific policy becomes ever more difficult to follow.

Units of analysis
Individual indicators

Health promotion evaluations typically use the individual as the unit of analysis, measuring personal changes in knowledge, attitudes, practices and sometimes risk-factor reduction. Policy-making evaluations focus on strategies, actions and organizational changes that contribute to or result from policy development.

Reviews of the most widely known, large-scale evaluations of community health promotion trials concluded that health benefits, especially over the long term, were meagre relative to effort *(36,37)*. Researchers recommended that future programmes include public policy initiatives and the social factors that influence the distribution of risk, using qualitative measures of individuals, organizations and environments *(38–40)*. The implication is that health promotion will become sustainable when institutionalized in policies and the organizations that promote and implement them. Second, evaluations should encompass this policy–organization–population web to learn what actions work and how they are accomplished.

The relatively few studies that evaluate organizational change also use measures of individuals, such as clients' records, participants' perceptions of benefits and costs, individuals' leadership characteristics and members' characteristics (41,42).

Measuring change in individuals poses a problem for drawing inferences to guide strategic action by policy proponents. That is, individual-level measures can suggest only that individuals in the organization must change – of necessity, a repetitive process with staff turnover. They do not illuminate what in the organization's structure, with its explicit and tacit incentives, produces certain patterns of behaviour in staff, clients or external relations.

For example, one well planned evaluation in a large community health promotion trial measured the impact on the health services delivery system by outputs (such as numbers of health promotion activities) and organization structure (defined as, for example, the existence of committees and coalitions). These were not anchored to the organization's core mission or budget. The measures did not have the potential to indicate long-term organizational change. Such process measures, like committee activities, do not address the longer-term interests of organizations, which are far more likely to explain decision-making about resource changes in health promoting directions. Health promotion evaluators concluded that institutionalization might be more likely to occur in organizations whose "current needs and interests fit the goals of the intervention activity", rather than as a result of anything a health promotion project does to encourage sustainability (43). This is useful strategic information for practitioners. It suggests the necessity to assess organizational interests as an element of long-term organizational change.

Organization indicators

When viewed as the creators and targets of policy-making processes, organizations become the units of analysis in local or national policy arenas. They may be measured and assessed for their effectiveness in achieving both their strategic and health objectives. This task is best served by empirical organizational indicators, supplemented by information drawn from the perceptions of key organization members.

Stakeholder interests and resource changes are critical factors in policy-making processes. The appropriate unit of analysis becomes the organization, or a subunit of the organization that has sufficient discretion to control decisions over a portion of the operating funds and other resources. Organization-level indicators are needed for policy evaluation. The most important are those that suggest the potential influence and power of organizations, including their:

* mission and specific objectives;
* age, connoting long-term relationships with economic resources and decision-makers;
* governance (for example, appointed or elected board or superior administrative unit);

- source of authority (such as law or community support); and
- size, implying actual or potential influence (for example, size of budget, staff and facilities; stability of funding sources, such as taxes, donations, member fees or sales revenues; and access to expert information, policy-makers and the media).

The impact made by organizations on policies or vice versa is evident from organization-derived measures of before-and-after changes in resource allocation in the administrative or strategic planning structure, the fiscal system and programmes, services or product systems, such as shifts in:

- budget priorities
- sources of financing
- personnel assignments
- clientele or market
- sites, products and services
- information types, uses and technologies.

Changes may also include spin-off effects on other organizations and environments, and public opinion about the organization and the issues it promotes *(44)* (Fig. 16.1).

Dissemination and use of evaluations
Only in recent years have public health workers again become aware of the importance of working more closely with policy-makers and the public to implement their findings in policy arenas *(45)*. Accordingly, the final step in the evaluation process should focus on dissemination: planned ways to convey applicable lessons, working hypotheses or rules of thumb, for the health community.

Findings must be translated into the organizational or political priorities of potential users *(11)*. They may have an influence early in policy development (before interest groups have developed around a substantive policy issue) or very much later (after the social environment has become favourable). Studies may stimulate new ways to conceive policy problems and solutions; more rarely, they may be incorporated into policy development, or simply be applied in an immediate, narrow setting, such as a particular organization, rather than across similar relevant organizations *(46)*.

In the past, the issue of dissemination of findings was discussed in the framework of diffusion studies. Newer forms of this discussion emphasize dissemination processes, implying a more purposeful set of actions *(47)*. Sustained dissemination and use of evaluations requires the commitment of resources for, for example, designated staff, continuing intergroup ties, prior involvement with prospective users, technical assistance or training funds for policy-makers, their aides, the press, relevant community groups or health promotion advocates as potential users.

Evaluation studies rarely include funds for planned dissemination of the policy implications outside professional circles: a disincentive to timely, user-friendly distribution. An exception here is some advocacy groups that employ staff to search for such studies and promote the distribution of their own studies in a variety of formats. Resources for knowledge transfer could support a range of channels, such as debriefing meetings, seminars, customized reports or talking points, public meetings and press conferences.

Conclusions

When the purpose of health promotion policy evaluation is to provide lessons applicable to policy and organizational changes that sustain health, a guiding conceptual framework can support this strategic goal. The policy-making framework illustrated here identifies processes and organizational players, their interests, strategies and effects. No matter what framework evaluators use, operational definitions of conceptual components are needed to guide data collection and methodologies and produce credible results for potential user groups.

Evaluations may be done of one or more phases of policy development, ranging from early initiation of the idea to adoption, implementation, assessment and reformulation, in any jurisdiction or among any set of organizations. Such knowledge can indicate how organizations can most effectively apply what is already known to be capable of promoting health, how they can work intersectorally toward these ends and how they can work in public and organizational policy-making arenas to encourage changes that will promote health.

As an applied field, evaluation studies can usefully include planned dissemination as a part of the process. Involving a wide range of public and private stakeholders in the process of formulating questions and discussing results will improve the timeliness and usefulness of such studies. This approach would answer the calls for practice-relevant research and policy intervention research to determine the conditions for policy successes and failures (48). A number of changes in the bodies that train, develop, fund and communicate evaluations could encourage these new foci: academic institutions, research funding bodies, national and regional departments funding health programmes, and journal publishers.

References

1. MILIO, N. A framework for prevention: changing health damaging to health generating life patterns. *American journal of public health*, **66**: 35–38 (1976).
2. MINKLER, M., ED. *Community organizing and community building for health*. New Brunswick, Rutgers University Press, 1997.
3. HU, T.-W. ET AL. Reducing cigarette consumption in California: tobacco taxes vs an anti-smoking media campaign. *American journal of public health*, **85**(9): 1218–1222 (1995).

4. LINENGER, J. ET AL. Physical fitness gains following simple environmental change. *American journal of preventive medicine*, **7**: 298–310 (1991).
5. PENTZ, M.A. ET AL. The power of policy: the relationship of smoking policy to adolescent smoking. *American journal of public health*, **79**(7): 857–862 (1989).
6. GLANTZ, K. ET AL. Environmental and policy approaches to cardiovascular disease prevention through nutrition: opportunities for state and local action. *Health education quarterly*, **22**(4): 512–527 (1992).
7. SCHMID, T. ET AL. Policy as intervention: environmental and policy approaches to the prevention of cardiovascular disease. *American journal of public health*, **85**(9): 1207–1211 (1995).
8. HEISER, P. & BEGAY, M. Campaign to raise the tobacco tax in Massachusetts. *American journal of public health*, **87**(6): 968–973 (1997).
9. LYNAGH, M. ET AL. School health promotion programs over the past decade: a review of the smoking, alcohol and solar protection literature. *Health promotion international*, **12**(1): 43–60 (1997).
10. MILIO, N. Case studies in nutrition policymaking: how process shapes product. *In*: Garza, B., ed. *Beyond nutrition information*. Ithaca, Cornell University Press, 1997.
11. BREWER, G. & DE LEON, P. *Foundations of policy analysis*. Homewood, IL, Dorsey, 1983.
12. BENJAMIN, K. ET AL. Public policy and the application of outcomes assessments: paradigms vs. politics. *Medical care*, **33**(4): AS299–AS306 (1995).
13. MILIO, N. *Nutrition policy for food-rich countries: a strategic analysis*. Baltimore, Johns Hopkins University Press, 1990.
14. MILIO, N. *Engines of empowerment: using information technology to create healthy communities and challenge public policy*. Chicago, Health Administration Press, 1996.
15. MILIO, N. US policy support for telehealth: organizational response to a new policy environment. *Telemedicine & telecare*, **1**(4): 1–6 (1996).
16. CAMPBELL, H.S. *Impact of scientific data on policy initiation* [Dissertation]. Chapel Hill, School of Public Health, University of North Carolina, 1990.
17. LAUMANN, E. & KNOKE, D. *The organizational state*. Madison, University of Wisconsin Press, 1987.
18. WALLECK, L. Media advocacy. *In*: Minkler, M., ed. *Community organizing and community building*. New Brunswick, Rutgers University Press, 1997, pp. 339–352.
19. CAPPELA, F. & JAMIESON, K. *Media in the middle: coverage of the health care reform debate of 1994*. Philadelphia, Annenberg School of Communication, University of Pennsylvania, 1996.
20. JACOBSON, P. ET AL. Politics of antismoking legislation. *Journal of health policy, policy and law*, **18**: 787–818 (1993).

21. ROCHEFORT, D. & COBB, R. Problem definition, agenda access, and policy choice. *Policy studies journal*, **21**(1): 56–71 (1993).

22. KESSLER, D. ET AL. The Food and Drug Administration's regulation of tobacco products. *New England journal of medicine*, **335**(13): 988–994 (1996).

23. FELDSTEIN, P. *The politics of health legislation. An economic perspective*. Chicago, Health Administration Press, 1996.

24. JASANOFF, S. *The fifth branch: science advisors as policymakers*. Cambridge, Harvard University Press, 1993.

25. GOODMAN, R. ET AL. A critique of contemporary community health promotion approaches: based on a qualitative review of six programs in Maine. *American journal of health promotion*, **7**(3): 208–220 (1993).

26. GOODMAN, R. ET AL. Development of level of institutionalization scales for health promotion programs. *Health education quarterly*, **20**(2): 161–78 (1993).

27. KEGLER, M. *Community coalitions for tobacco control: factors influencing implementation* [Dissertation]. Chapel Hill, School of Public Health, University of North Carolina, 1995.

28. WALKER, J. *Mobilizing interest groups in America: patrons, professions, and social movements*. Ann Arbor, University of Michigan Press, 1991.

29. LINDBLOM, C. & COHEN, D. *Usable knowledge*. New Haven, Yale University Press, 1979.

30. MILIO, N. Making healthy public policy; developing the science by learning the art: an ecological framework for policy studies. *In*: Badura, B. & Kickbusch, I. *Health promotion research: towards a new social epidemiology*. Copenhagen, WHO Regional Office for Europe, 1991 (WHO Regional Publications, European Series, No. 37).

31. *What shapes lawmakers' views? A survey of members of Congress and key staff on health care reform*. Washington, DC, Columbia Institute, 1995.

32. CAPPELA, F. & JAMIESON, K. *Public cynicism and news coverage in campaigns and policy debates: 3 field experiments*. Philadelphia, Annenberg School of Communication, University of Pennsylvania, 1994.

33. EDGAR, T. ET AL. *AIDS: a communication perspective*. Hillsdale, NJ, Lawrence Erlbaum, 1992.

34. MCCOMBS, M. & SHAW, D. The evolution of agenda-setting research. *Journal of communication*, **43**(2): 58–67 (1993).

35. ZERVIGON-HAKES, A.M. Translating research into large-scale public programs and policies. *Future of children*, **5**(3): 175–191 (1995).

36. FORTMANN, S. ET AL. Changes in adult cigarette smoking prevalence after 5 years of community health education: the Stanford Five-City Project. *American journal of epidemiology*, **137**: 1383–1393 (1993).

37. WINKLEBY, M.A. The future of community-based cardiovascular disease intervention studies. *American journal of public health*, **84**(9): 1369–1372 (1994).

38. LUEPKER, R. ET AL. Community education for cardiovascular disease prevention: risk factor changes in the Minnesota Heart Health Program. *American journal of public health*, **84**(9): 1383–1393 (1994).

39. MITTLEMARK, M. ET AL. Realistic outcomes: lessons from community-based research and demonstration programs for the prevention of cardiovascular diseases. *Journal of public health policy,* **14**(4): 437–462 (1993).

40. FISHER, E.B The results of the COMMIT trial. *American journal of public health*, **85**(2): 159–160 (1995).

41. SCHEIRER,M. & REZMOVIC, E. Measuring the degree of implementation: a methodological review. *Evaluation review*, 7: 599–633 (1983).

42. PRESTBY, J. ET AL. Benefits, costs, incentive management and participation in voluntary organizations. *American journal of community psychology*, **18**(1): 117–149 (1990).

43. WEISBROD, R. ET AL. Impact of a community health promotion program on existing organization: the Minnesota heart health program. *Social science and medicine*, **34**(6): 639–648 (1992).

44. CHEADLE, A. ET AL. Environmental indicators: a tool for evaluating community-based health-promotion programs. *American journal of preventive medicine*, **8**: 345–350 (1992).

45. STIVERS, C. The politics of public health: the dilemma of a public profession. *In*: Litman, T. & Robins, S. ed. *Health politics and policy*. Albany, NY, Delmar, 1991, pp. 356–369.

46. BRINT, S. Rethinking the policy influence of experts: from general characterizations to analysis of variation. *Sociological forum*, **5**(3): 361–385 (1990).

47. KING, L. ET AL. *A review of the literature on dissemination and uptake of new information and research related to health promotion and illness prevention activities. Report to the Department of Community Health and Family Services*. Canberra, Commonwealth of Australia, 1995.

48. GENERAL ACCOUNTING OFFICE. *Improving the flow of information to the Congress*. Washington, DC, US Congress, 1995.

17
Evaluation of countrywide health promotion policies: the Canadian experience

Reg Warren, Irving Rootman and Rick Wilson

Introduction

This chapter examines a variety of issues, constraints and complexities inherent in evaluating countrywide health promotion policies. Previous research has done an excellent job of identifying many of the major complexities involved in evaluating large, relatively controlled demonstration projects, such as those of the WHO countrywide integrated noncommunicable disease intervention (CINDI) programme, heart health programmes in the United States and the COMMIT smoking cessation initiative in Canada and the United States *(1–3)*. These problems are heightened considerably in evaluating national policies, of which large-scale demonstration projects constitute only one of many interrelated components.

We present our current approach to the evaluation and monitoring of countrywide health promotion policies, which attempts to address some of these limitations. This approach involves the implementation of dynamic evaluation and monitoring processes, the active participation of programme participants in developing performance indicators, the development of low-cost, targeted and integrated information systems, the implementation of practical, utilization-driven information collection and dissemination procedures, and the establishment of consensus-based assessments of programme performance.

Canada's health promotion programme

In 1978, Canada became one of the first countries in the world to establish a health promotion programme, as a response to a government discussion paper *(4)*. The federal health promotion programme focused heavily on a set of key health issues that were predominantly behavioural in nature, including alcohol, tobacco and drug use, nutrition and safety. It developed and delivered interventions, and supported community programmes linking these issues to a series of target groups, such as children, young people, women and elderly people. Programme delivery often took the form of delivery through key settings, such as homes, schools, workplaces and communities. The programme has been repositioned as a programme for population health in Health Canada.

The need for evaluation was recognized early in the development of this programme, and led to the development of a framework for evaluating it *(5)*. An evaluation of the programme, drawing information from the system that was established on the basis of the framework and from other sources, was conducted in 1989.

Information collection was extensive throughout the life of the health promotion programme. This included relatively detailed monitoring of inputs and expenditure; activities undertaken and outputs produced and/or delivered; a host of evaluation studies on programme delivery and short-term effects (including media tracking studies); in-depth outcome evaluation of selected key projects (such as the peer-assisted smoking prevention project); and a range of national surveys to monitor progress related to the key issues, target groups and settings. In fact, over the period in question, well over Can $10 million was devoted to monitoring and evaluation activities within the Health Promotion Directorate.

Nevertheless, these relatively extensive and proactive information collection activities fell far short of providing definitive evidence about the effectiveness of the federal health promotion programme. Although much information was collected and used as part of the evaluation process, the final evaluation required additional information, such as assessments by key informants and an expert panel, to ascertain programme effectiveness.

The study team for the 1989 evaluation employed:

- a general literature review;
- reviews of project evaluations carried out by the Health Promotion Directorate and of the programme's operations and implementation;
- surveys of 50 key informants (mainly provincial and nongovernmental representatives), 70 experts in the field of health promotion and 100 community groups receiving Health Canada funds and sponsoring health promotion projects; and
- an expert panel of seven people.

Given the relatively large-scale information collection already undertaken, it seems curious that the final evaluation project was forced to rely so heavily on qualitative data and the subjective judgements of partners, stakeholders, grant recipients and the expert panel to derive its final conclusions and recommendations. Some of the reasons for this are described below.

Evaluating Canada's health promotion programme: challenges and barriers

The administrative context

The 1989 evaluation was designed to evaluate the federal, not the national, health promotion programme. It largely focused on outcomes attributable to federal expenditure and related activities. In contrast, the national health promotion programme is the summation of all health promotion activities undertaken at all levels in Canada (federally, provincially and locally); federal activities constitute only one component. Assessing the extent to which federal activities contribute to the goals of the national programme is functionally impossible without evaluating the latter. Attributing results to specific programme components is difficult in view of the large number of intermediaries involved in programme delivery. Unfortunately, no agency has the cross-jurisdictional responsibility for undertaking such an evaluation. Future evaluations should ensure that processes are in place to monitor the larger national programme. This would, of course, require carefully negotiated agreements with partners, stakeholders and programmers.

The Canadian Public Health Association recognized the long-standing need for continuing monitoring of progress towards national health promotion goals in its *Action statement on health promotion (6)*. This document articulates a series of priorities for action that are firmly rooted in and derived from a vision statement and a clearly articulated set of core values. As a final note, the Association articulates its commitment "to working with a variety of organizational and community partners to facilitate action on the ideas presented in this statement and to monitor and report on our progress" *(6)*.

The political context: roles and responsibilities, and shifting priorities

One critical issue in Canada, and possibly in other countries with federal systems, is the importance of regional and local programming in the causal chain for intermediate and long-term outcomes. Constitutional and jurisdictional constraints dictate that programme implementation resides primarily at the provincial and local levels. Consequently, the federal programme was intended to consult with and obtain the agreement of government at other levels on mutual goals and the design of programmes. The attribution of outcomes tends to focus on questions about consultation and strategies, so the contributions of federal efforts to national health promotion objectives (particularly long-term behavioural change) were difficult to assess.

In addition, neither the provinces nor many of the other key players had direct reporting or accountability relationships with the federal Government. This rendered coordinated information collection an excessively complex undertaking. Future evaluations will require carefully negotiated partnerships and protocols for information sharing.

Further, political priorities change constantly, particularly with changes of government, and, more recently, with a renewed emphasis on expenditure reduction. Both affected the health promotion programme and its evaluation. During the course of the programme, a number of major, well funded national strategies were introduced to tackle alcohol and drug abuse, tobacco control, driving under the influence of alcohol or drugs, and child and family health, while cuts in expenditure continued to reduce the resources available to ad-

389

dress other issues. As a consequence, the emphasis of the programme changed markedly between the initial design and the evaluation. This raised a number of fundamental questions. In particular, should the indicators of accomplishment be based upon the programme as it was initially designed and implemented or as it had evolved? In this context, evaluation appears to need to evolve a more dynamic set of methods and procedures to reflect changes in the programme.

The socioeconomic context

As in much of the western industrialized world, the period covered by the national evaluation saw continued growth in percaput incomes and education levels in Canada, as well as important demographic shifts. Canada experienced some extremely positive shifts in relation to key health promotion outcomes (such as tobacco use, driving under the influence of alcohol or drugs and physical inactivity). Several other countries with rising education and income levels, however, also showed such progress. The initial evaluation design made no provision for incorporating the broader determinants of health into the information collection processes. As a result, it could not ascertain whether any desirable changes resulted from the programme or from broader socioeconomic and demographic changes. Comparisons with other countries have been made from time to time, but there is little logical or rational justification for using other countries as control groups, given their vast cultural, historical, sociopolitical and other differences.

Evolution of health promotion

From the start of the programme (1978) to its evaluation (1989), the field of health promotion evolved considerably. Several key events had a major influence on the evolution of the programme. These included the government paper on achieving health for all (7), the adoption of the Ottawa Charter for Health Promotion (8) and the WHO conference on healthy public policy (9). By 1989, the health promotion programme had evolved dramatically, to keep pace with current thinking in the field.

Differing resources and capacities

The resources and capacities to implement sophisticated evaluation studies or even rudimentary, continuing data collection vary dramatically between provinces and within communities. Within that context, the demand for evaluation studies and the burden of supplying information on a continuing basis must often compete with the demands of programme delivery. Resources are often devoted to monitoring and evaluation at the expense of enhanced programme delivery (opportunity cost). Consequently, information collection at the local level must often take a lowest-common-denominator approach, which is sensitive to the resource constraints of the least well equipped partner.

Data collected by communities often comprise narrative descriptions of events or processes. If data are provided or available, analytical capacity is

390

limited at best. Communities and, for that matter, voluntary NGOs or others rarely have the resources required to implement textbook evaluations. Impact evaluation studies at all levels are not usually available, or are available only for selected interventions.

Nevertheless, information generated from the continuing evaluation of specific health promotion projects remains the single most important input into monitoring and evaluation of a health promotion programme. Such information provides the critical linkage that allows the mapping and attribution of the contribution of programme activities (projects) to goal attainment. Much greater effort must therefore be devoted to enhancing community capacities in these areas if future monitoring and evaluation efforts are to succeed.

Coordination and integration
Information was collected at the federal, provincial and local levels, but there were little coordination across jurisdictional boundaries and little vertical flow of information. Administrators routinely collected considerable amounts of information on programme inputs, activities and outputs. These efforts are usually designed to meet administrative requirements; rarely are they sensitive to the need for such information as an input to programme monitoring and evaluation. Although programmes were often developed using a partnership approach, information flows tended to reflect the accountability requirements at each level of the system, rather than an organized, collaborative and comprehensive undertaking.

In addition, horizontal coordination and integration between researchers, programmers, policy-makers and administrators seemed to be lacking. The research conducted rarely addressed needs for national monitoring and evaluation information. For example, at one time four different national surveys and several provincial and local surveys were measuring smoking behaviour. Each employed different research designs and methodologies, and asked questions on smoking behaviour that were not comparable either between studies or over time. To be sure, the principal intent of these surveys was not to monitor or evaluate the tobacco component of the health promotion programme; with greater horizontal coordination and integration, however, these surveys could have made a much greater contribution in that regard.

Lack of control conditions
For a wide range of legal, administrative, technical and conceptual reasons, the lack of suitable control groups frequently hinders the evaluation of national programmes. Even when some semblance of control is feasible, it is difficult to protect against contamination resulting from the rapid movement and flow of ideas, information and people in modern societies. Even if some semblance of control of aspects of information could be introduced, national policy measures must of necessity be inclusive and comprehensive.

This lack of controls necessitated reliance upon key informants' judgements and expert panels to set standards for programme performance. While

391

such evaluation criteria are useful, their value and their legitimacy would be much greater if they were established at the outset of the process (rather than afterwards) and based on programme participants' consensus on what constitutes acceptable performance.

Timeliness
By the completion of the evaluation in 1989, the federal health promotion programme had changed so fundamentally that many of the results of the evaluation were irrelevant to the programme as it had evolved. The continuing provision of information on the programme must constitute a central element of future evaluations.

Seeking convergence from multiple sources
Over the course of ten years of activities evaluating the health promotion programme, a massive database was assembled. This included background theoretical and applied literature reviews relating to best practice; needs assessments and feasibility studies; administrative records relating to expenditure, inputs and outputs; studies of programme implementation, delivery and receipt; studies of the long- and short-term effects of specific projects or programme components (such as media campaigns); and a range of national surveys. Each of these information streams provided key aspects of the information required to inform judgements about the effectiveness of the programme, but also had important limitations that rendered it less than satisfactory. Thus, the final assessments of programme effectiveness were assigned to a panel of experts whose task was to review the body of evidence, and to seek convergence through triangulation.

The key lesson from this experience is that no single study or set of studies is likely to provide a sufficient basis for assessing the effectiveness of health promotion activities. Different research approaches are required, each of which provides different types of information characterized by strengths and limitations endemic to studies of that genre. Ultimately, different genres have complementary strengths and weaknesses. The triangulation of information sets reduces the level of uncertainty in judgements of programme effectiveness.

This is not unusual. To cite a specific example, there appears to be a reasoned consensus that some progress has been made to reduce deaths in Canada due to driving under the influence of alcohol or drugs. This did not result from a single study or genre of scientific inquiry, but from a multiplicity of studies using convergent methodologies and approaches, including: clinical research, driver simulations, a host of evaluation studies of specific initiatives (including behavioural and policy interventions), assessment of the experience of multiple jurisdictions, studies in real-world settings (including hospitals and crash sites), studies in psychopharmacology, toxicology and forensic sciences, and a wide range of surveys, longitudinal databases and related information sets.

392

Indeed, one can argue that many of the verdicts on the effectiveness of health promotion interventions have been based on consensus judgements arising from the triangulation of broad and disparate, but potentially complementary information sources, using a wide array of approaches, techniques and methodologies.

The Canadian experience: lessons learned

Our experience in evaluating Canada's health promotion programme has provided a number of lessons applicable to the evaluation of other countrywide health promotion initiatives. For example, such evaluations should:

- establish a robust information base, using a wide range of methodologies and approaches, as a basis for reducing uncertainties about the effectiveness of health promotion projects and programmes;
- take account of the political and sociocultural context within which large-scale health promotion programmes are implemented and evolve;
- develop partnerships to overcome administrative and jurisdictional barriers to the flow of information;
- develop dynamic procedures that are capable of monitoring and evaluating an evolving programme on a continuing basis;
- develop user-driven approaches to evaluation and in particular involve partners, stakeholders and other potential users at all stages of the process, especially in developing, adapting and reporting on performance indicators; and
- develop and nurture programme evaluation and monitoring capacities within various nodes of the programme delivery infrastructure.

In addition, there are needs for:

- greater coordination and integration of existing information systems for both collection and dissemination;
- more cost-effective use of research funds, through greater coordination, integration and involvement of stakeholders and other users;
- more timely access to relevant data on programme performance on a continuing basis;
- more utilization-driven approaches to the collection, analysis and dissemination of information about the programme; and
- stronger mechanisms to judge programme effectiveness, on the basis of triangulation of multiple information sets.

Many of these needs are intrinsic to the evaluation of health promotion programmes in real-world settings. Taken together, they indicate that a definitive evaluation of the effectiveness of health promotion programmes (conforming to classical evaluation research methods, techniques and criteria) seems unlikely (see chapters 1–3). Much of the evidence on effectiveness may have to be accumulated through triangulation. Key questions arise, however, about what information is needed, who should participate in such processes and how such judgements should be rendered in order to minimize uncertainty and to enhance credibility and perceived legitimacy.

The next section describes one approach to the generation of consensus-based judgements of programme efficacy. We illustrate this approach with examples drawn from the monitoring and evaluation of the Ontario Tobacco Strategy. An annual monitoring report produced by the Ontario Tobacco Research Unit *(10)* gives a relatively concise description of one application of this monitoring and evaluation process and its related outputs, and we use it to provide some practical examples of our approach.

Applying the lessons learned

The approach that we have adopted for monitoring health promotion programmes in Ontario is predicated on partnership with and full participation by stakeholders. The methodology is a hybrid of management science, systems analysis and evaluation research concepts, methods and techniques. It focuses on goal attainment, implementation and the consolidation and communication of available information from a wide variety of sources to produce an accurate assessment of outcomes at all levels, on a continuing basis and in a timely manner. It emphasizes consultation and partnerships with participants in identifying key indicators and providing relevant information. A unique aspect of the approach is that it is neither top down nor bottom up, but collaborative, participatory and voluntary.

The process draws heavily on the coordination and integration of information from a wide variety of sources. Massive amounts of information are already generated routinely, including administrative records; records of outputs produced, disseminated and received; formative, process and intermediate evaluation studies; periodic, in-depth, long-term outcome evaluations; demonstration projects with related evaluations; and a host of special studies, surveys and corollary information sets. Such information would appear to provide the ideal basis for the development of an inexpensive yet effective monitoring and evaluation system. We are attempting to coordinate, integrate and rationalize the various sources in the hope of eliminating redundant collection efforts, consolidating information from a wide variety of sources and making it readily available to a broad spectrum of users in a timely and cost-effective manner. This approach seeks to capitalize on the information already collected, to coordinate and integrate collection systems and to supplement them with information from special studies and corollary information collection systems. The approach reflects a number of key strategies:

1. implementing a user-driven approach
2. obtaining agreement on basic operating principles

3. building and nurturing partnerships
4. forging consensus on programme activities, outputs and intended effects
5. establishing criteria for accountability
6. involving users in the collection and interpretation of information
7. producing an annual monitoring report
8. disseminating and using the information
9. making a commitment to continuing improvement.

A user-driven approach

The general approach that we have used to monitor health promotion programming in Ontario is user driven. It proceeds from the notion that participants and users at all levels (administrators, policy-makers, programme designers and staff, and community practitioners) should be directly involved at all stages of the process. As such, the general approach draws heavily upon participatory action research *(11)* (see Chapter 4), transposing it from a local-level to a large-scale general monitoring and evaluation model, and using information not just for these purposes but also as an input into environmental scanning, strategic planning and programme development. Emphasis must be placed on determining what information users need. The information needs of a policy-maker who is attempting to decide whether to invest in health promotion may differ widely from those of a community programme staff person who is dealing with a pressing local health promotion issue, a programme administrator who must justify resource allocation decisions or a journalist who wishes to provide information to the general public.

The community of partners should influence decisions on all aspects of information collection and dissemination, including:

- what research is funded (through determining how research outputs are packaged);
- how availability is promoted; and
- how information is distributed, disseminated and used.

In particular, users must be directly involved in any discussion of accountability, including how standards are set, what performance indicators are meaningful and appropriate, and how the resulting information will be collected, analysed, interpreted and disseminated.

Agreement on basic operating principles

A series of operating principles has been integrated into the monitoring and evaluation methodology:

- ensuring that information is collected and communicated in a manner that is sensitive and responsive to the needs, requirements and values of a diversity of stakeholders;

- identifying core information requirements, with emphasis on collecting information not available from any other source;
- rationalizing existing information collection to minimize the response burden;
- ensuring the information is meaningful and useful at the local and provincial levels;
- ensuring the integration of existing information sources (to eliminate redundancy in data collection);
- enhancing the capacity of partners to participate in the monitoring and evaluation process; and
- identifying key information gaps and stimulating targeted research projects and evaluation studies to fill them.

Partnerships

Mechanisms are needed to promote and to nurture partnerships between researchers, programmer designers and staff, administrators, policy-makers, practitioners, communication specialists and user communities. The main features of this approach are:

- establishing and following the information collection principles identified above;
- clearly identifying information needs in close collaboration with programme participants;
- integrating with existing information sources;
- focusing new research on filling gaps left by existing information systems;
- ensuring the involvement of information users at all stages of the process;
- minimizing response burdens in the information collection process; and
- forming partnerships for collecting information and developing evaluation and monitoring frameworks.

Consensus on programme activities, outputs and intended effects

Users are involved in identifying the key components of the programme, including activities, outputs and expected effects. This enables all programme stakeholders to agree on the overall goals of the programme, and to situate their specific activities within it. Typically, this involves:

- developing a monitoring and evaluation framework in close consultation with stakeholders, users and participants (including narrative descriptions of objectives, activities, outputs, desired effects and indicators);
- defining all aspects of the programme through the use of logic models or a similar mapping procedure; and
- consulting and building consensus on the framework and/or logic model as an accurate description of programme operations.

Criteria for accountability

Stakeholders and practitioners are directly involved in building consensus on programme performance and accountability requirements. In that sense, the participants themselves decide the evaluation criteria against which their activities and those of the programme as a whole will be measured. They also are directly involved in deciding how, by whom, how often, in what formats and to whom this information will be collected and reported. This typically involves four tasks.

The first is standardizing information collection processes around identified needs and indicators. Those involved define and agree on these needs and indicators during the consultations on the monitoring framework and the logic model, and during independent consultation on standards for accountability. Second, they map current monitoring-related information collection, including what is being collected, by whom and in what formats.

Third is negotiating continuing arrangements for information collection and sharing. This focuses on ensuring the provision of needed raw data from existing and modified organizational or project information systems. Where feasible, this process seeks to coordinate the requirements for continuing administrative reporting with those for programme evaluation and monitoring to minimize the response burden. It also includes identifying evaluation studies required, completed or in progress, as well as appropriate data sources for secondary analysis and the procedures for obtaining access to them.

Fourth, specific evaluation research projects, monitoring surveys and special studies are conducted to address information needs identified in the framework and not suitably addressed by existing sources and systems. External funding and researchers are mobilized to reduce these information gaps.

Involving users in information collection and interpretation

Stakeholders are directly involved in interpreting the diverse sources of information, with special emphasis on the information sets most familiar to them, whether these be administrative records, evaluation studies, special studies, surveys or other sources. The participation of a variety of stakeholders with a broad range of expertise aids greatly in the triangulation of information from these multiple data sets, and gives further credibility and legitimacy to the inferences made. It further ensures that any assessment of effectiveness takes account of a rich diversity of perspectives.

Annual monitoring report

Stakeholders are directly involved in all stages of the production of an annual monitoring report on the programme. This and appropriate summary reports are produced to assist programme implementation and planning. They also provide an objective and agreed-on measure of progress. Mandatory cyclical evaluation reports are completed using all available information resulting from this process. To be sure, a host of other monitoring and evaluation publications are produced that focus on individual projects, components, strategies or goals.

These special reports provide the information base for the comprehensive annual report on the programme.

Users are involved in deciding what key issues and questions the monitoring reports are to address, providing data on their activities, interpreting the results of convergent sets of information on the collective effects of the programme, assessing the implications of these findings and making recommendations for further action. Thus, the stakeholders constitute not only an integral part of report production but also a key element of peer review. This lends not only credibility and legitimacy to the report but also commitment to follow up any recommendations. Typically, an annual monitoring report addresses at least the following sets of topics and issues, for both the programme as a whole and the projects or activities that comprise it:

1. what the project/programme is attempting to do (goals and objectives);
2. what key activities have been undertaken to date (activities, resources and functions);
3. what outputs and/or products have been produced (outputs);
4. how they have been used, by whom, etc. (receipt of intervention);
5. what effects have been obtained;
6. whether there has been progress towards the stated goals (goal attainment), and what sources of evidence are used to determine this; and
7. what has been the specific contribution of individual projects, components and/or strategies to the attainment of the programme' objectives, and what sources of evidence are used to determine this.

Disseminating and using the information

A chronic problem in health promotion is a lack of clear evidence of programme effectiveness. This is not surprising, given the barriers to conclusive evaluation outlined above. In the absence of conclusive evidence of effectiveness, the key requirement becomes the accumulation of evidence (ideally through triangulation from several independent sources). Fortunately, considerable evidence of this type is available. The long-term viability of health promotion, however, depends not only on evidence of its effectiveness but also on who has access to this information and the extent to which it meets their standards for acceptable performance. Accordingly, the requirements of decision-makers must play an important role in the establishment of evaluation and monitoring criteria, and this information must be communicated to them and other stakeholders as rapidly as it becomes available, and in a manner consistent with and responsive to their needs, expectations and values.

As such, stakeholders participate directly in the dissemination and utilization of the results of the annual monitoring report in two important ways. First, as key intermediaries, they disseminate the results to constituent or client groups, either directly or through repackaging the information in a manner that suits the needs of their audiences. Client groups include programme planners, managers and participants; administrators; community groups; local councils;

the media; health ministers and/or other decision-makers; and the general public.

Second, as key users, stakeholders use the information to change and improve the programme. The types of uses range from environmental scanning and strategic planning; programme planning, modification and design; accountability and justification processes; and organizational review to the generation of political and public support for continued health promotion activities as a central element of public policy.

Continuing improvement
All participants have a commitment to the continuous improvement of the quality, quantity, timeliness and relevance of the information produced as a result of the collective monitoring effort. Thus, on an annual basis, they make explicit efforts to enhance the information base referable to programme monitoring. Since this is a voluntary process from which participants stand to benefit, initial resistance to participation has dissipated considerably; users have actively suggested improvements to the product and the process.

Towards implementation: the Ontario Tobacco Strategy
The Ontario Tobacco Strategy is a comprehensive province-wide programme focusing on smoking prevention and cessation and the protection of the public from environmental tobacco smoke. Key components include: interministerial coordination; legislation; public information, awareness and education; community programmes; resource centres; and research. The implementation of the Strategy has required eight steps. The first was creating an independent, arm's-length agency to monitor and to report on programme performance. Recognizing this need, the designers of the Strategy created the Ontario Tobacco Research Unit. The agency funding such strategies requires independent monitoring, and continuing brokerage between the competing interests of various groups and partners.

Second, a wide range of stakeholders was involved in establishing the goals, objectives, key components and activity structures for the Strategy. This process produced clear consensus on and broad acceptance of the key aspects of the Strategy. Third, stakeholders also took part in establishing accountability standards and procedures for the Strategy as a whole and particularly aspects for which key stakeholder groups have accepted responsibility. As a result, the rate of participation in providing information referable to these standards of accountability has been extremely high.

Researchers and Strategy participants took the next three steps in partnership. They strengthened participants' capacities for information collection by working with stakeholders to identify core information needs, identifying and rationalizing existing collection efforts to reduce the response burden and strengthening skills. In many instances this has resulted in both a net reduction of the response burden and an extremely high rate of reporting, accompanied by continuing efforts to improve the quality of the information generated.

Next, they identified key information gaps, and focused resources on filling them. This has involved working with stakeholders to identify information requirements not currently met through existing information collection systems, and encouraging special studies and/or the establishment of appropriate data systems to address these needs.

Then they involved users in the collection and interpretation of the information. The assessment of programme effectiveness inevitably involves the triangulation and synthesis of a wide range of information sources. Involving the generators of information in its interpretation brings a broad array of expertise and experience to the process. This diversity of expertise is required to ensure serious consideration of alternative interpretations of the information from these sources. It lends credibility and legitimacy to subsequent interpretations, since these judgements reflect a consensus of the community of stakeholders.

The seventh step is producing, disseminating and using the results. This is accomplished in several ways, including: integrating the results into strategic planning processes, continuing the assessment of the Strategy's goals and activities, strengthening these activities by focusing attention on emerging needs, communicating with policy-makers through internal and external processes, and communicating through the media or other intermediaries with the broader community.

Eighth, in the same fashion that stakeholders agreed to standards of accountability, a team conducts regular evaluations of the monitoring processes and outputs to solicit advice on prospective improvements in the system. This ensures that the monitoring and evaluation system is accountable to partners and stakeholders.

Limitations of the process

This approach, like all others, has a number of limitations that must be considered. These include: voluntarism, self-report, so-called resistance to negative findings and, most important in our experience, issues of power and control. A reliance on voluntarism can cause problems for a number of reasons. Most partners and stakeholders already have a variety of reporting requirements and are reluctant to agree to further information collection demands. We have attempted to address this through the fourth step in Strategy implementation. Since the inception of the Strategy, both the quality and quantity of voluntarily provided information have continued to increase.

The obvious human tendency to focus upon positive results may raise problems with the reliance on self-report. This has been overcome in large measure by the agreements on accountability standards and reporting requirements. In addition, most Strategy partners carry out externally funded evaluations, and are accountable to their own advisory committees, boards, institutions and funding agencies. The clarification and streamlining of these accountability requirements has resulted in high rates of open participation.

While there is always resistance to negative findings, the involvement of a broad array of stakeholders and partners in the interpretation and triangulation of results ensures that the reports on the project reflect the diversity of viewpoints and expertise. Again, the objective is not to render unassailable judgements on effectiveness, but to reflect the diversity of community viewpoints and alternative explanations of the results. Thus, there may well be a community consensus that the programme is effective; equally plausible, however, would be a community consensus that such judgements are premature and further research is required.

Issues of power and control continue to be extremely multifaceted and complex, and one of the major barriers to monitoring. At the root of these issues, however, lies a fundamental debate on the identity and thus the methods of the final arbiters of the effectiveness of health promotion interventions. Should they be expert researchers, using criteria set outside the programme, or should they be the people involved in programme delivery, whose intended effects may be more difficult to measure quantitatively, and may need to be supplemented at least in part by qualitative research, administrative data sets and other data? While such tensions and debates can have benefits, their resolution is essential to any discussion of the fundamental issue of the effectiveness of health promotion interventions. In that regard, the advantages and limitations of an arm's-length research agency must inevitably be counterbalanced by some semblance of community control and involvement.

Conclusions

Our review of the 1989 evaluation of the Canadian federal health promotion programme and the application of lessons learned in the development of participatory monitoring and evaluation approaches in Ontario lead us to the following conclusions.

Health promotion evaluation requires the recognition of the need to emphasize the continuous collection of consistent and relevant information on programme performance to satisfy the information needs of a diverse group of stakeholders on a continuing basis and in a timely manner. The identification of these information needs and the concomitant early identification and integration of existing information collection and research processes in the design of an evaluation and monitoring system are essential to ensuring satisfactory outcomes. The emphasis is placed on consolidating and organizing all information collection activities at the start of the programme, with provision for continuing adaptation and continuous quality improvement.

The evaluation of countrywide health promotion programmes is a complex undertaking. Traditional approaches are expensive and have a low probability for success, unless complemented by a broad array of information sources, derived using a broad array of methodologies and approaches. The approach outlined here offers a new, cost-effective way to organize information and provide continuous monitoring data to assist programme planning, implementation and modification.

The continuing utilization of all existing information and research should be adopted as a prerequisite for the monitoring and evaluation of large-scale health promotion programmes. Detailed, specialized collection processes and extensive experimental processes remain useful in the evaluation of individual projects, strategies and/or specialized model projects and demonstrations. Thus, these studies remain an important contribution to the monitoring and evaluation of health promotion programmes, but other sources remain equally important and useful, including administrative records, records of outputs produced, disseminated and received, secondary data sources, large-scale and/or local health surveys, and special studies. They are most powerful and have great appeal to an extremely broad constituency when they are used in a complementary fashion.

Information on the expenditure of public resources, including what outputs were produced and disseminated, who received and benefited from them and how, and demonstrable evidence of value for money must be delivered to stakeholders and programme sponsors on a continuing and timely basis. In particular, the continuing provision of information on progress towards objectives (purportedly the prerequisite for continued funding) and the efficiency and effectiveness of implementation processes is now essential to the survival of health promotion programmes.

To the degree feasible, conclusions on programme effectiveness must be based on a broad array of information sets, considered within an equally broad context of community participation, including researchers, practitioners, stakeholders, partners, funding agencies and affected communities. To the degree feasible, these conclusions should reflect a consensus of the community (or the lack of it).

The new environment of economic constraint and political (public) accountability demands that evaluation itself become increasingly cost-effective. It seems reasonable to assume that demands to maximize the return on public investment in information collection, research and evaluation related to health promotion will continually increase.

References

1. NÜSSEL, E. &LEPARKSKI, E. CINDI. *Countrywide integrated noncommunicable disease intervention programme. Protocol and guidelines for monitoring and evaluation procedures.* Berlin, Springer, 1987.
2. MITTELMARK, M.B. ET AL. Realistic outcomes: lessons from community-based research and demonstration programs for the prevention of cardiovascular diseases. *Journal of public health policy*, **14**: 437–462 (1993).

3.   COMMIT RESEARCH GROUP. Community intervention trial for smoking cessation (COMMIT). I. Cohort results from a four-year community intervention. *American journal of public health*, **85**: 183–192 (1995).

4.   LALONDE, M. *A new perspective on the health of Canadians: a working document.* Ottawa, Canada Information, 1974.

5.   ROOTMAN, I. Developing a system for evaluating a national health promotion programme. *Health promotion*, **3**(1): 101–110 (1988).

6.   *Action statement on health promotion.* Ottawa, Canadian Public Health Association, 1996.

7.   EPP, J. *Achieving health for all: a framework for health promotion.* Ottawa, Health Canada, 1986.

8.   Ottawa Charter for Health Promotion. *Health promotion*, **1**(4): iii–v (1986).

9.   KICKBUSCH, I. ET AL. *Healthy public policy. Report on the Adelaide Conference. 2nd International Conference on Health Promotion, April 5–9, 1988, Adelaide, Australia.* Copenhagen, WHO Regional Office for Europe, 1988.

10. ONTARIO TOBACCO RESEARCH UNIT. *Monitoring the Ontario Tobacco Strategy: progress toward our goals: 1995/1996.* Toronto, Ontario Ministry of Health, 1996.

11. GREEN, L.W. ET AL. *Study of participatory research in health promotion. Review and recommendations for the development of participatory research in health promotion in Canada.* Ottawa, Royal Society of Canada, 1995.

18
Health impact assessment as a tool for health promotion and population health

C. James Frankish, Lawrence W. Green, Pamela A. Ratner,
Treena Chomik and Craig Larsen

Introduction

Government activities, policies and programmes seek to solve public problems and to serve the public good. With intractable debt and budgetary deficits, the public, perhaps more than ever, demands accountability and wants to know that policies and programmes fulfil their objectives. Such evaluation is not easy, however, when the relevant outcomes may result from numerous factors (related or unrelated to government activity) and the relevant programmes and policies may amass numerous outcomes, some undesired or unintended.

Pal *(1)* identifies four concepts of policy impact that may be included in an evaluation: direct, economic, social and political. A policy can be examined in relation to its intended target, the balance between its costs and benefits, its effect on the texture of social life and the government's political interests (re-election chances). These four concepts have underpinned most policy analysis debates.

Health advocates have recognized relatively recently that conventional policy analyses and evaluations have disregarded or neglected the impact of government policies on the population's health. The Ottawa Charter for Health Promotion *(2)* urges that the health of a population should be of concern to all policy-makers; regardless of their sector, they should be aware of the health consequences of their decisions. Saying this, however, is the easy part. The challenges are to determine how to realize this goal and then to do it. What procedures or methods must be in place to judge a policy or programme in the health sector for the effect(s) it may have on the population's health status?

There was a time when public health could easily track the impact of its programmes or its neglect of programmes. Systems for reporting communicable diseases and monitoring outbreaks provided a warning whenever a controlled disease threatened to become uncontrolled. The short incubation period

405

between infection and symptoms meant that cases could be traced quickly back to the probable source of infection, which could then be controlled.

Today's focus on population health is complicated by the facts of multicausality and long latency periods (sometimes decades) between the causes, sources or determinants of health and their effects. Health impact today becomes a matter of tracing single diseases, disabilities or deaths back to genetic factors, past or present living conditions or early environmental exposure. A further complication is that most of the leading causes of disease, disability and death are no longer discretely detected at a point in time. Chronic and degenerative diseases creep up on individuals and populations over long periods. They are not detectable or isolatable as outbreaks.

Criteria for the evaluation of health, social, environmental and economic policies and programmes are changing. This is particularly true in the health sector, as many governments are adopting an understanding of health that includes a focus on social and environmental determinants and the quality of life. They recognize that societal structures, attitudes and behaviour influence health profoundly, and that prevention is both better (or at least more timely) than cure and a way to reduce disability and social dependence. Consequently, how social, environmental and economic policies influence health and the prevention or production of ill health needs systematic monitoring at all levels of government.

Collins (3) noted that the mood for reform had enveloped the health sector in Canada; this was coupled with considerable interest in shifting emphasis from health care to disease prevention and health promotion, to address the determinants of health and illness (4). Collins (3) argued that health reform, in the absence of an explicit conceptual model of health, can focus only on parts of the problem, with little overall benefit. Further, models of health, without an explicit supporting text detailing their implications for policy, can be misunderstood and misused. In today's climate of fiscal restraint, they may be used to justify cutting costs.

Increasing official commitment to decentralization and community participation in decision-making and growing consideration of the social determinants of health leave some ambiguity and perhaps controversy about what impact on health this new perspective will have, what strategies will work to achieve beneficial outcomes, what criteria should be applied to judge health impact, how health impact assessment (HIA) can work to produce better decisions and what its ultimate influence on policies and programme decisions may be. Most calls for evidence-based decision-making offer little indication of how the use of HIA can lead to better health decisions. Without tools and methods to assess the health impact of policies and programmes, these questions cannot be answered, and health impact cannot be known. Developing healthy public policy requires concrete activities, particularly those that address the development of tools for HIA.

This chapter is based on a report for the Canadian Government (5) on a situational analysis of HIA strategies for public policy development and population health promotion in the 1990s. The overall objective was to report on the status of HIA, internationally, nationally, provincially and locally. We use regional, local and national examples of health impact assessment from Canada and other countries to identify key issues and challenges in undertaking HIAs.

This chapter defines key concepts and terms, considers the historical context of HIA and reviews current approaches to related forms of impact assessment, emphasizing the situation in Canada. This review leads to consideration of conceptual, methodological and analytic issues related to the measurement of the impact of public policy. Finally, we discuss the development of health objectives, goals and targets as a key strategy for HIA.

Key concepts and terms

The topic must be clear before debate can begin. Issues of definition are essential for the conceptual domains of health, health promotion, healthy public policy and HIA. The definitions and scope of these terms determine what constitutes challenges to human health and what solutions ought to be sought.

Health

Consistent with the work of Rootman & Raeburn (6), we define health from a health promotion perspective. That is, health is a multidimensional concept that goes far beyond the mere absence of disease or the effects of lifestyle and behaviour. It involves subjective and objective components, and environmental and policy components, as well as those that related to the individual, and must be assessed in qualitative as well as quantitative terms. Rootman & Raeburn (6) offer the following definition:

> Health ... has to do with the bodily, mental, and social quality of life of people as determined in particular by psychological, societal, cultural, and policy dimensions. Health is ... to be enhanced by sensible lifestyles and the equitable use of public and private resources to permit people to use their initiative individually and collectively to maintain and improve their own well-being, however they may define it.

More succinctly and specifically, we define health as the capacity of people to adapt to, respond to or control life's challenges and changes.

Our definition may seem considerably narrower than those in some health promotion documents, official and unofficial. For example, many rely on the WHO definition: "Health is a state of complete physical, mental and social well-being and not merely the absence of disease or infirmity" (7) or tautological definitions similar to that used by O'Donnell (8): "Optimal health ... [is] a balance of physical, emotional, social, spiritual and intellectual health".

Such definitions have been judged to be too idealistic at best, and inoperable, impractical and unattainable at worst. They tend to obfuscate distinctions between health and social development, conceptualize virtually all human activity as health related and associate all human and social values with health *(9–11)*. They place no boundaries on the health field and what it contains. Other sectors may interpret this as a form of professional imperialism or, at best, expansionism by the health sector. With no parameters for health planning, policy, expenditure, practice or science, the health field and therefore its expenditure are unbounded *(6,12)*.

Other definitions of health that encompass the determinants of health – such as education, income or lifestyle – mix cause and effect, making it difficult to use that concept of health as a dependent or outcome variable in HIA. This confounds health with its determinants and makes it immeasurable as the outcome of those determinants. Authorities that choose to use a broader or narrower definition of health will need to adjust their approach to HIA accordingly.

Quality of life

We make important distinctions between the quality of life and health. While discussions of wellness, wellbeing and the multidimensionality of health, including intellectual, spiritual and social pursuits, are more closely related to matters of quality of life, we view health as one of its many determinants (see Chapter 6). That is, health is an instrumental value rather than an end in itself *(13)*. As stated in the Ottawa Charter *(2)*: "Health is … seen as a resource for everyday life, not the objective of living". We agree that health is a resource for achieving an acceptable quality of life, but for HIA the concepts must be held apart.

Health impact versus health outcome

A distinction must be made between impact and outcome. The methods (and indicators) one would employ in an HIA depend on whether one is truly interested in impact, rather than outcome. A dictionary *(14)* defines *impact* as "an effect or influence, esp. when strong" and *outcome* as "a result", making the two terms indistinguishable. As Green & Kreuter *(13)* point out, however, usage varies among disciplines and professions; that of people in the health field is diametrically opposed to that of people conducting evaluations in other fields.

Impact, then, refers in the health field to the immediate effect of a health programme, process or policy, while outcome refers to the distant or ultimate effect. This issue becomes important when one realizes that those who coined the term *HIA* borrowed from the field of environmental impact assessment without acknowledging that the latter defines impact differently than the health field. We conform to current practice by using the term with the understanding that the impacts to which we refer are usually thought of as health outcomes.

Healthy public policy

Evans & Stoddard *(15)* criticize the WHO definition of health on the grounds that it is "difficult to use as the basis for health policy, because implicitly it includes *all* policy as health policy". For many proponents of health promotion, however, this seems to be precisely the point. Trevor Hancock *(16–18)*, a well known Canadian public health physician, coined the term *healthy public policy*

to describe policy enacted by the various levels of government that is characterized by explicit concern for health and equity, and by accountability for
health impact *(19–21)*. If equity is to be accommodated in HIA as an objective
of health policy, it must be seen as equity in health, or reductions in health gaps
between social groups, not the reduction of other inequities that cause or result
from health problems.

HIA

We define HIA as any combination of procedures or methods by which a proposed policy or programme may be judged as to the effect(s) it may have on
the health of a population.

Policies or programmes of any nature may affect the health of a population
directly or indirectly by altering, influencing or affecting the determinants of
health, and consequently will affect the quality of life. Fig. 18.1 shows these
relationships. We acknowledge that the health impacts of such policies or
programmes are only one of the many consequent effects. Such policies or
programmes may also be found to have economic, social or environmental impacts (Fig. 18.2).

Fig. 18.1. Influences of policies and programmes on health

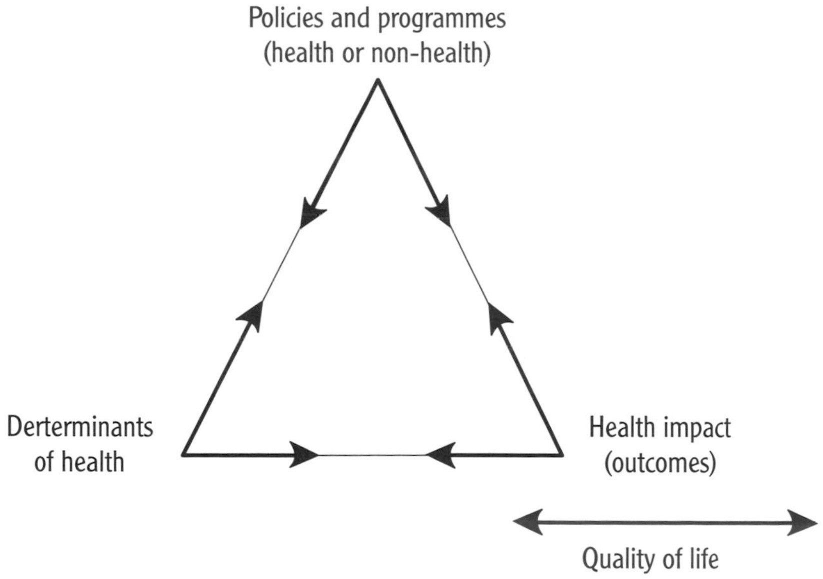

Source: Frankish, J. et al. *Health impact assessment as a tool for population health promotion and
public policy. A report submitted to the Health Promotion Development Division of Health Canada*
(http://www.hc-sc.gc.ca/hppb/healthpromotiondevelopment/pube/impact/impact.htm).
Ottawa, Health Canada, 1996 (accessed 21 February 2001). © Minister of Public Works and
Government Services Canada, 2001.

Fig. 18.2. Potential impact of policies and programmes

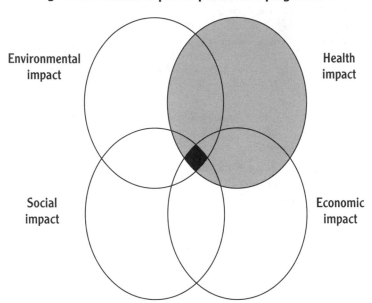

Source: Frankish, J. et al. *Health impact assessment as a tool for population health promotion and public policy. A report submitted to the Health Promotion Development Division of Health Canada* (http://www.hc-sc.gc.ca/hppb/healthpromotiondevelopment/pube/impact/impact.htm). Ottawa, Health Canada, 1996 (accessed 21 February 2001). © Minister of Public Works and Government Services Canada, 2001.

We limit our approach to HIA to the study of the outcomes that can be shown to be of a health nature, as defined above. In recognizing the complexity and potentially far-reaching effects of many policies and programmes, however, we note that, where such activities may potentially have impact beyond the health field, desirable assessments would involve intersectoral cooperation and collaboration.

We also limit our treatment of HIA to considerations of population health. Many policies and programmes potentially affect the delivery of health care services. Assessments of these may require indicators of, for example, medical, surgical and nursing outcome, quality assurance and service utilization. We have not included such considerations in our discussion of HIA.

Historical context
Healthy public policy
In its earliest manifestations, *healthy public policy* served as the heading for target 13 of the 1984 targets for health for all in the WHO European Region

410

(22–26), and was identified as the first of five key action areas for health promotion delineated in the 1986 Ottawa Charter *(2)*. The coordination of healthy public policy was conceived as a strategy to implement health promotion mechanisms. The notion is intended to imply that all public policies, regardless of their intended audience, should be examined for their impact on health; "policies which have a major impact on health are not limited to the delivery of health care services or even public health services" *(23)*. Rachlis & Kushner *(27,28)* define healthy public policy as "any policy that creates and encourages a context for health".

WHO and health promotion agencies use the concept to emphasize the need for governments to acknowledge and address the connections between health and the social, physical and economic environments *(29)*. In Canada, Epp's report *Achieving health for all: a framework for health promotion (30)* called for the coordination of all policies that have a bearing on the population's health, including those on income security, employment, education, housing, business, agriculture, transportation, justice and technology.

The concept, although widely accepted as a key component of health promotion, has not been operationalized in any appreciable way. Hancock *(31,32)* decried the lack of progress towards developing healthy public policy at the national level in Canada. At the provincial level, he found some evidence that healthy public policy was valued and that the need for evaluation was recognized, yet the extent to which the idea had been operationalized remained unclear. He noted that, in the province of Manitoba, a supportive structure was in place and a commitment was articulated in a document *(33)*: "Every major action and policy of government will be evaluated in terms of its implications for the health of Manitobans".

Hancock also noted a commitment to healthy public policy in the province of British Columbia, where the Royal Commission on Health Care and Costs *(34)* recommended that a set of measurable indicators be established that would be suitable for the planning and evaluation of public policies related to health, as well as for the evaluation of possible health effects of all proposed provincial programmes and legislation. The intent was to ensure that decision-makers considered health and wellbeing in policy-making based on the broad determinants of health, including economic, social and physical influences. In 1993, a new format for submissions to the Government was released that required ministries to discuss the health impact of policy and programme options as part of the process. An HIA tool was developed to assist ministries with this function, and HIA tools and processes in the province were revised to align evaluation better with recently developed population health goals *(35–37)*.

Hancock *(31)* suggested that the most likely place to witness healthy public policy was at the municipal level, for several possible reasons.

- The social networks and scale of operations within communities created stronger ties between policy-makers and those affected.

411

- Policy-makers lived where they worked; they were identifiable as well as affected by their own policies.
- The bureaucracies of communities were relatively small and there was a greater chance of intersectoral cooperation.

Further, healthy public policy may be more suited to regional application and implementation where multiple communities share geographic and population characteristics and a history of working together. A notable example comes from Catalonia, Spain; its health plan served as the instrument for healthy public policy, setting out goals, objectives and indicators for health and proposing strategies to meet them. The use of objectives and targets to monitor health in Catalonia demonstrated improvements in a number of the priority areas outlined in the plan, including maternal and infant mortality rates, chronic disease, cervical and breast cancer screening, and accident prevention (38).

Why, then, was the progress in the operationalization of healthy public policy so limited? Many factors may have hindered its development. These fell broadly under two categories: political and technical challenges. Political challenges included a lack of political will; a long tradition of minimal public participation, and underdeveloped mechanisms and incentives; lack of cooperation among departments and jurisdictions; and competing interests. Technical challenges included insufficient knowledge and expertise, underdeveloped science, underdeveloped measurement of health-related phenomena, uncertainties about the relative influence of some determinants of health and insufficient structures for managing relevant information and systems. Political schedules and cycles perpetuated both types of challenge.

Given the problems associated with recent concepts of health, everyone may not have recognized many existing policies as falling within the health domain. A publication from the health ministry of British Columbia included speed limits, seat-belt legislation, penalties for drink-driving, no-smoking by-laws, bans on cigarette and alcohol advertising, and rules requiring labelling of dangerous products as healthy public policies (21). These were perhaps the most obvious choices, but the document also included such policies as building codes that enhanced access by the disabled, federal child tax credits that provided support to poor children, literacy programmes, land-banking for affordable housing and economic policies that promoted full employment and equal opportunity. These may not have been conceived as health policies. Indeed, rather than simply fail to recognize such policies as pertinent to health, some sectors may have actively or passively resisted what they perceived as encroachment by the health sector.

Health field concept

In addition to the experience of the national, provincial and local authorities that applied various forms of HIA, a few theory- and research-derived models of planning emphasized health impact as part of their frameworks and pro-

412

cedures. Such models provided guidance to local, provincial and sometimes national health planners in developing programmes and policies, or in suggesting guidelines for others within their jurisdictions to set priorities and to develop proposals for grant funding.

The essential feature of such models was their suggestion of a particular order and direction of cause-and-effect relationships, linking programmes, policies and regulatory activities to processes of change and then to health outcomes. Without denying the circularity and feedback loops of cause-and-effect chains, they emphasized the order of relationships that leads most directly from input to health outcomes. The degree of detail they offered in the intermediate steps determined the types of users who apply these models and the extent of their use in planning.

Notable among such models was one presented in 1973 by H.L. Laframboise, then Director-General of the Long Range Health Planning Branch of Health and Welfare Canada. This simple model sought only to break health policy "down into more manageable segments" (39), but led in the following year to the landmark policy paper now called the Lalonde report (40). Laframboise laid out four primary divisions of influence on health: lifestyle, environment, health care organization and basic human biology. In his 1973 paper, he concluded that (39):

> The challenge, in the health *field* in Canada, is to maintain the present high level of health care and medical research, while bringing our efforts up to a similar level in the areas of lifestyle and environment, where our principal problems now appear to lie. If the conceptual approach proposed in this paper takes anyone even one step further along the path to a balanced view of the health *field* it will have served its purpose.

This simple delineation of the four main categories of factors influencing health outcomes had a momentous impact on Australian, Canadian, European and United States health planning in the years that followed its popularization in the Lalonde report. In all, new thinking increasingly focused on the neglected dimensions of lifestyle and the environment, although expenditure remained predominantly (over 90%) in the health care organization category. Events in the United States led over the next five years to the publication of the first Surgeon General's report on health promotion and disease prevention (41), which was the first major volley in the Healthy People initiative described below.

The elegant simplicity of Laframboise's health field concept was lost in the Canadian debate that followed the issuing of the Lalonde report. No significant shift in lifestyle and environmental determinants was made the aim of policy; no major shift in federal health resources followed the report, and little change in programme support for health promotion from the federal level was sustained beyond the development of the Health Promotion Directorate. Lavada Pinder (42) attributes this largely to the failure of both the Lalonde report (40) and its successor, the Epp framework *(30)*, to engage Health and Welfare Canada and other sectors of the federal Government in a substantial consultation or goal-setting process similar to the one used in the United States with the development of the objectives for the nation in disease prevention and health promotion *(42)*.

Changes of government and ministers left the internationally acclaimed concepts of both reports largely unsupported by policy or sustained programme funding. In short, the health field concept set in motion a train of subsequent policy documents and conceptual frameworks for planning or coordinating health programmes and public policy, but most of these lacked continuous funding and did not cause policy changes.

Health promotion, population health and population health promotion

Downplaying lifestyle as the pivotal point of the causal chain between programmes or policies and health impact, the Epp framework *(30)* added *for all* to *health* to emphasize attaining equity in health. The causal links to health were then arrayed in three tiers: health challenges (reducing inequities, increasing prevention and enhancing coping), health promotion mechanisms (self-care, mutual aid and healthy environments) and implementation strategies (fostering public participation, strengthening community health services and coordinating healthy public policy).

The Ottawa Charter *(2)* promulgates the most widely adopted definition of health promotion as essentially a statement of its goal of enabling people to gain control over and to improve their health (see Chapter 1). Its emphasis on empowerment shifted the spotlight away from health care services and towards other determinants of health in the environment and in living conditions and lifestyles. As mentioned, the Charter *(2)* also helped position health in this implicit causal chain as "a resource for living", referring to other qualities of life for which health is to be seen as a determinant.

As efforts to give the Ottawa Charter greater practicability, the Epp framework *(30)* and subsequent definitions placed more emphasis on the strategies and methods by which policy and practice from the national to local levels might achieve the Charter's goal. One methodologically and procedurally oriented definition of health promotion fit with the causal chain implied by the Ottawa Charter and the Epp framework: "the combination of educational and environmental supports for actions and conditions of living conducive to health" *(13)*. The Epp framework, subsequent formulations of health promotion and the Ottawa Charter detailed the actions implied here as both individual coping and actions by people themselves and a range of organizational, community and societal action related to policy, the environment and health services.

The health promotion perspectives described above were combined with the population health perspective adopted by federal, provincial and territorial health ministers *(43)* to outline strategies for action on the full range of health determinants at all levels, from individual to societal. Hamilton & Bhatti *(44)* formulated an integrated model of population health and health promotion that

414

combined the foregoing formulations to suggest a framework that could guide actions to improve health. They suggested a three-dimensional model for policy and practice (Fig. 18.3) that indicated an intersection of each of the determinants of health named above with each of the levels of population, and

Fig. 18.3. Model for population health promotion

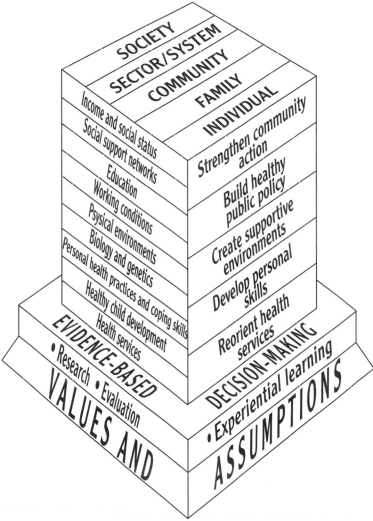

Source: Frankish, J. et al. *Health impact assessment as a tool for population health promotion and public policy. A report submitted to the Health Promotion Development Division of Health Canada* (http://www.hc-sc.gc.ca/hppb/healthpromotiondevelopment/pube/impact/impact.htm). Ottawa, Health Canada, 1996 (accessed 21 February 2001). © Minister of Public Works and Government Services Canada, 2001.

their intersections with the five strategies for health promotion of the Ottawa Charter and Epp framework. This model made more explicit the ecological perspective that has been a foundation of public health and health promotion from their earliest articulations *(45,46)*, but was only partially operationalized in most health promotion projects funded by federal and provincial agencies in Canada *(47)*. The three dimensions address the questions of who, what and how. The intersections of each set of three questions, or levels of population, determinants and strategies, ideally lend themselves to the formulation of goals and objectives.

Determinants of health

Emphasis on population health has given further attention to the delineation and documentation of evidence on the determinants of health *(48–50)*. The Canadian Federal, Provincial and Territorial Advisory Committee on Population Health *(51)* adopted these determinants as the targets for refocused national and provincial strategies for population health:

> **Income and social status**: not the amount of wealth but its relative distribution, together with the control it gives people over their life circumstances and capacity to take action.
>
> **Social support networks**: the help and encouragement people get (or know they can tap if needed) to cope with difficult situations and to maintain their sense of efficacy in dealing with life circumstances.
>
> **Education**: the combination of relevant and meaningful information with skills that equip people to cope with daily challenges and enable them to participate in their community through opportunities for employment and voluntary activities.
>
> **Employment and working conditions**: the conditions of meaningful employment, economic stability, and a work environment conducive to health.
>
> **Physical environment**: air, water, soil, housing, and food protection, combined with other conditions for safe living in communities.
>
> **Biology and genetic endowment**: the physiological, anatomical and mental capacities with which people are born and which naturally develop and decline over the life cycle.
>
> **Personal health practices and coping skills**: those actions by which individuals can prevent diseases and promote self-care, cope with challenges, and develop self-reliance, solve problems and make choices that enhance health.
>
> **Healthy child development**: positive prenatal and early childhood experiences.
>
> **Health services**: the linking of accessible preventive and primary care services, including well baby, immunization and health education programs.

Approaches to impact assessment
Environmental impact assessment

Environmental impact assessment (EIA) is a tool to examine the environmental and social implications of proposed development projects, and is required

416

by legislation in most of the provinces of Canada. EIAs that address health issues are a special case of HIA in that they are tools used to evaluate the health impact of planned developments. In 1992, Australia developed a national framework for HIA in EIA, which designates policy areas and types of development projects that are subject to HIA. In the Australian model, HIA and environmental HIA are twin elements of a single process. In many cases, consultation with health authorities is mandatory for planned development projects.

The HIA process parallels the standard EIA process, which includes screening for relevance, assessing the range of potential factors, profiling for baseline data, assessing and managing risks, implementation and decision-making, and monitoring and evaluation. Public participation, workforce training and accreditation for the implementation of HIA are key components of the Australian approach (52).

It is generally recommended that, when a proposed project may cause potentially significant health effects, the EIA should include an assessment of the risks to human health in its assessment of the potential environmental risks. In a report for the Canadian Environmental Assessment Research Council, Simon (53) acknowledged that EIA had the potential to assess the health impacts of proposed projects, and that, to some extent, such assessments were already being conducted in several countries, including Canada. Simon concluded that most Canadian provincial governments and federal ministries addressed health issues in EIAs sporadically, and lacked sufficient procedures and mechanisms to ensure their consistent and adequate consideration. She further concluded that most statutes and policies that formed the basis of the EIA mandates failed to require the consideration of health impact. She noted that weak links between environment and health ministries led to the allocation of insufficient resources to enable health professionals to participate in EIAs, and that, while some EIAs addressed human health risks, the proportion with health studies was low, and most of those were limited to qualitative analysis.

The health components usually addressed in the EIAs conducted in Canada include the impact of the proposed project on critical subpopulations, future generations, residents and workers during plant construction and operation; positive health effects; cumulative exposure; and impact on health care facilities, waste disposal methods and so forth. Simon (53) noted marked variations between the provinces and the federal Government. While Quebec had a mechanism for formal cooperation between its environment, health and social services ministries to ensure consultation, arrangements in Nova Scotia and Prince Edward Island were less formal. In the latter, EIAs were conducted on an *ad hoc* basis as part of permitting or licensing procedures, and health was rarely identified as a concern. Simon's definition of health impact is narrower than ours, which includes the determinants of health. She noted that Nova Scotia and Prince Edward Island paid greater attention to issues such as unemployment and the welfare of the fishing industry, factors that could be viewed as important determinants of health.

At the federal level, Simon *(53)* was critical of the lack of formal links between the ministries for the environment, health and welfare, and labour, and pointed to a lack of political will, personnel and financial resources to ensure and formalize communication between them. Additionally, the Canadian public, unlike that of the United States, cannot take government departments to court for poor performance. Simon suggested that public oversight ensures that EIAs in the United States are comprehensive; one cannot know the extent to which the lack of public accountability in Canada has limited the likelihood of health being considered in EIAs.

Simon's report *(53)* made a number of recommendations to the Canadian Environmental Assessment Research Council to improve the extent of HIA in EIA processes. These recommendations included:

- the development of a policy agreement between health and environment ministries requiring the consideration of health issues in EIAs when relevant;
- conducting a federal–provincial workshop to develop definitions of human health, human health impact and HIA;
- establishing a task group or sponsoring research projects to develop guidelines on screening, methodologies, HIA and industry-specific health issues, standards and objectives; and
- conducting research to identify agency procedures other than EIA (regulatory, licensing and permitting procedures) in which health components are already addressed.

Davies *(54)*, also for the Canadian Environmental Assessment Research Council, conducted a study to identify the factors that determined whether health was considered as a part of an EIA, and what typically comprised an HIA. She concluded that, although HIAs were usually conducted when there was a health concern, EIA legislation rarely required such assessments, so there were no guidelines to assist government reviewers in decision-making. Neither were there guidelines to determine the factors or indicators that should be included in HIAs, or the methods by which they should be made. Apart from these limitations, Davies *(54)* noted some common themes.

- HIAs were most likely to be done when the proposed development was near human settlements; southern urban centres were more likely than northern rural or remote areas to have HIAs completed.
- Developments with longer estimated lifetimes were more likely to have HIAs completed than those with relatively short estimated lifetimes; for example, oil and gas explorations planned to last 100–150 days were not likely to be assessed.
- The nature of the project was likely to be the strongest determinant of whether an HIA would be completed; if perceived or actual health impacts were likely, so was an HIA.

Further, Davies noted several barriers to the consideration of health in EIA, including: a shortage of knowledgeable health professionals familiar with EIA, inadequate communication between different departments and levels of government, and insufficient or conflicting scientific literature. Despite the limitations of the EIA approach to HIA, much of the current expertise in Canada rests within the environmental health sector.

Health risk assessment

Risk is a reality of everyday life. Determining how risks affect health and the quality of life is a central mandate of governments *(55–58)*. In this vein, health risk research, with a focus on disease prevention, is important for the development of rational and cost-effective health and regulatory policies *(59,60)*. Health risk assessment has been defined as "the qualitative or quantitative estimation of the likelihood of adverse effects from exposure to specified health hazards or from the absence of beneficial influences" *(58)*. Typically, health risk assessment involves four main steps: hazard identification, hazard characterization, exposure assessment and risk characterization.

Considerable progress has been made in integrating risk-related concerns into mainstream government policies and planning *(61)*. Progress has been much more rapid in EIA than in HIA, even though the rationale for environmental improvement is often ultimately related to human health and wellbeing *(62)*. Nevertheless, there remains considerable debate on risk assessment practices for estimating the impact of policies or programmes, rather than proposed projects *(63)*. Implicit in all risk assessment schemes is the need to extrapolate from high-exposure studies to low-exposure situations and from known to probable risks. Many schemes accommodate such uncertainty by incorporating arbitrary safety factors or other default approaches. Such factors are most often not experimentally derived, so they may over- or underestimate actual risks. Analogous procedures to estimate health impact have not been developed.

HIA can be distinguished from risk-related assessment in a number of ways. First, such assessment is most often concerned with minimizing the negative or harmful impact of specific activities on health, either directly or indirectly, as through environmental protection efforts. At best, many risk control efforts seek first to do no harm. In contrast, HIA is more concerned with maximizing the potential benefit to be gained from a given policy or programme.

Risk-related assessment is often tied to discrete projects, developments or activities *(56,57)*, while HIA may be associated with broader government initiatives. The scope of such policies or programmes makes it difficult to calculate the risk or benefit that can be directly linked to specific interventions *(64)*. Finally, work for risk reduction or control is often driven by efforts to improve the fairness of reimbursement or to provide risk-related adjustments for monitoring the outcomes of care. Given its focus on population health, rather than on health care, HIA cannot be driven by a bottom-line mentality that seeks first or only to reduce the costs of care.

Local environmental health programmes in Europe and North America face several related challenges. These include the need to demonstrate their effectiveness in improving the health status of the community they serve *(65,66)*. Using traditional health status measures to evaluate the impact of local environmental health programmes has serious limitations, including the long lag between many hazardous environmental exposures and ill health, and the lack of response to programme interventions of many environment-related diseases *(57)*.

In the face of these challenges, many Canadian authorities have attempted to develop models and delivery systems to meet environmental health objectives. In Alberta, a systematic framework was constructed to develop objectives for use by local environmental health programmes *(66)*. The Alberta framework involved the sequential development of process and structure objectives for health status and risk reduction. The intent was that local environmental health programmes would adapt a comprehensive provincial package of objectives to their own circumstances, and use the package to direct and monitor the effectiveness of their activities.

There is growing recognition that accurate and reliable exposure-related information is essential for informed decisions about protecting and promoting public health *(67)*. Approaches for undertaking exposure surveillance such as the National Human Exposure Assessment Survey (NHEXAS) in the United States have been suggested. NHEXAS has three purposes:

1. to establish a core set of approaches, methods and data;
2. to develop a strong and direct connection between science and policy decisions about assessment, management and communication of health risks; and
3. to create a connected group of researchers and regulators.

An information management tool was presented for the Assessment Protocol for Excellence in Public Health *(68)*: a software package (CDC-AIM) that could also be used to help provincial and local health departments work with communities to establish health programmes based on mortality, morbidity and risk factor data. McDonald et al. *(69)* discussed the process used to develop an environmental health addendum to the Assessment Protocol. The addendum included environmental exposure indicators as well as health status indicators. Similarly, strategies such as Oregon's Public Health Improvement Plan *(70)* defined specific standards for risk reduction, outcomes for improved health and performance measures for assuring accountability.

Finally, a presidential and congressional commission in the United States provided a new framework for risk assessment and risk management in regulatory decision-making *(71)*. Although this approach was limited in its focus on environmental issues and related regulatory processes, it provided a highly useful discussion of more general issues related to HIA. More important, the commission's process and framework highlighted the need for a collaborative,

420

participatory to approach to the framing and implementation of impact assessments.

Status of HIA in Canada

We discuss the Canadian experience as an example of the development of HIA. The application of HIA was highly variable across provinces, using no single process or model. Most of the provinces developed their own unique approaches, paying little or no attention to the others' initiatives. Some linked HIA to cabinet submissions and the policy development process; others coupled it with provincial health goals, and several considered it in the context of EIA. The following summarizes the situations in provinces.

In British Columbia, ministries required an HIA as part of the cabinet submission process. All proposed policies, regardless of the ministry of origin, must be reviewed for potential impact upon the health of British Columbians. HIA tools and guidelines were developed for policy-makers and programme developers. The tools were adjusted to converge with recently developed health goals.

Alberta linked HIA to healthy public policy, sustainable development and provincial health goals. *The rainbow report (72)* recommended that policies be reviewed and legislation, regulations and procedures introduced to ensure that the health of Albertans was given full and equal consideration in matters of economic development, diversification and job creation, and in determining the impact of environmental policies. Another report *(73)* outlined nine broad health goals and related objectives and strategies for improvement. The goals supported decision-making for resource investment in health.

Working together toward wellness (74) proposed a strategy for health reform that included a vision, principles and goals for wellness in Saskatchewan. Population health goals and measurable objectives were established. The Provincial Health Council recommended the adoption of an HIA process and tool to assist policy-makers in decision-making on health care. Applying HIA to proposed policies ensured that the Government's policies and programmes contributed to the ideals captured by the health goals for Saskatchewan.

The Manitoba action plan *(33)* outlines a strategy for health that includes a comprehensive system of health measurement within a framework of healthy public policy. A set of shared goals and objectives was developed to track the health status of Manitobans. All government programmes are being reviewed for their contribution to health, and every major action and policy of the Government is evaluated for its implications for people's health.

In Ontario, a process begun in 1987 led to the definition of five broad health goals in 1989 *(75)*. From 1991 to 1993, working groups of invited experts developed objectives and targets for each of the health goals. The objectives and targets were used to evaluate provincial health reform initiatives. In terms of HIA, the goals and targets influenced the direction and development process of policy in the province.

The policy in Quebec *(76)* outlined five general goals and ten specific objectives (related to four life-cycle stages) for health improvement. The goals were developed through a process in alignment with that described in the 1979 report of the US Surgeon General on health promotion and disease prevention *(42)*. The regions of Quebec were expected to translate provincial goals into regional plans, with an emphasis on health needs of citizens versus health services and resources.

The New Brunswick health strategy *(77)* defined health goals for the province and encouraged ministries, health care providers, community groups and consumers to transform the goals into objectives, targets and action strategies. A parallel initiative for the public health service *(78)* established goals by priority areas as a means to track and monitor people's health.

Health goals were developed as part of the comprehensive health policy of Nova Scotia. A discussion paper *(79)* presented health goals as a means to guide planning and policy decisions for improved health of Nova Scotians. As recommended by the Royal Commission on Health Care *(80)*, all initiatives proposed by the Government were considered for their impact on the health of Nova Scotians.

Newfoundland integrated HIA with community health. Communities assessed the potential impact of government policies against defining community characteristics, including: population groups, employment, economic conditions, social support, health services, basic services (for water, waste disposal, transportation and housing) and community resources (such as consumer organizations, voluntary organizations and clubs). Newfoundland also developed health goals as part of its provincial strategy for health *(81)*.

In Prince Edward Island, a health policy council, comprising community and professional representatives, was responsible for the development and monitoring of measurable health goals and objectives for the province. It developed a set of five broad goals to track and monitor people's health status.

Further, Canadian territories are setting goals. A Northwest Territories document outlined priority areas for health and supported the development of goals and objectives. Two earlier initiatives in the Yukon Territory, the *Health status report (82)* and the Yukon health promotion survey, served as the basis for goal development.

Measuring the impact of public policy: what is needed?
Health indicators

In a review of healthy public policy, Pederson et al. *(83)* identified a need for health indicators that could clarify the relationship between healthy public policy and health status. They stressed the significance of conspicuous indicators such as morbidity and mortality rates, as well as measures of health and wellbeing, which are more difficult to quantify. Most important, they claimed that indicators of events that are not always identified as health related but are causally linked to health, must be developed for policy and programme analysis. To this end, the recommendations of the 2nd International Conference on Health Promotion, in Adelaide, South Australia *(19)* called for the development of health information systems.

Relating this recommendation to HIA, we see such systems as useful in providing performance measures to be associated with health impact measures available from existing vital statistics systems, discharge records and billing systems for medical care, pharmacy record systems, tumour and other registers, and periodic population surveys. Indicators of the determinants of health can and should be used as benchmarks of progress towards improving health, but they cannot be taken as equivalent to health impact without stretching the definition of health beyond the credibility and tolerance of other sectors.

In 1984, the international Beyond Health Care Conference, on healthy public policy, was held in Toronto. Afterwards, a one-day workshop, called Healthy Toronto 2000, was held to examine how the broad themes of healthy public policy could be applied at the municipal level. So began the Healthy Cities movement in Canada *(29,84)*, where the Canadian Healthy Communities Project aimed to ensure that health was a "primary factor in political, social and economic decision making" at the municipal level *(84)*.

The Project had great promise, but a short life. Manson-Singer *(84)* gave many reasons for its failure, including inexperience, lack of resources, definitional problems, competition with other social movements and poor relationships with funding agencies. The problem most relevant to this discussion was the difficulty of arriving at a suitable definition of *healthy communities*. This problem parallels our caveats about defining health too broadly. In making a broad definition, the Project steering committee believed it was being inclusive, but people at the municipal level were concerned that the federal Government was passing on its constitutional responsibility for health to municipalities, and those providing federal health funding had difficulty justifying or defending the broad definitions as focusing sufficiently on health.

Rootman *(85)* examined whether indicators were required within the Project. His observations seem relevant to the broader notion of HIAs of all public policy and the search for appropriate indicators. First, he asked how one could know what indicators mean in the absence of a conceptual framework or theory to locate and explain them. Then he pointed to some methodological issues in identifying and developing appropriate indicators.

- Indicators are not currently available for the positive dimensions of health (those other than reductions in morbidity and mortality).
- It is difficult to develop holistic measures that combine objective and subjective dimensions of health.
- It is unclear how one would capture the contextual factors related to health status, and no indicators are targeted at the community level; they are based on the aggregation of individual measures.

423

The Healthy Communities strategy was played out in many communities in British Columbia, which created their own vision of a healthy community, developed community profiles that highlighted both needs and strengths, and forged coalitions and partnerships committed to improving the health of citizens. The British Columbia health ministry encouraged communities to develop indicators as a means to define and track progress towards improved health for people and communities. Using indicators to measure community health is a means by which communities can influence decision-makers and participate in the planning of programmes and development of policies that affect them (35–37).

Debate on the selection of suitable indicators has most often taken place within the forum of the Healthy Cities movement. Even there, knowledgeable and dedicated people seemed to be unable to develop an agreed set of indicators. The WHO Healthy Cities project sponsored a meeting in March 1987 to achieve consensus on what could and should be measured (86). The selection criteria chosen required indicators to be: relatively simple to collect and use; sensitive to short-term change; capable of analysis at the small-area level; related to health, the WHO policy for health for all, health promotion and the Healthy Cities project; able to carry social and political punch; limited to about 30 in number; concerned with all aspects of city life; and both subjective and objective (87).

In response to the meeting, a guide to assessing project cities (87) was developed. As O'Neill (86) noted, however, the plan could not be carried out because of its massive size; it included knowing everything from the geography of a city (including its topography, climate, natural resources, biological ecosystem and "urban form") to its history, demography, political structure (including jurisdiction and governance), economy, social issues and the influence of religion and the churches. This appears to be another instance of mixing performance indicators and background data with the need for health impact indicators. At a subsequent meeting on Healthy Cities evaluation, none of the reports presented offered concrete indicators for HIA (88).

The Healthy Cities and Shires Project in Australia, like the WHO Healthy Cities project, is a means to achieve health for all. Under the Australian Project, municipal governments develop a vision for their cities, identify needs, set priorities, define measurable health goals and targets, and monitor and evaluate progress towards them. In 1993, the Project was pilot-tested in three cities in the state of Queensland (89).

The WHO European Healthy Cities project seems to have altered its approach, acknowledging the pitfalls of seeking uniform or systematized indicators (see Chapter 14). Attempts made in other places, and reviewed by O'Neill and Cardinal (90,91), seem to have led to the same conclusion. There is no simple and uniform way to assess cities' health.

The mayors of Canada's 14 largest municipalities recommended that a quality-of-life index be developed to assess the effects of federal and provincial spending cuts on the liveability of cities. The proposed index would consider such factors as the proportion of people living under the poverty line, the numbers on welfare, food bank usage and the types of community services offered *(92)*. This mix of impact indicators did not include morbidity, disability or mortality, but it would amount to a combination of determinants and consequences of changes in health.

Determinants of health

As described earlier, the Lalonde report *(40)* introduced Laframboise's health field concept *(39)* in the first major policy document seeking to reorient the emphasis of government health policy from medical care to three other major determinants of health: lifestyle, the environment and human biology. The Canadian Institute for Advanced Research *(93)*, building on the work of others who provided evidence for the importance of the other determinants of health relative to medical care *(94–99)*, separated the environment into social and physical components, and human biology into genetic endowment as a primary determinant, and biological response to the environmental and genetic determinants as part of individual response, along with behavioural response as a secondary or more proximal determinant of health. The Institute further separated health into health and function, disease as immediate effects of these determinants, and wellbeing as a longer-term or secondary effect.

With more direct relevance to HIA, the Institute's formulation of population health determinants clearly disaggregates the concept of health. In search of more practical alternatives to "the all-encompassing definition of WHO, almost a Platonic ideal of 'the good'", Evans & Stoddardt *(49)* separated biological responses (which could be equated with physiological risk factors) from functional limitations, and health as capacity, from illness or disease and from wellbeing. They concluded that *(49)*:

> There are no sharply drawn boundaries between the various concepts of health in such a continuum, but that does not prevent us from recognizing their differences. Different concepts are neither right nor wrong; they simply have different purposes and fields of application.

Whatever the level of the definition of health employed, however, it should be distinguished from the question of the determinants of (that definition of) health.

These important distinctions by the progenitors of the population health model driving the current interest in HIA supports our conclusion that health impact must be assessed on the basis of measurable outcomes on this continuum of health and cannot be equated with impact on determinants or the presumed consequences of health (such as medical care and wellbeing, respectively).

Assessing the policy environment

In addition to the development of indicators to assess the health impact of policies, Pederson et al. *(83)* called for the development of specific indicators to

425

measure the presence of healthy public policy. In this way, researchers could track the various phases of policy-making, including: the identification of social organizations and institutions involved, the identification of processes and outcomes, a description of policy directions and an analysis of past, present, and future trends. This suggestion is consistent with the report of the Adelaide Conference *(100)*, which recommended facilitating healthy public policy through analyses of physical, social and economic factors, and political priorities and commitment. These analyses are important indicators of determinants and performance, but they cannot stand alone as HIA.

Health objectives, goals and targets as a strategy for HIA

One way to avoid the pitfalls associated with the adoption of expanded definitions of health and the confusion of determinants and outcomes is to articulate a health strategy or, more specifically, to specify health goals and objectives for a country and/or regions. This provides a framework for identifying relevant indicators or outcomes for the HIA process. While general policy directions are important, the setting of measurable objectives, with deadlines, is an important motivator for action. Such objectives obviate the need to assess the effectiveness of previous actions and the feasibility of future proposals *(101)*. In the absence of achievable objectives and targets for health, agreed on as policy, the relative potential health impact of other proposed policies can be argued endlessly. Goals and objectives provide the essential yardstick for assessment.

Goals and objectives in Canada

Although Canadian provinces have developed or are developing health goals, national goals have been elusive. Pinder *(39)* showed that different stakeholders have called in publications and speeches for the setting of national goals *(40,102–105)*.

At the national level, objective setting has been limited to priority areas such as tobacco and drug use, child health and injury control. For example, a symposium was held in May 1991 to establish a national strategy and to attempt to establish national objectives for injury prevention, based on the framework of the Healthy People initiative in the United States *(106)*. The symposium brought together representatives of government, public interest groups, professional associations, academia, standard-setting organizations, workers, employers, injury survivors and the general public, who developed injury control objectives for Canada in four settings: home and community, occupational health and safety, sport and recreation, and transport. A fifth group was convened to examine the feasibility of setting objectives related to violent and abusive behaviour. Setting injury control objectives is one of the few examples of a Canadian approach to setting targets by health priority area *(55)*.

Another notable example of national goal setting in Canada is *The national strategy to reduce tobacco use (107)*, whose goals are to help

426

nonsmokers to avoid tobacco use (prevention), to help smokers quit (cessation) and to protect the health and rights of nonsmokers (protection). The strategy outlines seven strategic directions to meet these goals, including legislation, access to information, availability of services and programmes, support for citizen action, message promotion, research and intersectoral policy coordination. The strategy is a collaborative initiative between the federal and provincial/territorial governments and various national health organizations, including the Canadian Council on Smoking and Health, the Lung Association, the Heart and Stroke Foundation and the Canadian Public Health Association.

Similarly, national goals have been developed for cardiovascular diseases in Canada. The Canadian Heart Health Initiative (see Chapter 20) links the federal health authority with all ten provincial/territorial health ministries and with communities where demonstration projects are conducted *(108)*. There is a national network of initiatives, characterized by shared responsibility among government jurisdictions. The national jurisdiction is responsible for technical support, the establishment of a national database on heart health risk factors and the provision of matching research funds for surveys and demonstration projects. Provincial governments are responsible for conducting baseline surveys of risk factors, developing action plans, and implementing and evaluating community-based demonstration projects.

The management-by-objectives approach to planning has been practised with increasing regularity across countries, and under WHO auspices and encouragement. The essential logic of this approach is that goals, objectives and targets can be specified with levels of achievement and deadlines projected from a current or recent starting point. This provides a clear road map for a policy or programme, indicating its expected pace of progress and health outcomes. A health objective takes the form of a single sentence that states who (usually expressed as a population group) will achieve how much (usually expressed as a morbidity or mortality rate or percentage target) of what change (usually expressed as the health problem or need) by when (usually expressed as a year within a ten-year time frame).

The process of developing health goals, objectives and targets will determine the extent of their support from various levels of government, sectors and organizations. The wider the participation in developing and ratifying the objectives, the greater can be the acceptance and active dedication of resources to their achievement by potential organizational partners at all levels in all relevant sectors.

Healthy People initiative in the United States
The most systematic and sustained process of HIA by a government in guiding health promotion and disease prevention policy has been the planning-by-objectives process that the Office of Disease Prevention and Health Promotion of the US Department of Health and Human Services has led since 1979. As a contribution to national and state health policy and programmes

427

in the United States, it is monumental among the federal Government's efforts. Its contribution to the changes in the population's health status can be debated, because so much else has happened in this period, but the 1995 review and revision reported measurable and undeniable progress *(106)*. Setting goals, objectives and targets as a strategy for HIA is the cornerstone of the Healthy People initiative. New goals and objectives for 2010 were launched in January 2000 (http://www.health.gov/healthypeople, accessed 21 February 2001).

How much credit can work on planning, policy-making, and programme and data development take for progress in reducing morbidity, disability and mortality? How much of the progress can be attributed to improved planning and policies at the national level, and how much to the secondary influence of improved planning and policies at the state and local levels? These questions will be debated for decades to come. At the very least, these debates can use the history documented by the midcourse reviews of 1985 and 1995 *(106)*. They are unsurpassed in rich detail on the historical linkages between policies, goals, objectives, programmes and services for health promotion and disease prevention, and the consequent risk reductions for the population and improvements in environmental and health outcomes.

The Healthy People initiative directly influenced or provided a model for action at the state and local levels, and in other countries. The diffusion effect from the national level in the United States stands out in some of the volumes documenting the Healthy People initiative *(109,110)*. One of the objectives for the year 2000, for example, was to increase to at least 90% the proportion of people served by a local health department carrying out the core functions of public health. The bottom-up influence from local and state constituencies in formulating the Healthy People 2000 objectives was impressive. The ripple effect outward to other countries counts as an additional, international contribution.

The success of the Healthy People initiative suggests some lessons for the content and particularly the development process of the documents that accompany a national initiative in HIA and policy. Central to the experience in the United States have been the work to build consensus, ensure wide-ranging consultation and build coalitions and, following each of these efforts, a willingness to revise and improve the objectives. The subtitle of the 1995 review *(106)* expresses the spirit and the substantive essence of the continuing process of needs assessment and planning by objectives: it is self-correcting and constantly improving in targeting efforts where they are needed most and demonstrating health impact.

WHO and country initiatives
The WHO policy for health for all, adopted in 1981, includes the setting of goals and targets. The WHO Regional Office for Europe issued a set of targets in 1985, updated them in 1991 and revised its policy for the year 2000 *(24–26)*, based on broad consultation with and among European Member States.

428

Setting national goals for health has become a feature of the United Kingdom. In England, *The health of the nation (111)* selected five priority areas for action, set national objectives and targets in the priority areas, outlined the action needed to achieve the targets, proposed implementation strategies and offered a framework for continuing monitoring and review. In setting health targets, an estimate of future trends was combined with an assessment of the potential impact of interventions, programmes or policies on the health of the population. Consequences for health were integrated into the policy formulation process. National goals and targets in England have been translated into regional and local goals, targets and action plans. Similar initiatives have been completed or are underway in Northern Ireland, Scotland and Wales.

Australia published its first national goals and targets for population health in 1988 *(112)*. Similarly to experience in the United States, goal setting at the national level in Australia influenced the development of goals and objectives for health promotion at the state level. Healthy Victorians 2000 *(113)* is an outgrowth of the Australian national strategy. It is a joint initiative between the Victorian Health Promotion Foundation and the Department of Health and Community Services, with the central aim of developing goals and targets for the population of Victoria. This is expected to increase the accountability if the health system and to improve the ability of decision-makers to assess the impact of programmes upon the health of its people. Four of the eight Australian states and territories have created health promotion foundations whose central function is to set state goals and targets to monitor and assess the impact of programmes on health.

Nutbeam and his colleagues at the University of Sydney *(114)* outlined the history and development of further goals and targets for the year 2000 and beyond in Australia, giving due credit to the model provided by the United States objectives. Reflecting on the Australian experience in setting national health goals and targets, Harris & Wise *(115)*, ascribed its significant impact on health policy to its:

- focusing the attention of the health system on the outcomes that it achieved, rather than the services it provided;
- providing an information base against which progress could be measured;
- highlighting the differences between the health outcomes of different groups within the community; and
- providing a way of thinking about what needed to be done if the health of Australians was to be improved and health inequality reduced, including the integral importance of health literacy and skills, and health promoting environments.

The national strategy in Australia defined goals and targets for four priority areas, including heart disease, cancer, mental health and injury. Strategies to achieve targets have been developed at the state and territorial level, and encompass all aspects of care, including health promotion and disease prevention, early intervention, treatment, rehabilitation, extended care and research. States and territories establish standards and systems for best practice and performance monitoring that facilitate regular reporting to the national Government. The framework for goals and targets was incorporated into the 1992 Medicare Agreement, which determines the health funding arrangements between the Commonwealth of Australia and the states and territories, and requires all states to participate in the goal-setting process.

The New Zealand experience presents a contrasting history in terms of the staying power of health policy and objectives promulgated at the national level *(116)*. The New Zealand Health Charter and model contract made area health boards accountable to the national Government for achieving objectives to justify their budgets. The United States and Australian approaches have been less directive, giving states and communities autonomy in deciding whether to adopt or adapt the national objectives in their own policies and plans. With the change in government in 1990, New Zealand abandoned the goals and targets; in contrast, the Healthy People process and objectives in the United States have been carried out through four presidents and six secretaries of health and human services without changing course. Although the White House made some notable modifications of the draft objectives for Healthy People 2000, each Government has honoured the process and the goals and targets.

Conclusion

Throughout the world, health reform is occurring at an unprecedented rate, and in an evolving context shaped by large-scale social trends that include greater demand for community control, diminishing resources, an aging population and recognition that health care delivery alone does not bring about health. We believe that such reform should not proceed in the absence of a conceptual or organizing framework that provides the requisite signposts: at a minimum, population health goals. Such goals ought to be operationalized in concrete, measurable objectives.

HIA offers an innovative approach to ensuring that governments' programme and policy initiatives align or are congruent with agreed health goals. It suggests that policies and programmes, regardless of the sectors from which they originate, should be assessed for their influence on health and the quality of life. Setting national health objectives and targets, and conducting HIAs in relation to them, requires the involvement of all sectors of government. The ideal role of the health sector is not only to take action but also to influence, enable and mediate partnerships for intersectoral collaboration.

References

1. PAL, L.A. *Public policy analysis: an introduction*, 2nd ed. Scarborough, Nelson Canada, 1992.
2. Ottawa Charter for Health Promotion. *Health promotion*, **1**(4): iii–v (1986).

430

3.   COLLINS, T. Models of health: pervasive, persuasive and politically charged. *Health promotion international*, **10**: 317–324 (1995).
4.   GREEN, L.W. Refocusing health care systems to address both individual care and population health. *Clinical investigative medicine*, **17**: 133–141 (1994).
5.   FRANKISH, J. ET AL. *Health impact assessment as a tool for population health promotion and public policy. A report submitted to the Health Promotion Development Division of Health Canada* (http://www. hc-sc.gc.ca/hppb/healthpromotiondevelopment/pube/impact/impact.htm). Ottawa, Health Canada, 1996 (accessed 21 February 2001).
6.   ROOTMAN, I. & RAEBURN, J. The concept of health. *In*: Pederson, A. et al. *Health promotion in Canada: provincial, national and international perspectives*. Toronto, W.B. Saunders, 1994, pp. 56–71.
7.   Constitution of the World Health Organization. *In*: *Basic documents*, 42nd ed. Geneva, World Health Organization, 1999.
8.   O'DONNELL, M.P. Definition of health promotion. Part III: expanding the definition. *American journal of health promotion*, **3**(3): 5 (1989).
9.   BERLIN, S. Current status and indicator needs of the Canadian Healthy Communities Project. *In*: Feather, J. & Mathur, B., ed. *Proceedings of an invitational workshop: indicators for Healthy Communities*. Winnipeg, Prairie Region Network on Health Promotion Knowledge Development, 1990, pp. 5–7.
10. CRAWFORD, R. You are dangerous to your health: the ideology and politics of victim blaming. *International journal of health services*, **7**: 663–680 (1977).
11. STRONG, P.M. A new-modelled medicine? Comments on the WHO's regional strategy for Europe. *Social science and medicine*, **22**: 193–199 (1986).
12. LABONTÉ, R. Death of program, birth of metaphor: the development of health promotion in Canada. *In*: Pederson, A. et al. *Health promotion in Canada: provincial, national and international perspectives*. Toronto, W.B. Saunders, 1994, pp. 72–90.
13. GREEN, L.W. & KREUTER, M.M. *Health promotion planning: an educational and environmental approach*, 2nd ed. Mountain View, Mayfield, 1991.
14. ALLEN, R.E., ED. *The concise Oxford dictionary of current English*, 8th ed. New York, Oxford University Press, 1990.
15. EVANS, R.G. & STODDARD, G.L. *Producing health, consuming health care*. Toronto, Canadian Institute of Advanced Research, 1990 (CIAR Population Health Working Paper No. 6).
16. HANCOCK, T. Beyond health care: creating a healthy future. *The futurist*, **16**(4): 4–13 (1982).
17. HANCOCK, T. Beyond health care: from public health policy to healthy public policy. *Canadian journal of public health*, **76**(Suppl. 1): 9–11 (1985).

18. HANCOCK, T. Health in transition. *Canadian home economics journal*, **35**(1): 11–13,16 (1985).

19. *Healthy public policy: Adelaide recommendations*. Geneva, World Health Organization, 1995 (document WHO/HPR/HEP/95.2).

20. *Healthy public policy*. Victoria, Office of Health Promotion, British Columbia Ministry of Health, 1991 (Health Promotion in Action, No. 7).

21. *A guide for communities to enact health-promoting policies*. Victoria, Office of Health Promotion, British Columbia Ministry of Health, 1991.

22. KICKBUSCH, I. Introduction: tell me a story. *In*: Pederson, A. et al. *Health promotion in Canada: provincial, national and international perspectives*. Toronto, W.B. Saunders, 1994, pp. 8–17.

23. PEDERSON, A. ET AL. Preface. *In*: Pederson, A. et al. *Health promotion in Canada: provincial, national and international perspectives*. Toronto, W.B. Saunders, 1994, pp. 1–7.

24. *Targets for health for all. Targets in support of the European regional strategy for health for all*. Copenhagen, WHO Regional Office for Europe, 1985 (European Health for All Series, No. 1).

25. *Health for all targets. The health policy for Europe*. Copenhagen, WHO Regional Office for Europe, 1993 (European Health for All Series, No. 4).

26. *HEALTH21. The health for all policy framework for the WHO European Region*. Copenhagen, WHO Regional Office for Europe, 1999 (European Health for All Series, No. 6).

27. RACHLIS, M. & KUSHNER, C. *Strong medicine: how to save Canada's health care system*. Toronto, HarperCollins, 1994.

28. RACHLIS, M. & KUSHNER, C. *Second opinion: what's wrong with Canada's health care system and how to fix it*. Toronto, HarperCollins, 1989.

29. The argument for healthy public policy. *In*: *Healthy public policy*. Victoria, Office of Health Promotion, British Columbia Ministry of Health, 1991 (Health Promotion in Action, No. 7), pp. 1–3.

30. EPP, J. *Achieving health for all: a framework for health promotion*. Ottawa, Health Canada, 1986.

31. HANCOCK, T. Public policies for healthy cities: involving the policy makers. *In*: Flynn, B.C., ed. *Proceedings of the Inaugural Conference of the World Health Organization Collaborating Center in Healthy Cities*. Indianapolis, Institute of Action Research for Community Health, Indiana University School of Nursing, 1992, pp. 33–41.

32. HANCOCK, T. Health promotion in Canada: did we win the battle but lose the war? *In*: Pederson, A. et al. *Health promotion in Canada: provincial, national and international perspectives*. Toronto, W.B. Saunders, 1994, pp. 350–373.

33. *Quality health for Manitobans: the action plan*. Winnipeg, Manitoba Health, 1992.

34. *Closer to home*. Victoria, Royal Commission on Health Care and Costs, 1991.

432

35. *Health impact assessment guidelines.* Victoria, Population Health Resource Branch, British Columbia Ministry of Health, 1995.

36. *Health impact assessment tool kit.* Victoria, Population Health Resource Branch, British Columbia Ministry of Health, 1994.

37. *Health indicator workbook: a tool for healthy communities.* Victoria, Population Health Resource Branch, British Columbia Ministry of Health, 1995.

38. *Working together for health gain at a regional level: the experience of Catalonia.* Barcelona, Department of Health and Social Security, Autonomous Government of Catalonia, 1994.

39. LAFRAMBOISE, H.L. Health policy: breaking the problem down into more manageable segments. *Canadian Medical Association journal,* **108**: 388–393 (1973).

40. LALONDE, M. *A new perspective on the health of Canadians: a working document.* Ottawa, Canada Information, 1974.

41. *Healthy people: the Surgeon General's report on health promotion and disease prevention* Washington, DC, US Department of Health, Education, and Welfare, 1979 (PHS Publication No. 79–55071).

42. PINDER, L. The federal role in health promotion: art of the possible. *In*: Pederson, A. et al. *Health promotion in Canada: provincial, national and international perspectives.* Toronto, W.B. Saunders, 1994, pp. 92–106.

43. FEDERAL, PROVINCIAL AND TERRITORIAL ADVISORY COMMITTEE ON POPULATION HEALTH. *Strategies for population health: investing in the health of Canadians.* Ottawa, Ministry of Supply and Services, 1994.

44. HAMILTON, N, & BHATTI, T. *Population health promotion: an integrated model of population health and health promotion.* Ottawa, Health Promotion Development Division, Health Canada, 1996.

45. GREEN, L.W. ET AL. Ecological foundations of health promotion. *American journal of health promotion,* **10**: 270–281 (1996).

46. WORLD HEALTH ORGANIZATION MONICA PROJECT. Ecological analysis of the association between mortality and major risk factors of cardiovascular disease. *International journal of epidemiology,* **23**: 505–516 (1994).

47. RICHARD, L. ET AL. Assessment of the integration of the ecological approach in health promotion programs. *American journal of health promotion,* **10**: 318–328 (1996).

48. DRUMMOND, M. & STODDART, G. Assessment of health producing measures across different sectors. *Health policy,* **33**: 219–231 (1995).

49. EVANS, R.G. & STODDART, G.L. Producing health, consuming health care. *Social science and medicine,* **31**(12): 1347–1363 (1990).

50. EVANS, R.G. ET AL., ED. *Why are some people healthy and others not? The determinants of health of populations.* New York, Walter de Gruyter, 1994.

51. DIANE MCAMMOND & ASSOCIATES. *Analytic review towards health goals for Canada.* Ottawa, Federal, Provincial, and Territorial Advisory Committee on Population Health, 1994.

52. *National framework for health impact assessment in environmental impact assessment.* Wollongong, University of Wollongong, 1992.

53. SIMON, J.S. *Health aspects of environmental impact assessment. Vol. 1. Overview of current practice, findings, and recommendations.* Hull, Canadian Environmental Assessment Research Council, 1988.

54. DAVIES, K. Health and environmental impact assessment in Canada. *Canadian journal of public health,* **82**: 19–21 (1991).

55. SAUNDERS, L.D. & STEWART, L.M. *A safer Canada: year 2000 injury control objectives for Canada. Proceedings of a National Symposium. Edmonton, Alberta. May 21–22, 1991,* Ottawa, Health Canada, 1991.

56. ALDRICH, T. & GRIFFITH, J. *Environmental epidemiology and risk assessment.* New York, Van Nostrand Reinhold, 1993.

57. BAILAR, J. ET AL. *Assessing risk to health: methodological approaches.* London, Auburn House, 1993.

58. US DEPARTMENT OF HEALTH AND HUMAN SERVICES TASK FORCE ON HEALTH RISK ASSESSMENT. *Determining risk to health: government policy and practice.* Dover, Auburn House, 1986.

59. MARINKER, M. *Controversies in health care policies.* London, BMJ Books, 1994.

60. OLDEN, K. & KLEIN, J. Environmental health science research and human risk assessment. *Molecular carcinogenesis,* **14**(1): 2–9 (1995).

61. WIGLE, D. Canada's health status: a public health perspective. *Risk analysis,* **15**: 693–698 (1995).

62. WARFORD, J. Environment, health, and sustainable development: the role of economic instruments and policies. *Bulletin of the World Health Organization,* **73**: 387–395 (1995).

63. IEZZONI, L. *Risk adjustment for measuring health outcomes.* Ann Arbor, Health Administration Press, 1994.

64. SCHMID, T. ET AL. Policy as intervention: environmental and policy approaches to the prevention of cardiovascular disease. *American journal of public health,* **85**: 1207–1211 (1995).

65. KOTCHIAN, S. Environmental health services are prerequisites to health care. *Family & community health,* **18**(3): 45–53 (1995).

66. SAUNDERS, L. ET AL. Measurable objectives for local environmental health programs. *Journal of environmental health,* **58**(6): 6–12 (1996).

67. SEXTON, K. ET AL. Informed decisions about protecting and promoting public health: a rationale for a national human exposure assessment survey. *Journal of exposure analysis and environmental epidemiology,* **5**: 233–256 (1995).

68. VAUGHN, E. ET AL. An information manager for the Assessment Protocol for Excellence in Public Health. *Public health nursing,* **11**: 399–405 (1994).

69. McDONALD, T. ET AL. Development of an environmental health addendum to the Assessment Protocol for Excellence in Public Health. *Journal of public health policy*, **15**: 203–217 (1995).

70. BERKOWITZ, B. Improving our health by improving our system. *Family and community health*, **18**(3): 37–44 (1995).

71. PRESIDENTIAL/CONGRESSIONAL COMMISSION ON RISK ASSESSMENT AND RISK MANAGEMENT. *Risk assessment and risk management in regulatory decision-making.* Washington, DC, Environmental Protection Agency, 1997.

72. PREMIER'S COMMISSION ON FUTURE HEALTH CARE FOR ALBERTANS. *The rainbow report: our vision for health.* Edmonton, Alberta Ministry of Health, 1989.

73. *Health goals for Alberta: progress report.* Edmonton, Alberta Ministry of Health, 1993.

74. *Working together toward wellness: a Saskatchewan vision for health.* Regina, Saskatchewan Health, 1992.

75. PREMIER'S COUNCIL ON HEALTH, WELL-BEING AND SOCIAL JUSTICE. *A vision for health: health goals for Ontario.* Toronto, Ontario Ministry of Health, 1989.

76. *The policy on health and well-being.* Quebec, Quebec Ministry of Health and Social Services, 1992.

77. *Health 2000: toward a comprehensive health strategy.* Fredericton, New Brunswick Government, 1990.

78. *Public health service: vision, mission, goals and objectives.* Fredericton, New Brunswick Government, 1993.

79. *Developing health goals and a comprehensive health strategy for Nova Scotia.* Halifax, Nova Scotia Provincial Health Council, 1992.

80. *The Report of the Nova Scotia Royal Commission on Health Care.* Halifax, Nova Scotia Government, 1989.

81. *Provincial health goals.* St John's, Newfoundland Department of Health, 1994.

82. *Health status report.* Whitehorse, Yukon Health and Social Services, 1992.

83. PEDERSON, A.P. ET AL. *Coordinating healthy public policy: an analytic literature review and bibliography.* Toronto, Department of Behavioural Science, University of Toronto, 1988 (HSPB Publication No. 88-1).

84. MANSON-SINGER, S. The Canadian Healthy Communities Project: creating a social movement. *In*: Pederson, A. et al. *Health promotion in Canada: provincial, national and international perspectives.* Toronto, W.B. Saunders, 1994, pp. 107–122.

85. ROOTMAN, I. Current issues in indicator development. *In*: Feather, J. & Mathur, B., ed. *Proceedings of an invitational workshop: indicators for healthy communities.* Winnipeg, Prairie Region Network on Health Promotion Knowledge Development, 1990, pp. 9–19.

435

86. O'NEILL, M. Healthy Cities indicators: a few lessons to learn from Europe. *In*: Feather, J. & Mathur, B., ed. *Proceedings of an invitational workshop: indicators for healthy communities*. Winnipeg, Prairie Region Network on Health Promotion Knowledge Development, 1990, pp. 33–38.

87. WHO HEALTHY CITIES PROJECT. *A guide to assessing Healthy Cities*. Copenhagen, FADL, 1988 (WHO Healthy Cities Papers, No. 3).

88. DE LEEUW, E. & O'NEILL, M. *Towards a Healthy Cities research agenda*. Maastricht, Department of Health Ethics and Philosophy, School of health Sciences, University of Limburg, 1992.

89. *Municipal public health planning: resource guide*. Brisbane, Health Advancement Branch, Queensland Health, 1995.

90. O'NEILL, M. & CARDINAL, L., ED. *Des indicateurs pour évaluer les projets québécois de villes et villages en santé: la nécessité de faire des choix*. Québec, Groupe de recherche et d'intervention en promotion de la santé de l'Université Laval (GRIPSUL), 1992.

91. CARDINAL, L. & O'NEILL, M. Building information partnerships with communities: the necessity of strategic choices. *In*: Scott, L.R., ed. *Building partnerships in community health through applied technology. Proceedings of the fourth national and second international conferences on information technology and community health (ITCH)*. Victoria, University of Victoria, 1992, pp. 245–248.

92. MUNRO, H. Mayors propose quality-of-life index. *The Vancouver sun*, 27 February 1996, p. B1.

93. EVANS, R.G. & STODDART, G.L. *Producing health, consuming health care*. Toronto, Canadian Institute for Advanced research, 1990 (CIAR Population Health Working Paper No. 6).

94. DUTTON, D.B. Social class and health. *In*: Aitken, L.H. & Mechanic, D., ed. *Application of social science to clinical medicine and health policy*. New Brunswick, Rutgers University Press, 1986, pp. 31–62.

95. LEVINE, S. & LILLIENFELD, A. *Epidemiology and health policy*. London, Tavistock Press, 1987.

96. MARMOT, M.G. Social inequalities in mortality: the social environment. *In*: Wilkinson, R.G., ed. *Class and health: research and longitudinal data*. London, Tavistock Press, 1986, pp. 21–33.

97. MCKEOWN, T. *The role of medicine: dream, mirage or nemesis?* 2nd ed. Oxford, Basil Blackwell, 1979.

98. MCKINLAY, J.B. ET AL. A review of the evidence concerning the impact of medical measures on recent mortality and morbidity in the United States. *International journal of health services*, **19**: 181–208 (1989).

99. TOWNSEND, P. & DAVIDSON, N., ED. The Black report. *In*: *Inequalities in health*. Harmondsworth, Penguin, 1992.

100. KICKBUSCH, I. ET AL. *Healthy public policy. Report on the Adelaide Conference. 2nd International Conference on Health Promotion, April 5–9,*

1988, Adelaide, Australia. Copenhagen WHO Regional Office for Europe, 1988.

101. ASVALL, J. *Healthy public policy: stimulating health for all development.* Copenhagen, WHO Regional Office for Europe, 1988 (document).
102. *Report of the Ad Hoc Committee on National Health Strategies.* Ottawa, Health Canada, 1982.
103. CANADIAN PUBLIC HEALTH ASSOCIATION. CPHA 1984 resolutions and motions. *CPHA health digest,* **8**(4): 61 (1984).
104. CANADIAN PUBLIC HEALTH ASSOCIATION. CPHA 1987 position paper/resolutions and motions. *CPHA health digest,* **11**(3): 19 (1987).
105. *Caring about health. Issue paper on federal/provincial/territorial arrangements for health policy.* Ottawa, Canadian Public Health Association, 1992.
106. US DEPARTMENT OF HEALTH AND HUMAN SERVICES. *Healthy People 2000: midcourse review and 1995 revisions.* Boston, Jones & Barlett, 1996.
107. *The national strategy to reduce tobacco use in Canada.* Ottawa, Health Canada, 1995.
108. *Canadian heart health initiative.* Ottawa, Health Canada, 1992.
109. CENTERS FOR DISEASE CONTROL. *Profile of state and territorial public health systems: United States, 1990.* Atlanta, US Department of Health and Human Services, 1991.
110. *Healthy Communities 2000: model standards. Guidelines for community attainment of the Year 2000 national health objectives,* 3rd ed. Washington, DC, American Public Health Association, 1991.
111. SECRETARY OF STATE FOR HEALTH. *The health of the nation.* London, H.M. Stationery Office, 1992.
112. COMMONWEALTH DEPARTMENT OF HUMAN SERVICES AND HEALTH. *Goals and targets for Australia's health in the year 2000 and beyond.* Canberra, Australian Government Publishing Service, 1993.
113. *Healthy Victorians 2000 – Towards Victorian health promotion goals and targets.* Melbourne, Victorian Health Promotion Foundation. 1995.
114. NUTBEAM, D. ET AL. *Goals and targets for Australia's health in the year 2000 and beyond.* Canberra, Australian Government Publishing Service, 1993.
115. HARRIS, M. & WISE, M. Can goals and targets set a radical agenda? *Health promotion international,* **11**: 63–64 (1996).
116. *New Zealand health goals and targets for the year 2000.* Wellington, New Zealand Department of Health, 1989.

19
Social capital: evaluation implications for community health promotion

Marshall W. Kreuter, Nicole A. Lezin,
Laura Young and Adam N. Koplan[5]

Introduction

The terms *community* and *community-based* have become virtual shorthand for a number of basic tenets of health promotion. Grounded in principles of collaboration and participation, community-based health promotion places primary emphasis on the health of populations and, in so doing, implicitly acknowledges that the physical and social infrastructure of daily life strongly influences individual health behaviour *(1)*. Even the most casual examination of the health issues so often addressed by a community-based approach – such as infant mortality rates, HIV infection, and smoking and unplanned pregnancy in teenagers – quickly reveals the complexity of and connections between health problems and their social determinants – poverty, housing, and education – which tend to cluster by neighbourhood or community *(2,3)*.

Community health promotion: the conundrum of mixed results

Research providing evidence that community-based health promotion programmes can yield positive effects supports their compelling philosophical and intuitive appeal *(4–10)*. Accounts of intervention strategies applied in these

[5] We gratefully acknowledge the contributions of colleagues who reviewed drafts of this chapter and struggled with us to make potential measures of social capital more concrete and measurable. We are indebted to: Beth Baker, St Louis University School of Public Health, United States; David Cotton, Macro International, United States; Robert Goodman, Wake Forest University, United States; Larry Green, University of British Columbia, Canada; Pamela Gillies and Moira Kelly, HEA, United Kingdom; Donna Higgins and David McQueen, CDC, United States; Richard Levinson, Emory University, United States; Irving Rootman, University of Toronto, Canada; and Gerry Veenstra, McMaster University, Canada. We also thank Nathan Jones and Lisa Powell, Health 2000 Inc., United States, for their diligent efforts in tracking down existing social capital indicators and references.

studies also support the assumption that much is known about the theory, process and methods required to implement community-based health promotion programmes that work *(11)*. We use the phrase *programmes that work* rather than *efficacy*, because in public health parlance the latter implies a precise level of outcome that is often unrealistic for community-based interventions. In spite of this evidence, however, findings from research aimed at assessing the effectiveness of community-based health promotion are mixed and somewhat equivocal, even when appropriate standards for planning and implementation have been applied *(12,13)*. A community-based health promotion strategy meets such standards when it:

1. adheres to sound theories of community engagement and participation;
2. employs methods that are grounded in sound theory and have been shown effective in similar settings;
3. addresses the sociopolitical system, as well as environmental and behavioural forces that influence health;
4. is managed by capable, competent staff;
5. has adequate financial, administrative and organizational support; and
6. is deemed appropriate for the problem, circumstances and audience in question.

The measurement challenge

One possible explanation for this inconsistency may lie in the complexity of the measurement challenge. Measuring the effectiveness of community-based health promotion has been widely debated in the literature. Several authors *(14–16)* provide thoughtful commentary. McKinley *(17)* has argued that much greater consideration needs to be given to the matter of the appropriateness of health promotion research methodology:

> The appropriateness of any research methodology, to the extent that it is important, is a function of the phenomenon under study, its magnitude, the setting, the current state of theory and knowledge, the availability of valid measurement tools, and the appropriate uses of the information to be gathered. The utility of any methodological approach is, in large part, a function of the load you are asking it to carry, and who it's being delivered to.

The issue of appropriateness often surfaces in discussions about the designs used for assessing the effectiveness of community-based health promotion. For example, while the randomized clinical trial has been the gold standard for determining the effectiveness of public health interventions, several scholars, including Pearce *(18)*, have questioned its application in ecological community studies (see also chapters 1, 10 and 11):

> ... the randomized clinical trial may be an appropriate paradigm in many epidemiologic studies of specific risk factors, but it often is inappropriate in studies

that require a consideration of the historical and social context. The danger is that attempting to eliminate the influence of all other causes of diseases – in an attempt to control confounding – strips away the essential historical and social context, as well as the multiple moderating influences that constitute true causation. Thus, the tendency to only study factors that fit the clinical trial paradigm should be resisted, and appropriate study designs should be chosen (or developed) to fit the public health question that is being addressed.

Mediating factors

Clearly, academics and practitioners should give priority to reaching some consensus on what constitutes an appropriate and coherent methodology for assessing the impact and effectiveness of community-based health promotion strategies. Unlike vaccines, which are developed to act on biological properties that are predictable and consistent, community-based health promotion interventions are expected to have an effect in spite of the dynamic social, cultural, and political factors that are idiosyncratic to that community. Strong social, cultural and political forces operate within but vary between communities. As discussed in Chapter 1, the failure to take account of social and political context is a major factor in making community health interventions particularly difficult to evaluate.

Thus, another possible explanation for the lack of reported effectiveness of community-based health promotion may lie in the inherent, often hidden complexities of community life. In reviewing 20 years' experience of community-based cardiovascular disease prevention in Finland, Puska and his colleagues *(19,20)* concluded that even programmes employing the best methods and practices, and managed by the most capable practitioners, face substantial resistance in the absence of community participation and collaboration. The notion that the willingness and capacity to collaborate may mediate the effectiveness of a health promotion programme is supported by studies investigating community competence *(21)*, community readiness *(22,23)*, empowerment *(24)* and participatory research *(25)*.

Purpose and assumptions

The theory of social capital suggests that levels of trust, civic participation and organizational cooperation mediate collective action requiring collaborative effort. Since such participation and cooperation are key aspects of community health promotion programmes, it seems appropriate to ask whether variations in the levels of social capital mediate the effects of these programmes. Addressing this question requires the asking of three prior questions.

1. Can social capital be feasibly measured at the community level?
2. If so, is there any evidence that variance in levels of social capital is associated with the effectiveness of health promotion programmes?
3. If social capital can be measured and is found to be associated with health promotion effectiveness, can it be created or modified?

This chapter raises and discusses some of the salient challenges that researchers and evaluators are likely to address as they pursue answers to these questions.

Social capital: an overview
The concept

In the context of community-based health promotion, *social capital* refers to those specific processes among people and organizations, working collaboratively in an atmosphere of trust, that lead to accomplishing a goal of mutual social benefit. This interpretation incorporates James Coleman's emphasis on social relations within and among organizations and structures that people build themselves *(26)*. It also highlights Robert Putnam's notion of mutual interest *(27)*. Social capital does not refer to individuals, the implements of production or the physical infrastructure, but is a relational term that connotes interaction among people through systems that enhance and support that interaction.

In the United States, social capital has recently been catapulted from its somewhat obscure academic origins to much broader discussion and dissent in the mainstream media, notably through the popular interpretation of Putnam's research on the evolutionary patterns of local government in Italy *(28)* and his related inquiry in the United States. Over two decades, Putnam studied the performance of regional governments in Italy and, not surprisingly, discovered that some performed better than others. More importantly, Putnam concluded that the regions with superior governance had more social capital, as manifested by citizens' public spirit, higher levels of civic engagement and tendency to form collaborative, often non-political, associations. Putnam also suggested that the core elements of social capital – trust and cooperation – could develop over time from the repeated interaction of people involved in long-term relationships that are supported by community institutions. As such, these core elements are learned behaviour.

Coleman, generally recognized as the scholar who formally introduced the term into social theory, argued that social capital has the potential to produce a stronger social fabric because it builds bonds of information, trust and solidarity between people, most often as by-products of other activities *(29)*. Trust is an especially salient factor in virtually all conceptualizations of social capital. Figuratively speaking, one can see trust in the making of a judgement that a particular event will occur, when relationships with others could put that event at risk. A statement such as "I feel safe in this neighbourhood because I know the people here and have a good relationship with them" is an example of trust.

As a construct of social capital, especially in the context of community health promotion, the perception of trust should be assessed at the level of institutions and organizations, as well as individuals. For example, selecting and buying food are easier when people trust the private and public institutions

442

responsible for food safety. Outbreaks of foodborne disease or the erosion of confidence in government, however, can compromise that trust.

Robert Wuthnow at Princeton University (personal communication, July 1998) describes trust as fundamental to the effectiveness of democratic societies in so far as the fate of those societies lies in the hands of the people. He points out that conditional levels of trust are more consistent with most theories of democracy than overly optimistic, blind, universal ideals of trust that may encourage faith in totalitarian leaders and not ensure the operation of effective checks and balances. These subtleties increase the complexity of the challenge to measure trust.

Putnam's assertion that key elements of social capital are learned behaviour provides hope that social capital can be created. According to Coleman, however, increases in social capital do not come easily. Paradoxically, the property that distinguishes social capital from other forms of capital – a commitment to public good – may act as a barrier for some. Because social capital implicitly constitutes an investment, Coleman notes that many individual actors (as either individuals or members of organizations) who invest in the betterment of the whole community personally capture only a small portion of the benefits. For some, the realization of this fact can lead to underinvestment in social capital *(30)*. Scholars generally agree that social capital increases when people spend it – the more they use, the more they produce *(31)*. In this sense, social capital functions much as wisely invested financial capital does – by generating further production.

The production of social capital appears to be related to reciprocity: the act of making arrangements, establishing relations or initiating exchanges for the purpose of cooperation or some form of sharing. According to Taylor *(32)*, reciprocity is:

> usually characterized by a combination of short-term altruism and long-term self interest: I help you now in the (possibly vague, uncertain and uncalculating) expectation that you will help me out in the future.
>
> Reciprocity is made up of a series of acts, each of which is short-run altruistic (benefitting others at a cost to the altruist) but which together typically make every participant better off.

The notion of reciprocity is especially relevant to the interactions and exchanges among the multiple organizations that are inevitably called on to cooperate for the promotion of public policy and programmes to address such tasks as preventing alcohol and drug use, injuries and teenage pregnancy, and ensuring immunization and child safety and welfare.

Popularization of social capital

In the United States, Putnam's application of social capital to contemporary life triggered mainstream attention to the concept and, in its wake, criticism of his methods and conclusions. In Putnam's original work on regional differences in

443

Italian political and civic life, his central thesis was that "good government in Italy is a by-product of singing groups and soccer clubs" *(28)*. Turning his attention to the United States, Putnam suggested that citizens' participation in such groups had declined, and that the civic and political fabric had suffered as a result. This thesis has yielded three main areas of disagreement:

1. a methodological disagreement that Putnam's measures do not accurately reflect social capital;
2. a related disagreement with his conclusion that social capital is in decline; and
3. a sense that, whether or not social capital is in decline, little can be done about it.

The article that moved social capital from academia to *People* magazine was called "Bowling alone" *(33)*. Its title and that of the book developing its theme *(34)* are derived from Putnam's observation that, although the number of individual bowlers in the United States rose by 10% between 1980 and 1993, league bowling (bowling in groups) declined by 40%. Putnam also offered a number of other measures to bolster the argument that an increasingly atomized, isolated public was retreating from the civic social bonds that fueled "the vibrancy of American civil society" and its participatory democratic traditions. These include declines in voter turnout, church attendance, membership in everything from unions to volunteer organizations, and overall trust in government.

Critics have asserted that these measures do not reflect a true picture of civic connections. Bowling alone instead of in a league, for example, does not necessarily imply that solitary bowlers fill the bowling alleys. Instead, bowling continues as a more informal social event; people still bowl in groups, but the sport perhaps takes a back seat to general camaraderie. Further, while membership has decreased in the organizations Putnam cites, it has increased dramatically in others (such as young people's soccer teams) *(35)*.

Some critics have also protested that all types of membership should not be counted equally. For example, trust and collaboration related to governance may be more likely (or more profound) by-products for organizations devoted to solving some type of community problem, such as substance abuse coalitions, rather than more social or recreational groups *(36)*.

In addition, membership alone may not reflect the intensity of civic activity. For example, some individuals' church membership may in fact reflect a high degree and variety of voluntarism through a variety of church-sponsored events (such as building houses through Habitat for Humanity), which are not reflected accurately in the single count of one individual's church affiliation. Similarly, membership in associations does not necessarily translate into interaction that benefits the broader community. Extremist groups, for example, may exhibit high levels of social connectedness within their ranks, but their actions may be destructive to outsiders.

444

Measuring social capital in a public health context

The constructs or components of social capital (trust, civic participation, social engagement and reciprocity) have been independently measured in several health-related studies. For example, using selected data from the 1990 United States census and state-level population surveys to examine the relationships among income inequity, mortality and social capital, Kawachi et al. *(37)* concluded that income inequality leads to increased mortality through the reduction of social capital. An important implication of this study is its assertion that positive reserves of social connectedness – an ecological, health promoting force – can exist in communities where economic capital appears to be low or depleted.

Sampson et al. *(38)* studied the relationship between "collective efficacy" and evidence of violence in young people as measured by crime rates in multiple neighbourhoods of inner-city Chicago. They used two dimensions of social capital: trust and social engagement. They measured social engagement by asking neighbourhood residents to declare their willingness to intervene if they observed children in any of the following circumstances: not attending school, engaged in spray-painting graffiti on property, being disrespectful to an adult or fighting. The study revealed that neighbourhoods demonstrating higher levels of collective efficacy had the lowest levels of crime and violence.

In a study of over 600 children aged 2–5 years and their care givers (all of whom were participants in a longitudinal study of child abuse and neglect), Runyan et al. *(39)* found that only 13% of the children were classified as "doing well", based on measures from the Battelle Developmental Inventory and the Child Behaviour Checklist. Their analysis revealed that the factors that best discriminated between a child who functioned well and those not doing well were: church attendance, mother's perception of personal social support and support within the community.

Project Northland is a community-wide demonstration research project designed to be conducted in multiple school districts in Minnesota *(40)*. Perry and her colleagues designed the Project to determine whether active coordination of a theoretically sound school curriculum, parental involvement and community task force support could affect young people's alcohol consumption. Differences between the intervention and control districts after three years reveal that Project Northland was effective in reducing alcohol use. In an editorial independently critiquing Project Northland, Wechsler & Weitzman *(41)* called attention to the possible role of social capital – manifested by patterns of trust, mutual obligation and supportive informal and formal social networks – in this success. They hypothesize "that it is the accrual and expenditure of social capital through sharing responsibility, resources, and roles to achieve reductions in youth substance use that will, in the end, achieve sustained reductions in the extent of use and the progression to abuse" *(41)*.

Higgins *(42)* conducted a study to determine how individual perceptions of social capital were associated with selected actions taken by low-income, vol-

445

unteer peer educators working in HIV prevention projects in Denver, Colorado and New York City. She found that those with high scores in social capital also had higher involvement in the community, were more apt to seek screening themselves and had enlarged their social networks through participation in the project. Interestingly, the study findings also provide some modest evidence that participation in a community-based intervention may itself further or foster social capital.

Measurement caveats and clues

The literature offers some important cautionary notes for those attempting to measure social capital at the community level. For example, some scholars have observed that the assessment of social capital runs the risk of being tautological – that is, identifying the success or failure of a given community *a posteriori* with the presence or absence of social capital. For example, Portes & Landoldt *(43)* imply that Putnam was tautological in his comparisons of well governed communities in the north of Italy versus the poorly governed ones in the south:

> In [Putnam's] words "Civic communities value solidarity, civic participation and integrity, and here democracy works. At the other pole are uncivic regions like Calabria and Sicily, aptly characterized by the French term *incivisme*. The very concept of citizenship is stunted here." If your town is "civic," it does civic things; if it is "uncivic," it does not.

Nevertheless, the literature offers some important clues on how to approach the task of ascertaining which constructs or indicators would provide a valid indication of the degree to which social capital is operational in a community. For example, Carr *(44)* suggests that social capital appears in three forms:

1. dense horizontal networks and associations of community involvement;
2. high levels of information about the trustworthiness of individuals involved in the networks; and
3. effective norms and sanctions (shared values) built up through past successes in collaboration to achieve common goals.

Goodman, in exploring ways to assess the capacity of communities to implement complex community-based programmes, has identified ten general domains for assessing community capacity. One is called "rich social networks" and is characterized by several factors, including *(45)*:

• reciprocal links throughout the community network
• frequent supportive interactions
• the ability to form new associations
• trust and cooperation

446

- more horizontal than vertical ties and relationships
- cooperative decision-making processes
- the existence of similar network properties within and between organizations and groups.

Some community-level measures have been obtained from surveys that assess levels of intersectoral collaboration towards a common benefit and similar indicators under the rubric of civic engagement. For example, under contract from the California Center for Health Improvement, Louis Harris and Associates conducted 1338 telephone interviews with California residents aged 18 and older to determine how citizens want to lend their energies and apply their voting power toward improving the health of their communities *(44)*. The survey addressed the following topics:

- ratings of communities as places to live, and possible improvements to them;
- views on the overall health of people in a community and ratings on a variety of factors that contribute to health and quality of life;
- community involvement, voluntary work and the experience gained from it, voting participation and attitudes to improving community health;
- attitudes towards the role of the mass media in community involvement;
- views on the power and control of state and local government; and
- ratings of local health organizations, businesses and employers.

Designing a measurement protocol for social capital

The pursuit of a valid community-level measure of social capital raises several formidable design and measurement challenges, many of which are familiar to evaluators of community interventions. This section describes the challenges we encountered in carrying out a pilot project to develop a valid process to assess social capital in small communities. Our general tasks included:

- determining the measurable constructs within the theory of social capital;
- addressing the question of community size;
- determining the appropriate units of measurement (individual and/or organizational);
- developing and applying a protocol to estimate existing levels of social capital, and selecting comparison sites;
- developing a protocol and instruments for a qualitative assessment to verify or reject estimated levels of social capital; and
- developing and administering a questionnaire on social capital to a random sample of residents in the two comparison sites.

Each is described below.

Measurable constructs

Constructs are the concepts that collectively provide a causal explanation or underlying theory. For example, "perceived susceptibility" is one of several constructs in the Health Belief Model (46) and "precontemplation" is a construct in the Stages of Change Model (47). To develop an instrument to measure social capital, we identified and defined four constructs: trust, civic involvement, social engagement and reciprocity.

Trust is the belief that an individual, group or organization can be relied on to act in a consistent, fair, rational and predictable manner – criteria that are of course shaped by the individual's values and beliefs. As used here, trust is defined not as a general sentiment, but rather as a specific trust in something or someone, such as the government, family members or friends, the educational system, etc.

Civic involvement comprises participation in activities that directly or indirectly contribute to a community's overall wellbeing. These include solitary activities such as voting or reading newspapers, as well as interactive activities such as joining organizations that have civic improvement agendas. An informed, active population that contributes time and effort to activities benefiting the entire community would reflect high levels of civic involvement or engagement. A related subcategory might be civic consciousness, expressed in activities that are altruistic and take account of the common good. Markers of civic consciousness would include cleaning up after one's dog during walks in the neighbourhood or supporting recycling efforts.

Social engagement refers to the interactions that foster connections among community members or organizations. These connections include not only the organized groups that characterize many types of civic involvement but also informal connections that have no organized or defined purpose. Knowing or socializing with one's neighbours is one example of social engagement.

Reciprocity refers to the expectation of a return on one's investment: the faith that one's good deeds will be returned in some form. The exchange of resources, good deeds or support need not be immediate or perfectly matched in order to be mutually satisfactory. In fact, a defined exchange may not occur. Indeed, reciprocity may not be an explicit motivator for a person's generous actions. Rather, the expectation that such an exchange would occur if necessary is the important (and measurable) feature of reciprocity. This expectation can be based on one-time or repeated previous experience, or can be a by-product of trust – a belief that a specific individual or organization will act honourably.

Community size

Community health promotion practitioners are familiar with the problems of defining communities. The most natural definition relies on geographical boundaries – post codes, neighbourhoods, school districts and political precincts – that vary in size and homogeneity. In an extensive discourse defining the characteristics of community, Taylor (32) observes:

If community is characterized by shared values and beliefs, direct and many-sided relations, and the practice of reciprocity, then it is clear that communities must be relatively small and stable. In a large and changing mass of people, few relations between individuals can be direct or many-sided, and reciprocity cannot flourish on a wide scale, since its continuation for any length of time requires *some* actual reciprocation, which in turn requires stable relations with known individuals.

Taylor seems to be saying that, if smaller is not better, it is certainly more feasible. Since feasibility was a key factor in this exploratory pilot study, we sought to work with smaller communities with populations of about 20 000.

Units of measurement

Social capital's definition carries within it one of the methodological hurdles for evaluation: the processes among individuals that foster mutual benefit. From an evaluation perspective, this opens a Pandora's box of measurement problems. For example, at what point does individual action yield a measurable outcome at the community level? How do these two measures interact? What is the role of institutions and social networks in generating social capital? From a community health standpoint, each of these – individuals, communities, institutions and social networks – is important to the success of health promotion efforts. As the literature in social capital emphasizes the dual importance of individual and organizational perceptions of social capital, we concluded that exploring measurement strategies for both domains was critical.

Estimating existing levels of social capital

To estimate existing levels of social capital within potential target communities, we tested the following procedure as part of this protocol. We contacted senior officials in a Midwestern health department, and they agreed to be participants and facilitators in the study. They reviewed the theory of social capital and its operational constructs, and were then asked to designate communities that were either high or low in social capital. When the matter of common demographic characteristics was taken into account, two communities were left in the cluster with high social capital, and four remained in the low cluster. We considered this judgement to represent what we call *prima facie* social capital. The local health officers in each of the remaining six communities were asked to ascertain their communities' willingness to participate in a research project to measure social capital. All agreed. Ultimately two communities with similar demographic characteristics were chosen, one with high and one with low *prima facie* social capital.

Verifying the estimates

In an effort to confirm the *prima facie* estimate of social capital, we triangulated data from three sources: structured interviews with key informants and leaders in each community, structured interviews with ten county cooperative extension agents (people employed by a county to provide grassroots technical assistance to local organizations and businesses on agricultural, business and health matters), who served as external observers, and a content analysis assessing the constructs of social capital reported in selected newspapers in the two communities.

We conducted face-to-face, structured interviews with 25 stakeholders in each community. Identified by the directors of the local health departments, the stakeholders were people recognized as community leaders representing the following sectors: business, health, news media, religion, social and health services (private, public and voluntary) and local government. The Appendix lists the general questions used. In addition, most of the questions in the structured interview guide were also asked of five cooperative extension agents from the two counties in which the communities were located.

The content analysis was purely quantitative. Front-page and editorial articles were read and coded according to the presence or absence of mentions of the four social capital constructs and code counts were generated for each construct in each paper.

We analysed the data generated from these three assessments to ascertain whether the selected communities varied in their levels of social capital in the direction predicted by the *prima facie* estimates.

Designing a questionnaire

To assess individual levels of social capital, a quantitative questionnaire was designed using a modification of the protocol recommended by Windsor et al. *(48)*. First, a pool of 40 questions was created. These questions were linked conceptually to the four constructs of social capital and were based either on previous questionnaires or on theoretical assumptions underlying social capital. Measurement examples frequently cited in the literature included: voter turnout; newspaper readership; the number of social action groups, youth groups and day-care centres in a community; perceptions of trust in institutions and people; personal commitment to the common good; and the perceived strength of social networks in families.

We convened a panel of international experts in behavioural science and health promotion to review and critique the questions, and used the panel's recommendations to make additions, deletions and revisions. These collective steps provided a level of content validity for the questionnaire *(49)*.

The scale was field-tested in the two selected communities. Random-digit dialling was used to contact 400 respondents (18 years or older) in each community.

Fig. 19.1 provides a schematic outline of the research design used in this study. The triangles marked A and B represent the combined findings through triangulation from the structured interviews and the newspaper content analysis in the two study towns. Findings from telephone surveys in the two communities are labelled C and D. A comparison of data from A and B addresses the first research question, verifying differing levels of *prima facie* social capital.

450

It also reveals perceptions of social capital at the organizational level in the two communities. Comparison of A with C and of B with D addressed the second research question: whether the population-level measure of social capital reflected the *prima facie* and organization-level assessments of social capital.

Fig. 19.1. Measuring social capital in two Midwestern communities

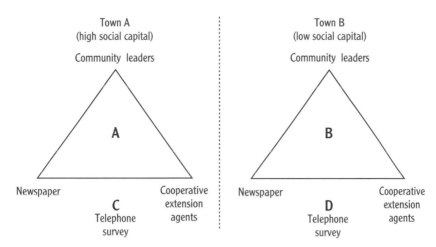

Town A
(high social capital)

Community leaders

A

Newspaper

C
Telephone
survey

Cooperative
extension
agents

Town B
(low social capital)

Community leaders

B

Newspaper

D
Telephone
survey

Cooperative
extension
agents

Findings and implications

In general, the data triangulation used to verify the estimates of social capital confirmed the hypothesized difference between the communities. Interview data provided the strongest confirmatory evidence. Although evidence from the newspaper content analysis was less confirmatory, there was a statistically significant difference confirming the estimate for one construct of social capital: trust.

Comparison of findings from the data triangulation and the telephone survey was the primary method used to assess the survey's validity. This comparison was inconclusive in that the results of the survey did not reflect the differences shown by the interview data.

Notes on content analysis

The newspaper content analysis confirmed the estimates for trust, but not for the other three constructs of social capital. While the analysis provided some useful insights, its overall value for assessing social capital at the community level remains in question. Because the constructs are inherently complex and difficult to define, reliability between coders, an essential aspect of any valid content analysis, was difficult to establish.

Further, we discovered that newspapers rarely report on certain constructs, such as social engagement and reciprocity. This reduces the validity of content

451

analysis as a method to assess them. Finally, newspapers as data sources are especially prone to historical effects. The time period of sampling can lead to a biased data pool. These factors made it difficult to use content analysis for a valid assessment of social capital levels in this study.

Explaining the results of the telephone survey

One of the central questions explored in this study was, if the level of social capital in a given community were known, whether the mean responses to a valid questionnaire, administered to a random sample of a community's population, would serve as a proxy indicator of this level. As stated earlier, the differences revealed by the structured interviews with community leaders were not reflected in the telephone surveys assessing the attitudes of community members. Among several possible explanations for this finding, we highlight two.

First, the population questionnaire might have consisted of items that were not sufficiently discriminating. Item selection was based on three criteria: content validity confirmed by the expert panel, adaptation of most of the items from previously published and tested instruments, and confirmation by those administering the telephone interviews that the process was going smoothly with no indication of confusion among interviewers or respondents. In retrospect, these criteria may have been insufficient. More extensive pre-testing of the instrument might have eliminated this problem before survey administration.

Observations by Tourangeau & Rasinski (50) provide added perspective on this issue. They note that, when people are asked to respond to attitude questions using a framework that they rarely use or that is not strongly formed, strong context effects and measurement error are introduced. The towns selected for this study are well defined, stable communities with rich cultural histories. Visitors frequenting local shops and restaurants would discover the residents to be friendly, pleasant and engaging; they would probably notice nothing unusual about either community. From a pragmatic perspective, residents of these two towns are not likely to consider issues of trust, reciprocity, etc. on a daily basis. Thus, they probably have not made fully formed judgements on these issues; this makes their responses more context sensitive. In contrast, community leaders, actively involved in the day-to-day operation of community organizations and government, must continually adjust their attitudes about social capital according to their experiences interacting with other leaders and their respective organizations. Thus, their responses may be less prone to context effects, as their judgements are more readily used and more strongly formed.

Measures of social capital at the population level may require that questions be framed within the context of a specific issue, rather than the more general approach used in our study. For example, Sampson et al. (38) examined the association between a dimension of social capital (community efficacy) in a neighbourhood setting with a specific dependent variable: violence by young people. At a minimum, this raises concerns about the universality of social capital constructs.

452

A second possible explanation for the lack of association between the interview and the survey results is that organization- and population-level social capital are interdependent parts of a larger model of social capital. Temkin & Rohe *(51)* propose a model of neighbourhood change that highlights two operational levels of social capital: sociocultural milieu and institutional infrastructure. They define sociocultural milieu as the manifestation of three characteristics: residents' identity with their neighbourhood, neighbours' degree of social interaction and residents' links with people outside the neighbourhood. Institutional infrastructure is defined as the degree to which local organizations work to benefit the neighbourhood. In our study, findings revealing differences between perceptions of social capital at the organizational and population levels can be interpreted in a model similar to that described by Temkin & Rohe.

Fig. 19.2 presents a social capital model for community-based health initiatives extrapolated from the empirical observations made in our study. Several assumptions were made in constructing this model.

1. The ultimate outcome (indicator of success) of community-based health promotion programmes is evidence of improvement in health and the quality of life in the community.
2. The presence of high trust and cooperation between organizations strengthens the probability that a community based-health promotion programme will succeed.
3. Collaboration among organizations varies across communities.
4. The population's perceptions of social capital vary across communities.

Fig. 19.2. A social capital model of community change

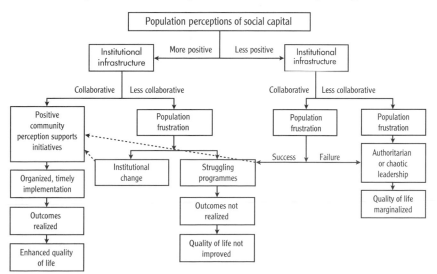

The flow of the model (Fig. 19.2) follows these assumptions in reverse. It begins with the notion that the level of a community's social capital, as perceived by the residents, may be high or low. In either case, that perception is affected by the extent to which the community's institutional infrastructure (its public, private and voluntary organizations) shows trust and cooperation in efforts to address issues of mutual interest. The model suggests that, when the community's perception of social capital is positive and the organizational infrastructure is cooperative (as in the left side of the chart), the probability for successful implementation of a community-based initiative is substantially increased. It follows that well planned community initiatives ultimately enhance the quality of residents' lives.

If the community's perception of social capital is positive and the organizational infrastructure is less cooperative, however, the dissonance creates a level of frustration that, if not addressed, can hamper programmes, making them struggle, fail to reach their goals or do little to improve the quality of life. Thus, community-based initiatives are at risk in the absence of either a positive perception of social capital or a cooperative organizational infrastructure (centre or right side of the chart). Communities capable of acknowledging low reserves of social capital can take the planning and organizational steps needed to make positive changes.

Conclusions

Our practical and research experience with community-based public health interventions, combined with our understanding of social capital theory, lead us to the following interrelated conclusions.

1. Community-based intervention is an inherently interdependent concept; that is, theoretically sound intervention methods and tactics, properly administered, will be effective to the extent that the community has organizational entities and systems supportive of the enterprise and that those entities and systems are activated.
2. This activation depends in part on the extent to which relevant community entities and systems trust and collaborate with one another and to which the community (individuals and organizations) is aware of, values and trusts the proposed intervention.
3. Because the notions of activated organizational entities and trust are fundamental constructs of social capital theory, measures of social capital within the context of community-based intervention may reveal important insights into questions of the feasibility, timing, methodology and effectiveness of intervention.

Intuitively, trust, civic involvement, social engagement and reciprocity are principles common to both community health promotion and social capital. Although the measurement of these constructs must be adapted to the cultural nuances of a given region, the principles of social capital appear to operate irrespective of geography, culture, language or socioeconomic status. This may in part explain the emergence of a cross-national agenda for social capital research manifested by preliminary studies of the relationships between social capital and community health strategies that are now underway in Australia, Canada, Spain, the United Kingdom and the United States. We have made contact and started collaboration with scholars and practitioners in all these countries.

From an evaluation research perspective, the pilot study described above focuses on the notion of social capital primarily as an independent variable: that is, exploring the extent to which it may influence the effectiveness of community health promotion programmes. One could, however, investigate social capital as a dependent variable; that is, examining the extent to which action for health promotion promotes, enhances or creates social capital as a legitimate outcome. Regardless of the tack one takes, measurement is the critical task at this stage.

Measuring social capital: policy implications

Globally, most of the funding to support the application of community-based health promotion strategies continues to be tied to a specific health category: heart disease, asthma, tobacco, HIV/AIDS, domestic violence, etc. In these instances, with the notable exception of forming coalitions and organizational partnerships, the implicit funding policy is that resources are justifiable to the extent that they will be spent on action directly linked to the resolution of the health problem in question. In spite of the extensive literature pointing to the social, economic and political determinants of contemporary health problems, resources are rarely earmarked for building or strengthening the community capacity that appears to be so crucial to the effective implementation of community health promotion. This is somewhat akin to the label "batteries not included": selling a functional product without the energy source essential to its use.

Two possible explanations for this situation come to mind. Funding agencies either are not aware or do not believe that such capacity is needed, or believe that such activity is inappropriate for health funding. If valid measurement can show that social capital or some aspect of community capacity is clearly linked to the effective application of community-based public health programmes, funding agencies would have valuable information justifying a re-examination of current policies. Specifically, public, private and philanthropic funding agencies would be able to make more informed decisions about the most productive ways to contribute health-related funding to a given community – either to bolster the capacity required for successful interventions or to move directly to the interventions themselves.

References

1. GREEN, L.W. & KREUTER, M.M. *Health promotion planning: an educational and environmental approach*, 2nd ed. Mountain View, Mayfield, 1991.
2. EVANS, R.G. ET AL. *Why are some people healthy and others not? The determinants of health of populations.* New York, Aldine de Gruyter, 1994.
3. GERSTEIN, R. ET AL. *Nurturing health: a framework on the determinants of health.* Toronto, Premier's Council on Health Strategy, 1991.
4. KREUTER, M.W. Human behaviour and cancer: forget the magic bullet! *Cancer,* **72**(3): 996–1001 (1993).
5. KOTCHEN, J.M. ET AL. The impact of a high blood pressure control program on hypertension control and CVD mortality. *Journal of the American Medical Association,* **257**: 3382–3386 (1987).
6. CENTERS FOR DISEASE CONTROL. Increasing breast cancer screening among the medically underserved, Dade County, FL. *Morbidity and mortality weekly report,* **40**(16): 261–263 (1991).
7. PUSKA, P. ET AL. The community-based strategy to prevent coronary heart disease: conclusions from the ten years of the North Karelia Project. *Annual review of public health,* **6**: 147–193 (1985).
8. VARTIAINEN, E. ET AL. Prevention of non-communicable diseases: risk factors in youth – the North Karelia Youth Project (1984–1988). *Health promotion,* **1**(3): 269–283 (1986).
9. LANDO, H.A. ET AL. Community impact of a localized smoking cessation contest. *American journal of public health,* **80**: 601–603 (1990).
10. PIERCE, J.P. ET AL. Long-term effectiveness of mass media led antismoking campaigns in Australia. *American journal of public health,* **80**: 565–569 (1990).
11. FISHBEIN M. Great expectations, or do we ask too much from community-level interventions? *American journal of public health,* **86**(8): 1075–1076 (1996).
12. HANCOCK, L. ET AL. Community action for health promotion: a review of methods and outcomes. *American journal of preventive medicine,* **13**: 229–239 (1992).
13. COMMIT RESEARCH GROUP. Community intervention trial for smoking cessation (COMMIT). II. Changes in adult cigarette smoking prevalence. *American journal of public health,* **85**: 193–200 (1995).
14. SCHWAB, M. & SYME, S.L. On paradigms, community participation, and the future of public health. *American journal of public health,* **87**(12): 2050 (1997).
15. WINKELSTEIN, W. Editorial. Eras, paradigms and the future of epidemiology. *American journal of public health,* **86**: 621–622 (1996).
16. SUSSER, M. The logic in ecological. II. The logic of design. *American journal of public health,* **84**: 830–835 (1994).

17. McKINLEY, J.B. The promotion of health through planned socio-political change: challenges for research and policy. *Social science and medicine*, **36**: 109–117 (1993).
18. PEARCE, N. Traditional epidemiology, modern epidemiology, and public health. *American journal of public health*, **86**: 678–683 (1996).
19. PUSKA, P. ET AL. *The North Karelia Project: 20 year results and experiences.* Helsinki, National Public Health Institute, 1995.
20. PUSKA, P. ET AL. Use of lay opinion leaders to promote the diffusion of health innovations in a community programme: lessons learned from the North Karelia project. *Bulletin of the World Health Organization*, **64**(3): 437–446 (1986).
21. ENG, E. & PARKER, E. Measuring community competence in the Mississippi Delta: the interface between program evaluation and empowerment. *Health education quarterly*, **21**(2): 199–220 (1994).
22. Creating capacity: a research agenda for public education. *Health education quarterly*, **22**(3) (1995).
23. BOWEN, D.J. ET AL. Analyzing communities for readiness to change. *American journal of health behavior*, **21**: 289–298 (1997).
24. WALLERSTEIN, N. & BERNSTEIN, E. Introduction to community empowerment, participatory education and health. *Health education quarterly*, **21**(2): 141–148 (1994).
25. GREEN, L.W. ET AL. *Study of participatory research in health promotion. Review and recommendations for the development of participatory research in health promotion in Canada.* Ottawa, Royal Society of Canada, 1995.
26. COLEMAN, J. *Foundations of social theory.* Cambridge, Harvard University Press, 1990.
27. PUTNAM, R.D. The prosperous community: social capital and public life. *The American prospect*, **13**: 33–42 (1993).
28. PUTNAM, R.D. *Making democracy work: civic traditions in modern Italy.* Princeton, Princeton University Press, 1993.
29. COLEMAN, J. & HOFFER, T. *Public and private high schools: the impact of communities.* New York, Basic Books, 1987.
30. COLEMAN, J.S. Social capital in the creation of human capital. *American journal of sociology*, **94**(Suppl.): 95–120 (1988).
31. COX, E. *A truly civil society. 1995 Boyer Lectures.* Sydney, Australian Broadcasting Company Books, 1995.
32. TAYLOR, M. *Community, anarchy and community.* London, Cambridge University Press, 1982.
33. PUTNAM, R.D. Bowling alone: America's declining social capital. *Journal of democracy*, **2**: 65–78 (1995).
34. PUTNAM, R.D. *Bowling alone: the collapse and revival of American community.* New York, Simon and Schuster, 2000.
35. LEMANN, N. Kicking in groups. *Atlantic monthly*, April 1996.

36. SCHUDSON, M. What if civic life didn't die? *American prospect*, **25**: 17–20 (1996).
37. KAWACHI, I. ET AL. Social capital, income inequality, and mortality. *American journal of public health*, **87**(9): 1491–1498 (1997).
38. SAMPSON, R.J. ET AL. Neighbourhoods and violent crime: a multilevel study of collective efficacy. *Science*, **277**: 918–924 (1997).
39. RUNYAN, D.K. ET AL. Children who prosper in unfavourable environments: the relationship to social capital. *Pediatrics,* **101**: 12–18 (1998).
40. PERRY, C.L. ET AL. Project Northland: outcomes of a community-wide alcohol use prevention program during early adolescence. *American journal of public health*, **86**: 956–965 (1996).
41. WECHSLER, H. & WEITZMAN, E.R. Editorial. Community solutions to community problems: preventing adolescent alcohol abuse. *American journal of public health*, **86**: 923–925 (1996).
42. HIGGINS, D.L. *Social capital and HIV intervention* [Thesis]. Nottingham, University of Nottingham, 1997.
43. PORTES, A. & LANDOLDT, P. The downside of social capital. *American prospect*, **26**: 18–21 (1996).
44. CARR, M. *Social capital, civil society, and social transformation.* Vancouver, British Columbia, 1996.
45. GOODMAN, R.M. ET AL. An attempt to identify and define the dimensions of community capacity to provide a basis for measurement. *Health education and behavior*, **25**(3): 258–278 (1998).
46. ROSENSTOCK, I.M. & KIRSCHT, J.P. The Health Belief Model and personal health behavior. *Health education monographs*, **2**: 470–473 (1974).
47. PROCHASKA, J.O. ET AL. In search of how people change: applications to addictive behaviors. *American psychologist,* **47**: 1102–1114 (1992).
48. WINDSOR, R.A. ET AL. *Evaluation of health promotion programs.* Mountain View, Mayfield Publishing, 1984, pp. 205–212.
49. GREEN, L.W. & LEWIS, F.M. *Measurement and evaluation in health education and health promotion.* Mountain View, Mayfield Publishing, 1986, pp. 106.
50. TOURANGEAU, R. & RASINSKI, K.A. Cognitive processes underlying context effects in attitude measurement. *Psychological bulletin*, **103**(3): 299–314 (1988).
51. TEMKIN, K. & ROHE, W. Neighborhood and urban policy. *Journal of planning education and research*, **15**: 159–170 (1996).

Appendix. Community key informant structured interview: general

Make appropriate introduction.

We are conducting a study to help us better understand how people and organizations in communities work together and _____ is one of the study communities. Because of your position or reputation as someone whose opinion is important in this community, we are interested in your insights about the institutions and people in _____.

The information we obtain from these interviews **will not** be coded by your name. Once we complete approximately 25 interviews, we will aggregate the information and report it as the general perspective "key informant leaders in the community".

Before any data are formally presented for academic purposes, we will report our findings back to leaders in _____ in a meeting with community members.

Interview questions

1. First I'd like to get your thoughts on children growing up in _____. What would you say are the *best* things about this area for raising kids? PROBE UP TO THREE: (Is there anything else?)

_____

_____

2. What would you say are the *worst* things about _____ for raising kids? PROBE UP TO THREE: (Is there anything else?)

_____

_____

To what extent do you agree or disagree to the following statements?

3. The faith community (religious organizations) in _____ is really active in providing programs and offering support for youth in trouble and helping those in need.
   SA   A   NS   DA   SDA
   [SA = strongly agree, A = agree, NS = not sure, DA = disagree, SDA = strongly disagree]
   Comment?

4. There is really no problem getting people to do volunteer work in _____ .
   SA   A   NS   DA   SDA
   Comment?

459

Now I am going to ask about contacts you may have had with some officials in _____ *during the last year*, that is, from about February 1997 to now. For each position I ask you about, please tell me if you have had *direct contact* with any person holding that position during the last year. **I'm interested in contact you've had "officially" – as a member of one organization to another, and related to some aspect of community life in _____ . By direct contact we mean contact by telephone, in writing, or in person.**

5. A school principal?
   YES   NO   DON'T KNOW   REFUSED
   If yes, nature of contact? Results?

6. A chair of a local school board?
   YES   NO   DON'T KNOW   REFUSED
   If yes, nature of contact? Results?

7. During the last year, have you had any direct contact with a director of a neighborhood business association or local Chamber of Commerce in _____ ? **Again, by direct contact we mean contact by telephone, in writing, or in-person.**
   YES   NO   DON'T KNOW   REFUSED
   If yes, nature of contact? Results?

8. An owner or manager of a realty company in _____ ?
   YES   NO   DON'T KNOW   REFUSED
   If yes, nature of contact? Results?

9. An officer of a bank or savings and loan?
   YES   NO   DON'T KNOW   REFUSED
   If yes, nature of contact? Results?

10. The editors of either of the papers in _____ ?
    YES   NO   DON'T KNOW   REFUSED
    If yes, nature of contact? Results?

11. A director of a hospital or medical clinic?
    YES   NO   DON'T KNOW   REFUSED
    If yes, nature of contact? Results?

12. The director of a social service agency or organization?
    YES   NO   DON'T KNOW   REFUSED
    If yes, nature of contact? Results?

13. The mayor (or city manager) himself or herself or a high-ranking mayoral staff member?
    YES   NO   DON'T KNOW   REFUSED
    If yes, nature of contact? Results?

14. The local Chief of Police or another high-ranking Police Department official?
    YES   NO   DON'T KNOW   REFUSED
    If yes, nature of contact? Results?

15. During the last year, have you had any direct contact with an official from the _____ County Health Department?
    YES   NO   DON'T KNOW   REFUSED
    If yes, nature of contact? Results?

16. A state representative or legislator from _____ ?
    YES   NO   DON'T KNOW   REFUSED
    If yes, nature of contact? Results?

17. Throughout history we have used many different indicators to assess the quality of life of the places where we live. For example, the mortality rate, maternal mortality rate, percent of people who are employed, access to health services, levels of pollution, quality of the weather, and so on.
    Let's say we added another indicator that measured the three factors: (1) the level of trust people had in one another, (2) the level of trust people have in their community institutions, and (3) the willingness of people to work collaboratively to get things done for the mutual benefit of the community.
A. On a scale of 1–5 where 5 = a high level of trust among people, and 1 = a low level of trust, what number would you assign for _____ ?_____
B. On a scale of 1–5 where 5 = a high level of trust people have for their community institutions, and 1 = a low level of trust for those institutions, what number would you assign for _____ ? _____
C. On a scale of 1–5 where 5 = a high level of willingness to work collaboratively, and 1 = a low level willingness to work collaboratively, what number would you assign for _____ ? _____

18. To what extent do people in _____ trust local government to:

		Very much				Not at all	
a.	respond to community needs	5	4	3	2	1	R
b.	be free from corruption	5	4	3	2	1	R
c.	try to be fair	5	4	3	2	1	R
d.	keep citizens informed	5	4	3	2	1	R

19. With respect to news and "goings on" in _____ , how accurate is the coverage by the _____ ?

VA   SA   NVA   R

(VA = very accurate; S = somewhat accurate; NVA = not very accurate; R = refused)

20. Now I am going to describe a hypothetical community called Roseville.
"In Roseville, folks may not always agree with one another but, when there's an important issue or problem facing the town, community organizations and the people are willing to pitch in and get the job done."
To what extent do you *agree* with the following statement?

"_____ is a lot like Roseville."   SA   A   NS   D   SD
Note to Interviewer: Score 5 = strongly agree; 4 = agree; 3 = not sure; 2 = disagree; and 1 = strongly disagree. If response is a "4" or "5", ask 20A and 20B. If response is less than "4", skip to 20C.

20A. Please give an example of how _____ is like the hypothetical community of Roseville:

20B. Why do you think the people of _____ are so willing to pitch in and work collaboratively on a problem of mutual concern?

20C. What do you think it might take to enable you to respond a higher number?

20
Case study: the Canadian Heart Health Initiative

Sylvie Stachenko

Introduction

This chapter provides a practical evaluative description of a multilevel, multi-component health promotion strategy to prevent cardiovascular diseases (CVD) in Canada. The context of the evaluation is the Canadian Heart Health Initiative, initiated in 1988 as a systematic, organized approach to CVD prevention that links policy, implementation, research and action to build capacity among numerous partners: the federal and provincial departments of health; voluntary, professional and academic organizations; and the private sector. The aim was to implement a national CVD prevention policy through a combination of:

- research to develop practical knowledge in health promotion through implementing community-based heart health demonstration programmes; and
- work to build capacity for implementation in provinces and communities.

CVD are the main cause of mortality and health care costs in Canada *(1)*, and present an opportunity to make major health gains through organized community prevention initiatives *(2)*. The Canadian approach to CVD prevention follows a public health or population health model *(3)*, and has been built into the existing health system. In this sense, the design of the Initiative differs from demonstration projects for CVD prevention implemented in other countries in the late 1970s and 1980s *(4–7)*. Most of these projects were intended to demonstrate the effectiveness and feasibility of community intervention to prevent CVD, based in universities and funded to support extensive outcome and process evaluations. In contrast, the provincial heart health projects in the Canadian Heart Health Initiative were set up in the public health branches of provincial departments of health, with links to university departments; the evaluation focused on the process of implementing the five-year demonstration programme.

The account of the evaluation process given here refers to the demonstration phase of the federal and provincial heart health programmes, which was completed in 1997. The decentralized management approach and the diversity of provincial heart health protocols presented special methodological challenges, as well as opening avenues of implementation research on health promotion programmes on other topics. The current phase of the Canadian Heart Health Initiative focuses on the dissemination and deployment of successful interventions.

The Canadian Heart Health Initiative

The hallmark of CVD is their multifactorial nature; lifestyles, socioeconomic environment and genetic–environmental interactions influence the major risk factors: smoking, high blood pressure, dyslipidaemias, obesity, diabetes and physical inactivity. This has two key implications for policy development. First, dealing with CVD, whether at the individual or at the population level, requires attention to the various risk factors and their determinants. Second, mounting interventions that address the lifestyle and environmental determinants and provide access to preventive health services requires action by both the health and non-health sectors. For these reasons, heart health exemplifies a challenge that needs to be addressed by combining health promotion and disease prevention.

The Initiative systematically implements a multilevel (national, provincial and community) strategy to build capacity to prevent CVD. It may be described as a linkage system that relates the national, provincial and community levels *(8,9)*. It was conceived in five phases, from policy development to dissemination and deployment, over a period of 15 years. The Initiative is co-funded by Health Canada, through the National Health Research Development Program, and by the ten provincial departments of health. The Heart and Stroke Foundation of Canada and its provincial affiliates are key partners. The Initiative aims to exploit the synergies between the health promotion and disease prevention approaches that are most useful in reducing CVD risk and its determinants *(10)*.

Policy consensus

The Initiative originated in the commissioning in 1986, by the Provincial Conference of Deputy Ministers of Health, of a strategy for CVD prevention and control. Contrary to some policy development exercises, which focus on the writing of a report (sometimes by a consultant), in this case the Federal–Provincial Working Group on Cardiovascular Disease Prevention and Control consulted extensively across the country. Its membership represented Health Canada, three provincial departments of health and the Heart and Stroke Foundation. During 1986 and 1987 the Group visited all provincial and territorial capitals and elicited comments on the issues to be addressed and strategies to be followed, using as a backdrop a presentation on the epidemiology of CVD, the case for prevention, potential strategies and potential stakeholders. During the consultation period, the Group met with representatives of over 100 stakeholder health agencies and organizations in the private and public sectors. On

464

the basis of this work, the Group prepared the report *Promoting heart health in Canada (11),* which was approved by the Conference of Deputy Ministers of Health. In a sense, the consultation process pre-sold the key recommendations to the stakeholders that had been involved.

CVD risk factor database
The federal–provincial partnership enabled the implementation of standardized provincial heart health surveys, leading to the Canadian Heart Health Database on CVD risk factors. In 1985, Nova Scotia became the first province to carry out the survey *(12).* The protocol from this survey was made available to other provinces, and public health personnel from Nova Scotia helped to support their surveys. The key, consistent finding from each province was that about two thirds of adults had one or more of the risk factors for CVD. This provided a scientific base for the proposition that CVD prevention ought to be considered a public health matter that primarily needed a health promotion approach. Obviously, an issue affecting most of the population could not be addressed through a clinical preventive approach alone; hence the strong community orientation of the provincial demonstration programmes for heart health that followed *(13).*

Commitment of the public health system
The implementation of the provincial heart health surveys by the public health system was significant for policy and subsequent partnership development. The public health nurses who were trained to carry out the surveys acquired practical knowledge about heart health, and were sensitized to prevention issues. Many of them later championed the programme in the demonstration phase. Because provincial departments of health carried out their surveys with limited coordination from Health Canada, provinces took ownership of the results and ran with the ball, so to speak. The survey results were submitted for public review by independent scientific panels that built bridges between health care practitioners and the scientific community. After the surveys were completed, heart health demonstration programmes were launched with much publicity in all provinces. Thus, the surveys' implementation methods, their results and the review process strengthened the consensus on a public health approach to CVD prevention, facilitated the development of partnerships for heart health and created commitment in the public health system to the prevention of chronic disease, in addition to traditional programmes to control communicable diseases.

All the provinces had completed the provincial surveys by 1992; the results were subsequently integrated into the Canadian Heart Health Database in the Department of Community Health at Memorial University, in St John's, Newfoundland. The data were published in 1992 *(14).* Federal–provincial cooperation had made possible the creation of a national database in a way that linked policy, epidemiological research and political support to follow through with intervention programmes.

The demonstration phase and development of partnerships

The provincial heart health demonstration programmes, co-funded by the federal and provincial departments of health, were the key instrument for translating policy into practice. The demonstration phase spanned the years 1989–1997, and provinces joined at different times. The provincial programmes built on the good will and epidemiological information base created by the provincial surveys. The federal and provincial departments of health established the following conditions for funding the provincial programmes:

- a focus on a public health approach;
- the setting up of provincial intersectoral coalitions to support programme development and implementation;
- evaluation of the process of intervention as an essential component; and
- review of the intervention and the evaluation protocols by a scientific team in site visits arranged by the National Health Research and Development Program of Health Canada.

In retrospect, the decision to put limited but concrete financial resources on the table to follow through on *Promoting heart health in Canada (11)* seems to have been instrumental in ensuring that the policy document did not gather dust, but served as a catalyst for provincial action. In addition, the provinces' freedom to join the Initiative when they deemed it appropriate was significant for the quality of the partnerships built. The co-funding arrangements and flexibility in the definition of the project intervention mix of the provincial programmes contributed to the good functioning of the national coalitions. The Conference of Principal Investigators of Heart Health is one such coalition, which also includes representatives of the Heart and Stroke Foundation of Canada. Typical components of the various provincial heart health programmes have been documented, and include strategies for public education, community mobilization, healthy public policy and preventive services *(13)*.

The conditions for funding had two important implications for implementation. First, they created focal points with clear responsibility for the continued development and implementation of the heart health policy: the provincial departments of health. Second, they encouraged the process of partnership development from the beginning. While the terms and conditions for the provincial coalitions varied, the partnership approach became the *modus operandi* of heart health programmes in the provincial and the community demonstration areas.

Evaluation approach

The main aim of the Initiative is to develop provincial- and community-level capacity to address CVD prevention through health promotion. Accordingly, the provincial heart health demonstration programmes concentrated on feasibility and capacity building. Following a model proposed by Nutbeam *(15)*, the evaluation of the Canadian Hearth Health Initiative focused on process, rather than on outcome, an approach endorsed by others working for CVD prevention in communities *(16,17)*. Evaluation took place at both the national and provincial levels.

Provincial evaluation protocols and information gathering

The principal investigators of the provincial programmes jointly adopted process guidelines for evaluation, with some coordination from the national level and technical consultation of academic experts as needed *(18)*. The guidelines proposed goals for health, as well as health systems, and served as a basis for the preparation of the provincial evaluation protocols that were reviewed in site visits by Canadian and foreign scientists. The guidelines offered a menu of process indicators for the key strategies that had been identified in *Promoting heart health in Canada (11)*.

The guidelines were structured as goals of various types (for health, environmental change and the health system). A key tenet was to keep the evaluation practical and affordable: no more than 3–6 indicators for any one project were envisaged to be tackled. While this was to be the norm for most projects, the guidelines recognized that the provincial programmes might wish to conduct evaluation research on certain projects. Thus, a two-tier system was adopted that provided for in-depth evaluation of some projects and a simpler tracking system for most.

Consistent with the guidelines *(18)*, each of the provincial heart health programmes developed its own evaluation plans, typically involving stakeholders in defining the indicators for the projects that were subject to review by scientific teams. While following the guidelines, the provincial programmes collected information for process evaluation according to different schemes and sets of indicators. Nevertheless, provinces shared considerable information on approaches to evaluation. This resulted in the selection of a range of common indicators to document and track the projects in the Initiative.

The evaluation information for provincial and community projects came from a variety of sources: instruments designed *ad hoc*, minutes of meetings, quarterly reports, informant interviews, surveys (to track social marketing campaigns, for example) and administrative and financial records. Some provinces established computerized databases to handle qualitative information, a development that added considerable capacity for generating reports and providing quick feedback to communities and stakeholders. In addition to project-related process indicators data, the provincial programmes carried out a series of provincial and community needs assessments and community resource inventories. These were used to identify contextual factors and to determine changes in the social and policy environments of the programmes.

Core evaluation: Canadian process evaluation database

With a decentralized process evaluation of the provincial heart health programmes for the demonstration phase, the challenge was to aggregate the information gathered at the provincial level so as to create a national picture of the Initiative as a whole. The provincial programmes adopted different sets of process evaluation indicators, as their protocols had different intervention mixes. This necessitated the retrospective identification of core indicators, common to all provinces, to establish a basis for documenting the type, extent and nature of the projects implemented by the provincial programmes.

In a consensual, participatory two-year process, the principal investigators agreed on a set of core process indicators that were meaningful in describing inputs, processes and intermediate outcomes (outputs). All the provinces collected data on them. Training manuals were prepared and training sessions were offered to all the provincial heart health coordinators who served as information collectors. The core process evaluation data were collected between 1994 and 1996, and the period for which activities were documented and information obtained was 1989–1995.

The data were collected, verified and assembled in a qualitative evaluation database located at Memorial University. The database contains information on inputs and processes, and selected impact indicators such as programme outreach. Programme inputs included: information on project costs (direct and indirect) and types (financial and in-kind) and sources of contributions (public, private and voluntary sectors; health and non-health sectors). The information obtained on process indicators was categorized according to the strategies used: public education, enhancing access to appropriate health services, community mobilization, public health system leadership and healthy public policy.

In addition to the core process indicators, the principal investigators were asked to reflect on various aspects of the implementation. In consultation with their teams, they prepared written responses on the following topics:

- contextual influences, such as political climate, economy and health care reform;
- resources, including volunteers, staff and resource mobilization;
- organization and management, including leadership and functioning of coalitions;
- processes, including the selection of demonstration communities, integration of strategies, linkage with other health issues, strategic and operational planning, and partnership development;
- evaluation, including experience with process evaluation in provinces and communities;
- technical support;
- perceptions of success and barriers to implementation, and reference to the most and least successful projects; and
- the legacy of the demonstration projects.

Telephone interviews were conducted with the principal investigators to clarify the written submissions.

Analysis of the process evaluation information

While the data gathered at the national, provincial and community levels were being analysed, a preliminary report was presented at the 4th International Conference on Preventive Cardiology in 1997 for the core indicators gathered from 302 projects between 1989 and 1995. It identified public education and community mobilization as the most commonly used strategies, and noted that the projects overwhelmingly focused on determinants of behavioural risk factors (such as poor diet and physical inactivity) rather than biological risk factors (such as hypertension and diabetes).

Projects set goals for both behaviour and systems; the latter included the establishment of coalitions, implementation, organizational capacity, infrastructure, sustainability and the dissemination and institutionalization of interventions. The vast majority of the projects involved action on more than one risk factor and had more than two partners, attesting to the integrated approach that heart health is supposed to bring to risk reduction and to the intersectoral and partnership model for implementation.

The resource inputs indicated that provincial departments of health contributed 44% of the resources (financial or in-kind); Health Canada, 26% (mostly financial); and voluntary agencies and the private sector, the remaining 30%. Of the total funds allocated to the Canadian Heart Health Initiative, 30% was directed to evaluation.

The qualitative database has been analysed, but no report has yet been made. The treatment of the information in the database, however, proved to be a challenge that showed the need to acquire capacity to analyse and aggregate qualitative information from process evaluation.

Conclusions

The Canadian Heart Health Initiative has followed a participatory model of evaluation, focusing on process and the acquisition of practical knowledge to implement integrated approaches to health promotion and disease prevention.

The multilevel organization of the Initiative, made possible by the federal–provincial partnership, has provided a context for policy-makers, health professionals and community coalitions to work together on the systematic implementation of the cardiovascular health policy. Coalitions and networks have proved to be a significant asset in obtaining policy support, access to target populations and resources from various sectors.

There is evidence that the linkage of the provincial heart health programmes to the provincial public health systems supports the sustainability and institutionalization of interventions. The maintenance of the co-funding arrangements by the provincial departments of health, over ten years after their inception and despite economic constraints, reflects the value that the departments place on the Initiative as an instrument to enhance capacity in health promotion.

While the long-term impact of the Initiative cannot be foreseen, some factors have favoured the development and implementation of the policy and attendant partnerships.

1. A broad consensus on health policy was developing in Canada in 1986, when consultation on the CVD policy started. The Ottawa Charter for Health Promotion *(19)* and the framework for achieving health for all in Canada *(20)* were published at that time, and set the scene for the type of intersectoral approaches needed to implement the CVD population strategy.
2. CVD are an entry point to demonstrate the value of joint work by health promotion and disease prevention. The scientific basis for CVD prevention, at the clinical and population levels, is strong. Descriptive and interventional epidemiology in CVD supports evidence-based decision-making.
3. The consultative approach followed in the development of *Promoting heart health in Canada (11)* built consensus among and commitment in all public health departments that participated in the heart health surveys and in the subsequent demonstration and dissemination phases of the Initiative.
4. The federal initiative to allocate some financial resources, to follow up this report, was probably a key factor in the provincial buy-in and will continue to be crucial in ensuring sustainability.
5. The development of a national database through individual provincial surveys gave ownership of the Initiative to the provinces, and facilitated the follow-up demonstration phase in each province.
6. Partnership became the *modus operandi* of the Initiative at the national, provincial and community levels. Partnerships have also been developed at the international level.
7. The flexibility offered to the provinces in designing the demonstration and dissemination programmes has provided a rich variety of interventions, which are being analysed and should provide a valuable knowledge base to support health promotion interventions. The Initiative now serves as a platform for dissemination research.
8. The decentralization and flat organizational structure of the Initiative have minimized administrative barriers and enabled flexibility in and rapid transfers of knowledge across provincial heart health programmes.
9. A most important component has been the attention given to technology transfer through site visits by and consultations with Canadian and other scientists.
10. The co-funding arrangements have ensured commitment to and the sustainability of the partnerships, and considerably enhanced the resources available.
11. The core evaluation of the Initiative has shown a dearth of literature on the evaluation of multilevel initiatives that combine health promotion and disease prevention strategies. Methodology needs to be developed to study

linkage systems, the sustainability of partnerships and the dissemination of interventions and implementation processes.

The provincial heart health programmes have entered the dissemination research phase, in keeping with the prevalent policy view that knowledge of CVD is sufficient for prevention and that the challenge is implementation *(21)* and making use of best practices *(22)*. The dissemination phase of the Initiative was launched in 1995, at the time of the first Canadian conference on dissemination research. Dissemination research was defined as the study of variables and processes that mediate the uptake of heart health programmes by jurisdictions, organizations and communities *(23)*. The study of processes of capacity building figures prominently in the dissemination protocols, other issues for study are:

1. the economics of delivery of interventions;
2. the development of models and interventions that can be widely deployed at reasonable cost; and
3. the identification of the organizational configurations that best support wide implementation of good health promotion practices *(24–27)*.

The research platform built by the Initiative provides a context for pursuing the study of the implementation, dissemination and deployment of health promotion and disease prevention interventions.

References

1. REEDER, B. ET AL., ED. *Heart disease and stroke in Canada*. Ottawa, Heart and Stroke Foundation of Canada, 1997.
2. VARTIAINEN, E. ET AL. Changes in risk factors explain changes in mortality from ischaemic heart disease in Finland. *British medical journal*, **309**: 23 (1994).
3. ROSE, G. *The strategy of preventive medicine*. Oxford, Oxford University Press, 1992.
4. FARQUHAR, J.W. ET AL. Community studies of cardiovascular disease prevention. *In*: Kaplan, N.M. & Stamler, G., ed. *Prevention of coronary heart disease: practical management of risk factors*. Philadelphia, Saunders, 1983.
5. LEFEBVRE, R.C. ET AL. Theory and delivery of health programming in the community: the Pawtucket Heart Health Program. *Preventive medicine*, **16**: 80–95 (1987).
6. PUSKA, P. ET AL. The community based strategy to prevent coronary heart disease: conclusions from ten years of the Karelia Project. *Annual review of public health*, **6**: 147–163 (1985).
7. SCHOOLER, C. ET AL. Synthesis of findings and issues from community prevention trials. *In*: Pearson, T.A. & Stone, E., ed. Community trials for

cardiopulmonary health: directions for public health practice, policy and research. *Annals of epidemiology,* 7(Suppl.): S1–S3 (1997).

8. ORLANDI, M.A. Promoting health and preventing disease in health care settings: an analysis of barriers. *Preventive medicine,* **16**: 119–130 (1987).

9. ORLANDI, M. Health promotion technology transfer: organizational perspectives. *Canadian journal of public health,* **87**: S28–S33 (1996).

10. STACHENKO, S. The Canadian Heart Health Initiative: a countrywide cardiovascular disease prevention strategy. *Journal of human hypertension,* **10**(Suppl. 1): S5–S8 (1996).

11. *Promoting heart health in Canada. Report of the Federal–Provincial Working Group on Cardiovascular Disease Prevention and Control.* Ottawa, Department of National Health and Welfare, 1988.

12. MACLEAN, D. & PETRASOVITS A. The prevalence of hyperlipidemia in Nova Scotia. *Nova Scotia medical journal,* **67**(5): 144–147,151 (1988).

13. HEALTH AND WELFARE CANADA. The Canadian Heart Health Initiative: a policy in action. *Health promotion,* **30**(4): 1–19 (1992).

14. SURVEYS RESEARCH GROUP. Canadian heart health surveys. *Canadian Medical Association journal,* **146**(Suppl.): S1969–S2029 (1992).

15. NUTBEAM, D. ET AL. Evaluation in health education: a review of progress, possibilities, and problems. *Journal of epidemiology and community health,* **44**: 83–89 (1990).

16. NUTBEAM, D. & CATFORD, J. The Welsh heart programme evaluation strategy: progress, plans and possibilities. *Health promotion international,* **2**: 5–18 (1987).

17. MITTELMARK, M.B. ET AL. Realistic outcomes: lessons from community-based research and demonstration programs for the prevention of cardiovascular diseases. *Journal of public health policy,* **14**: 437–462 (1993).

18. STACHENKO, S. *Evaluation guidelines for heart health programs.* Ottawa, Department of National Health and Welfare, 1991.

19. Ottawa Charter for Health Promotion. *Health promotion,* **1**(4): iii–v (1986).

20. EPP, J. *Achieving health for all: a framework for health promotion.* Ottawa, Health Canada, 1986.

21. ADVISORY BOARD FOR THE INTERNATIONAL HEART HEALTH CONFERENCE. *The Victoria Declaration on Heart Health.* Ottawa, Health and Welfare Canada, 1992.

22. *The Catalonia declaration – Investing in heart health. Declaration of the Advisory Board of the Second International Heart Health Conference.* Barcelona, Department of Health and Social Security, Autonomous Government of Catalonia, 1995.

23. JOHNSON, J.L. ET AL. A dissemination research agenda to strengthen health promotion and disease prevention. *Canadian journal of public health,* **87**(Suppl. 2): S5–S10 (1996).

24. STACHENKO, S. The Canadian Heart Health Initiative: dissemination perspectives. *Canadian journal of public health*, **87**(Suppl. 2): S57–S59 (1996).

25. ELLIOTT, S.J. ET AL. Assessing public health capacity to support community based heart health promotion: the Canadian Heart Health Initiative, Ontario Project (CHHIOP). *Health education research*, **13**(4): 607–622 (1998).

26. TAYLOR, S.M. ET AL. Heart health promotion: predisposition, capacity and implementation in Ontario public health units, 1994–96. *Canadian journal of public health*, **89**(6): 406–409 (1998).

27. CAMERON, R. ET AL. The dissemination of chronic disease prevention programs: linking science and practice. *Canadian journal of public health*, **87**(Suppl. 2): S50–S53 (1996).

21
Issues in evaluating mass-media health communication campaigns

Vicki Freimuth, Galen Cole and Susan D. Kirby [6]

Introduction

Most premature deaths in developed countries can be linked to the action or inaction of individuals and/or communities *(1)*. As a result, public health practitioners have developed interventions to promote healthful attitudes and actions and to suppress harmful ones. Health communication, which we define as the study and use of strategies to inform and influence individual and community decisions that improve health, plays an increasingly central role in these interventions.

Communication may play a dominant or a supporting role in an intervention. Some roles may include communication strategies such as public relations, whose objective is to get a health issue on the public agenda; entertainment education, in which an entertainment programme models desired behaviour; and media advocacy, which entails using the mass media as an advocacy tool to achieve policy change. All of these strategies may include a range of communication activities at the individual, small-group or mass-media level. This chapter addresses only the last category and, more specifically, the issues surrounding the evaluation of the development, implementation and effects of mass-media health communication campaigns. We discuss these evaluation issues under the commonly known headings of formative, process and summative evaluation.

Health communication campaigns

Rogers & Storey *(2)* maintain that health communication campaigns have four defining characteristics. They strive to generate specific outcomes or effects in a relatively large number of people, usually within a specified period of time and through an organized set of communication activities. Health communication campaigns that rely on mass-media outlets frequently consist of a series of television and radio public service announcements (PSAs), or paid commercials with collateral print materials such as posters, booklets and brochures.

---

[6] We thank Carole Craft and Linda Cockrill, CDC, United States for editing this text.

Most health communicators would agree that a common set of variables is considered in the development of a mass-media campaign and that one can expect a common set of outcomes as a result of a communication experience. Communication development or independent variables can be categorized into four broad areas:

- the psychosocial attributes of the receiver;
- the source or spokesperson;
- the settings, channels, activities and materials used to disseminate the message; and
- the message itself, including content, tone, type of appeal, audio characteristics and visual attributes.

Taken together, any combination of these independent variables constitutes what we call the communication strategy *(3–10)*. The outcomes or dependent variables of a mass health communication effort may be categorized into six broad areas: exposure, attention, comprehension, yielding, attitude change and behaviour *(4,5,11,12)*. These outcomes are not exhaustive, and we do not mean to imply that they progress in a linear way. We believe, however, that these terms provide a common language pertinent to this discussion.

Formative research and evaluation issues

The research carried out before the implementation of a health communication campaign in the mass media is often called formative research or evaluation. It assists planners of interventions in understanding and developing effective communication strategies and tactics to mitigate or eliminate problems *(6,9,13–15)*.

This section discusses issues related to the formative research and evaluations carried out during the developmental stages of mass communication strategies and tactics. These issues pertain to the data required to understand and profile the receiver characteristics of target audiences, and the evaluation or testing of strategies and tactics before their implementation.

Data issues

The strategic development of a health communication campaign targeting an entire society requires descriptive and analytic epidemiological data to understand the nature and extent of the health problem addressed as a basis for determining: whether mass communication is an appropriate intervention, which audiences are the most appropriate targets of such intervention and what the overall goal of the communication should be. In addition to relying on traditional epidemiological data, health communicators also need data required to characterize potential audiences according to the independent variables that have the most bearing on how one communicates with them *(6,9,13,14)*. This includes data on the four independent variables listed above. These data allow the communicator to disaggregate the population of interest into homogeneous subgroups or audience segments. Health-related audience segments are usually defined as being alike in one of two ways: predictors of behaviour (such as similar levels of self-efficacy, social norms or knowledge) or factors in communication strategy (for example, motivation by a fear-based message or a preference for a lay person to communicate the message).

Despite the number of sources of data on health and on consumers (used for marketing purposes), to our knowledge only one (14) provides national data generated in the United States that combine health behaviour predictors with communication variables. The lack of data forces communication planners to collect primary data, merge or retrofit epidemiological and marketing data, or plan interventions without a clear understanding of possible communication-relevant differences in their target populations. Obviously, if adequate time and other resources are available, the first option is preferred. People working on a short deadline with a limited budget, however, would find multivariate data sets (16–24) a helpful source of information on salient health-related and communication variables. Thus, we recommend that researchers take steps systematically to link or create databases that provide:

- the etiological data required to understand health behaviour incidence and prevalence, such as those from the Behavioral Risk Factor Surveillance Study (25), which can help communicators understand what drives health problems that can be addressed by mass communication interventions; and
- the communication data that can help planners understand how to tailor mass communication strategies to the receiver characteristics of homogeneous segments of the population.

Pre-testing communication strategies and tactics
Once an audience is segmented into groups sharing similar characteristics that are important to the communication process, specific communication strategies and tactics can be crafted for each segment. Providing those responsible for developing such a strategy with a creative brief – a profile of the health-relevant knowledge, attitudes, actions and communication-related characteristics of each target audience – facilitates their task. While existing research may provide much guidance on each variable in the communication strategy at this point in the communication planning process, research on how to put those variables together most effectively for a particular audience segment is rare. Thus, health communication planners rely on a type of formative evaluation called pre-testing.

In short, pre-testing is a process for systematically determining which combination of options represented by each communication variable (that is, communication strategy) tends to be most effective in achieving the communication objectives. This type of formative research resembles both process and summative research in that it can be designed to examine both the simulated

477

delivery and the effects of a communication strategy and its tactics. At the same time, pre-testing differs from such evaluation research in that it is carried out before the final production and execution of a communication strategy, to determine whether each element in the mix helps achieve the communication objectives of the project and meets the information needs of the intended audience (26,27). Because directly attributing changes in individuals to a mass communication intervention is so difficult, pre-testing a strategy should have high priority. It can ensure that the strategy is feasible, produces intended cognitive effects in a sample of individuals representative of each target audience and does no harm.

While pre-testing is considered an indispensable formative evaluation method, there are some questions about its implementation: namely, the rigour of the research methods employed and comparison data for decision-making. This is particularly true with focus group interviews, which have steadily increased in the non-profit and health community (28). A simple search of MEDLINE® indicated a 266% growth in reported focus group studies, from 45 in 1988–1991 to 165 in 1992–1995. Although all research methods have inherent advantages and disadvantages, the potentially inappropriate use of focus groups can pose problems.

This method comprises conducting discussions with small groups from the intended audience segment. A series of groups is recommended because the unit of analysis is the group itself, not its members. Owing to various constraints, programme planners often address too few groups for each segment of interest. This tendency can result in conducting only one session for each segment type (for example, one group each of black women, white women and Asian women), which is inadequate for drawing research conclusions and particularly for finding any differences between groups (28). Another problem in using focus groups is the temptation to quantify participants' answers (for example, by asking for a show of hands on agreement), which leads others to believe that the data may adhere to the rules for quantitative data integrity, such as independent observation or central limit theorem. Authors have long cautioned practitioners not to quantify such results (28–30) because it misleads readers and destroys the true value of qualitative research, which is to gain a richer and deeper understanding of a topic, not a more precise or accurate measurement. Health communication planners need to be able to use focus groups to their best advantage while maintaining a high level of confidence in the findings. Focus groups, not to be confused with group interviewing, should not be used for pre-testing messages, except to explore answers to quantitative questions.

Researchers can use several other qualitative research methods, along with quantitative methods, to gather information when pre-testing messages. These include case studies, one-on-one interviews and record abstraction (31–33). In most instances, we prefer one-on-one interviews (or central intercept interviews, as they are often called in communication research) to test messages. They offer several advantages:

- easier connections with harder-to-reach respondents in locations convenient and comfortable for them;
- access to an increased number of respondents within the intended population if an appropriate location is selected;
- cost-effective and relatively speedy data collection; and
- use of a larger sample size than focus groups, and a tendency to eliminate the group bias that is possible in focus groups.

Finally, once formative researchers have some pre-test data in hand, few comparison data are available to help decide whether the pre-tested materials performed well enough to create change in the real world. Aside from the Health Message Testing Service *(34)*, few health communication programmes have conducted quantitative message pre-testing, published their findings or related pre-testing data to outcome evaluation data. Without knowledge of pre-testing data and actual communication outcomes, health communication planners cannot forecast how well a communication strategy will help reach objectives. The advertising world, which refers to message pre-testing as copytesting, may have some useful models that can be adopted to help overcome this lack of data.

Most advertising agencies employ some method of copytesting *(35)* and have established marketing surveillance systems for the consistent collection, analysis and cataloguing of the data generated by the copytesting process. The 1982 Positioning Advertising Copytesting (PACT) agreement *(36)*, prepared by 21 leading advertising agencies, demonstrates the rigour and systematic collection of these data. The PACT document *(36)* articulates nine principles that target multiple measures, representative samples, reliability and validity. Since the agreement was published, a plethora of research firms has been established to help deliver on these principles *(37)*. These firms research, track and collect copytesting data for primary purchasing and reselling to retail organizations. These data help identify the most effective and efficient communication strategy for the marketing communication dollar.

While outcomes such as consumer recall and purchase data are easily assessed and collected in the world of retail marketing, the cognitive and behavioural outcomes of health communication activities are not as easily assessed. Thus, health communication campaigns that rely on mass-media outlets are usually challenged with making formative decisions based on relatively little data and, even in the best conditions, without up-to-date information or comparison data. As noted above, however, health communication planners need timely comparison data systems, not unlike those established by the private sector, to identify and improve weak and inadequate programmes before implementation, if they are to bring the best messages to the prevention marketplace to attack the causes of today's health problems.

Process evaluation issues

In general, process evaluation determines whether a programme is delivered as planned *(27)*: in this case, how well and under what conditions a mass-media health communication campaign was implemented, and the size of the audience exposed to the message. The planning and implementation of such an evaluation should address a number of issues, including the utility of the evaluation, theoretical considerations and attributions of cause and effect, and whether to change an intervention during the course of an evaluation.

Utility

Stakeholders' clamour for data on the intended effects of campaigns has led many evaluators to become preoccupied with programme outcomes *(38–40)*, and thus to rely heavily on controlled experimental methods (see chapters 1–3). An enticing feature of these methods is that they can be used to estimate a campaign's net effects without an understanding of how the campaign works *(41)*. Thus, evaluators can satisfy the demand for effects without carefully considering, through process evaluation, the programme mechanisms that produce them.

The disadvantage of working this way is that stakeholders receive very little information on which to act *(38)*. That is, even though an experimental evaluation may demonstrate that an intervention produces intended effects, if a formal process evaluation does not account for the implementation processes, there is very little basis for action to improve a programme because stakeholders lack information about what produced the observed outcomes *(38)*. For example, if an evaluation of a PSA campaign to increase moderate physical activity among adults in a particular community does not include surveillance to determine what proportion of the target audience is exposed to the PSA, it is impossible to attribute observed effects to the intervention. Weiss *(42)* makes this point:

> Does it make any difference ... whether the program is using rote drill, psychoanalysis, or black magic? There are evaluators who are sympathetic to such an approach. They see the program as a "black box," the contents of which do not concern them; they are charged with discovering effects. But, if the evaluator has no idea of what the program really is, s/he may fail to ask the right questions.

Without process evaluation, one cannot differentiate between a bad campaign and a poorly implemented one. This is particularly true if one is trying to improve effects through modifying, enhancing and, if necessary, eliminating campaign processes. In sum, the best evaluation considers both processes and effects.

Theoretical considerations and attributions of cause and effect

Although many recognize the importance of both process and summative

480

evaluation, these assessments are sometimes conducted independently, as if they had no connection. This results in a *post hoc* cut-and-paste job: after collecting data on both process and outcome markers, the evaluators attempt to link effects with specific processes. To prevent this, evaluators should clearly delineate, in advance, linkages between programme processes and intended outcomes. Explaining the importance of this, Patton *(38)*, Weiss *(40)* and Chen *(41)* state that evaluators should define a campaign's theory of action before initiating evaluation. Before beginning an evaluation, evaluators should explicitly link each important intervention process (independent variable) with each desired outcome (dependent variable). This approach is often called theory-based evaluation *(41)* (see Chapter 4).

In theory-based evaluation, the standard for comparison is the programme's theory, or subtheories, if the evaluation is aimed at examining subcomponents of the programme. Thus, the first phase in such evaluation is theory construction. This requires an understanding of what programme theories are and how best to develop them. If one wants to know about different subcomponents – domains of the programme theory, as Chen *(41)* calls them – such as its development, delivery, cost or effects, a separate subtheory must be constructed for each programme domain to be evaluated. Chen *(41)* notes that programme theory domains can be considered independently (as basic types) or in some combination (as composite types). In short, the evaluator must construct a separate theory for each basic and/or composite domain selected for a theory-based evaluation, with each theory serving as a standard of comparison.

The idea of comparing what should happen to what does happen, in terms of programme, and/or comparing a theory of a problem against the reality discovered by a theory-based evaluation is rather simple. Less straightforward is determining how to construct a problem theory or an expected programme theory of action (the standard of comparison) that accurately reflects how a programme is supposed to perform and the nature of the problem(s) it is designed to overcome. Fortunately, various strategies have been developed to assist with this process *(40,43,44)*. They help users systematically to construct theories and subtheories of programme development, implementation and cause–effect relationships that serve as standards against which evaluation data can be compared to identify the extent of discrepancy or congruence between how the campaign activities are supposed to bring about intended effects and what actually happens *(44)*.

Changing an intervention during the evaluation

Evaluation is an iterative process designed to enable to stakeholders to make decisions to improve a programme. The implicit assumption is that, if this feedback dictates the need for change, the programme should be changed, particularly social marketing programmes, which aim to respond rapidly to feedback. Changing a programme, however, contradicts the scientific maxim to standardize or keep an intervention constant throughout the course of an evaluation.

To resolve this dilemma, evaluators and programme implementation staff should agree, from the outset, to make a schedule for reporting feedback and, if appropriate, to make changes in the programme. Threats to the validity of the findings can be minimized by ensuring that: changes in the campaign processes are documented, process evaluation tracking protocols are modified to account for these changes and measurements are taken on key outcome variables both before and after important changes in the implementation process. This will ensure the consistency needed to pick up effects that may result from changes in the campaign processes, while allowing planners to use timely and relevant feedback to improve the programme.

Summative evaluation issues

Summative evaluation assesses whether a mass-media health communication programme reached the intended audience and achieved its impact and outcome objectives to the satisfaction of the stakeholders. This section discusses issues around both of these aspects.

Issues in assessing reach

For a message to have a desired influence, receivers must first attend to it (5). Thus, a summative evaluation must seek an early effect of communication: whether the intended audience paid attention to the desired message. Even if a programme is implemented as planned and desired effects result, these effects cannot be attributed to the intervention without evidence that the campaign reached the intended audience.

A necessary first step in answering this question is to determine whether and how many times a message is aired. This is greatly simplified if one can afford paid advertising, because the time, place and frequency of airing can be controlled. For a number of reasons, however, particularly cost, public-sector health communicators seldom use paid advertising.

When paid advertising is not an option, health communicators often rely on PSAs, which are aired at no cost to the producer. Unfortunately, PSAs are aired in the United States at the discretion of public service directors at the various television and radio stations, making the tracking of airing difficult. Attempts to overcome these difficulties have included relying on services that monitor commercials and PSAs. For example, one media service operates an electronic tracking service that detects the airing of PSAs in over 1100 broadcast stations (including 40 Spanish-language stations) in all 211 designated market areas of the United States, plus 28 national cable networks. This service ascertains the number of times a PSA plays, the market(s) where it played, the station call letters, air date and air time. This monitoring goes on 24 hours a day, 7 days a week.

To get some idea about the extended reach of broadcast and print media that may have been triggered by our CDC mass-media campaigns, we consistently track both. We use one service to track broadcast media and another for print. The first monitors news and public affairs programming in 46 of the top media markets, including 300 local television stations and 50 network and cable channels. It also monitors selected news radio programming generated by 60 radio stations in 15 of the top media markets. The second service continually updates and maintains a regional news library consisting of a combination of news sources grouped together by geographical area. It contains more than 125 full-text regional news sources in the United States, selected documents, abstracts from two newspapers in different cities and material from a wire service.

Together, these three services allow us to estimate the overall reach of both broadcast and print media. Although these data satisfy the need to determine whether, when and where a PSA is aired, along with the extended reach of collateral media that the campaign may have triggered, these services and the data they generate do not show who attended to, comprehended and yielded to the key messages of a campaign. This requires further audience research.

In the United States, to determine who was watching or whether those who were watching were attending to a central message broadcast on television as a part of a national health communication campaign, one can rely on services such as the Nielson Station Index, which generates information on the viewing behaviour of individuals (over 100 000) living in randomly selected households in each television market. The Index characterizes viewers demographically by their age and gender. Participants keep diaries for each television in their homes, recording the programmes they watch and for how long, the station on which the programme was aired, and the date and time of airing. Data from set meters that electronically capture household viewing events in a sample of television markets are used to verify and adjust the diary data.

To further characterize the audiences who may have viewed a particular message, Index data can be merged with geographical and psychographic data aggregated into neighbourhood clusters that represent demographic and/or psychographic profiles of people living in different neighbourhoods in various locations across the United States. Merging these data with Index data allows for the indirect approximation of the psychographic characteristics of those who view a message in question. For example, through a cluster analysis system, a corporation – perhaps the most prominent vendor of geo-psychographic data clusters – provides information on households categorized to 1 of 62 neighbourhood audience segments based on 6 criterion factors: social rank, household composition, residential mobility, ethnicity, urbanization and types of housing. This database also includes information on media habits, patterns of small and large purchases, political beliefs, geographic location and demographic factors. Merging a variety of data sets allows for an indirect approximation of who is watching what and when.

What is still unknown, however, is whether these audiences attended to and comprehended the messages. Some approaches to determining this include: conducting a general population survey to determine audience awareness of a campaign, adding specific relevant questions to an omnibus survey, relying on data collected in national probability sample surveys and/or adding tags to a televised message that is designed to motivate viewers to call a particular number for more information, on the assumption that a burst of calls just after the airing of a tagged message almost certainly indicates that the audience attended to it. Questions directed at those who call can help further to determine whether those who attended to the message actually understood it. CDC has used all of these summative evaluation approaches in attempts to monitor the reach of our HIV/AIDS health communication efforts, which were carried out by what was the National AIDS Information and Education Program at CDC (45).

As with tracking electronic media, one must be highly creative in determining who is exposed to messages in newspapers or magazines, particularly with collateral materials such as brochures, flyers, posters and billboards. This often entails high financial and labour costs.

Assessing intended effects

Flay & Cook (46) have identified three models used to conduct summative evaluations of the effects of health communication programmes: advertising, impact monitoring and experimental. The first is the most frequently used and consists of a baseline survey, before the programme is implemented, and another survey at the end of the programme. The evaluation of the Cancer Prevention Awareness Campaign (47) is a representative example of this approach. National probability surveys were conducted before the launch of a multichannel cancer prevention campaign and a year later, after it was implemented. Materials included booklets, radio and television PSAs, and special events. The evaluation compared knowledge of risk factors and concern about cancer before and after the campaign. This evaluation model is simple, and often criticized because the lack of a control group prohibits establishing a direct cause-and-effect relationship between the campaign and its outcomes.

The impact-monitoring model uses routinely collected data from a management information system to monitor the effects and outcomes of a health communication campaign. For example, as part of its evaluation of the campaign against AIDS in the United States, CDC examined knowledge, attitude and behaviour measures from its annual national health interview surveys. This method is easy and cost-effective, but it usually measures behavioural outcomes only and often fails to provide information that can explain successes and failures.

The experimental model contrasts two or more equivalent groups, one of which is a control group. An antismoking campaign, designed to recruit women cigarette smokers with young children to call for information on quitting, used this evaluation model (48). The campaign included a mix of professionally produced broadcast and print materials encouraging mothers who were smokers to call the National Cancer Institute's Cancer Information Service for information on quitting. The use of paid advertising enabled the

484

careful placement of media messages. Fourteen media markets in the states of Delaware, New York and Pennsylvania were paired off according to size, and one of each pair was randomly assigned to the experimental and control groups. Response to the campaign was gauged by monitoring calls to the area offices of the Cancer Information Service from smokers residing in the media markets. This model is usually considered the most rigorous, but has been challenged as inappropriate for evaluating what is essentially a messy social process *(49)*.

The choice of an appropriate model of evaluation depends on an understanding of the way health communication campaigns work. Hornick *(49)* presents a compelling argument against the randomized controlled experimental design. He contrasts the limited effects attributed to such well known community-based health promotion efforts as the Stanford three- and five-city studies, the Minnesota and Pawtucket heart health programmes and COMMIT with the impressive evidence of behavioural change from the National High Blood Pressure Education and Control Program, the original campaign of smoking counter-advertising televised between 1967 and 1970, the public communication about the AIDS epidemic in the United States and an antismoking campaign underway in California. He attributed this surprising contrast in effectiveness to the constraints imposed by the research design itself. Thinking that no background communication on a health issue occurs in control communities is quite misleading; treatment communities may have only slightly more exposure to messages about these issues. Stanford, for example, claimed that it provided 25 hours of exposure on average to heart disease messages over 5 years in its treatment communities. This estimate suggests that most people only received one hour of messages per year on each of the five types of behaviour promoted. Hornick *(49)* contrasts this limited exposure to the more intense scale of the National High Blood Pressure Education and Control Program, which represents the complex social diffusion process: deliberate communication messages, the conversations that ensue, the coverage by other media sources and the resulting demands on institutions, which then respond. Health institutions offer different advice and treatments. Businesses provide new products and advertise different benefits. Political institutions change public policy to support health behaviour. Hornick argues that communication is a social process, not a pill, and should be evaluated as such.

Hornick's reasoning also reinforces the difficulty in disentangling communication effects from those of other intervention components or disentangling the effects of several communication activities. Assuming that a complex process of social change has occurred, one must either develop more sophisticated tools for measuring this diffusion process and disentangling its separate components, or be content with assessing overall effects without attribution to individual components of the intervention. It may be reasonable to expect practitioners to do only the latter in routine evaluations of campaigns, but to ask health communication researchers to design studies to capture this

485

complex social diffusion process and discover how individual communication components contribute to it.

Above all, one must resist the effort to design rigorous, controlled experimental studies that strive to compare the effects of individual communication products such as pamphlets, PSAs and posters with the goal of discovering which product is the most effective to use in all situations. That kind of evaluation is inconsistent with the research and practice literature, which recommends multiple messages and channels, and cautions that formative research, conducted early in campaign development, is the best way to find the right channels to reach the right audiences with the right messages, delivered by the right sources at the right times.

Even after an appropriate evaluation design is selected, summative evaluations of health communication campaigns face some serious methodological issues. Measuring and sampling problems are the most common.

Measurement problems

The health communication components of interventions often have several objectives. One of the most critical measurement problems involves determining which effects to measure. Does the evaluator measure comprehension, attitude change or behaviour change? One might argue that, the further along this chain the measurement takes place, the more important the effects. As one measures further along the chain, however, the potential effects of the messages and the ability to control for extraneous variables decrease. For example, is it realistic to assume that the direct cause of a smoker quitting is an antismoking PSA? Undoubtedly, the causal chain is more complicated than that. In addition, many behavioural changes advocated in health messages are impossible to observe directly. For example, how can hypertensives' use of medication or a woman's breast self-examination be observed? In such cases, self-reported behaviour is measured. Such measurement is subject to error because of the tendency to overreport socially desirable behaviour. Some evaluations can validate self-report measures with behavioural or physiological data. For example, smoking cessation studies often validate a percentage of their self-report measures with saliva continine testing and proxy data from people who are willing to observe the smoking behaviour of participants in the cessation programme.

Most summative evaluations of health communication programmes attempt to measure exposure to messages by asking respondents what they recall of the messages. Unaided recall generally produces an artificially low estimate of audience exposure. Most evaluators use some form of aided recall: providing the respondent with some information about the message and then asking if the respondent remembers hearing or seeing it. With the use of aided recall, however, some overreporting of exposure occurs because respondents acquiesce or try to help by giving what they think is the desired answer. In an attempt to avoid overreporting, evaluators often request verbatim descriptions of the messages. Only respondents whose descriptions can be clearly tied to the message are identified as having been exposed. This approach requires rigorous coding procedures to classify the respondents.

We suggest a measurement compromise: the use of unaided questions followed by a series of aided questions. Estimates of the magnitude of error due to overreporting can be calculated based on measurement of (spurious) reported awareness among respondents not exposed to the ads (in a control condition) or on reported awareness to bogus messages.

Sampling problems

While most mass-media health communication campaigns target a specific segment of the audience, the evaluation frequently is not limited to that segment. When sampling for a post-campaign evaluation, how does one find women who have not had a mammogram, people who do not take their hypertension medication regularly or drivers who do not wear seat belts? At best, some demographic data are available, but these are far from perfectly descriptive of the target group. Low exposure to many of these messages (often as low as 10%) compounds the difficulty in identifying the target group. Consequently, every random sample of 1000 may only yield 100 people who remember seeing the message, among whom, for example, there are even fewer women who have not had a mammogram but recall seeing messages recommending them. Most surveys used to measure the effectiveness of health messages need to screen respondents carefully, a time-consuming and costly process.

Discussion

Communication's varied roles in public health interventions raise a number of issues in evaluating health communication campaigns. This chapter has highlighted these issues and provided a number of ways to resolve them through formative, process and summative evaluation.

Formative evaluation of health communication campaigns helps to develop the most effective communication strategies and then test them to forecast their effectiveness. This entails breaking the audience into homogeneous segments and then characterizing or profiling them to tailor campaign messages and implementation more closely. These profiles can best be made with the benefit of data sets that include both etiological data on the distribution and determinants of health problems that may be mitigated by mass communication, and information on variables that allows planners to understand how to best communicate with each audience targeted by the communication strategy (50).

Formative evaluation before implementation helps to ensure that a communication strategy is feasible, produces the intended effects in each target audience and does no harm. While pre-testing is indispensable, there are some questions about its use: which research methods should be employed and how. We recommend that formative evaluators judiciously select the quantitative and qualitative methods that are best suited to pre-testing and that employ them in a technically acceptable manner.

Once a mass-media health communication campaign is underway, process evaluation begins to assess how the programme is working. Without this knowledge, one cannot determine whether the programme brought about the desired effects, and thus what aspects, if any, should be changed or eliminated. We recommend applying the principles of theory-based evaluation to construct models that explicitly state how the programme will bring about intended effects, to provide a basis for comparison with actual performance. Further, health communication researchers should design studies to capture the complex social diffusion process that occurs in and around a mass-media campaign. This can help them systematically to discover how individual communication components contribute to the campaign process as a basis for explaining and replicating those that work.

Process evaluation can be used to determine a programme's effectiveness while it is underway. This allows for changes to be made midstream to increase the likelihood of desired outcomes. The implementers and evaluators of a programme should agree from the outset on a schedule for reporting feedback and making informed changes to ensure maximum relevance, efficiency and effectiveness.

Summative evaluation determines whether a mass-media health communication campaign reached the intended audience and achieved its objectives. Several factors, however, complicate this type of evaluation.

First, while one can monitor whether messages were disseminated, assessing audience exposure and attendance to them is more difficult. In the case of PSAs in a national media campaign, for example, a broadcast verification company can help determine exposure to the messages. Finding out whether the audience attended to those messages often requires conducting surveys, relying on data collected in national probability sample surveys or using tags on PSAs that are designed to motivate viewers to call a particular number for more information.

One can employ the advertising, impact-monitoring or experimental models to determine whether the campaign messages had the intended effects. The advertising model, with its two surveys, is the most frequently used, but draws criticism for lacking a control group. The impact-monitoring model uses routinely collected data from a management information system to monitor behavioural effects. This method, while easy and cost-effective, fails to provide information that explains success or failure. The experimental model contrasts two or more equivalent experimental and control groups. This method is imperfect because it assumes that no background communication is going on in control communities, a belief that is unrealistic.

Even after a summative evaluation design is selected, a number of concerns arise. When using surveys, overreporting can result, especially when dealing with socially desirable behaviour. For example, will drivers who say they saw PSAs on safety belts admit not using them? There is also difficulty in identifying the target audience after the campaign. Exposure may be low; many people may have forgotten seeing a message, and some may not admit seeing a message if they have not adopted the encouraged behaviour.

We have identified and discussed issues that are important to consider in the conduct of formative, process and summative evaluations of mass-media health communication campaigns. These issues and our recommendations on their resolution should provide a basis for further improvements in conceptualizing, planning, implementing and reporting feedback on evaluations aimed at improving mass-media health communication campaigns to promote health-enhancing behaviour and environments.

References

1. McGinnis, J.M. & Foege, W.H. Actual causes of death in the United States. *Journal of the American Medical Association*, **270**(18): 2207–2212 (1993).
2. Rogers, E.M. & Storey, J.D. Communication campaigns. *In*: Berger, C. & Chaffee, S., ed. *Handbook of communication science*. Newbury Park, Sage Publications, 1987.
3. Flora, J.A. & Maibach, E.W. Cognitive responses to AIDS information: the effects of issue involvement and message appeal. *Communication research*, **17**(6): 759–774 (1990).
4. Flay, B.R. et al. Mass media in health promotion: an analysis using extended information-processing model. *Health education quarterly*, **7**(2): 127–147 (1980).
5. McGuire, W.J. Theoretical foundations of campaigns. *In*: Rice, R.E. & Atkin, C.K., ed. *Public communications campaigns*, 2nd ed. Newbury Park, Sage Publications, 1989, pp. 43–65.
6. Sutton, S.M. et al. Strategic questions for consumer-based health communications. *In*: *5 a day for better health: NCI media campaign strategy*. Washington, DC, National Cancer Institute, 1993, pp. 1–12.
7. Gorn, G.J. The effects of music in advertising on choice behavior: a classical conditioning approach. *Journal of marketing*, **46**: 94–101 (1982).
8. Messaris, P. *Visual persuasion*. Thousand Oaks, Sage Publications, 1997.
9. Donohew, L. et al. Sensation seeking and targeting of televised anti-drug PSAs. *In*: Donohew, L. et al., ed. *Persuasive communication and drug abuse prevention*. Hillsdale, NJ, Lawrence Earlbaum Associates, 1991, pp. 209–226.
10. Prochaska, J.O. et al. *Changing for good*. New York, Avon Books, 1994, pp. 287–289.
11. Backer, T.E. et al. Generalizations about health communication campaigns. *In*: *Designing health communication campaigns. What works?* Newbury Park, Sage Publications, 1992, pp. 30–32.

12. PETTY, R.E. ET AL. Central and peripheral routes to advertising effectiveness: the moderating role of involvement. *Journal of consumer research*, **10**(2): 135–146 (1983).

13. ATKIN, C.K. & FREIMUTH, V. Formative evaluation research in campaign design. *In*: Rice, R. & Atkin, C.K., ed. *Public communication campaigns*, 2nd ed. Newbury Park, Sage Publications, 1989, pp. 131–150.

14. MAIBACH, E.W. ET AL. Translating health psychology into effective health communication. The American Healthstyles audience segmentation project. *Journal of health psychology*, **1**(3): 261–277 (1996).

15. SLATER, M.D. Theory and method in health audience segmentation. *Journal of health communication*, **1**: 267–283 (1996).

16. SLATER, M.D. Choosing audience segmentation strategies and methods for health communication. *In*: Maibach, E.W. & Parrott, R. L., ed. *Designing health messages: approaches from communication theory and public health practice*. Thousand Oaks, Sage Publications, 1995, pp. 169–185.

17. SLATER, M. & FLORA, J.A. Health lifestyles: audience segmentation analysis for public health interventions. *Health education quarterly*, **18**(2): 221–233 (1991).

18. PATTERSON, R.E. ET AL. Health lifestyle patterns of U.S. adults. *Preventive medicine*, **23**: 453–460 (1994).

19. MAIBACH, E.W. *Psychobehavioral segmentation: identifying audiences and tailoring cancer prevention programs*. Washington, DC, Porter Novelli Public Relations, 1996.

20. MAIBACH E.W. & COTTON, D. Moving people to behavior change: a staged social cognitive approach to message design. *In*: Maibach, E.W. & Parrott, R. L., ed. *Designing health messages: approaches from communication theory and public health practice*. Thousand Oaks, Sage Publications, 1995.

21. VELICER, W.F. ET AL. An empirical typology of subjects within stage of change. *Addictive behaviors*, **20**(3): 299–320 (1995).

22. WILLIAMS, J.E. & FLORA, J.A. Health behavior segmentation and campaign planning to reduce cardiovascular disease risk among Hispanics. *Health education quarterly*, **22**(1): 36–48 (1995).

23. MORRIS, L.A. ET AL. A segmentation analysis of prescription drug intervention-seeking motives among the elderly. *Journal of public relations and marketing*, **11**: 115–125 (1992).

24. ALBRECHT, T.L. & BRYANT, C. Advances in segmentation modeling for health communication and social marketing campaigns. *Journal of health communication*, **1**: 65–80 (1996).

25. POWELL-GRINER, E. ET AL. State- and sex-specific prevalence of selected characteristics – Behavioral Risk Factor Surveillance System, 1994 and 1995. *Morbidity and mortality weekly report*, **46**(3):1–31 (1997).

26. FREIMUTH, V. Developing public service advertisement for nonprofit contexts. *In*: Belk, R.W., ed. *Advances in nonprofit marketing*. Greenwich, CT, JAI Press, 1985, pp. 55–94.

27. COLE, G. ET AL. Addressing problems in evaluating health-relevant programs through a systematic planning and evaluation model. *Risk: issues in health, safety and environment*, **6**(1): 37–57 (1995).

28. KRUEGER, R.A. *Focus groups: a practical guide for applied research*, 2nd ed. Thousand Oaks, Sage Publications, 1994.

29. STEWART D.W. & SHAMDASANI, P.N. *Focus groups: theory and practice*. Newbury Park, Sage Publications, 1990 (Applied Social Science Research Methods Series, Vol. 20).

30. TEMPLETON, J.F. *The focus group (revised edition)*. Burr Ridge, IL, Irwin Professional Publishing, 1994.

31. CRABTREE, B.F. & MILLER, W.L. *Doing qualitative research*. Newbury Park, Sage Publications, 1992, pp. 3–28 (Research Methods For Primary Care, Vol. 3).

32. *Making health communication programs work*. Washington, DC, US Department of Health and Human Services, 1992 (NIH Publication No. 92-1493).

33. PATTON, M.Q. *How to use qualitative methods in evaluation*. Newbury Park, Sage Publications, 1987.

34. *Pretesting in health communications: methods, examples, and resources for improving health messages and materials*. Washington, DC, US Department of Health and Human Services, 1984 (NIH Publication No. 84-1493).

35. SHIMP, T.A. *Promotion management and marketing communications*, 2nd ed. Chicago, Dryden Press, 1990, pp. 428–432.

36. PACT document. *Journal of advertising*, **11**(4): 4–29 (1982).

37. STEWART, D.W. ET AL. *A guide to commercial copytesting services. In*: Leigh, J.H. & Martin, C.R., Jr, ed. *Current issues and research in advertising*. Ann Arbor, MI, Division of Research, Graduate School of Business, University of Michigan, 1983, pp.1–44.

38. PATTON, M.Q. *Utilization-focused evaluation*, 2nd ed. Beverly Hills, Sage Publications, 1986.

39. GARDNER, D.E. Five evaluation frameworks. *Journal of higher education*, **48**(5): 571–593 (1977).

40. WEISS, C.H. Nothing as practical as good theory: exploring theory-based evaluation for comprehensive community initiatives for children and families. *In*: Connell, J.P. et al., ed. *New approaches to evaluating community initiatives: concepts, methods and contexts*. New York, Aspen Institute, 1995, pp. 65–92.

41. CHEN, H.T. *Theory-driven evaluation*. Thousand Oaks, Sage Publications, 1990.

42. Weiss, C.H. *Evaluation research. Methods for assessing program effectiveness*. Englewood Cliffs, Prentice Hall, 1972.

43. Shern, D.L. et al. The use of concept mapping for assessing fidelity of model transfer: an example from psychiatric rehabilitation. *Evaluation and program planning*, **18**(2): 143–153, 1995.

44. COLE, G.E. Advancing the development and application of theory-based evaluation in the practice of public health. *American journal of evaluation*, **20**(3): 453–470, 1999.

45. NOWAK, G.J. & SISKA, M.J. Using research to inform campaign development and message design: examples from the "America Responds to AIDS" campaign. *In*: Maibach, E.W. & Parrott, R. L., ed. *Designing health messages: approaches from communication theory and public health practice*. Thousand Oaks, Sage Publications, 1995.

46. FLAY B.R. & COOK, T.D. Three models for summative evaluation of prevention campaigns with a mass media component. *In*: Rice, R. & Atkin, C., ed. *Public communication campaigns*, 2nd ed. Newbury Park, Sage Publications, 1989, pp. 175–196.

47. US DEPARTMENT OF HEALTH AND HUMAN SERVICES. *Technical report on cancer prevention awareness survey wave II*. Bethesda, MD, National Institutes of Health, 1986.

48. CUMMINGS, K.M. ET AL. Results of an antismoking campaign utilizing the Cancer Information Service. *Monographs – National Cancer Institute*, **14**: 113–118 (1993).

49. HORNICK, R. *Public health communication: making sense of contradictory evidence*. Philadelphia, University of Pennsylvania, 1997.

50. CHERVIN, D.D. ET AL. Using audience research in designing public health initiatives at the federal level. *Social marketing quarterly*, **5**(3): 34–39 (1999).

22

Investment for health: developing a multifaceted appraisal approach

Erio Ziglio, Spencer Hagard and Lowell S. Levin

Introduction

A sound and credible strategy for health promotion requires the concerted efforts of a variety of players at all levels of government. The concept and principles of health promotion must influence sectors such as health care, social services, education, the environment and economic and social development. Public and private offices, the mass media, NGOs and all other institutional arrangements crucial to social cohesion, social justice and human rights must be involved (1–4). With so many interests visibly involved, the strategy required to implement health promoting programmes and policies is bound to be intersectoral, involve multiple levels of policy-making in economic and social development (local, regional, national and in several instances supranational) and use a wide range of measures (educational, legislative, fiscal, etc.).

We believe this multifaceted strategy can be implemented through investment for health: the explicit dedication of resources to the production of health. Thus, multifaceted approaches are required to evaluate policy decisions influencing economic and social development and their effect on a population's health.

This chapter describes a new service of the WHO Regional Office for Europe to its Member States – appraisal of investment for health – which has been developed, tested and refined since 1995. Working at the national or subnational level, it:

- assesses a country's, region's or locality's current efforts, both within and outside the health sector, to promote the health of its population; and
- advises on the construction of a strategy that strengthens population health through selective investment (both within and outside the health sector) while supporting the country's key economic and social priorities.

This chapter examines the rationale for and development of investment for health, reviews the learning process of appraising investment for health, describes how the task has been carried out so far and concludes with some reflections on experience to date.

The changed context

The modern era of public health in Europe and North America is barely a century old. To a large extent, it began when the one-on-one clinical experience of medicine was applied to the community as a whole (5–8). By the 1940s, the inclusion of epidemiological principles strengthened this approach and, for the first time, provided a basis for rational planning of both local programmes and national policies (9). In many instances, the public health enterprise developed a sophisticated operational infrastructure at local, regional, national and international levels.

Until quite recently, evidence drawn from classical epidemiology has almost exclusively guided public health practice, including the range and selection of interventions (2,4). Little attention was given to the effect of economic and social development on a population's health. The notion that public health decisions must be profoundly linked to wider social and economic goals to ensure sustainable benefits is, in many cases, still not well appreciated. An expanding literature is making a powerful case for the relationship between health and economic development (10–20).

In modern societies, the public health enterprise must lose its isolation and become a full partner in economic and social development (21–23). Public health brings unique analytic capacities to social and economic development, but must accommodate economic development strategies calling on the skills and responsibilities of other disciplines (policy analysis, organization and management) and subject areas normally outside the purview of public health (transport, housing, income maintenance, tourism, agriculture, etc.) (24–26).

Rationale for investment for health

Investment for health is an approach for improving population health, with its roots in the observations, theories and commentaries on health, social welfare, and economic and social development published in the last 20 years. Many authors (8,12,15,24,27–35) have put forward a common thesis: social, demographic and economic factors and public policies, well beyond the traditional remit of medicine or public health, by and large determine population health (3,36,37). Together, these studies and commentaries provide a coherent framework that compels a reassessment of the role of traditional public health. The Ottawa Charter for Health Promotion (2) provides a framework for organizing public health priorities and refocusing its strategies to promote population health. Investment for health is instrumental in implementing such a reorientation (38).

In May 1998, the World Health Assembly affirmed its will to promote health by addressing the basic determinants and prerequisites for health (39). The ultimate aim of economic and social development is people's health and wellbeing, and health targets, such as those set for the WHO European Region (22), must be viewed within their economic and social contexts. Health is a crucial social and personal resource that needs nurturing, that needs investment. If government invests in securing health and wellbeing, it also contributes to economic and social benefits for the whole society *(38)*. Not all economic and social investments promote health *(22)*; the key is to identify those that do.

Investment for health is a deliberate attempt to strengthen the main causes of health in a credible, effective and ethical manner *(38)*. The approach develops strategies that are based on and address key determinants of health. Such determinants are mainly linked to economic and social factors. Thus, life conditions heavily influence the patterns of behaviour that determine lifestyles.

A credible approach to promoting health involves a pragmatic framework for implementing health promotion, including programmes on behaviour and lifestyle resting on a foundation of policies on settings and life conditions. For robust implementation, a health promotion strategy needs to be based on a good balance of programmes and policies that constitute an investment portfolio (Table 22.1). Some of the biggest returns will come from adopting a strategy that, in addition to benefiting a population's health, contributes to healthy economic and social returns for society in a sustainable and equitable way. This message is embodied in the Jakarta Declaration on Leading Health Promotion into the 21st Century, adopted at the Fourth International Conference on Health Promotion, in Jakarta in 1997, *(4)* and has found its place in HEALTH21, the health for all policy framework for the WHO European Region *(22)*.

Table 22.1. Relevant types and areas of investment for health

Types of investment	Life conditions	Settings	Lifestyles	Behaviour
Public/Private development measures	✓✓✓✓	✓✓✓	✓✓	✓
Individual measures	✓	✓	✓✓	✓✓✓

Kickbusch *(26)* argues that at least three key questions need to be addressed in developing a strong and credible health promotion strategy.

* Where is health promoted and maintained in a given population?
* Which investments and strategies produce the largest population health gains?
* Which investments and strategies help reduce health inequities and are in line with human rights?

These questions are at the heart of investment for health *(40)*. The approach also poses and seeks to answer a fourth question. Which investments contribute to economic and social development in an equitable and sustainable manner and result in high health returns for the overall population *(38)*?

495

Very few of the health-sector reforms underway in many countries address these four questions *(40,41)*. Investment for health is a practical attempt to tackle them by: identifying relevant policy attributes, considering factors that may encourage or inhibit policy change, assessing options that benefit both health and a specific policy sector, and planning the political process of achieving the necessary legislative, regulatory, financial, organizational or educational changes *(38)*. Optimizing the health promoting effects of development involves various government and private-sector initiatives in policy sectors such as education, labour, income maintenance, health care, housing, agriculture, tourism and transport.

Clearly, investment for health is not a new concept. It is a powerful approach for implementing a robust health promotion strategy. When different policy sectors achieve mutual benefits, population health becomes a socially useful value, rather than an isolated goal. Investment for health can therefore attract and hold a variety of political allies whose agendas are compatible with promoting the public's health. Indeed, this mutuality is a factor in sustaining collaborative public policies that strengthen overall economic and social development.

The challenges of appraising of investment for health

Public health's role in working with multiple public and private policy sectors is new. Pressure is mounting for public health entities to work with sectors that are involved in economic and social development and affect public health. Housing policy needs to be adjusted to the factors that affect the health of residents. Pension planners need help to create progressive support programmes that reduce poverty among elderly people. Tourism authorities are concerned with tourists' effects on public-health-related infrastructures. Agriculturists seek input into effective alternatives to chemical fertilizers and pesticides. Communication bodies need advice on the validity of and access to health information. Each of these policy areas might be willing to develop strategies that would support public health, if these strategies would not adversely affect the policy areas' primary aims.

Investment for health is in an early stage of development. There is no signpost pointing to an optimum operating strategy for public health's role in intersectoral investment. How should this new role be developed? What are the conceptual, strategic, tactical and logistical barriers? What criteria of success should be applied, and how? Given the lack of precedent, appraising investment for health is easier said than done. Common sense would argue that evidence of impact should include:

- legislative initiatives or specific regulatory adjustments;
- the creation or adaptation of planning and implementation infrastructures;
- the secondary consequences – positive and negative – of a change in investment patterns; and
- the benefits to client groups directly affected by specific policies.

496

The last item is, of course, the most difficult to assess because public policies tend to have long-term and diffuse effects on client groups and because these effects become particularly complex if the group is affected by several policy areas. We are not discussing the simple input–throughput–output model of organizational productivity, and no possibility exists for applying experimental designs.

Evaluation schemes appropriately applied to situations where independent and dependent variables are clearly defined simply do not fit the circumstances of health investments in public policies and private-sector initiatives linked to economic and social development. In general, standard systems analysis methodology or traditional health impact methods are not appropriate to appraise investment for health. Most existing methods need to be adapted to this approach, rather than inflexibly applied. The work to be done is more that of a craftsman than a laboratory scientist or clinical epidemiologist.

As part of a group of experts, we have had to design and test a rather eclectic appraisal scheme suitable to investment for health and its outcomes. The group has borrowed some evaluative tools from anthropology (participant observation), economics (fiscal feasibility and cost–benefit and cost–effectiveness ratios) operations research (management by objectives), systems engineering (monitoring) and business (investment analysis, portfolio balancing and market analysis). Our task is not to reinvent established methodologies that can be useful in enhancing the health gains from public policies, but to test new applications of them. The group cannot simply theorize how these new applications may be achieved; they must be undertaken in the messy realities of a country's, region's or local area's economic, social and political environment.

The appraisal of investment for health is necessarily both systems based and all encompassing. The appraisal team takes account of the full range of available evaluation techniques (systems), most of which are discussed in this book, but also focuses on a country's economic, social and health development as a whole. It treats the roles of health and other sectors as a single system, and systematically assesses the integrity, power and potential of that system *(42)*. The appraisal team, with the participation of stakeholders, constructs recommendations – educational, fiscal, regulatory, managerial, organizational and legislative – on future strategy, investment characteristics and supportive infrastructures. The team also advises on measures to support the recommended investment-for-health strategy. This work links the recommended investment-for-health strategy to the overall economic and social development agenda of the country.

Appraisal tools and methodologies

Most communities can agree on the major issues affecting their health and sense of wellbeing. Employment, education, financial and physical security and housing will usually top the list, with transportation, urban cleanliness and access to health care following closely. Moving from general agreement on issues to operational strategies, however, is seldom simple.

Investment for health constitutes a complex independent variable whose integrity is damaged by separating its essential elements. For example, various changes in transportation policy (reducing fares for off-peak hours, redesigning vehicles to accommodate elderly and disabled people and changing transport mode (from buses to minivans) to allow greater access to remote dwellings) can reduce the isolation of elderly people. Each change links to other elements of the transport policy so that the effect of changes in one domain is evaluated in terms of the effect on other domains. Similarly, the effect of health investment on transport policy must be measured against its effect on other policy areas, which may complement the change in transport policy. Finally, one must account for how the investments in health gain contribute to community development in broader social and perhaps even economic terms. An evaluation of such impact requires continuous monitoring and sensible criteria to avoid becoming enmeshed in tracking trace elements of effect.

One can assume that all policy areas influence, to some degree, a population's health and welfare. The impact of public policy on health must be assessed both qualitatively and quantitatively. A map of health gain or other inventory of the impact of public policies, private initiatives, regulations and programmes could form a baseline as well as a continuing accounting system *(43,44)*. Table 22.2 comprises a sample; more or different groups and sectors could be covered.

Table 22.2. Sample map of health gain

Population groups	Gains in sectors				
	Health services	Education	Transport	Social care	Environment
1	✓✓✓	✓	✓✓✓	✓	✓✓
2	✓✓	✓✓✓✓✓	0	✓	✓✓✓

Various methodologies can be used to create a map of health gain for a particular community or geographical area. These include typical HIA methods *(45,46)* (see Chapter 18), policy analysis *(47–50)* and simulations *(51)*. Important information can be gathered by involving the community in the appraisal. Nominal group techniques, focus groups and other methods have proven valuable here *(52,53)*.

These techniques, along with decision analysis *(54–57)*, sensitivity analysis *(55,58)* and multiattribute value analysis *(59–61)*, are particularly useful in identifying the potential contribution to health of various policy sectors in a health-gain matrix. This matrix is used when different investment-for-health options have to be weighed according to a number of criteria. Fig. 22.1 shows a health gain matrix with four criteria (C1–C4) that have been agreed for appraising the options. These criteria could be, for example: equity, sustainability, empowerment and the overall resources needed.

The above-mentioned techniques are helpful in weighing the relative importance attributed to these criteria by various segments of the community, policy-makers and other stakeholders. Sensitivity analysis, in particular, can be useful in appraising the degree of variation in the weights given to the various criteria and how this affects the final selection of the investment-for-health option.

Fig. 22.1. A health gain matrix (including criteria)

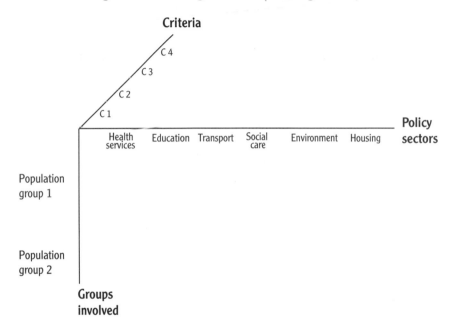

Policy sectors are not waiting to be reformed or even advised by health experts *(62)*. Motivation for strengthening the health impact of a policy area must exist or be fostered to be sufficient to encourage the sharing of data and exploration of options that fit a sector's culture. In addition, the proposed strategy should try to avoid negative consequences (such as additional cost, loss of jobs or jurisdictional conflicts).

The appraisal team learned these lessons in a demonstration project carried out in southern Spain by the WHO Regional Office for Europe in cooperation with the Institute for Public Health of Valencia *(63)*. The main goal of the demonstration was to explore the possibility of developing investment-for-health alliances with sectors crucial to the economic, social and health development of the Valencian Community: health, tourism (which represents a major proportion of the region's gross domestic product – GDP) and agriculture (historically a very important sector for both culture and productivity and still one of the largest economic domains).

The demonstration identified shared goals and policy decisions among the three sectors (area D in Fig. 22.2) that would result in gains for all three. The common agenda for investment for health could be achieved only through negotiated prioritization and a search for win–win solutions. Decisions on this agenda often need to be placed within a bargaining policy environment. Thus, the health sector would be prepared to support win–win decisions for agriculture and tourism (area B, with no effect on health) as long as the agriculture sector was prepared to support win–win decisions for health and tourism (area A) and the tourism sector was willing to support win–win decisions for agriculture and health (area C).

Fig. 22.2. Goals and policy decisions shared by three sectors in the Valencian Community

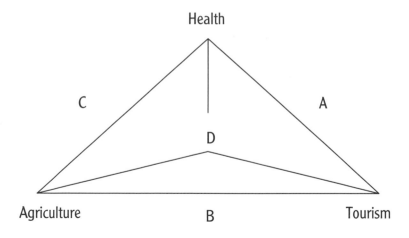

Policy sectors can use many tools and techniques when they revisit their development priorities and establish new and shared ones, thereby setting a common agenda for investment for health. These tools include opportunity appraisals, conflict assessment analysis, multiattribute modeling, stakeholder analysis and behavioural and organizational simulations *(61)*. Theories of institutional change, such as Malinowski's seven notions of value exchange, may contribute to this bargaining process, but concrete case studies and anecdotal material remain the most helpful guidance *(64)*. We hope that a larger number of practical applications of investment for health will culminate in a body of experience-based observation sufficient to form a validating framework for assessing future effects in health investment *(65)*.

A more immediate option for applying investment for health and concomitantly developing a useful evaluation scheme would be to approach investments that minimize the negative health effects of public policies. Literature on the issue and methods of HIA is already substantial (see Chapter 18) *(45,46)*. In contrast to health-enhancement investments that require substantial analysis of health promoting options and weighing of their relative benefits, a pre-emptive focus on first doing no harm seeks policy compliance with a set of prescribed values and specific protections for health. This focus is comparable to the well tested environmental impact statements that accompany various public laws and policies that do or may affect the environment *(66)*. Another example is the social clause; if adopted by international trade negotiators, this would require specific protections for the health and welfare of vulnerable groups in the developing world *(62)*. Appraisal of investment-for-health action taken in these circumstances would focus on each point (or directive) in the policy that prohibits any action that could be detrimental to the health of a vulnerable population. In this approach, both the independent and dependent variables are clear. Measures of these variables would be proxies for measures of ultimate benefits for population health, on the hypothetical grounds of a strong and predictable association between a given legislative initiative to avoid a harmful practice and a specific health benefit to the population.

Clearly, much remains to be learned about the efficacy of the investment-for-health process and the composition of an appropriate menu of factors to be appraised *(38)*. Only through actual field trials can one begin to identify and order the variables that contribute to effective processes and outcomes of health investment. Living laboratories are needed, where the flow of the investment process can be observed and appropriate adjustments made in policy targets, administrative and logistical support, and action strategies. These trials are of particular importance when the aim is maximizing community health assets, rather than minimizing or alleviating the negative impact of public- and private-sector policies and programmes.

Maximizing health assets: learning to appraise investment for health

The WHO Regional Office for Europe has, since 1995, undertaken a series of advisory service activities at the request of several Member States in the spirit of mutual learning about how health investments can be decided, implemented and evaluated *(23,42,67)*. The experience has shown the necessity of taking account of the whole of a country's health promoting assets to locate the increments of development needed, whether substantial policy investments, regulatory changes, nurturing of nongovernmental resources and programme initiatives, strengthening of health promoting infrastructures and decision-making, refocusing on research, training in requisite health promotion skills or environmental improvement.

Indeed, the identification and strengthening of assets are at the heart of investment for health. Such assets can be operationalized according to the priorities and unique opportunities of a given country, region or community. They could include a community's willingness to change and improve its living conditions, the beauty of the physical environment, the level of social capital (see Chapter 19) or any other collective resource that could be used to promote and gain more control over the determinants of population health.

Thinking in terms of assets for health does not come naturally. Most appraisals focus on the needs or problems of a population. Although appraisals take account of health needs, need reduction is not the primary objective of implementing investment for health. The main focus is the status and potential of health assets (resources) (Fig. 22.3).

Fig. 22.3. Needs and assets for health

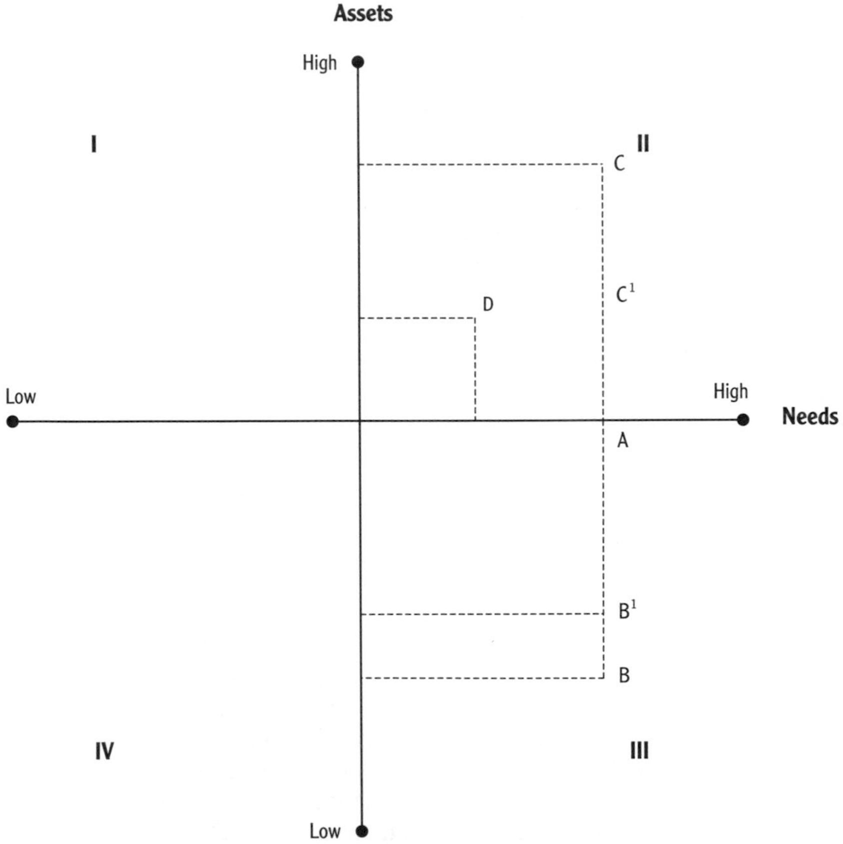

If one assumes that a community's level of need is A on the need axis, the type of strategy for investment for health depends on the community's level of

502

assets: low (B) or high (C). If the chosen strategy has no effect on need (for example, from B to B^1), traditional epidemiological or other need-based indicators would suggest that health promotion has no effect at all, when in fact the strategy increases the community's assets for health. Similarly, if the initial condition of a community is C and, as a result of a given strategy that community moves to C^1, according to conventional need-based evaluation there is no effect, but in practice C^1 is worse than the initial C overall. Further, if a community moves from C to D, D is not necessarily a better condition, because the reduction in need comes with a drop in assets for health.

Appraisal of investment for health involves accounting and searching for asset maximization, not only need reduction. Further, appraisal helps identify different health promotion strategies when a country, region or community belongs to different quadrants in the need–assets grid (see Fig. 22.3). Assets for health can be appraised using the same community participation techniques as those mentioned earlier for the health gain map.

In investment-for-health appraisals (see Appendix), one must take a whole-systems approach to enable policy-makers to comprehend the big picture, identify priorities for investment and create the most appropriate infrastructure and decision-making process to sustain effective investment. Only this all-encompassing approach can optimally deploy the battery of evaluative approaches cited in other chapters of this book. The multitude of factors – economic, social, cultural and political – that interact and form the context for the appraisal of a given health investment at the policy level substantially muddy the waters for evaluators who are used to more orderly traditions of measuring the impact of behaviour change/interventions (see Chapter 16).

WHO has also focused attention on the nature of the direct and indirect contributions of investment for health to economic and social development. These contributions are not a trivial issue in the appraisal plan. At both the government and parliamentary levels, priority-setting values are geared to favour proposals and programmes that will clearly improve the general quality of life and economic prosperity. These goals are more than indications of economic growth; they are indicators of economic development. Economic development implies sustainable growth, the equitable distribution of benefits, quality of life and conservation of resources, both human and environmental.

Health is both a product of and a resource for economic and social development. This relationship is self-evident, but policy-makers do not always act on it. Links between health investment and economic development must be forged. Accounting for these links is a major aspect of evaluating health investments.

A closely related issue is parsimony. Like financial investments, health investing usually seeks the minimum necessary outlay of resources for the largest proportionate benefit. Thus, investments that blend well into existing legislation, cause little or no displacement of resources and have a long shelf-life before requiring revision are favoured. Health investments ideally complement, not supplement, the central thrust of the public policy involved.

That is, they contribute to the central policy goals while achieving health benefits.

In some circumstances, however, investment for health will require substantial policy change, possibly involving major financial, institutional, regulatory or educational efforts. Managing these changes is a key part of investment for health.

Brief reflections on experience to date

Evaluating the health investment process is a formidable task. To be useful, evaluation requires a dedicated and continuing centre for development. The expertise needed may not be available in most countries, even those whose expenditure on health services forms a substantial percentage of GDP. Using appropriate expertise to carry out and sustain an investment-for-health appraisal is a key challenge for implementing the concept and principles of health promotion effectively and credibly.

Investment for health, with its sectoral and intersectoral components, can become a powerful tool for modern public health practice. The technology required for its effective growth, however, is far from fully formed. A general sense of what is required is now emerging through the field consultations and services of the programme on health promotion at the WHO Regional Office for Europe.

Early reviews of the usefulness of investment for health have been positive and suggest exciting new options for improving population health equitably and sustainably, often without additional stress on national budgets. Indeed, such investments are often consistent with announced economic and social goals.

We invite scholars and practitioners in health promotion and allied disciplines to contribute their expertise and experience in applying and testing the efficacy of the Ottawa Charter's challenge to build healthy public policy, create supportive environments, strengthen community action, develop personal skills and reorient health services (2). We strongly believe that these goals can be met pragmatically and effectively through investment for health.

References

1. *Discussion document on the concept and principles of health promotion.* Copenhagen, WHO Regional Office for Europe, 1984 (document).
2. Ottawa Charter for Health Promotion. *Health promotion*, **1**(4): iii–v (1986).
3. *Intersectoral action for health: addressing health and environment concerns in sustainable development.* Geneva, World Health Organization, 1997 (document WHO/PPE/PAC/97.1).
4. *Jakarta Declaration: on leading health promotion into the 21st century. Déclaration de Jakarta sur la promotion de la santé au XXIe siécle*

(http://www.who.int/hpr/docs/index.html). Geneva, World Health Organization, 1997 (document WHO/HPR/HEP/4ICHP/BR/97.4) (accessed on 22 November 2000).

5. ROSEN, G. *A history of public health*. New York, MD Publications, 1958.
6. ROSEN, G. The evolution of social medicine. *In*: Freeman, H.E. et al., ed. *Handbook of medical sociology*. Englewood Cliffs, Prentice Hall, 1979.
7. DUBOS, R. *Mirage of health*. New York, Anchor Books, 1959.
8. POWELS, J. On the limitations of modern medicine. *Science, medicine and man*, **1**: 1–30 (1973).
9. RESEARCH UNIT IN HEALTH AND BEHAVIOURAL CHANGE. *Changing the public health*. Edinburgh, University of Edinburgh, 1989.
10. McKEOWN, T. & RECORD, D. Reasons for the decline of infant mortality in England and Wales during the 20th century. *Population studies*, **16**: 94–122 (1962).
11. McKEOWN, T. A historic appraisal of the medical task. *In*: McLachlan, C. & McKeown, T., ed. *Medical history and medical care: a symposium of perspectives*. London, Oxford University Press, 1971.
12. McKEOWN, T. *The role of medicine: dream, mirage or nemesis?* London, Nuffield Provincial Hospital Trust, 1976.
13. LALONDE, M. *A new perspective on the health of Canadians: a working document*. Ottawa, Canada Information, 1974.
14. DRAPER, P. ET AL. Health and wealth. *Royal Society of Health journal*, **97**(3): 121–126 (1977).
15. OMRAN, A.R. Changing patterns of health and disease during the process of national development. *In*: Albrecht, G.L. & Higgins, P.C., ed. *Health, illness and medicine: a reader in medical sociology*. Chicago, Rand McNally, 1979.
16. POPAY, J. ET AL. The impact of industrialization on world health. *In*: *Through the '80s: thinking globally acting locally*. Washington, DC, World Future Society, 1980.
17. DRAPER, P. & SMART, T. *Health in the economy – The NHS crises in perspective*. London, Unit for the Study of Health Policy, Guy's Hospital Medical School, 1984.
18. MARMOT, M. Improving the social environment to improve health. *Lancet*, **351**(1): 57–60 (1998).
19. MAKARA, P. The effect of social changes on the population's way of life and health: a Hungarian case study. *In*: Levin, S.L. et al., ed. *Economic change, social welfare and health in Europe*. Copenhagen, WHO Regional Office for Europe, 1994 (WHO Regional Publications, European Series, No. 54).
20. WILKINSON, R.G. *Unhealthy societies*. London, Routledge, 1996.
21. LEVIN, S.L. ET AL., ED. *Economic change, social welfare and health in Europe*. Copenhagen, WHO Regional Office for Europe, 1994 (WHO Regional Publications, European Series, No. 54).

505

22. *HEALTH21: an introduction to the health for all policy framework for the WHO European Region.* Copenhagen, WHO Regional Office for Europe, 1998 (European Health for All Series, No. 5).

23. *Public health in Latvia with particular reference to health promotion.* Copenhagen, WHO Regional Office for Europe, 1998 (document EUR/ICP/IVST 04 03 02).

24. MILIO, N. *Promoting health through public policy.* Ottawa, Canadian Public Health Association, 1986.

25. WHITEHEAD, M. Counting the human costs: opportunities for and barriers to promoting health. *In*: Levin, S.L. et al., ed. *Economic change, social welfare and health in Europe.* Copenhagen, WHO Regional Office for Europe, 1994 (WHO Regional Publications, European Series, No. 54).

26. KICKBUSCH, I. Think health: what makes the difference? *In: New players for a new era: leading health promotion into the 21st century: 4th International Conference on Health Promotion, Jakarta, Indonesia, 21–25 July 1997.* Geneva, World Health Organization, 1998 (document).

27. DREZE, J. & SEN, A. *Hunger and public action.* Oxford, Oxford University Press, 1989.

28. CHU, C. Integrating health and environment: the key to an ecological public health. *In*: Chu, C. & Simpson, R., ed. *Ecological public health: from vision to practice.* Brisbane, Queensland, Watson Ferguson & Company, 1994.

29. EVENS, R.G. ET AL., ED. *Why are some people healthy and others not?* New York, Aldine de Gruyter, 1994.

30. SEN, A. *Mortality as an indicator of economic success and failure.* Florence, UNICEF International Child Development Centre, 1995.

31. CORNIA, G.A. & PANICCIA, R. *The demographic impact of sudden impoverishment: eastern Europe during the 1989–94 transition.* Florence, UNICEF International Child Development Centre, 1995.

32. BLANE, D. ET AL. *Health and social organization – Towards a health policy for the 21st century.* London, Routledge, 1996.

33. MUSTARD, J.F. *Health and social organization in health and social capital.* London, Routledge, 1996.

34. CORNIA, G.A. *Labour market shocks, psychosocial stress and the transition's mortality crisis.* October. Helsinki, World Institute for Development of Economic Research, United Nations University, 1997 (Research in Progress 4).

35. BARTLEY, M. ET AL. Socioeconomic determinants of health: health and the life course: why safety nets matter. *British medical journal,* **314**(4): 1194–1196 (1997).

36. *Health in social development. WHO position paper. World Summit for Social Development, Copenhagen, March 1995.* Geneva, World Health Organization, 1995 (document WHO/DGH/95.1).

37. *The world health report 1998. Life in the 21st century: a vision for all. Report of the Director-General.* Geneva, World Health Organization, 1998.
38. ZIGLIO, E. *Producing and sustaining health: the investment for health approach.* Copenhagen, WHO Regional Office for Europe, 1998 (document).
39. *World Health Assembly resolution WHA51.12 on health promotion* (http://www.who.int/hpr/docs/index.html). Geneva, World Health Organization, 1998 (accessed on 8 December 2000).
40. ZIGLIO, E. Key issues for the new millennium. *Promoting health: the journal of health promotion for Northern Ireland,* **2**: 34–37 (1998).
41. SALTMAN, R. & FIGUERAS, J. *European health care reform, analysis of current strategies.* Copenhagen, WHO Regional Office for Europe, 1997 (WHO Regional Publications, European Series No. 79).
42. *Investment for health in Hungary.* Copenhagen, WHO Regional Office for Europe, 1997 (document EUR/ICP/IVST 04 02 03).
43. *Securing investment in health: Report of a demonstration project in the provinces of Bolzano and Trento. Final report. June 1995.* Trento, Autonomous Province of Trento, 1995.
44. ZIGLIO, E. How to move towards evidence-based health promotion interventions. *Promotion and education,* **IV**(2): 29–33 (1996).
45. Assessing health and monitoring progress in populations. *In*: Abelin, T. et al., ed. *Measurement in health promotion and protection.* Copenhagen, World Health Organization, 1987, pp. 389–531 (WHO Regional Publications, European Series, No. 22).
46. SWEDISH NATIONAL INSTITUTE OF PUBLIC HEALTH. *Determinants of the burden of disease in the European Union.* Stockholm, National Institute of Public Health, 1997 (F series No. 24).
47. BREWER, G. & DE LEON, P. *Foundations of policy analysis.* Homewood, IL, Dorsey, 1983.
48. WILDAVSKI, A. *Speaking truth to power. The art and craft of policy analysis.* Boston, Little Brown & Co., 1979.
49. VEDUNG, E. *Public policy and programme evaluation.* London, Transnational, 1997.
50. WEISS, C.H. *Methods for studying programmes and policies.* Upper Saddle River, Prentice Hall, 1998.
51. MCMAHON, L. Learning from the future – Using behavioural simulations for management learning. *Future management,* **1**: 4–5 (1995).
52. DELBECQ, A.L. ET AL. *Group techniques for program planning: a guide to nominal group and Delphi processes.* Glenview, IL, Scott-Foreman and Co., 1975.
53. ZIGLIO, E. The Delphi method and its contribution to decision-making. *In*: Adler, M. & Ziglio, E., ed. *Gazing into the oracle: the Delphi method and its application to social policy and public health.* London, Jessica Kingsley Publishers Ltd, 1996.

507

54. GUSTAFSON, D.H. & HOLLOWAY, D. A decision theory approach to measuring severity of illness. *Health services research*, **10**: 97–196 (1975).

55. PHILLIPS, L.D. A theory of requisite decision models. *Acta psychologica*, **56**: 29–48 (1984).

56. LINSTONE, H.A., ED. *Multiple perspectives for decision-making: bridging the gap between analysis and action*. Amsterdam, North Holland, 1984.

57. LINSTONE, H.A. & MELTSNER, X. Guidelines for users of multiple perspectives. *In*: Linstone, H.A., ed. *Multiple perspectives for decision-making: bridging the gap between analysis and action*. Amsterdam, North Holland, 1984.

58. ALEMI, F. ET AL. How to construct a subjective index. *Evaluation and health professions*, **9**(1): 45–52 (1986).

59. COOK, R.L. & STEWART, T.R. A comparison of seven methods for obtaining subjective description of judgmental policy. *Organizational behavior and human performance*, **12**: 31–45 (1975).

60. KEENEY, R.L. The art of assessing multi-attribute utility functions. *Organizational behavior and human performance*, **19**: 267–310 (1977).

61. GUSTAFSON, D.H. ET AL. *Systems to support health policy analysis: theory, models and uses*. Ann Arbor, Health Administration Press, 1992.

62. LABONTÉ, R. Healthy public policy and the World Trade Organization. *Health promotion international*, **13**(3): 245–256 (1998).

63. *Investment for health in the Valencia Region: mid-term report*. Copenhagen, WHO Regional Office for Europe, 1996 (document).

64. MALINOWSKI, B. The group and individual in functional analysis. *American journal of sociology*, **44**: 938–964 (1939).

65. LEVIN, S.L. & ZIGLIO, E. Health promotion as an investment strategy: a perspective for the 21st century. *In*: Sidell, M. et al., ed. *Debates and dilemmas in promoting health*. London, Macmillan, 1997.

66. MACARTHUR, I. & BONNEFOY, X. *Environmental health services in Europe 2. Policy options*. Copenhagen, WHO Regional Office for Europe, 1998 (WHO Regional Publications, European Series, No. 77).

67. *Investment for health in Slovenia*. Copenhagen, WHO Regional Office for Europe, 1996 (document).

Appendix. The appraisal process

Here we outline the process of the investment-for-heath appraisal service developed by the WHO Regional Office for Europe.[7] This process necessarily differs from those used in the demonstration projects mentioned above. The appraisal of investment for health, as so far practised, has operated at a country level, and been initiated by a WHO Member State's national parliament and supported by the health ministry. The process comprises: initiation, preparation, team briefing, fieldwork, report writing and submission, and longer-term follow-up.

Initiation

Typically, parliamentary, government, professional or other officials of a Member State will initiate discussions with Regional Office staff about policy-making, organizational or other aspects of their health promotion arrangements that cause them concern. Such discussions often evoke the possibility of WHO's offering assistance through the new service for appraisal of investment for health. Its applicability to a Member State's situation is normally judged by the following criteria.

1. The Member State has already taken some important steps in developing health promotion.
2. Before drafting a service agreement with WHO, relevant officials understand the investment appraisal service and its implications for government decision-makers.
3. The service is provided at the joint invitation of the government and parliament.
4. The Member State demonstrates its commitment to the service by agreeing to provide some of the necessary resources for its operation.
5. Senior officials are assigned responsibility for ensuring that terms of the service agreement are fulfilled, including commitment to longer-term follow-through work with the WHO Regional Office for Europe.

The Member State's priority statement and the intended response of the appraisal service comprise the heart of the service agreement. Typical examples of priority statements include:

• increasing understanding of some of the opportunities to strengthen health, taking into account relevant economic, social, cultural and psychological factors;
• strengthening integration of existing health promotion activities;

---

[7] ZIGLIO, E. & HAGARD, S. *Appraising investment for health opportunities.* Copenhagen, WHO Regional Office for Europe, 1998.

- creating greater awareness in government and parliament of the importance of health promotion and the need to take appropriate action; and
- strengthening the basis for sound decision-making and choice of priorities, in the light of current economic circumstances, to optimize the return on investment.

The appraisal service provides an expert international team, experienced in the priority areas raised by the Member State, to appraise and report to both the health ministry and parliament on:

- the strategy needed to improve the health status of the population
- the potential for investment for health in the country
- the infrastructure needed to build, support and sustain investment for health.

Preparation

When the Regional Office for Europe and the Member State have made an agreement to proceed with the appraisal service, a detailed service planning process begins. The senior officials named in the service agreement and the expert appraisal team leader and secretariat (from the Regional Office) do this planning in the country. This preparatory phase includes:

1. briefing the health minister and senior representatives of parliament;
2. briefing all parties involved in the organizational arrangements for the service and assigning them specific tasks;
3. agreeing on dates for fieldwork by the appraisal team;
4. considering the range of skills and experience the team will need, which the team leader should take into account in selecting members;
5. meeting and briefing members of a multidisciplinary local resource group, appointed by the country, to provide technical assistance to the team;
6. preparing specific analyses of a wide range of policy sectors;
7. agreeing on a schedule and location for interviews and for individual and group meetings of team members with key representatives of relevant organizations and with other people within and outside the health sector;
8. before the fieldwork, planning the content and assembly of a resource pack to brief team members, and preparing a written presentation of the appraisal process for all parties involved; and
9. developing a process within which the tasks described above can be fulfilled in a participatory and transparent manner involving a wide range of the country's institutions, professionals, nongovernmental organizations, lay community representatives and others.

Team briefing

At least four weeks before the fieldwork is due to start, team members receive their resource packs. These packs include documents about the country's:

510

- history and geography
- constitution and governance system
- laws most directly affecting health
- key economic and health-related budgetary data
- demographic, social, health and morbidity/mortality data
- relevant structural, organizational and institutional information, including nongovernmental resources affecting health.

Having read the resource packs, team members assemble in the Member State for 2–3 days of detailed briefing, analysis and fieldwork planning.

Fieldwork

Fieldwork usually extends over two weeks, and has five purposes:

- to recognize the potential contribution of different elements in the country to promoting health and identify the practical steps for activating these elements (accomplished through interviews and semistructured discussions with key individuals and groups, both government and nongovernmental);
- to assess and analyse the country's economic, social, institutional, legislative and other potential strengths and weaknesses as these may affect the promotion of health;
- to begin formulating conclusions and an outline of the main elements of a potential investment-for-health strategy, including proposals for the essential development and reform of legislative, institutional, organizational and professional arrangements and processes;
- to stimulate and sustain learning by and political consensus on aims, methods and strategy among leaders whose future day-to-day collaboration will be essential for successful investment for health; and
- to provide an outline to the country's government and parliament of the main elements of an investment for health strategy for their country.

Report writing and submission

As fieldwork draws to a close, the appraisal team increasingly directs its attention to the construction of its report to the country's relevant minister (usually the health minister) and parliament. The appraisal team's leader and rapporteur facilitate the work by agreeing on the report's overall structure, broad conclusions and recommendations. Then the full team reviews their work. The local resource group has a major role at this stage: acting as a sounding board before the main elements of the report are discussed with the minister and parliament.

The rapporteur is responsible for writing, consulting with the other team members and clearing a draft report with the team leader within four weeks. The team submits the draft report to the minister and parliament for comments and the verification of facts. With these, the rapporteur completes the report, and the team leader formally submits it.

In doing so, the team leader aligns the report with the central aim of the investment-for-health appraisal process by pointing out that the report, itself the result of a wide-ranging and participatory process, has assembled the results in a format to be used to enhance discussion, foster consensus, stimulate synergy and direct the action of both government and parliament. Thus, the report is not a static document, but an important instrument to facilitate progress in formulating, implementing and sustaining an innovative and effective investment strategy for promoting the population's health.

The WHO Regional Office for Europe offers its support to the country in acting on the recommendations. This support has taken the forms of participation in parliamentary discussions, advice about implementation and structured capacity-building activities.

Presenting the appraisal report
The team's appraisal has three parts:

1. the overall situation in the country;
2. sector-by-sector analysis (industry and commerce as a whole; financial services; tourism and catering; agriculture horticulture, and the food industry; transport; education; health care; and the mass media) and policy options for intersectoral consideration; and
3. structural, organizational, intersectoral and institutional issues.

The appraisal of the first and second items identifies the perceived strengths and weaknesses in policy development of current investment-for-health practice, followed by an assessment of future opportunities and threats. The third part addresses issues related to both sectoral and intersectoral development. Each part of the appraisal identifies the opportunities to promote health more effectively through key policy features of economic and social development and through the corresponding opportunities to strengthen such development through investment for health.

The third part of the appraisal requires a little more discussion. Reporting on structural, organizational, intersectoral and institutional issues focuses on the extent to which the policy environment is sufficiently conducive to investment for health. The policy environment must be able to develop and sustain:

1. consensual policy-making (favouring sustainable medium- and long-term commitments from government) and consistent, well informed support from parliament and other policy-making bodies for the approach and implications of investment for health;
2. a fully coherent and enabling infrastructure to assist policy formulation and ensure its implementation;
3. an appropriate focus and sufficient capacity at national and subnational levels;
4. evidence-based local health promotion practices;

5. incentives for alliance building at all levels;
6. skilled survey, research and evaluation practice;
7. education and training for all aspects of health promotion practice, especially advocacy, mediation, and community participation and empowerment; and
8. long-term resources and their flexible and sustainable use.

The appraisal team presents practical recommendations on fundamental issues, and offers WHO advice and assistance with implementation. Typically, the team's presentation includes:

1. advice to the government and parliament for drawing up an investment-for-health strategy;
2. recommendations identifying specific deficiencies in the current health promotion infrastructure and the steps needed to repair them;
3. procedures to establish secure and robust long-term funding of investment for health; and
4. plans to devise and implement robust measures for the development and deployment of sufficient numbers of the appropriately skilled personnel necessary for successful investment for health.

In focusing on an overall systems view of the task, the recommendations on infrastructure call for structural changes based on sound functional analyses, adapting and modifying wherever possible. They suggest new structures only if adaptation is impossible.

Part 5
Synthesis and conclusion

23

Evaluation in health promotion: synthesis and recommendations

Michael S. Goodstadt, Brian Hyndman, David V. McQueen, Louise Potvin, Irving Rootman and Jane Springett

From its inception, a clear and specific goal has guided the development of this book *(1)*:

> To stimulate and support innovative approaches to the evaluation and practice of health promotion, by reviewing the theory and best practice of evaluation and by producing guidelines and recommendations for health promotion policy-makers and practitioners concerning evaluation of health promotion approaches.

This chapter revisits and examines the work of the WHO European Working Group on Health Promotion Evaluation from two perspectives. First, the Group can ask how well it has accomplished the specific tasks set in its two objectives: examining the current range of quantitative and qualitative evaluation methods and providing guidance to policy-makers and practitioners. Success is essential to fostering the use of appropriate methods for health promotion evaluation and increasing the quality of such evaluations *(1)*.

An examination of the Group's work suggests that it has achieved its objectives. The chapters of this book comprise an extensive compilation and discussion of the theory, methodologies and practice of evaluating health promotion initiatives. Further, the document *Health promotion evaluation: recommendations to policy-makers (1)* provides general but seminal recommendations to guide policy-makers and others involved in decisions that affect the evaluation of health promotion practice. To this extent, the Working Group is confident that its work will have a positive impact on the quantity and quality of health promotion evaluation. Nevertheless, it must assess its work more critically. The Working Group has much to gain from examining its fidelity to the original conceptual framework (see Chapter 1) by synthesizing what it has learned, probing unanswered questions and outstanding issues, and suggesting an action plan for improving the future evaluation of health promotion.

Revisiting a framework for health promotion evaluation

Chapter 1 has two objectives: attempting to capture the Working Group's initial

517

perspectives on the evaluation of health promotion and acting as a reference point for the development of the project and the remaining chapters. As to its first objective, after clarifying the understanding of health promotion and evaluation, Chapter 1 presents three distinct, interrelated dimensions of the Group's thinking about health promotion evaluation. First, it identifies five overriding issues that are fundamental to, though often left latent in, any discussion of health promotion evaluation: social programming; knowledge construction, valuing and use; and evaluation itself. Then it discusses eight challenges faced in evaluating health promotion: philosophical (including epistemological) issues; conceptual ones related specifically to health promotion (empowerment, capacity building and control); issues related to the role of theory in health promotion and its evaluation and to the appropriateness of methodologies; and ethical, political and other types of issues related to evaluating health promotion. Last, it provides a more specific framework that outlines the principles and the seven steps involved in undertaking health promotion evaluation.

A book of this kind cannot be expected to meet the needs of all readers: a single volume cannot do justice to the range and depth of issues associated with health promotion evaluation. An examination of the topics covered, as well as the manner in which issues are discussed, suggests that the book possesses both strengths and weaknesses, depending on the reader's point of view.

This volume has many strengths. It covers a wide range of both general and specific topics related to the evaluation of health promotion. At the more general level, most of the chapters comprising Part 2 (and especially Chapter 3) deal with generic issues related to the nature and meaning of evidence in evaluating health promotion initiatives, and how this evidence can/should be obtained. Other chapters address issues of general relevance to health promotion evaluation, such as qualitative versus experimental methodologies, and participatory research and evaluation (see chapters 2 and 5).

Dealing with more specific issues, the present volume makes a strong contribution by providing detailed discussions of and guidance on health promotion evaluation in the community in general and three settings in particular: schools, the workplace and urban areas (chapters 10–14). In addition, chapters 15–18 deal with issues in evaluating policies in general or those intended to promote health or support other health initiatives at the community, national and international levels. Chapters 19–21 provide insights into issues related specifically to the evaluation of health communication, health systems and the emerging field of social capital's contributions to the development and maintenance of health in communities. In summary, the Working Group feels justified in concluding that its attention to many of the general and specific issues involved in evaluation both makes a contribution to the field of health promotion and is faithful to the discussion of the five fundamental issues set out in Chapter 1.

While many readers may benefit from this book's guidance on these issues, some might be less satisfied with the level of detail and direction it provides on how to conduct evaluations of health promotion initiatives. Early in the life of the project, however, the Working Group decided that the creation of a recipe book for evaluation should not be the priority. It had two reasons for this decision. First, a vast library of manuals can provide step-by-step guidance on how to conduct evaluations. The challenges faced by health promotion emanate from the goals, values, principles and strategies that are particularly characteristic of health promotion practice, such as those set out in the Ottawa Charter for Health Promotion *(2)*. At each step of the evaluation process, such as the seven steps set out in Chapter 1, practitioners must ask what innovative evaluation methodologies or modifications to standard procedures are required to address the unique issues and challenges involved in evaluating health promotion initiatives.

Second, until those in health promotion have developed a clear scientific foundation, and dealt with broad, often difficult and sometimes value-laden questions, evaluation will remain *ad hoc* and sometimes incoherent and unconvincing. The authors have therefore struggled with and, they hope, clarified the larger questions about the nature of the phenomena to evaluate (that is, the ontological question), what knowledge means with respect to the effectiveness of health promotion (the epistemological question) and how this knowledge might be acquired through evaluation of health promotion (see Chapter 3).

By way of conclusion, this final chapter addresses three questions.

1. What has been learned about the evaluation of health promotion?
2. What issues and questions still need resolution?
3. What is needed to foster more appropriate evaluations of health promotion?

A detailed analysis of how the chapters in this volume might answer these questions indicates that the three are closely related; for example, outstanding issues relate both to what those in health promotion have learned and to what they need to do in the future. For simplicity and clarity, the next two sections give a detailed analysis of the first two questions and then focus on recommendations for the future of health promotion evaluation. The chapter concludes by presenting a generic model to assist in planning and evaluating health promotion initiatives.

Lessons about the evaluation of health promotion
The Working Group has identified at least nine important principles; evaluation in health promotion:

1. is an evolving field
2. can make a major contribution to practice
3. suffers from a shortage of evidence on the effectiveness of initiatives

4. involves a wide range of approaches and models
5. offers legitimate roles for both qualitative and quantitative methodologies
6. employs a wide range of social science disciplines and approaches
7. builds on a range of planning models
8. requires theory and other conceptualizations to be effective
9. offers many potential roles to evaluators/researchers.

An evolving field

The discussion contained in many chapters shows that health promotion is an evolving field. Paradoxically, while people have been doing health promotion for many years, if not centuries, only in the last few decades have health promotion practitioners begun to identify a coherent set of values, goals, principles, strategies and practices that offers a more comprehensive and potentially more effective approach to health-related problems in communities. Although many of the approaches taken by previous generations to prevent health problems and strengthen health are compatible with recent developments in health promotion, the principles and strategies – as set out in documents such as the Ottawa Charter for Health Promotion *(2)* and the Jakarta Declaration on Leading Health Promotion into the 21st Century *(3)* – reflect a rapid development in the understanding of health, the broad set of social, environmental and individual factors that affect it, and the complex array of approaches required for effective action (see Chapter 22).

Not surprisingly, however, the evolving nature of health promotion presents many challenges. First, the conceptual challenge is to provide a clear, coherent and convincing statement of what constitutes health promotion. The second challenge is to identify and conceptually organize the full range of approaches, strategies and interventions (programmes, policies and services) that constitute health promotion's repertoire of activities. The third challenge is to select and implement the coordinated subset of strategies most likely to have the desired effect. The final challenge is to address issues and problems involved in evaluation, as discussed in this book.

Increasing pressure for evaluation is another feature of the developing field of health promotion. This has several origins, resulting in evaluation's taking several forms. First, health promotion practitioners and stakeholders often experience self-imposed internal pressure. Professional and other stakeholders frequently have a strong personal investment in their health promotion interventions, resulting in a natural desire to know whether their time, energy and other resources are well spent. They often want to know not only whether their efforts have had a positive effect (outcome or impact evaluation) but also the reasons why (process evaluation). A second and increasing demand for evaluation of health promotion has its roots in the external pressure imposed by government and nongovernmental funding agencies' demand for accountability (see Chapter 8). Understandably, they want reassurance that their increasingly scarce financial resources are being appropriately used. Funding agencies most commonly require:

520

- evidence of effectiveness and particularly cost-related effectiveness (cost–effectiveness, cost–benefit or cost–utility analyses); and/or
- evidence that interventions have been, or are being, implemented as originally intended.

While not wanting to appear defensive about the state of health promotion and health promotion evaluation, the Working Group could argue that an emerging field is not expected to be as sophisticated as those with longer histories. In addition, health promotion reflects the state of development in the many disciplines from which it draws. That is, the challenges faced in evaluating health promotion initiatives are similar, if not identical, to those faced in the evaluation of initiatives in related fields, including education, social work, psychology, sociology, urban planning and public health. As these disciplines develop and evaluate programmes and policies that address the needs of communities, they face the same four challenges as health promotion. The Working Group therefore expects that health promotion in general and its evaluation in particular will continue to evolve, and that the latter will continue to benefit from developments in its parent disciplines.

Major contribution to practice

One of the most powerful conclusions drawn from the chapters in this publication is the special value of evaluation to health promotion practice. Many authors deal at length with the multiple approaches to and benefits of evaluation. In summary, evaluation can increase the quality and effectiveness of any initiative by contributing to the processes of its planning, development and implementation. Several chapters argue that appropriate evaluation procedures contribute to health promotion in two general ways. First, they can help to develop knowledge valuable at the local level and can be applicable to initiatives in other settings and circumstances. Second, procedures can contribute to the central mechanism of health promotion – the empowerment of individual and community stakeholders to exercise control over the factors affecting their health – by:

1. providing the knowledge base that allows stakeholders to exercise control in identifying issues and making informed decisions on actions that affect their wellbeing;
2. promoting appropriate expectations for responsibility and accountability among partners; and
3. strengthening the capacity of marginalized groups to understand and control their own affairs.

Shortage of evidence on effectiveness

Relatively few evaluations of health promotion have been undertaken, at least as shown by the published literature; systematic reviews of health promotion are in particularly short supply. The paucity of evaluations is less disheartening, however, when one understands the difficulties in undertaking and publishing them, and compares the state of evaluation in health promotion and other fields.

Various chapters identify three groups of factors that contribute to the lack of access to evaluations of health promotion. First, some factors relate to the ability to undertake health promotion evaluations. These include the inherent difficulty of evaluating complex interventions that involve multilevel, multistrategy interventions, have an extended time frame and have poor control over the implementation of health promotion initiatives. In addition, funding for appropriate kinds of evaluation is limited; relatively few resources have historically been invested in the evaluation of the complex interventions that characterize health promotion. A second set of factors relates to the criteria for assessing effectiveness. This challenge has two aspects: the great debate over appropriate methodologies, variables, measures and criteria for evaluating individual initiatives, and the considerable disagreement about appropriate methods (for example, randomized controlled trials versus community stories – analysing narratives provided by the people involved in or affected by an issue) for synthesizing the evidence on the effectiveness of health promotion in general. The influence of evidence-based medicine creates pressure to measure effectiveness against the so-called gold standard of randomized controlled trials, which are held to be a prerequisite criterion for inclusion in reviews of the literature. Finally, some factors limit the ability to know about (and learn from) the evaluations that are undertaken, including the limited outlets for publishing health promotion evaluations and the difficulty of identifying the grey or fugitive evaluations that are not published in accessible journals and books.

As discussed, the low number and methodological limitations of health promotion evaluations reflect the current phase in the evolution of both health promotion and evaluation. Again, one should recognize that many related fields face the same evaluation challenges, with similar meagre outcomes. For example, reviews of the literature on the effectiveness of initiatives related to nutrition, drug use, physical activity and teenage pregnancy have identified few well conducted evaluations or consistent findings. The Working Group hopes that health promotion evaluations will continue to grow in quantity and quality, with a corresponding increase in the number of comprehensive reviews of the health promotion literature.

Use of a wide range of approaches and models

Many in the health promotion community question traditional assumptions about evaluation goals and research paradigms, methodologies, designs and methods. At the same time, they are uncertain or confused about the utility and appropriateness of the alternatives. This debate has many aspects, including: the appropriateness of traditional evaluation methodologies based on a positivistic research paradigm, the identification and/or development of alternative approaches and the possible dominance of a limited subset of professional fields (and their particular areas and methods of research) in health promotion research and evaluation (in particular, the weight given to epidemiological and biomedical research).

Legitimate roles for qualitative and quantitative methodologies[8]
A recurring, highly contentious issue encountered in many chapters relates to the appropriateness of quantitative and qualitative approaches. Four questions need to be asked about the latter.

1. What is qualitative research in health promotion terms?
2. How appropriate is it to the evaluation of health promotion initiatives?
3. How useful is it in such evaluations?
4. What do evaluators need to know about applying qualitative research methods in such evaluations?

The chapter authors generally agree that qualitative research is useful and appropriate in the evaluation of most health promotion initiatives, except in economic evaluation. They also appear to agree that such evaluations require the use of both qualitative and quantitative methods.

The authors seem to be less united, however, in defining qualitative research in health promotion terms, using *qualitative* to refer to an evaluation approach or design, the type of data collected, data-collection techniques or a form of analysis. *Qualitative research* can therefore be considered a paradigm, a methodology and/or a method. These different perspectives raise a number of issues, including: which paradigm is best for health promotion, which methodology is most consistent with the chosen paradigm and which specific methods, qualitative or otherwise, are best suited to answer the questions posed by an evaluation in particular circumstances and a particular context.

Finally, while a great deal is known about the use of qualitative research in health promotion evaluation, more skill and knowledge are required. Examples of areas requiring further exploration include: how to combine qualitative with quantitative research methods, what procedures to follow to ensure confidence in the results, how best to provide further training and education for health promotion evaluators in the use of qualitative research and how to address ethical issues.

Use of a wide range of social science disciplines and approaches
As already indicated, health promotion frequently involves multistrategy interventions in complex community settings that do not lend themselves to the kind of (and standards for) control favoured by traditional research and evaluation methodologies. In addition, health promotion is ideologically committed

---

[8] This section summarizes the conclusions of an analysis by Barbara Kahan *(The role of qualitative research in the evaluation of health promotion initiatives: an examination of a collection of papers written for WHO.* Toronto, University of Toronto, 1998 (document)).

to promoting empowerment and community ownership of all aspects of an intervention's development and evaluation. For these reasons, the range of approaches available to evaluators must be broad enough to permit the selection of methodologies that are appropriate to the breadth of issues and settings in which they will be used.

In addition, health promotion initiatives are typically complex responses to problems or issues that have been identified through a variety of data sources (such as community stories) and epidemiology and population surveys. These responses depend for their effectiveness on the use of a broad array of social sciences, such as psychology, sociology, political science, anthropology and economics. The evaluation of health promotion initiatives should therefore pay attention to the psychosocial and cultural factors and theoretical variables underlying initiatives, rather than merely assessing initiatives' impact on outcomes such as the incidence or prevalence of health problems.

Use of a range of planning models

Many have observed that the process of evaluation is integrally related to the process of planning. The two can be seen as mirror images; planning, implementation and evaluation are often portrayed as components of an iterative cycle, whereby planning leads to implementation, which leads to evaluation, which in turn can lead to a further development in planning, etc. Not surprisingly, therefore, several chapters discuss the planning and implementation of health promotion initiatives. Part of this discussion elaborates a number of models. Issues particularly relevant for health promotion evaluation include: the differences between community and other health promotion programmes (especially in their complexity and extended time frames), large- versus small-scale community programmes, the influence of environment on programme impact and the differing functions of evaluation as a programme progresses through development, implementation and conclusion. Each of these stages poses different evaluation questions.

Role of theory and other conceptualizations in effective evaluation

Many chapters emphasize the important contributions made by theory and related conceptualizations to the processes of evaluation. Theory, as well as more limited concepts and assumptions, contributes to evaluation in two important ways; they provide a framework for planning and implementing evaluation and are essential to understanding why and how an initiative succeeds or fails to produce its desired effects. Although whether there is a theory of health promotion is not yet clear (just as it is not clear that theories of public health or education exist), theory can contribute to health promotion practice in a number of ways. For example, theories and concepts help to describe and explain the nature and etiology of issues. Abundant theories and concepts drawn from the social sciences help in developing and implementing effective ways of responding to issues. In addition, health promotion concepts incorporated into frameworks such as the Ottawa Charter for Health Promotion (2) provide

524

a foundation and process for developing these responses. Finally, evaluation is always embedded in the theoretical and conceptual perspectives of evaluators; hence the importance of a careful and critical analysis of evaluators' values and interests.

Roles of evaluators/researchers
In addition to evaluators and researchers' obvious role in assessing the effectiveness of initiatives, this book identifies their other important contributions to health promotion in general (see chapters 4, 10 and 11). Evaluators can provide added value through two particular aspects of their work. In their primary role as knowledge developers, evaluators are in a powerful position to reduce barriers and resistance to knowledge development, to encourage the sharing of knowledge among all stakeholders and to foster the use of evaluation results. In fostering the principle of participatory evaluation, evaluators are able to promote stakeholders' participation in all elements and stages of the health promotion initiative, and to increase their capacity to plan and carry out evaluations and to identify and make use of their implications.

Recommendations to foster more appropriate evaluations of health promotion

All chapters make recommendations on what is needed to improve health promotion evaluation. A detailed analysis of these recommendations clustered them into three major categories: philosophical and conceptual needs, methodological needs and other practical, political and ethical needs. Not surprisingly, these categories and their constituent recommendations closely correspond to the conclusions and recommendations for policy-makers developed by the WHO European Working Group on Health Promotion Evaluation (1). For reasons of coherence and symmetry, the authors of this chapter summarize this book's recommendations within the context of the recommendations to policy-makers. The recommendations given here provide the basis for a comprehensive plan of action to foster more appropriate evaluations of health promotion. While some f the tasks listed would fall to other groups, policy-makers would be responsible for enabling them to be accomplished.

1. Policy-makers should "encourage the adoption of participatory approaches to evaluation that provide meaningful opportunities for involvement by all of those with a direct interest in health promotion initiatives" (1) by:

   - increasing public and private stakeholders' participation in evaluations, to increase timeliness and usefulness;
   - studying the impact of community participation on the validity of the research;
   - identifying local assets; and
   - identifying and working with new partners, such as economists.

2. Policy-makers should "require that a minimum of ten percent of the total financial resources for a health promotion initiative be allocated to evaluation" *(1)*; they should provide funds to support participatory evaluation and to disseminate reports of policy implications outside professional circles.
3. Policy-makers should "ensure that a mixture of process and outcome information is used to evaluate all health promotion initiatives" *(1)* by:

   - widening definitions of outcome to include the processes and outcomes identified or implied in the Ottawa Charter for Health Promotion *(2)*;
   - designing outcome measures that are practical, while capturing the full impact of health promotion interventions;
   - using indicators at various levels, including the community level;
   - providing a full account of proximal and distal outcomes;
   - judging each project against its own aims and objectives;
   - articulating specific national and regional health goals and objectives;
   - developing indicators that could clarify the relationship between healthy public policy and health status;
   - using indicators of important determinants of health as benchmarks of progress;
   - developing methods for process evaluation to assess partnerships, and tools for monitoring the long-term sustainability of collective action;
   - emphasizing the continuous collection of consistent and relevant information on programme performance;
   - assessing health impact using measurable outcomes based on a continuum of health; and
   - adding quality assurance to discussions of effectiveness and efficiency.

4. Policy-makers should "support the use of multiple methods to evaluate health promotion initiatives" and "further research into the development of appropriate approaches to evaluating health promotion initiatives" *(1)*. To address philosophical and conceptual needs, they should:

   - redefine rigour in evaluation;
   - question randomization and the randomized controlled trial as requirements for adequate evaluation;
   - develop appropriate theory and methods of evaluation;
   - develop and use an interdisciplinary science of population health;
   - understand both qualitative and quantitative approaches;
   - make explicit the theoretical links related to initiatives;
   - increase the transparency of conflicting interests and give greater attention to epistemology;
   - articulate the purposes underlying projects and activities;
   - accept that participatory evaluation is political; and
   - place more emphasis on concepts such as quality of life and social capital.

526

As to evaluation and research designs and methodologies, they should:

- make evaluation an internal part of every programme;
- develop and use a wider range of designs;
- employ multiparadigm designs;
- encourage the use of alternative methodologies;
- adapt methods from other disciplines;
- use an action research approach;
- develop a more dynamic set of methods and procedures to reflect changes in a programme over time;
- strengthen mechanisms that triangulate multiple information sets;
- use strategically oriented analyses of the policy-making process;
- focus on policy analysis that is theoretically informed about the structure and dynamics of the policy-making process;
- complement economic evaluations with other kinds;
- incorporate less formal economic appraisals into the planning process;
- use more partial evaluations;
- critically analyse the use of auditing methods in international health promotion partnerships.

5. Policy-makers should "support the establishment of a training and education infrastructure to develop expertise in the evaluation of health promotion initiatives" *(1)* by:

- making changes in bodies that train, develop, fund and disseminate evaluations to encourage a new focus on policy evaluation;
- providing skills training for researchers and practitioners, including the use of both qualitative and quantitative research methods;
- enhancing community capacities by mapping them and identifying the connection between them and the attainment of programme goals;
- increasing the number of skilled researchers available; and
- incorporating an understanding and appreciation of health communication research methods into graduate training (of epidemiologists and health professionals, for example).

6. Policy-makers should "create and support opportunities for sharing information on evaluation methods in health promotion through conferences, workshops, networks and other means" *(1)* by:

- facilitating the alignment of evaluation findings with the priorities of the organizations with which potential users are associated;
- disseminating information in a planned and systematic fashion;
- strengthening countries' information on health and risk factors by providing reports from different sectors; and

527

- identifying and using innovative examples of more effective ways of communication through conventional and electronic media.

7. Policy-makers should also build a strong infrastructure for evaluation by ensuring funding, training, organizational development and networking to support:

- determining how information on risk factors can best be compiled, assessed and synthesized;
- identifying information needs and organizing information collection activities from the beginning of a programme;
- creating national data sets that provide information on the most effective audience segments to address for the wide variety of public health issues;
- encouraging efforts to evaluate community health promotion programmes;
- ensuring that stakeholders' needs and expectations are met in a timely and cost-efficient way;
- increasing research into the quality of international cooperation;
- launching international research on global cooperation in health promotion training and research;
- undertaking studies designed to capture the complete social diffusion process of mass-media campaigns; and
- providing better descriptions of interventions.

Generic model for planning and evaluating health promotion

A number of models, differing in purpose and content, have relevance to the evaluation of health promotion initiatives. Some models, the prime example of which is the Ottawa Charter for Health Promotion *(2)*, are largely conceptual in nature and recommend broad goals, values, principles and general strategies for health promotion. Others, such as PATCH *(4,5)* and MATCH (the multilevel approach to community health *(5)*), have been developed to assist in the operational planning of initiatives. Few, if any, of these models, however, address the planning of initiatives under the guidance of the goals, values, principles and strategies contained in frameworks such as the Ottawa Charter. The general evaluation literature is replete with a third group of models, which suggest structures and flow for evaluation processes; similarly, however, few of these address the issues and challenges of evaluating initiatives grounded in the Ottawa Charter or similar frameworks. A fourth group focuses on the interrelationships between conceptual, planning and evaluation elements, such as PRECEDE/PROCEED *(5)*, but they are not grounded in health promotion principles as reflected in the Ottawa Charter and similar frameworks.

Thus, a model needs to be developed that incorporates three elements:

- the principles and strategies in the Ottawa Charter;
- a structure and sequence of components that can be used in planning health promotion initiatives and that are consistent with the Ottawa Charter; and
- a corresponding structure and sequence of steps that can be used in evaluating the effectiveness of initiatives that have conceptual and operational roots in the Ottawa Charter.

For this purpose, this chapter presents the generic model shown in Fig. 23.1.

Components

The upper portion of Fig. 23.1 identifies the key elements of the Ottawa Charter for Health Promotion *(2)*. In particular, according to this model, health promotion initiatives should:

1. have goals that extend beyond reducing and preventing ill health to include improving health and wellbeing;
2. focus on positive health, holistic health, social justice, equity and participation;
3. use empowerment as a core mechanism;
4. address the determinants of (or prerequisites for) health: macro-level factors that include those shown in Fig. 23.1; and
5. take action in the areas given priority by the Ottawa Charter: strengthening community action, building healthy public policy, creating supportive environments, developing personal skills and reorienting health services.

These principles and elements suggest that the objectives of health promotion might be stated as: empowerment and the development and fostering of institutional and physical environments that support the goals, values, principles and strategies identified above.

The lower portion of Fig. 23.1 identifies and lists examples of the elements involved in the operational planning of health promotion initiatives. This planning includes decisions related to:

1. the objectives, processes and outcomes that are instrumental in achieving the goals and objectives of health promotion;
2. the strategy or combination of strategies needed, which are not unique to health promotion but originate in other disciplines such as education, psychology, sociology and political science; and
3. the activities, products, outputs, etc. that result from using the selected strategies and will be instrumental in achieving the identified health promotion goals and objectives.

Fig. 23.1. Generic logic model for planning and evaluating health promotion

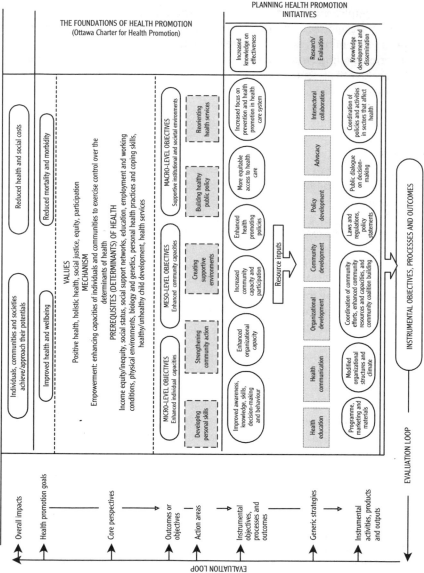

As suggested by this discussion, the planning of health promotion initiatives should reflect the conceptual framework that underlies: the understanding of the nature and origins of health issues/problems of concern, and the understanding of how one might influence these (by prevention, for example). Health promotion is likely to be more effective if practitioners plan initiatives within the context of an explicitly stated framework such as the Ottawa Charter.

Implications of the model for evaluation

The proposed generic model has several important implications for the evaluation of health promotion. First, evaluation is inextricably related to and depends on both a clear understanding of the conceptual framework underlying the initiative and the processes and elements involved in planning it. It is not an exaggeration to state that the evaluation of health promotion initiatives will only be as good as the preceding planning. Again, planning, implementation and evaluation are often portrayed as equally important parts of an iterative cycle, a relationship shown by the evaluation loop included in Fig. 23.1.

Second, evaluation involves an assessment of each of the elements emanating from the various planning steps. In this way, evaluation should examine an initiative with respect to:

1. its success in achieving the goals and objectives identified in planning, which requires paying attention to the achievement of all levels of goals and objectives, including the overall health promotion goals, as well as the instrumental objectives, processes, outcomes, products and other outputs;
2. the extent to which the initiative employed/reflected the values identified as its guiding principles;
3. its success in implementing the core mechanism of health promotion: individual and community empowerment;
4. its success in addressing the determinants of health, identified through the planning process as being relevant to the issue/problem of concern (such as employment opportunities and economics-based access issues); and
5. the way in which the initiative worked in one or more of the general health promotion action areas and used the strategies identified in planning.

Evaluation can include an assessment of the range of action areas and strategies employed, the appropriateness of the strategies included or excluded, and the synergy or mutual support among strategies.

Third, evaluation involves retracing the steps taken in planning, usually in reverse order: that is, assessing first the most specific activities and components, then the intermediate or instrumental effects and finally the overall outcomes and impact. This temporal approach to evaluation offers three advantages: it systematizes and simplifies the evaluation process, and goes beyond a simple description of the intervention and its effects to an understanding of the reasons for success or failure.

Fourth, the logic underlying this evaluation model is that each step in both implementing and evaluating a planned initiative builds on the contributions of the previous steps. For this reason, in addition to assessing an initiative's success in achieving its planned effects (as discussed above), evaluation of health promotion initiatives should include an assessment of the contributions made by each element to the achievement of the higher-order elements of the initiative. For example, in addition to assessing success in achieving tangible outcomes, evaluation should also examine the contributions these make (or fail to make) to the achievement of the initiative's instrumental and intermediate objectives. Similarly, in addition to assessing an initiative's success in addressing poverty as a determinant of health, evaluation should also examine how the initiative contributed (or failed to contribute) to improvements in health.

Finally, the proposed model implies that evaluations of health promotion:

- can serve a number of functions, including assisting in the formative development and implementation of initiatives, and in assessing an initiative's outcomes and summative impact;
- can and probably should employ a variety of methodologies and procedures, depending on their purposes;
- should give attention to the assessment of processes, as well as outcomes and impacts;
- should focus on a variety of variables, which are related to goals, mechanisms, instrumental objectives, activities and outputs; and
- should occur at a variety of levels related to the sequence or hierarchy of elements included in the planning process.

In conclusion

This book has taken three perspectives in examining the issues related to the evaluation of health promotion. It includes a retrospective examination of the evolution of health promotion evaluation; this provides the context for assessing and understanding its current state. Finally, the many recommendations provide a look into the future.

The WHO European Working Group on Health Promotion Evaluation and the other contributors to this book believe that, in spite of the many ideological and practical challenges it faces, the field of health promotion is in a period of accelerated development. This development is spurred and fostered by a growing understanding that most of the world's health and social problems have their roots in an array of social and economic conditions, and that these broad determinants of health cannot be effectively addressed through interventions focused narrowly on individual lifestyles. Recent evidence indicates that policy-makers, professionals of all kinds and the general public are increasingly aware that poverty and wealth inequity, among other factors, are particularly important health determinants, but their willingness to tackle these problems or their effects on health is not yet clear. This book provides a solid foundation for understanding how to respond to these challenges. More particularly, it indicates how a health promotion approach, as set out in the Ottawa Charter for Health Promotion (2), offers a comprehensive framework for planning and implementing the interventions that are more likely to be effective in addressing today's major health-related problems.

532

In addition to making the case for taking a health promotion approach, the contributors to this book hope that their work and the voluminous literature and experience on which it is based make the case for a more concerted and intensive investment in the evaluation of health promotion. In this volume, authors have not been shy in identifying the collective and individual weaknesses of previous health promotion efforts; they have given special attention to the challenges of increasing the quantity and quality of evaluations. In response to these challenges, they have provided a wealth of guidance on how to undertake appropriate evaluations of health promotion initiatives. Perhaps their greatest contribution, however, lies in the case they make for the added value that good evaluation brings to the field of health promotion, and the achievement of the goals to which it aspires.

Finally, the reader should recognize that this book represents only one of many current attempts to address the issue of evidence on the effectiveness of health promotion. Moreover, being an early attempt to bring together the issues involved in the evaluation of health promotion, its chapters represent work in progress, rather than a definitive end-point in the evolution of the field. The contributors hope that their work will stimulate policy-makers and practitioners to invest in and undertake good evaluation of good health promotion. This is their commitment; they hope that readers share it.

References

1. *Health promotion evaluation: recommendations to policy-makers: report of the WHO European Working Group on Health Promotion Evaluation.* Copenhagen, WHO Regional Office for Europe, 1998 (document EUR/ICP/IVST 05 01 03).
2. Ottawa Charter for Health Promotion. *Health promotion*, **1**(4): ii–v (1986).
3. *Jakarta Declaration: on leading health promotion into the 21st century. Déclaration de Jakarta sur la promotion de la santé au XXIe siécle* (http://www.who.int/hpr/docs/index.html). Geneva, World Health Organization, 1997 (document WHO/HPR/HEP/4ICHP/BR/97.4) (accessed on 22 November 2000).
4. SIMONS-MORTON, B.G. ET AL. *Introduction to health education and health promotion*, 2nd ed. Prospect Heights, Waveland Press, Inc, 1995.
5. GREEN, L.W. & KREUTER, M.W. *Health promotion planning: an educational and ecological approach*, 3rd ed. Mountain View, Mayfield, 1999.